THERAPEUTIC STRATEGIES IN THROMBOSIS

THERAPEUTIC STRATEGIES IN THROMBOSIS

Edited by

Steen Dalby Kristensen,
Raffaele De Caterina and David J. Moliterno

CLINICAL PUBLISHING

OXFORD

Clinical Publishing
an imprint of Atlas Medical Publishing Ltd

Oxford Centre for Innovation
Mill Street, Oxford OX2 0JX, UK

Tel: +44 1865 811116
Fax: +44 1865 251550
Web: www.clinicalpublishing.co.uk

Distributed by:

Marston Book Services Ltd
PO Box 269
Abingdon
Oxon OX14 4YN, UK

Tel: +44 1235 465500
Fax: +44 1235 465555
E-mail: trade.orders@marston.co.uk

A catalogue record for this book is available from the British Library

ISBN 1 904392 34 2

The publisher makes no representation, express or implied, that the dosages in this
book are correct. Readers must therefore always check the product information and
clinical procedures with the most up-to-date published product information and data
sheets provided by the manufacturers and the most recent codes of conduct and safety
regulations. The authors and the publisher do not accept any liability for any errors in
the text or for the misuse or misapplication of material in this work.

Project manager: Gavin Smith
Typeset by Mizpah Publishing Services Private Limited, Chennai, India
Printed in Spain by T G Hostench s.a., Barcelona, Spain

Contents

Contributors

WALTER AGENO MD, Associate Professor of Internal Medicine, Department of Clinical Medicine, University of Insubria University of Insubria, Varese, Italy

JOHN H. ALEXANDER MD, MS, FACC, Assistant Professor of Medicine in Cardiovascular Medicine, Duke Clinical Research Institute, Durham, North Carolina, USA

HENNING RUD ANDERSEN MD, DMSc, Associate Professor of Cardiology, University Department of Cardiology, Skejby Hospital, Aarhus University Hospital, Aarhus, Denmark

LINA BADIMON PhD, FESC, FAHA, Professor and Director of Cardiovascular Research Center, Hospital de Santa Cruz y Pablo, Barcelona, Spain

SHANNON M. BATES MDCM, MSc, FRCP(C), Associate Professor, Department of Medicine, McMaster University Medical Centre, Hamilton, Ontario, Canada

DEEPAK L. BHATT MD, FACC, FSCAI, FESC, Director, Interventional Cardiology Fellowship, Cleveland Clinic Foundation, Cleveland, Ohio, USA

M. A. BROUWER MD, Heartcenter, Department of Cardiology, Nijmegen, The Netherlands

BRANDON E. BROWN MD, Fellow in Cardiovascular Medicine, Gill Heart Institute, University of Kentucky, Lexington, Kentucky, USA

ERIC GORDON BUTCHART FRCS, FETCS, FESC, Senior Consultant Cardiothoracic Surgeon, University Hospital of Wales, Cardiff, Wales, UK

MARC COHEN MD, Professor of Medicine, Mount Sinai School of Medicine, Chief of Cardiology, Newark Beth Israel Medical Center, Newark, New Jersey, USA

JACQUELINE CONARD PhD, Unite Hemostase-Thrombose, Hotel Dieu University Hospital, Paris Notre-Dame, Paris, France

ERON D. CROUCH MD, Cardiology Fellow, University of North Carolina at Chapel Hill, Chapel Hill, North Carolina, USA

RAFFAELE DE CATERINA MD, PhD, Professor of Cardiology, Institute of Cardiology, "G. d'Annunzio" University – Chieti, Ospedale San Camillo de Lellis, Chieti, Italy

ROBERT B. FATHI MB BS, PhD, Staff, Cardiac, Peripheral and Carotid Intervention, Cleveland Clinic Foundation, Cleveland, Ohio, USA

VALENTIN FUSTER MD, PhD, Professor of Cardiology, Mount Sinai Medical Center, New York, USA

CHRISTA GOHLKE-BAERWOLF MD, Cardiologist and Senior Staff Physician, Herz-Zentrum Bad Krozingen, Bad Krozingen, Germany

ROBERT A. HARRINGTON MD, FACC, FSCAI, Professor of Medicine, Director, Cardiovascular Clinical Trials, Duke Clinical Research Institute, Durham, North Carolina, USA

JACK HIRSH CM, MD, FRCP(C), FRACP, FRSC, DSc, Professor Emeritus, McMaster University, Henderson Research Centre, Hamilton, Ontario, Canada

KURT HUBER MD, FESC, FACC, Professor of Cardiology and Internal Medicine, 3rd Medical Department (Cardiology and Emergency Medicine), Wilhelminenhospital, Vienna, Austria

STEEN HUSTED MD, DMSc, Head of Department, University Department of Medicine-Cardiology, Aarhus Hospital, Aarhus, Denmark

VIDYASAGAR KALAHASTI MD, Staff, Department of Cardiovascular Medicine, Cleveland Clinic Foundation, Cleveland, Ohio, USA

STEEN DALBY KRISTENSEN MD, DMSc, Head of Cardiology, University Department of Cardiology, Skejby Hospital, Aarhus University Hospital, Aarhus, Denmark

JENS FLENSTED LASSEN MD, PhD, Consultant Cardiologist, Associate Professor, Department of Cardiology, Skejby Hospital, Aarhus University Hospital, Aarhus, Denmark

A. MICHAEL LINCOFF MD, FACC, FESC, Professor of Medicine, Cleveland Clinic Lerner College of Medicine of Case Western Reserve University, Cleveland, Ohio, USA

VENUGOPAL MENON MD, MBBS, FACC, Director, Coronary Care Unit, Assistant Professor of Medicine and Emergency Medicine, University of North Carolina at Chapel Hill, Chapel Hill, North Carolina, USA

DAVID J. MOLITERNO MD, Chief of Cardiovascular Medicine, Professor and Vice Chair of Medicine, Gill Heart Institute, University of Kentucky, Lexington, Kentucky, USA

DEBRABRATA MUKHERJEE MD, Associate Professor of Medicine, Director of Peripheral Interventional Programs, Gill Heart Institute, University of Kentucky, Lexington, Kentucky, USA

MARTIN JAMES O'DONNELL MB, MRCPI, Assistant Professor, Department of Medicine, Henderson Research Centre, Hamilton, Ontario, Canada

E. MAGNUS OHMAN MD, FACC, Ernest and Hazel Craige Professor of Cardiovascular Medicine, Chief, Division of Cardiology and Director, University of North Carolina Heart Center, Chapel Hill, North Carolina, USA

CARLO PATRONO MD, Professor of Pharmacology, Università di Roma "La Sapienza", Ospedale Sant' Andrea, Rome, Italy

L. Creed Pettigrew MD, MPH, Professor of Neurology and Director, University of Kentucky Stroke Program, Department of Neurology, University of Kentucky Chandler Medical Center, Lexington, Kentucky, USA

Giulia Renda MD, PhD, Associate in Cardiology, "G. d'Annunzio" University – Chieti, Ospedale San Camillo de Lellis, Chieti, Italy

Meyer Michel Samama MD, PharmD, Professor Emeritus of Haematology, Hotel Dieu University Hospital, Paris Notre-Dame, Paris, France

Kiran Y. Saraff MD, Cardiovascular Medicine Fellow, Gill Heart Institute, University of Kentucky, Lexington, Kentucky, USA

Peter R. Sinnaeve MD, PhD, Professor, Department of Cardiology, University Hospital Gasthuisberg, Leuven, Belgium

Gregg W. Stone MD, FACC, Professor of Medicine, Columbia University Medical Center, Director of Cardiovascular Research and Education, Center for Interventional Vascular Therapy, Columbia University Medical Center, Vice-chairman, The Cardiovascular Research Foundation, New York, USA

Eric J. Topol MD, Chief Academic Officer, Cleveland Clinic Foundation, Provost, Cleveland Clinic Lerner College of Medicine of Case Western Reserve University, Chairman, Department of Cardiovascular Medicine and Professor of Medicine and Genetics, Cleveland Clinic Foundation, Cleveland, Ohio, USA

Peirluigi Trioci MD, Cardiology Fellow, Duke Clinical Research Institute, Durham, North Carolina, USA

Alexander G. G. Turpie MD, FRCP, FRCPC, FACC, Professor of Medicine, McMaster University, HHS-General Hospital, Hamilton, Ontario, Canada

Anand G. Vaishnav MD, Associate Professor of Neurology, Department of Neurology, University of Kentucky Chandler Medical Center, Lexington, Kentucky, USA

Frans J. Van de Werf MD, PhD, Chairman, Department of Cardiology, University Hospital Gasthuisberg, Leuven, Belgium

Freek W. A. Verheugt MD, Professor of Cardiology, Heartcenter, Department of Cardiology, Nijmegen, The Netherlands

Lars C. Wallentin MD, PhD, Professor of Cardiology, University Hospital, Uppsala, Sweden

1

Arterial thrombosis: a brief overview

L. Badimon, V. Fuster

INTRODUCTION

Arterial thrombosis comprises four basic pathways: platelet activation and aggregation, blood coagulation with fibrin formation, inflammation and fibrinolysis. These pathways interact with each other and with the vessel wall in special regulatory conditions set by the local blood flow to form a thrombus with a determined growth rate, mass and stability on top of an atherosclerotic plaque [1, 2]. Numerous pathological and angiographic and several angioscopic and intravascular ultrasound reports have documented the presence of intraluminal thrombi both in unstable angina and in acute myocardial infarction. In contrast with the very high incidence of thrombi in acute myocardial infarction (MI), the incidence in unstable angina varied significantly among different studies, related in part to the interval between the onset of symptoms and the angiographic study. Accordingly, when cardiac catheterisation was delayed for weeks, the incidence of thrombi was low; on the other hand, angiography early after the onset of symptoms revealed the presence of thrombi in approximately two-thirds of cases. Presumably, the thrombus is occlusive at the time of anginal pain and later may become subocclusive and slowly lysed or digested. Local and systemic 'thrombogenic risk factors' at the time of coronary plaque disruption may influence the degree and duration of thrombus deposition and hence the different pathological and clinical syndromes [3, 4].

The concept of vascular injury and local geometry as triggers and modulators of a thrombotic event is relevant to the pathogenesis of different cardiovascular disorders, including the initiation and progression of atherosclerosis, acute coronary syndromes (ACS), vein graft disease and restenosis following coronary angioplasty. The unveiling of the molecular interactions prevalent in thrombosis will serve development of more accurate strategies of pharmacological intervention (Figure 1.1).

PATHOGENESIS OF ARTERIAL THROMBOSIS

The endothelium has a central role in the preservation of vascular homeostasis and haemostasis. The endothelium, the inner layer of blood vessels, is a dynamic autocrine and paracrine organ that regulates contractile, secretory and mitogenic activities in the vessel wall, and the haemostatic process within the vessel lumen, by producing several local active substances. Vascular haemostasis, defined as the ability of the vascular system

Lina Badimon, Professor and Director of Cardiovascular Research Center, Hospital de Santa Cruz y Pablo, Barcelona, Spain.

Valentin Fuster, Professor of Cardiology, Mount Sinai Medical Center, New York, USA.

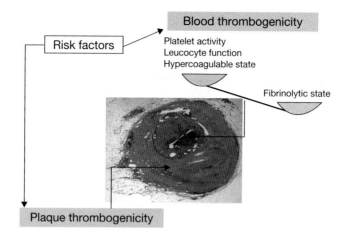

Figure 1.1   Diagram of atherothrombosis and pathways involved in thrombus formation.

to maintain blood fluidity and vascular integrity, is achieved by the interaction between the endothelium and blood cells. In physiological conditions, the normal endothelium actively supports the fluid state of flowing blood and prevents activation of circulating cells. In this context, of all the endothelial-borne agents, nitric oxide (NO) and prostacyclin (PGI_2) are the most efficacious platelet inhibitors. Endothelial dysfunction, as well as a breach of the endothelial integrity, triggers a series of biochemical and molecular reactions aimed at blood arresting and vessel wall repair. Vasoconstriction, platelet adhesion and fibrin formation at the place of injury aimed to form a haemostatic aggregate, are the first steps of the vessel wall repair and prevent excessive loss of blood. A few scattered platelets may interact with subtly injured, dysfunctional endothelium and contribute, by the release of growth factors, to very mild intimal hyperplasia. In contrast, with endothelial denudation and mild intimal injury, from a monolayer to a few layers of platelets may deposit on the lesion, with or without mural thrombus formation. The release of platelet growth factors may contribute significantly to an accelerated intimal hyperplasia, as it occurs in the coronary vein graft within the first postoperative year. In severe injury, with exposure of components of deeper layers of the vessel, as in spontaneous plaque rupture or in angioplasty, marked platelet aggregation with mural thrombus formation follows. Vascular injury of this magnitude also stimulates thrombin formation through both the intrinsic (surface-activated) and extrinsic (tissue-factor-dependent) coagulation pathways, in which the platelet membrane facilitates interactions between clotting factors. This concept of vascular injury as a trigger of the thrombotic response is important in understanding the pathogenesis of various vascular diseases associated with atherosclerosis in contrast to venous thrombosis.

Growing thrombi may locally occlude the lumen, or embolise and be washed away by the blood flow to occlude distal vessels. However, thrombi may be physiologically and spontaneously lysed by mechanisms that block thrombus propagation. Thrombus size, location and composition are regulated by haemodynamic forces (mechanical effects), thrombogenicity of exposed substrate (local molecular effects), thrombogenicity of the fluid phase and cellular blood components (local cellular effects), and the efficiency of the physiological mechanisms of control of the system, mainly fibrinolysis [5]. The inflammatory pathways triggered both by the underlying atherosclerotic lesion and the evolving thrombus contribute to the general risk of the patient and the progression of the disease (Figure 1.2).

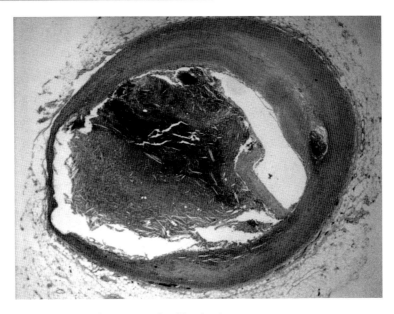

Figure 1.2   Coronary thrombus from a case of sudden death.

PLATELETS

After plaque rupture, the exposed vessel structures induce platelet aggregation and thrombosis by mechanisms, in some instances, different from those prevalent in haemostatic plug formation. The ulcerated atherosclerotic plaque may contain a disrupted fibrous cap, a lipid-rich core, abundant extracellular matrix and inflammatory cells. Such structures exhibit a potent activating effect on platelets and coagulation. Exposed matrix from the vessel wall and thrombin generated by the activation of the coagulation cascade, as well as circulating epinephrine, are powerful platelet agonists. Adenosine diphosphate (ADP) is a platelet agonist that may be released from haemolysed red cells and other platelets in the area of vessel injury. Each agonist stimulates the discharge of calcium from the platelet-dense tubular system and promotes the contraction of the platelet, with the subsequent release of its granule contents. Arachidonate, which is released from the platelet membrane by the stimulatory effect of collagen, thrombin, ADP and serotonin, is another platelet agonist. Arachidonate is converted to thromboxane A_2 by the sequential effects of cyclooxygenase and thromboxane synthetase. Thromboxane A_2 not only promotes further platelet aggregation, but is also a potent vasoconstrictor [2].

Signal transduction mechanisms initiated upon binding of agonists to membrane-spanning receptors on the platelet surface have been partially elucidated [2]. The initial recognition of a damaged vessel wall by platelets involves (a) adhesion and activation; (b) spreading of the platelet on the surface and (c) aggregation of platelets with each other to form a platelet plug or white thrombus. The efficiency of the platelet recruitment will depend on the underlying substrate and local geometry. A final step of recruitment of other blood cells also occurs; erythrocytes, neutrophils and occasionally monocytes are found on evolving mixed thrombus.

Platelet function depends on adhesive interactions, and most of the glycoproteins on the platelet membrane surface are receptors for adhesive proteins. Many of these receptors have been identified, cloned, sequenced and classified within large gene families that mediate a variety of cellular interactions. The most abundant is the integrin family, which includes GPIIb/IIIa, GPIa/IIa, GPIc/IIa, the fibronectin receptor, and the vitronectin receptor, in decreasing order of magnitude. Another gene family present in the platelet membrane glycocalyx is the leucine-rich glycoprotein family represented by the GPIb/IX complex, receptor for von Willebrand factor (vWF) on unstimulated platelets that mediates adhesion to subendothelium and GPV. Other gene families include the selectins (such as GMP-140) and the immunoglobulin domain protein (HLA class I antigen and platelet/endothelial cell adhesion molecule 1, PECAM-1). Unrelated to any other gene family is the GPIV (IIIa) [6].

The GPIb/IX complex consists of two disulfide-linked subunits (GPIbα and GPIbβ) tightly (not covalently) complexed with GPIX in a 1:1 heterodimer. GPIbβ and GPIX are transmembrane glycoproteins and form the larger globular domain. The elongated, protruding part of the receptor corresponds to GPIbα. The major role of GPIb/IX is to bind immobilised vWF on the exposed vascular subendothelium and initiate adhesion of platelets. GPIb does not bind soluble vWF in plasma; apparently it undergoes a conformational change upon binding to the extracellular matrix and then exposes a recognition sequence for GPIb/IX. The vWF-binding domain of GPIb/IX has been narrowed to amino acids 251–279 on GPIbα. The GPIbα-binding domain of vWF resides in a tryptic fragment extending from residue 449 to 728 of the subunit that does not contain an Arg-Gly-Asp (RGD) sequence. The cytoplasmic domain of GPIb/IX has a major function in linking the plasma membrane to the intracellular actin filaments of the cytoskeleton and functions to stabilise the membrane and to maintain the platelet shape.

Randomly distributed on the surface of resting platelets are about 50 000 molecules of GPIIb/IIIa. The complex is composed of one molecule of GPIIb (disulfide-linked large and light chains) and one of GPIIIa (single polypeptide chain). It is a Ca^{2+}-dependent heterodimer, non-covalently associated on the platelet membrane. Calcium is required for maintenance of the complex and for binding of adhesive proteins. On activated platelets, the GPIIb/IIIa is a receptor for fibrinogen, fibronectin, vWF, vitronectin and thrombospondin. The receptor recognition sequences are localised to small peptide sequences (RGD) in the adhesive proteins. Fibrinogen contains two RGD sequences in its α chain, one near the N-terminus (residues 95–97) and a second near the C-terminus (residues 572–574). Fibrinogen has a second site of recognition for GPIIb/IIIa, i.e., the 12-amino acid sequence located at the carboxyl-terminus of the γ chain of the molecule. This dodecapeptide is specific for fibrinogen and does not contain the RGD sequence, but competes with RGD-containing peptides for binding to GPIIb/IIIa [6, 7].

Thrombin plays an important role in the pathogenesis of arterial thrombosis. It is one of the most potent known agonists for platelet activation and recruitment. The thrombin receptor has 425 amino acids with seven transmembrane domains and a large NH_2-terminal extracellular extension that is cleaved by thrombin to produce a 'tethered' ligand that activates the receptor to initiate signal transduction [8]. Thrombin is a critical enzyme in early thrombus formation, cleaving fibrinopeptides A and B from fibrinogen to yield insoluble fibrin, which effectively anchors the evolving thrombus. Both free and fibrin-bound fibrin thrombin are able to convert fibrinogen to fibrin, allowing propagation of thrombus at the site of injury.

Therefore, platelet activation triggers intracellular signalling and expression of platelet membrane receptors for adhesion and initiation of cell contractile processes that induce shape change and secretion of the granular contents. The expression of the integrin IIb/IIa (αIIbβ₃) receptors for adhesive glycoprotein ligands (mainly fibrinogen and vWF) in the circulation initiates platelet-to-platelet interaction. The process becomes perpetuated by the arrival of platelets brought by the circulation. Most of the glycoproteins in the platelet membrane surface are receptors for adhesive proteins or mediate cellular interactions. Ligand binding to the different membrane receptors triggers platelet activation with different relative potencies. A lot of interest has been recently generated among the platelet ADP-receptors ($P2Y_{AC}$, $P2y_{1R}$, $P2X_{1R}$) because of available pharmacological inhibitors and new research is being generated in relation to PARs (protease-activated receptors).

COAGULATION SYSTEM

During plaque rupture, in addition to platelet deposition in the injured area, the clotting mechanism is activated by the exposure of the de-endothelialised vascular surface. Tissue factor (TF) may be exposed upon vessel injury and it directly contributes to triggering thrombosis. The activation of the coagulation cascade leads to the generation of thrombin, which, as mentioned before, is a powerful platelet agonist that contributes to platelet recruitment in addition to catalysing the formation and polymerisation of fibrin. Fibrin is essential in the stabilisation of the platelet thrombus and its withstanding of removal forces by flow, shear and high intravascular pressure. These basic concepts have clinical relevance in the context of ACS, where plaque rupture exposes vessel wall matrix and plaque core materials, which by activating platelets and the coagulation system results in the formation of a fixed and occlusive platelet-fibrin thrombus. The efficacy of fibrinolytic agents pointedly demonstrates the importance of fibrin-related material in the thrombosis associated with myocardial infarction. The proteins, which compose the clotting enzymes do not collide and interact on a random basis in the plasma, but interact in complexes in a highly efficient manner on platelet and endothelial surfaces. The major regulatory events in the coagulation (activation, inhibition, generation of anticoagulant proteins) occur on membrane surfaces.

The blood coagulation system involves a sequence of reactions integrating zymogens (proteins susceptible to be activated to enzymes *via* limited proteolysis) and cofactors (non-proteolytic enzyme activators) in three groups: (a) the contact activation (generation of factor XIa *via* the Hageman factor), (b) the conversion of factor X to Xa in a complex reaction requiring the participation of factors IX and VIII and (c) the conversion of prothrombin to thrombin and fibrin formation [9].

The TF pathway, through the TF/factor VIIa complex in the presence of Ca^{2+} induces the formation of Xa. A second TF-dependent reaction catalyses the transformation of IX into IXa. TF is an integral membrane protein that serves to initiate the activation of factors IX and X and to localise the reaction to cells on which TF is expressed. Other cofactors include factor VIIIa, which binds to platelets and forms the binding site for IXa, thereby forming the machinery for the activation of X, and factor Va, which binds to platelets and provides a binding site for Xa. The human genes for these cofactors have been cloned and sequenced. In physiological conditions, no cells in contact with blood contain active TF, although cells such as monocytes and polymorphonuclear leucocytes can be induced to synthesise and express TF [9].

Activated Xa converts prothrombin into thrombin. The complex which catalyses the formation of thrombin consists of factors Xa and Va in a 1:1 complex. The activation results in the cleavage of fragment 1.2 and formation of thrombin from fragment 2. The interaction of the four components of the 'prothrombinase complex' (Xa, Va, phospholipid and Ca^{2+}) yield a more efficient reaction.

Activated platelets provide a procoagulant surface for the assembly and expression of both intrinsic Xase and prothrombinase enzymatic complexes. These complexes respectively catalyse the activation of factor X to Xa and prothrombin to thrombin. The expression of activity is associated with the binding of both the proteases, factor IXa and factor Xa, and the cofactors, VIIIa and Va, to procoagulant surfaces. The binding of IXa and Xa is promoted by VIIIa and Va, respectively, such that Va and likely VIIIa provide the equivalent of receptors for the proteolytic enzymes. The surface of the platelet expresses the procoagulant phospholipids that bind coagulation factors and contribute to the procoagulant activity of the cell.

Blood clotting is blocked at the level of the prothrombinase complex by the physiological anticoagulant-activated protein C and oral anticoagulants. Oral anticoagulants prevent post-translational synthesis of γ-carboxyglutamic acid groups on the vitamin K-dependent clotting factors, preventing binding of prothrombin and Xa to the membrane surface. Activated protein C cleaves factor Va to render it functionally inactive. Loss of Va decreases the role of thrombin formation to negligible levels [10].

Thrombin acts on multiple substrates, including fibrinogen, factor XIII, factors V and VIII and protein C, in addition to its effects on platelets. It plays a central role in haemostasis and thrombosis. The catalytic transformation of fibrinogen into fibrin is essential in the formation of the haemostatic plug and in the formation of arterial thrombi. It binds to the fibrinogen central domain and cleaves fibrinopeptides A and B, resulting in fibrin monomer and polymer formation [11]. The fibrin mesh holds the platelets together and contributes to the attachment of the thrombus to the vessel wall.

The control of the coagulation reactions occurs by diverse mechanisms, such as haemodilution and flow effects, proteolytic feedback by thrombin, inhibition by plasma proteins (such as antithrombin III, ATIII) and endothelial cell-localised activation of an inhibitory enzyme (protein C), and fibrinolysis. Although ATIII readily inactivates thrombin in solution, its catalytic site is inaccessible while bound to fibrin, and it may still cleave fibrinopeptides even in the presence of heparin. Thrombin has a specific receptor in endothelial cell surfaces, thrombomodulin, that triggers a physiological anticoagulant system. The thrombin–thrombomodulin complex serves as a receptor for the vitamin K-dependent protein C which is activated and released from the endothelial cell surface. Activated protein C blocks the effects of factors V and VIII and limits thrombin effects. Endogenous fibrinolysis represents a repair mechanism, such as endothelial cell regrowth and vessel recanalisation. Fibrinolysis involves catalytic activation of zymogens, positive and negative feedback control and inhibitor blockade [12].

EFFECTS OF THE SEVERITY OF VESSEL WALL DAMAGE AND LOCAL GEOMETRY ON THE THROMBOTIC RESPONSE TO ATHEROSCLEROSIS

The dynamics of platelet deposition and thrombus formation following vascular damage are modulated by the type of injury and the local geometry at the site of damage (degree of stenosis) [13, 14]. Overall, it is likely that when injury to the vessel wall is mild, the thrombogenic stimulus is relatively limited, and the resulting thrombotic occlusion is transient, as occurs in unstable angina. On the other hand, deep vessel injury secondary to plaque rupture or ulceration results in exposure of collagen, TF, and other elements of the vessel matrix, leading to relatively persistent thrombotic occlusion and myocardial infarction [3, 4].

It is likely that the nature of the substrate exposed after spontaneous or angioplasty-induced plaque rupture is one factor determining whether an unstable plaque proceeds rapidly to an occlusive thrombus or persists as non-occlusive mural thrombus. The analysis of the relative contribution of different components of human atherosclerotic plaques (fatty streaks, sclerotic plaques, fibrolipid plaques, atheromatous plaques, hyperplasic cellular plaque and normal intima) to acute thrombus formation showed that the atheromatous core was up to 6-fold more active than the other substrates, in triggering thrombosis [15]. Therefore, plaques with a large atheromatous core content are at high risk of leading to ACS after spontaneous or mechanically induced rupture due to the increased thrombogenicity of their contents [16]. As proof of concept, we showed that local tissue blockade of TF, by treatment with tissue factor pathway inhibitor (TFPI), significantly reduces thrombosis [17]. Recently the use of active site-inhibited recombinant FVIIa (FF-rFVIIa), has been shown to significantly reduce thrombus growth on damaged vessels devoid of TF indicating that blockage of blood-borne TF at the site of a growing thrombus has therapeutic implications [18].

Platelet deposition is directly related to the degree of stenosis in the presence of the same degree of injury, indicating a shear-induced platelet activation [13, 14]. In addition, analysis of the axial distribution of platelet deposition indicates that the apex, and not the flow recirculation zone distal to the apex, is the segment of greatest platelet accumulation. These data suggest that the severity of the acute platelet response to plaque disruption depends in part on the sudden changes in geometry following rupture [1].

Spontaneous lysis of thrombus does occur, not only in unstable angina, but also in acute MI. In these patients, as well as in those undergoing thrombolysis for acute infarction, the presence of a residual mural thrombus predisposes to recurrent thrombotic vessel occlusion [19, 20]. Two main contributing factors for the development of re-thrombosis have been identified. First, a residual mural thrombus may encroach into the vessel lumen resulting in increased shear rate, which facilitates the activation and deposition of platelets on the lesion. Second, the presence of a fragmented thrombus appears to be one of the most powerful thrombogenic surfaces. rHirudin, a recombinant molecule that blocks both the catalytic site and the anion-exosite of the thrombin molecule, inhibited secondary growth significantly. Thus, following lysis, thrombin becomes exposed to the circulating blood, leading to activation of the platelets and coagulation, further enhancing thrombosis.

Thrombin generated at the site of injury binds to thrombomodulin, an endothelial surface membrane protein, initiating activation of protein C, which in turn (in the presence of protein S) inactivates factors Va and VIIIa. Thrombin stimulates successive release of both tissue plasminogen activator (tPA) and plasminogen-activator inhibitor type 1 from endothelial cells, thus initiating endogenous lysis through plasmin generation from plasminogen by tPA with subsequent modulation through plasminogen-activator inhibitor type 1. Thrombin therefore plays a pivotal role in maintaining the complex balance of initial prothrombotic reparative events and subsequent endogenous anticoagulant and thrombolytic pathways [21].

INFLAMMATION IN ARTERIAL THROMBOSIS

Atherothrombosis, the leading cause of mortality in the Western world, is a systemic disease involving the intima of large- and medium-sized arteries including the aorta, the carotids, coronaries and peripheral arteries that is characterised by intimal thickening due to cellular- and lipid-accumulation. Endothelial dysfunction and inflammation are the major facilitators of atherothrombotic disease. When fatty streaks progress to fibroatheroma, they develop a cap of smooth muscle cells (SMCs) and collagen, and when this plaque is disrupted, the subsequent thrombus formation brings about the onset of the ACS and strokes. Importantly, the culprit lesions leading to ACS are usually mildly stenotic, and therefore barely detected by angiography [22]. The composition of the plaque, rather than the percent stenosis, appears to be the main determinant of risk of plaque rupture and following thrombogenicity. High-risk rupture-prone lesions usually have a large lipid core, a thin fibrous cap, high density of inflammatory cells (particularly at the shoulder region, where disruptions most often occur) and high TF content [16]. Inflammatory processes also contribute decisively to atherosclerosis and its acute thrombotic complications, as is shown by the fact that many inflammatory mediators can augment TF gene expression by endothelial cells, thus triggering the coagulation cascade [23]. Due to the baffling heterogeneity in the composition of atherothrombotic plaques even within the same individual, a reliable, non-invasive imaging tool able to detect early atherosclerotic disease and characterise lesion composition would be clinically advantageous. Indeed, it would improve our understanding of the pathophysiological mechanisms of atherothrombosis and help in patient risk-stratification [24]. Atherothrombosis is also triggered by hyperthrombogenicity due to systemic factors, the so-called 'high-risk blood', with inflammatory mediators. As such, platelets have emerged as a source of inflammatory mediators. For example, they can both produce and respond to chemoattractant cytokines [25], or express CD154 (CD40 ligand), the molecule which regulates TF gene expression in the macrophage and SMCs [26]. Similarly P-selectin, a transmembrane protein present in the α granules of platelets can quickly move to the platelet surface after activation. It interacts with the P-selectin glyco-protein ligand-1 on leucocytes, forming aggregates and upregulating TF formation. It also enforces platelet aggregates through interaction with platelet sulfatides. This might explain why P-selectin expression in platelets has been linked to arterial thrombosis and coronary artery disease [27]. P-selectin is also present on activated endothelial cells, where it helps in the recruitment of leucocytes [28]. Indeed, selectins are specialised in lymphocyte homing and are involved in inflammation processes. In case of plaque rupture we also find that endothelial cells, vascular SMCs and especially foam cells also express TF [16], the latter two through the CD40 ligand [29], whereas the former are also notably affected by soluble lig-ands such as IL-1 and tumour necrosis factor [30]. The importance of TF is underscored by the fact that high levels in circulation have been linked to coronary artery disease patients most prone to thrombotic complications, such as diabetics, smokers and dyslipidaemics. This blood-borne TF is a key determinant in thrombi by incorporation to platelets in the growing thrombus [18].

TF synthesis is a rapid consequence of endotoxin infusion, which is a strong inflamma-tory stimulus, and this is followed by TF expression on inflammatory cells and on micropar-ticles, inducing thrombin and fibrin generation [31]. Interleukin (IL)-6 is a dominant cytokine in this process, but IL-1β and tumour necrosis factor-α are also involved. Atherosclerosis as a chronic (or recurrent) inflammatory condition and the recurrent inflammatory drive leads to recurrent induction of TF (with intermediate phases of hypo-responsiveness to stimu-lation) and assembly of catalytic complexes on aggregated cells and on microparticles, main-taining a certain level of thrombin production and fibrin formation [32]. The increased level of fibrinogen and fibrin monomers may enhance the uptake by the vessel wall of lipid-loaded particles and macrophages. In the vessel wall, further fibrin polymerisation can occur due to local thrombin or the activity of other proteases.

There seems to be an increased generation of thrombin and fibrin in the blood circulation due to increased presence of inflammatory cytokines and proteins, but this does not neces-sarily lead to increased free thrombin in plasma.

SUMMARY

Arterial thrombus formation seems to be an important factor in the conversion of chronic to acute atherosclerotic coronary events after plaque rupture, in the progression of coron-ary disease, and in the acute phase of revascularisation interventions. Disruption of a vulnerable or unstable plaque (type IV and Va lesions of the AHA classification) with a subsequent change in plaque geometry and thrombosis may result in an ACS. The high-risk plaques tend to be relatively small, but soft or vulnerable to 'passive' disruption because of high lipid content. Inflammatory processes are important components of all stages of atherosclerotic development, including plaque initiation and disruption. The knowledge gained (and studies now in progress) on the mechanisms of platelet activa-tion, signal transduction, receptor binding, zymogen activation and function, substrate recognition and adhesive events will help to design promising approaches for interven-tion. Receptors originally thought to be involved only in anchoring functions are also important factors in the transduction of information from the extracellular compartment to the inner cell and they are involved in governing cell function, shape, proliferation and differentiation. Inflammatory mediators and triggers directed to or originating in the platelet and in the coagulation pathway are being identified and their prognostic value is being analysed. These studies together with those to find the most prevalent agonist and substrate to trigger and perpetuate a thrombotic event in every clinical situation will help to establish strategies of prevention of clinical events and to reduce their associated mor-bidity and mortality.

ACKNOWLEDGEMENTS

Part of original contributions mentioned in the article are the product of a long-standing collaboration with Dr. V. Fuster from the Cardiovascular Institute, Mount Sinai Medical Center. Dr. L. Badimon is supported by grants from FIS C-03/01, FIS G-03/181, FIS PI020361, PN SAF2003-03187, FISPI042371, MSD unrestricted grant, Freedom to Discover BMS Program, Cardiovascular Research Foundation-Catalana Occidente, Spain.

The authors are indebted to many investigators whose work in basic biochemistry has served to advance our knowledge in thrombosis and because of space limits cannot be listed in the references.

REFERENCES

1. Badimon L, Chesebro JH, Badimon JJ. Thrombus formation on ruptured atherosclerotic plaques and rethrombosis on evolving thrombi. *Circulation* 1992; 86(suppl III):III-74–III-85.
2. Badimon L, Fuster V, Corti R, Badimon JJ. Coronary thrombosis: local and systemic factors. In: Fuster V (ed.). *Hurst's the Heart*, 11th edition. McGraw-Hill, New York, 2004, pp 1141–1151.
3. Fuster V, Badimon L, Badimon JJ, Chesebro JH. The pathogenesis of coronary artery disease and the acute coronary syndromes. (Part I). *N Engl J Med* 1992; 326:242–250.
4. Fuster V, Badimon L, Badimon JJ, Chesebro JH. The pathogenesis of coronary artery disease and the acute coronary syndromes. (Part II). *N Engl J Med* 1992; 326:310–318.
5. Badimon JJ, Fuster V, Chesebro JH, Badimon L. Coronary atherosclerosis. *Circulation* 1993; 87(suppl II): II-3–II-16.
6. Kieffer N, Phillips DR. Platelet membrane glycoproteins: functions in cellular interactions. *Annu Rev Biol* 1990; 6:329–357.
7. Ginsberg MH, Xiaoping D, O'Toole TE, Loftus JC, Plow EF. Platelet integrins. *Thromb Haemost* 1993; 70:87–93.
8. Coughlin SR. Thrombin receptor structure and function. *Thromb Haemost* 1993; 70:184–187.
9. Nemerson Y. Mechanism of coagulation. In: Williams WJ, Beutler E, Erslev AJ, Lichtman MA (eds). *Hematology*. McGraw-Hill, New York, 1990, pp 1295–1304.
10. Comp PC. Kinetics of plasma coagulation factors. In: Williams WJ, Beutler E, Erslev AJ, Lichtman MA (eds). *Hematology*. McGraw-Hill, New York, 1990, pp 1285–1290.
11. Nemerson Y, Williams WJ. Biochemistry of plasma coagulation factors. In: Williams WJ, Beutler E, Erslev AJ, Lichtman MA (eds). *Hematology*. McGraw-Hill, New York, 1990, pp 1267–1284.
12. Collen D, Lijnen HR. Molecular and cellular basis of fibrinolysis. In: Hoffman R, Benz EJ, Jr, Shattil SJ, Furie B, Cohen HJ (eds). *Hematology: Basic Principles and Practice*. Churchill Livingstone, New York, 1991, pp 1232–1242.
13. Badimon L, Badimon JJ. Mechanism of arterial thrombosis in non-parallel streamlines: platelet grow at the apex of stenotic severely injured vessel wall. Experimental study in the pig model. *J Clin Invest* 1989; 84:1134–1144.
14. Lassila R, Badimon JJ, Vallbhajosula S, Badimon L. Dynamic monitoring of platelet deposition on severely damaged vessel wall in flowing blood. Effects of different stenosis on thrombus growth. *Arteriosclerosis* 1990; 10:306–315.
15. Fernández-Ortiz A, Badimon JJ, Falk E *et al*. Characterization of the relative thrombogenicity of atherosclerotic plaque components: implications for consequences of plaque rupture. *J Am Coll Cardiol* 1994; 23:1562–1569.
16. Toschi V, Gallo R, Lettino M *et al*. Tissue factor modulates the thrombogenicity of human atherosclerotic plaques. *Circulation* 1997; 95:594–599.
17. Badimon JJ, Lettino M, Toschi V *et al*. Local inhibition of tissue factor reduces the thrombogenicity of disrupted human atherosclerotic plaques. Effects of TFPI on plaque thrombogenicity under flow conditions. *Circulation* 1999; 99:1780–1787.
18. Sánchez-Gómez S, Casani L, Vilahur G, Badimon L. FFR-rFVIIa inhibits thrombosis triggered by ruptured and eroded vessel wall. *Thromb Haemost* 2001; OC999.
19. Van de Werf F, Arnold AER, and the European Cooperative Study Group for Recombinant Tissue-Type Plasminogen Activator (rt-PA). Effect of intravenous tissue plasminogen activator on infarct size, left ventricular function and survival in patients with acute myocardial infarction. *Br Med J* 1988; 297:374–379.

20. Badimon L, Fuster V, Badimon JJ. Interaction of platelet activation and thrombosis. In: Fuster V, Topol EJ, Nabel EG (eds). *Atherosclerosis and Coronary Artery Disease*, 2nd edition. Lippincott-Raven Publishers, Philadelphia, 2004, chap. 41, pp 583–597.
21. Badimon L, Meyer BJ, Badimon JJ. Thrombin in arterial thrombosis. *Haemostasis* 1994; 24:69–80.
22. Ambrose JA, Weinrauch M. Thrombosis in ischemic heart disease. *Arch Intern Med* 1996; 156:1382–1394.
23. Libby P, Simon DI. Inflammation and thrombosis. The clot thickens. *Circulation* 2001; 103:1718–1720.
24. Fuster V, Corti R, Fayad ZA, Schwitter J, Badimon JJ. Integration of vascular biology and magnetic resonance imaging in the understanding of atherothrombosis and acute coronary syndromes. *J Thromb Haemost* 2003; 7:1410–1421.
25. Abi-Younes S, Sauty A, Mach F *et al*. The stromal cell-derived factor-1 chemokine is a potent platelet agonist highly expressed in atherosclerotic plaques. *Circ Res* 2000; 86:131–138.
26. Henn V, Slupsy JR, Grafe M *et al*. CD40 ligand on activated platelets triggers an inflammatory reaction of endothelial cells. *Nature* 1998; 391:591–594.
27. Merten M, Thiagarajan P. P-selectin in arterial thrombosis. *Z Kardiol* 2004; 93:855–863.
28. Vandedries ER, Furie BC, Furie B. Role of P-selectin and PSGL-1 in coagulation and thrombosis. *Thromb Haemost* 2004; 92:459–466.
29. Balasubramanian V, Vele O, Nemerson Y. Local shear conditions and platelet aggregates regulate the incorporation and activity of circulating tissue factor in ex-vivo thrombi. *Thromb Haemost* 2002; 88:822–826.
30. Mach F, Schoenbeck U, Bonnefoy J-Y *et al*. Activation of monocyte/macrophage functions related to acute atheroma complication by ligation of CD40: induction of collagenase, stromelysin, and tissue factor. *Circulation* 1997; 96:396–399.
31. Spronk HM, van der Voort D, Ten Cate H. Blood coagulation and the risk of atherothrombosis: a complex relationship. *Thromb J* 2004; 2(1):12.
32. Corti R, Hutter R, Badimon JJ, Fuster V. Evolving concepts in the triad of atherosclerosis, inflammation and thrombosis. *J Thromb Thrombolysis* 2004; 17(1):35–44.

2

Aspirin: a risk-based strategy

C. Patrono

Acetylsalicylic acid was first marketed as aspirin in 1899 and used extensively over the next decades as a prototypic non-steroidal anti-inflammatory drug (NSAID). Following the seminal discoveries made by the late Sir John Vane and Bengt Samuelsson in the early 1970s on the biochemistry and pharmacology of arachidonic acid metabolism, the molecular mechanism of action of aspirin in inhibiting platelet function was elucidated by the elegant studies of Philip Majerus [reviewed in ref. 1]. The development of whole blood thromboxane (TX)B$_2$ production as a mechanism-based biochemical endpoint for human studies allowed the characterisation of the dose- and time-dependence of the antiplatelet effect of aspirin in the early 1980s [2–4]. This in turn provided the rationale for a new wave of randomised clinical trials employing daily doses 10- to 50-fold lower than those used empirically in the past [reviewed in ref. 5]. A large database of placebo-controlled, randomised clinical trials of low-dose aspirin in a wide range of vascular disorders now provides solid grounds for assessing the balance between benefits and risks in the whole spectrum of atherothrombosis [6, 7].

MECHANISM OF ACTION OF ASPIRIN IN INHIBITING PLATELET FUNCTION

The best characterised mechanism of action of aspirin is related to its capacity to inactivate permanently the cyclooxygenase (COX) activity of prostaglandin H-synthase (PGHS)-1 and -2 (also referred to as COX-1 and COX-2) [reviewed in ref. 8]. These isozymes catalyse the first committed step in prostanoid biosynthesis, i.e., the conversion of arachidonic acid to PGH$_2$. PGH$_2$ is the immediate precursor of PGD$_2$, PGE$_2$, PGF$_{2\alpha}$, PGI$_2$ and TXA$_2$. COX-1 and COX-2 are homodimers of a ~72 kDa monomeric unit. Within the enzymatic domain, there is a peroxidase catalytic site and a separate, but adjacent, site for COX activity at the apex of a long, hydrophobic channel. There are a number of important differences between COX-1 and COX-2, some of which may contribute to variable COX-isozyme selectivity of the inhibitors [8].

The molecular mechanism of permanent inactivation of COX activity by aspirin is through blockade of the COX channel as a consequence of acetylation of a strategically located serine residue (Ser529 in the human COX-1, Ser516 in the human COX-2), that prevents access of the substrate to the catalytic site of the enzyme [9]. Because aspirin has a short half-life (15–20 min) in the human circulation and is approximately 50-fold more potent in inhibiting platelet COX-1 than monocyte COX-2 [10], it is ideally suited to act on anucleate platelets, inducing a permanent defect in TXA$_2$-dependent platelet function that cannot be repaired during a 24-hour dosing interval [2–4]. Moreover, since aspirin probably also inactivates COX-1 in relatively mature megakaryocytes, and only 10% of the platelet pool is replenished each day, once-a-day dosing of aspirin is able to maintain virtually

Carlo Patrono, Professor of Pharmacology, Università di Roma "La Sapienza", Ospedale Sant' Andrea, Rome, Italy.

complete inhibition of platelet TXA_2 production [3]. In contrast, inhibition of COX-2-dependent processes (e.g., inflammation) requires larger doses of aspirin (because of lower sensitivity of COX-2 to aspirin) and a much shorter dosing interval (because nucleated cells rapidly resynthesise the enzyme). This results in markedly different benefit/risk profiles of the drug, depending on the clinical indication and its variable dose requirements [5, 6].

PHARMACOKINETICS

Aspirin is rapidly absorbed in the stomach and upper intestine. Peak plasma levels occur 30 to 40 min after aspirin ingestion, and inhibition of platelet function is evident by 1 h. In contrast, it can take up to 3 to 4 hours to reach peak plasma levels after administration of enteric-coated aspirin. The oral bioavailability of regular aspirin tablets is approximately 40 to 50% over a wide range of doses [11]. A considerably lower bioavailability has been reported for enteric-coated tablets and sustained-release, microencapsulated preparations. Because platelet COX-1 is acetylated in the presystemic circulation, the antiplatelet effect of aspirin is largely independent of systemic bioavailability [11]. Both a controlled-release formulation [12] and a transdermal patch [13] with negligible systemic bioavailability have been developed in an attempt to achieve selective inhibition of platelet TXA_2 production without suppressing vascular PGI_2 synthesis. However, the clinical relevance of preparations relatively selective for the presystemic circulation remains to be established (see below).

PHARMACODYNAMICS

EFFECTS ON TXA_2 AND PGI_2 BIOSYNTHESIS

Human platelets and vascular endothelial cells process PGH_2 to produce TXA_2 and prostacyclin (PGI_2), respectively [1]. TXA_2 induces platelet aggregation and vasoconstriction, while PGI_2 inhibits platelet aggregation and induces vasodilation. Moreover, TXA_2 promotes and PGI_2 prevents the initiation and progression of atherogenesis through control of platelet activation and leukocyte-endothelial cell interaction [14]. Aspirin is antithrombotic in a wide range of doses inhibiting TXA_2 and PGI_2 [5–7] (Figure 2.1). While TXA_2 is largely a COX-1 derived product (mostly from platelets) and thus highly sensitive to aspirin inhibition, vascular PGI_2 can derive from both COX-1 (short-term changes in response to agonist stimulation, e.g., bradykinin; sensitive to transient aspirin inhibition) and COX-2

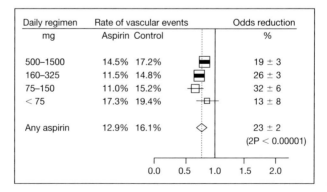

Figure 2.1 Indirect comparison of mean (±SE) odds reductions in important vascular events (non-fatal myocardial infarction, non-fatal stroke or vascular death) in placebo-controlled aspirin trials using different daily regimens in high-risk patients. Redrawn with permission from [7]

(long-term changes in response to laminar shear stress and inflammatory cytokines; largely insensitive to aspirin inhibition at conventional antiplatelet doses) [8, 15, 16]. This may account for the substantial residual COX-2-dependent PGI_2 biosynthesis *in vivo* at daily doses of aspirin in the range of 20 to 80 mg [17], despite transient suppression of COX-1-dependent PGI_2 release [12].

It is not convincingly established that more profound suppression of PGI_2 formation by higher doses of aspirin is responsible for blunting of the antithrombotic effect, as suggested by indirect comparisons of trials using higher doses vs. lower doses of aspirin (Figure 2.1). However, the evidence from direct randomised comparisons of different aspirin regimens is quite limited [6, 7]. Studies with mice deficient in the gene encoding the PGI_2 receptor support the importance of this prostanoid in the prevention of arterial thrombosis [18].

EFFECTS OF ASPIRIN NOT RELATED TO COX-1 INACTIVATION

Aspirin has been reported to have effects on haemostasis that are unrelated to its ability to inactivate platelet COX-1. These include dose-dependent inhibition of platelet function, enhancement of fibrinolysis, and suppression of plasma coagulation [reviewed in ref. 6]. In contrast to the well-characterised and saturable inhibition of COX-1 (nanomolar aspirin concentration, rapid time-course, physiologic conditions, single serine modification), the putative mechanisms underpinning the 'nonprostaglandin' effects of aspirin on haemostasis are dose-dependent and less clearly defined [6].

A subgroup analysis of the Physicians' Health Study, based on *post hoc* measurements of baseline plasma C-reactive protein (CRP) performed in 543 apparently healthy men who subsequently developed myocardial infarction (MI), stroke or venous thrombosis, and in 543 study participants who did not report vascular complications, found that the reduction in the risk of a first MI associated with the use of aspirin (325 mg on alternate days) appeared to be directly related to the level of CRP, raising the possibility of anti-inflammatory as well as antiplatelet effects of the drug in cardiovascular prophylaxis [19]. The anti-inflammatory effects of aspirin and other NSAIDs are largely related to their capacity to inhibit COX-2 activity induced in response to inflammatory cytokines, as these clinical effects can be fully reproduced by highly selective COX-2 inhibitors (coxibs) in patients with rheumatoid arthritis [reviewed in ref. 20]. The dose- and time-dependence of the effects of aspirin on nucleated inflammatory cells expressing COX-2 vs. anucleated platelets expressing COX-1 are markedly different, thus making an anti-inflammatory effect of the drug at 325 mg every other day pharmacologically implausible, given its very short half-life in the human circulation [6]. On the other hand, inhibition of TXA_2-dependent platelet activation at sites of vascular injury may have pleiotropic effects related to reduced release of other platelet products, including pro-inflammatory prostanoids and cytokines, oxygen radicals and growth factors [21].

Finally, aspirin has been reported to modify the way in which neutrophils and platelets or erythrocytes and platelets interact, to protect endothelial cells from oxidative stress and to improve endothelial dysfunction in atherosclerotic patients. However, neither the molecular mechanism(s) nor the dose-dependence of these effects have been clearly established [6].

DRUG INTERACTIONS

In contrast to the vast majority of COX-inhibitors, low-dose aspirin, 75 mg daily, does not affect blood pressure control or the need for antihypertensive therapy in intensively treated hypertensive patients [22]. This finding is consistent with its lack of effect on renal PG synthesis [3, 23] that is dependent on constitutively expressed COX-2 in the human kidney [20]. The suggestion that the use of aspirin is associated with reduced benefit from therapy with enalapril in patients with left ventricular systolic dysfunction [24] was not supported by the results of a large meta-analysis of MI trials [25]. Similarly, no negative interaction occurs between angiotensin-converting enzyme (ACE) inhibition and the cardioprotection afforded by low-dose aspirin in hypertensive patients [26]. The ACE Inhibitors Collaborative Group has carried out a systematic overview of data for 22,060 patients from six long-term randomised trials of ACE inhibitors to assess whether aspirin altered the effects of ACE inhibitor therapy on important clinical outcomes [27]. Even though results from these analyses cannot rule out the possibility of some sort of interaction, they show unequivocally that even if aspirin is administered, the addition of ACE inhibitor therapy produced substantial additional benefits on all vascular outcomes [27].

A pharmacodynamic interaction potentially interfering with the antiplatelet effect of aspirin is related to the two-step mechanism of COX-1 inactivation by the drug [8, 9]. Concomitant administration of reversible COX-1 inhibitors, such as ibuprofen [28] and naproxen [29], may prevent the irreversible acetylation of platelet COX-1 by low-dose aspirin. This is due to competition between these NSAIDs and aspirin for a common docking site within the COX-1 channel (Arginine-120), which aspirin binds to with weak affinity prior to acetylation of Serine-529. This pharmacodynamic interaction does not occur with coxibs or NSAIDs endowed with some degree of COX-2 selectivity, such as diclofenac [28]. Whether this interaction results in attenuation or loss of the cardioprotective benefit of low-dose aspirin is currently uncertain [30].

Low-dose aspirin therapy is a risk factor for upper gastrointestinal bleeding complications [6], and the concomitant use of aspirin and coxibs may amplify the risk of ulcer complications associated with the latter, apparently to a larger extent than the combination of aspirin and traditional NSAIDs [31, 32]. It should be emphasised that this finding derives from subgroup analyses of two gastrointestinal outcome trials [31, 32], neither of which was powered to examine this interaction.

INTERINDIVIDUAL VARIABILITY IN RESPONSE TO LOW-DOSE ASPIRIN

Practising physicians have long recognised that individual patients show quite substantial variability in response to the same drug treatment. Important sources of variability have been characterised, as outlined in Figure 2.2.

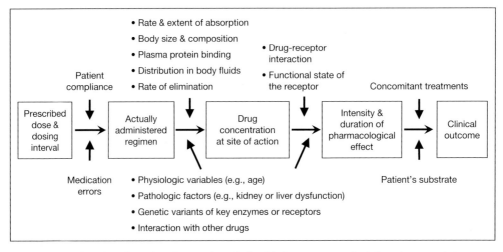

Figure 2.2 Variables that determine the complex relationship between prescribed drug dosage and drug effects on clinical outcome. Reproduced with permission from [34]

Table 2.1 Main determinants of the interindividual variability in the antiplatelet effects of aspirin and clopidogrel

Determinant	Aspirin	Clopidogrel
Dependence on systemic bioavailability	Largely independent	Completely dependent
Influence of liver metabolism	Partially inactivates active moiety	Converts pro-drug to active moiety
Influence of pharmacokinetic interactions	Not relevant	Lipophilic statins and other drugs may reduce formation of the active metabolite
Influence of pharmacodynamic interactions	Some NSAIDs prevent irreversible inactivation of COX-1	Unknown
Alternative sources of the platelet agonist	Monocyte and platelet COX-2 can produce TXA_2	Not relevant
Ratio of recommended dose to minimum effective dose for full pharmacodynamic effect	2–3	≤ 1?

The term 'aspirin resistance' has been used to describe a number of different phenomena, including the inability of aspirin to: i) protect individuals from thrombotic complications; ii) cause a prolongation of the bleeding time; iii) inhibit TXA_2 biosynthesis; or iv) produce an anticipated effect on one or more *in vitro* tests of platelet function [33]. The fact that some patients may experience recurrent vascular events despite long-term aspirin therapy should be properly labeled as 'treatment failure'. This is a common phenomenon occurring with any drug (e.g., lipid-lowering or antihypertensive drugs). Given the multifactorial nature of atherothrombosis, it is not surprising that only a fraction (usually one-quarter to one-third) of all vascular complications can be prevented by any single preventive strategy.

Similarly, the term 'clopidogrel resistance' has been used to denote non-responsiveness of ADP-induced platelet aggregation following standard clopidogrel therapy [34].

The term 'resistance' is uninformative of the mechanism(s) underlying interindividual variability in response to aspirin or clopidogrel, and is potentially misleading. Thus, it implies that something can be measured that has direct bearing on clinical efficacy and, depending on its results, may lead to a change in antiplatelet treatment. In fact, the relevance of the various functional indexes of platelet capacity that can be measured *ex vivo* to the actual occurrence of platelet activation and inhibition *in vivo* is largely unknown [33, 34]. Thus, the term 'resistance' should be avoided in order to advance our understanding of the distinct factors contributing to the interindividual variability in response to aspirin or clopidogrel (Table 2.1).

A test of platelet function should not be performed simply because an assay is available. In fact, no test of platelet function is currently recommended to assess the antiplatelet effects of aspirin or clopidogrel in the individual patient [6, 35]. At present, 'resistance' to aspirin or clopidogrel should not be looked for in the clinical setting, because there is no convincing evidence for an association with clinical events conditioning cost-effective changes in antiplatelet therapy [34, 35].

Increased awareness of the distinct factors potentially interfering with the desired antiplatelet effects of aspirin or clopidogrel, particularly avoidable drug interactions, may ultimately result in better patient management than requesting unnecessary, costly tests of platelet function.

As with any drug (antithrombotic, lipid-lowering or antihypertensive) used to prevent atherothrombosis, treatment 'failure' can occur with aspirin or clopidogrel, perhaps not surprisingly given the multifactorial nature of atherothrombosis. There is no scientific basis to change antiplatelet therapy in the face of a treatment 'failure', as we cannot be sure whether a second vascular event occurring in the same patient will reflect the same pathophysiological event that led to the first. Moreover, we have no controlled evidence that changing therapy is a more effective strategy than maintaining an evidence-based therapy.

Because we have a pretty detailed molecular understanding of how aspirin and clopidogrel work in preventing arterial thrombosis [6], new studies addressing the interindividual variability in response to these antiplatelet agents should rely upon mechanism-based biochemical endpoints rather than platelet aggregation measurements [34, 35].

Serum TXB_2 and urinary 11-dehydro-TXB_2 provide reliable information on the maximal biosynthetic capacity of circulating platelets *ex vivo* and on the actual rate of TXA_2 biosynthesis *in vivo*, respectively [36]. These measurements have been used extensively to characterise the clinical pharmacology of aspirin as an antiplatelet drug [5]. In patients treated with low-dose aspirin, serum TXB_2 levels reflect the adequacy of platelet COX-1 inhibition and its duration, while urinary TX-metabolite excretion provides a non-invasive, time-integrated index of aspirin-insensitive sources of TXA_2 biosynthesis [6, 37].

Reliable assessment of the adequacy and persistence of the expected pharmacodynamic effect of aspirin on platelet COX-1 would require a long-term, controlled study comparing aspirin to another antiplatelet drug in a sizeable group of stable patients requiring antiplatelet therapy. Clopidogrel would be an ideal comparator, because of remarkable similarities in the mechanism of action (permanent inactivation of a platelet protein), pharmacokinetics (short half-life of the active moiety) and dosing regimen (once daily).

Finally, given the size of the relative risk reduction (typically, 25 to 30% in high-risk patients) associated with long-term antiplatelet prophylaxis, novel studies aiming to detect an attenuation or loss of this protective effect, as a function of specific causes of interindividual variability in response to aspirin or clopidogrel, should have both the sensitivity and specificity necessary to detect such a small 'signal'. None of the studies published so far meets these requirements, and estimates of relative risk of recurrent atherothrombotic events associated with aspirin [38] or clopidogrel [39] 'resistance' are simply unrealistic.

Similarly, because of limitations with *post hoc* analyses and observational studies of drug interactions (e.g. between ibuprofen and aspirin or between atorvastatin and clopidogrel), well-designed clinical trials are needed to specifically evaluate the clinical read-outs of these interactions.

EFFICACY AND SAFETY OF LOW-DOSE ASPIRIN IN THE PREVENTION AND TREATMENT OF ATHEROTHROMBOSIS IN HIGH-RISK PATIENTS

The efficacy and safety of aspirin has been evaluated in patients covering the whole spectrum of atherothrombosis, from apparently healthy low-risk individuals to patients presenting with an acute MI or an acute ischaemic stroke. Among patients with occlusive vascular disease, both individual studies [reviewed in ref. 6] and a meta-analysis of trials of antiplatelet therapy [7] have shown that low-dose aspirin reduces the risk of a serious vascular event by approximately one quarter. This represents a composite of one-third reduction in non-fatal MI, one-quarter reduction in non-fatal stroke and one-sixth reduction in death from a vascular or unknown cause [6, 7]. Since each of these proportional reductions applies similarly to all categories of patients with vascular disease, the absolute benefits of aspirin in the individual patient can be estimated by applying a one-third reduction to her/his absolute risk of non-fatal MI, a one-quarter reduction to the risk of non-fatal stroke, and one-sixth reduction to the risk of vascular death [6, 7]. Thus, among a wide range of patients with vascular disease, in whom the annual risk of a serious vascular event ranges from 4% to 8%, aspirin typically prevents at least 10 to 20 fatal and non-fatal vascular events for every 1000 patients treated for one year [6, 7] (number needed to treat: 50 to 100).

Table 2.2 High-risk vascular disorders for which aspirin has been shown to be effective and lowest effective daily dose

Disorder	Lowest effective dose (mg)
Chronic stable angina	75
Unstable angina	75
Acute myocardial infarction	160
Transient ischaemic attack and ischaemic stroke	50
Severe carotid artery stenosis	75
Acute ischaemic stroke	160
Atrial fibrillation	325

Observational studies [40] and a meta-analysis [7] of trials among high-risk patients have demonstrated that long-term therapy with low-dose aspirin is associated with around a two-fold increased risk of major extracranial (mostly, upper gastrointestinal) bleeding, and this proportional excess hazard appears similar regardless of the variable underlying cardiovascular risk of the patient. In middle-aged patients, this corresponds to an estimated absolute excess of approximately 1 to 2 major bleeding complications per 1000 patients treated with low-dose aspirin for one year (number needed to harm: 500 to 1000). Therefore, for most high-risk patients using low-dose aspirin, the expected number avoiding a serious vascular event clearly outweighs the number experiencing major bleeding, unless there is some particular reason for an increased susceptibility to bleeding, such as advanced age, history of prior ulcer or concomitant treatment with other drugs interfering with primary haemostasis. Such a favourable benefit/risk balance of low-dose aspirin in high-risk patients has resulted in consistent level 1 recommendations by both North-American [6] and European [41] consensus documents and in regulatory approval of practically all vascular indications except for peripheral arterial disease. More aggressive antiplatelet regimens (e.g., the combination of low-dose aspirin and clopidogrel) may result in improved efficacy at the expense of increased bleeding complications. The benefit/risk profile of combined antiplatelet strategies are discussed elsewhere in the volume.

Thus, aspirin is recommended in all clinical conditions in which antiplatelet prophylaxis has a favourable benefit/risk profile. In consideration of dose-dependent gastrointestinal toxicity and its potential impact on compliance, physicians are encouraged to use the lowest dose of aspirin that was shown to be effective in each clinical setting (Table 2.2). The available evidence supports daily doses of aspirin in the range of 75 to 100 mg for the long-term prevention of serious vascular events in high-risk patients [6, 41]. In clinical settings where an immediate antithrombotic effect is required (such as in acute coronary syndromes or in acute ischaemic stroke), a loading dose of 160–200 mg should be given at diagnosis in order to ensure rapid and complete inhibition of thromboxane-dependent platelet aggregation.

EFFICACY AND SAFETY OF LOW-DOSE ASPIRIN IN PATIENTS AT INTERMEDIATE RISK OF VASCULAR COMPLICATIONS

As can be seen in Figure 2.3, depicting the absolute benefit and hazard produced by aspirin in six primary prevention trials [42–47], the number of major vascular events avoided does not clearly outweigh the number of major bleeds caused in most of these trials, and the two lines only begin to separate from each other above an annual baseline risk of 1.5%. Because at least three of these trials (Hypertension Optimal Treatment [HOT], Thrombosis Prevention

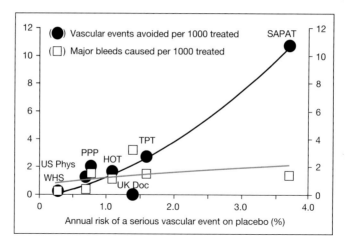

Figure 2.3 Benefits and risks of low-dose aspirin in primary prevention trials. Vascular events (●) avoided and major bleeds (□) caused per 1000 treated with aspirin per year are plotted from individual placebo-controlled aspirin trials in different patient populations characterised by variable cardiovascular risk, as noted on the abscissa. For each of the seven trials, a couple of symbols describe the absolute benefit (●) and hazard (□) associated with one year of aspirin therapy in 1000 subjects.

WHS = Womens' Health Study; US Phys = US Physicians' Health Study; PPP = Primary Prevention Project; HOT = Hypertension Optimal Treatment; UK Doc = British Doctors Trial; TPT = Thrombosis Prevention Trial; SAPAT = Swedish Angina Pectoris Aspirin Trial. Modified from [41]

Trial [TPT] and Primary Prevention Project [PPP]) were carried out in people selected for being at 'high' cardiovascular risk, it is perhaps surprising that the actual rate of vascular events in these 'high-risk' subjects was not markedly higher than that of unselected, apparently healthy subjects (e.g., compare the rate of events in TPT and in the British Doctors Study). Risk prediction algorithms employ multiple risk factors which are individually weak screening tools, so that their combination in a risk prediction algorithm is also weak and lacks adequate sensitivity and specificity.

Since disease rates rise exponentially above 60 years, and since demographic changes will result in large increases in the elderly population in the coming years, the potential for prevention in this group is substantial. However, the balance of risk and benefit is uncertain in older individuals (in whom the bleeding risks also increase) because the amount of randomised evidence in those aged 70 or over is limited (around 10% of the primary prevention trial population). Further randomised trials among elderly individuals would therefore help to strengthen the evidence in this important group.

Another important category of individuals without known vascular disease for whom aspirin might be considered is those with diabetes mellitus. Despite current guidelines on the routine use of aspirin in these patients, evidence that the benefit of antiplatelet prophylaxis outweighs the risk of major bleeding complications in this setting is largely inadequate. Thus, only one trial of aspirin vs. placebo has been conducted among diabetic patients. In the Early Treatment Diabetic Retinopathy (ETDRS) trial [48], diabetic patients were eligible if they had mild or moderate retinopathy, and were randomised to aspirin 650 mg daily vs. placebo. Among 3711 randomised patients, only 6% had a history of MI, and the mean annual risk of a major coronary event was 2.5%. However, although there was a marginally significant 17% reduction ($P = 0.04$) in major coronary events among them, there was no significant effect on stroke or vascular death. Consequently, there remains considerable uncertainty about the benefits and risks of aspirin among diabetic patients with no known vascular disease, and this is another area where further trials would be useful. One

Table 2.3 Primary prevention trials of low-dose aspirin vs. placebo

Trial	Subjects (n)	Follow-up (yrs)	Placebo event rate % per year	Aspirin RR
UK doctors	Healthy men (5139)	5.8	1.4	1.03
US physicians	Healthy men (22 071)	5.0	0.7	0.82
Thrombosis Prevention Trial (TPT)	High-risk men (5085)	6.3	1.6	0.83
Hypertension Optimal Treatment (HOT)	Hypertensive patients (18 790)	3.8	1.1	0.85
Primary Prevention Project (PPP)	High-risk men and women (4495)	3.6	0.8	0.71
Women's Health Study (WHS)	Healthy women (39 876)	10.1	0.3	0.91

such trial, ASCEND (A Study of Cardiovascular Events in Diabetes), is currently ongoing in the UK.

Another interesting paradigm of 'intermediate-risk' patients is that provided by myeloproliferative disorders, a heterogeneous group of diseases involving clonal haematopoietic stem cells that includes polycythaemia vera, essential thrombocythaemia, idiopathic myelofibrosis and chronic myelogenous leukaemia. In both polycythaemia vera and essential thrombocythaemia, thrombotic complications are a major cause of illness and death in untreated patients [49]. In the former condition, a recently completed placebo-controlled randomised trial of aspirin 100 mg daily has demonstrated that this regimen of antiplatelet therapy can safely prevent both arterial and venous thrombotic complications [50]. Interestingly, despite the lack of any evidence for the efficacy and safety of low-dose aspirin in essential thrombocythaemia, all such patients recruited in a recently published randomised trial of hydroxyurea vs. anagrelide were treated with aspirin 75–100 mg daily [51].

EFFICACY AND SAFETY OF LOW-DOSE ASPIRIN IN LOW-RISK SUBJECTS

Although the benefits of low-dose aspirin are clear among patients with vascular disease, the benefit/risk profile of the same preventive strategy is substantially uncertain in low-risk individuals with no clinically apparent vascular disease. The decision to prescribe low-dose aspirin in a person with no history of vascular disease must rely on an individual judgment that the likely benefits of aspirin will exceed any risks. On the basis of the available evidence from six primary prevention trials [42–47] (Table 2.3), low-dose aspirin therapy for 4 to 10 years prevents non-fatal MI by one-quarter, but it has no clear protective effect against ischaemic stroke or vascular death. Therefore, assessing the benefits and risks of low-dose aspirin requires balancing any absolute reduction in non-fatal MI (1 to 3 per 1000 treated for one year) against an increased risk of major gastro-intestinal bleeding (1 to 2 per 1000) and haemorrhagic stroke (0.1 to 0.2 per 1000).

It has been suggested that low-dose aspirin may be appropriate for individuals whose estimated annual risk of a coronary event, based on a risk prediction algorithm, exceeds a particular threshold [52, 53]. Various guidelines have adopted this approach [54–56] using risk thresholds for coronary events ranging from 0.6% to 1.5% per year. In particular, the suggestion [57] that aspirin therapy is safe and worthwhile at coronary event risk equal to or greater than 1.5% per year is potentially attractive. However, as shown in Figure 2.3, we lack clinical trial data in the area of cardiovascular risk that is intermediate between the observed risk in the placebo arm of the Thrombosis Prevention Trial [44] (approximately 1.5%) and that of the Swedish trial in patients with chronic stable angina [58] (approximately 3.5%).

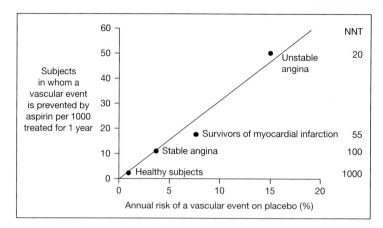

Figure 2.4 The absolute risk of vascular complications is the major determinant of the absolute benefit of antiplatelet prophylaxis. Data are plotted from placebo-controlled aspirin trials in different clinical settings. For each category of patients, the abscissa denotes the absolute risk of experiencing a major vascular event as recorded in the placebo arm of the trial(s). The absolute benefit of antiplatelet treatment is reported on the ordinate as the number of subjects in whom an important vascular event (non-fatal myocardial infarction, non-fatal stroke, or vascular death) is actually prevented by treating 1000 subjects with aspirin for 1 year.
NNT = number needed to treat.
Modified from [6].

Moreover, it should be emphasised that current estimates of the absolute excess of major bleeding complications associated with low-dose aspirin therapy are likely to underestimate the potential harm in individuals at increased risk of bleeding complications, who were typically excluded from aspirin trials [21]. Although many gastroenterologists would recommend the use of proton-pump inhibitors to reduce such risk, the best strategy to minimise the burden of gastrointestinal toxicity associated with low-dose aspirin is currently uncertain and more studies are needed to resolve this uncertainty.

CONCLUSIONS

Inhibition of TXA_2-dependent platelet function by aspirin may lead to prevention of thrombosis as well as to excess bleeding. Assessing the net effect requires an estimation of the absolute thrombotic vs. haemorrhagic risk of the individual patient. In individuals at very low risk for vascular occlusion, a very small absolute benefit may be offset by exposure of very large numbers of healthy subjects to undue bleeding complications. As the risk of experiencing a major vascular event increases, so does the absolute benefit of antiplatelet prophylaxis with aspirin, as shown in Figure 2.4, for a number of clinical settings in which the efficacy of the drug has been tested in randomised clinical trials [6]. Based on the results of such trials, the antithrombotic effect of aspirin does not appear to be dose-related, over a wide range of daily doses (30 to 1300 mg), an observation consistent with saturability of platelet COX inhibition at very low doses. In contrast, gastrointestinal toxicity of the drug does appear to be dose-related, consistent with dose- and dosing interval-dependent inhibition of COX activity in the nucleated lining cells of the gastrointestinal mucosa. Thus, aspirin once daily is recommended in all clinical conditions in which antiplatelet prophylaxis has a favourable benefit/risk profile. Because of gastrointestinal toxicity and its potential impact on compliance, physicians are encouraged to use the lowest dose of aspirin shown to be effective in each clinical setting [6, 41].

REFERENCES

1. Majerus PW. Arachidonate metabolism in vascular disorders. *J Clin Invest* 1983; 72:1521–1525.
2. Patrono C, Ciabattoni G, Pinca E *et al*. Low-dose aspirin and inhibition of thromboxane B2 production in healthy subjects. *Thromb Res* 1980; 17:317–327.
3. Patrignani P, Filabozzi P, Patrono C. Selective cumulative inhibition of platelet thromboxane production by low-dose aspirin in healthy subjects. *J Clin Invest* 1982; 69:1366–1372.
4. Patrono C, Ciabattoni G, Patrignani P *et al*. Clinical pharmacology of platelet cyclooxygenase inhibition. *Circulation* 1985; 72:1177–1184.
5. Patrono C. Aspirin as an antiplatelet drug. *N Engl J Med* 1994; 330:1287–1294.
6. Patrono C, Coller B, FitzGerald GA, Hirsh J, Roth G. Platelet-Active Drugs: The relationships among dose, effectiveness, and side effects. *Chest* 2004; 126(suppl 3):234S–264S.
7. Antithrombotic Trialists' (ATT) Collaboration. Collaborative meta-analysis of randomised trials of antiplatelet therapy for prevention of death, myocardial infarction, and stroke in high risk patients. *BMJ* 2002; 324:71–86.
8. Smith WL, Garavito RM, DeWitt DL. Prostaglandin endoperoxide H synthases (cyclooxygenases)-1 and -2. *J Biol Chem* 1996; 271:33157–33160.
9. Loll PJ, Picot D, Garavito RM. The structural basis of aspirin activity inferred from the crystal structure of inactivated prostaglandin H_2 synthase. *Nature Struct Biol* 1995; 2:637–643.
10. Cipollone F, Patrignani P, Greco A *et al*. Differential suppression of thromboxane biosynthesis by indobufen and aspirin in patients with unstable angina. *Circulation* 1997; 96:1109–1116.
11. Pedersen AK, FitzGerald GA. Dose-related kinetics of aspirin: presystemic acetylation of platelet cyclooxygenase. *N Engl J Med* 1984; 311:1206–1211.
12. Clarke RJ, Mayo G, Price P, FitzGerald GA. Suppression of thromboxane A_2 but not systemic prostacyclin by controlled-release aspirin. *N Engl J Med* 1991; 325:1137–1141.
13. McAdam B, Keimowitz RM, Maher M, Fitzgerald DJ. Transdermal modification of platelet function: an aspirin patch system results in marked suppression of platelet cyclooxygenase. *J Pharmacol Exp Ther* 1996; 277:559–564.
14. Kobayashi T, Tahara Y, Matsumoto M *et al*. Roles of thromboxane A_2 and prostacyclin in the development of atherosclerosis in apoE-deficient mice. *J Clin Invest* 2004; 114:784–794.
15. Topper JN, Cai J, Falb D, Gimbrone MA, Jr. Identification of vascular endothelial genes differentially responsive to fluid mechanical stimuli: cyclooxygenase-2, manganese superoxide dismutase, and endothelial cell nitric oxide synthase are selectively up-regulated by steady laminar shear stress. *Proc Natl Acad Sci USA* 1996; 93:10417–10422.
16. McAdam BF, Catella-Lawson F, Mardini IA, Kapoor S, Lawson JA, FitzGerald GA. Systemic biosynthesis of prostacyclin by cyclooxygenase (COX)-2: the human pharmacology of a selective inhibitor of COX-2. *Proc Natl Acad Sci USA* 1999; 96:272–277.
17. FitzGerald GA, Oates JA, Hawiger J *et al*. Endogenous biosynthesis of prostacyclin and thromboxane and platelet function during chronic administration of aspirin in man. *J Clin Invest* 1983; 71:676–688.
18. Murata T, Ushikubi F, Matsuoka T *et al*. Altered pain perception and inflammatory response in mice lacking prostacyclin receptor. *Nature* 1997; 388:678–682.
19. Ridker PM, Cushman M, Stampfer MJ, Tracy RP, Hennekens CH. Inflammation, aspirin, and the risk of cardiovascular disease in apparently healthy men. *N Engl J Med* 1997; 336:973–979.
20. FitzGerald GA, Patrono C. The Coxibs: Inhibitors of cyclooxygenase-2. *N Engl J Med* 2001; 345:433–442.
21. Patrono C, García Rodríguez LA, Landolfi R, Baigent C. Low-dose aspirin for the prevention of atherothrombosis. Submitted for publication.
22. Hansson L, Zanchetti A, Carruthers SG *et al*. Effects of intensive blood-pressure lowering and low-dose aspirin in patients with hypertension: principal results of the Hypertension Optimal Treatment (HOT) randomised trial. *Lancet* 1998; 351:1755–1762.
23. Pierucci A, Simonetti BM, Pecci G *et al*. Improvement of renal function with selective thromboxane antagonism in lupus nephritis. *N Engl J Med* 1989; 320:421–425.
24. Al-Khadra AS, Salem DN, Rand WM, Udelson JE, Smith JJ, Konstam MA. Antiplatelet agents and survival: a cohort analysis from the Studies of Left Ventricular Dysfunction (SOLVD) trial. *J Am Coll Cardiol* 1998; 31:419–425.
25. Latini R, Tognoni G, Maggioni AP *et al*. Clinical effects of early angiotensin-converting enzyme inhibitor treatment for acute myocardial infarction are similar in the presence and absence of aspirin: systematic overview of individual data from 96,712 randomized patients;

Angiotensin-converting Enzyme Inhibitor Myocardial Infarction Collaborative Group. *J Am Coll Cardiol* 2000; 35:1801–1807.

26.   Zanchetti A, Hansson L, Leonetti G *et al*. Low-dose aspirin does not interefere with the blood pressure-lowering effects of antihypertensive therapy. *J Hypertens* 2002; 20:1015–1022.

27.   Teo KK, Yusuf S, Pfeffer M *et al*; ACE Inhibitors Collaborative Group. Effects of long-term treatment with angiotensin-converting-enzyme inhibitors in the presence or absence of aspirin: a systematic review. *Lancet* 2002; 360:1037–1043.

28.   Catella-Lawson F, Reilly MP, Kapoor SC *et al*. Cyclooxygenase inhibitors and the antiplatelet effects of aspirin. *N Engl J Med* 2001; 345:1809–1817.

29.   Capone ML, Sciulli MG, Tacconelli S *et al*. Pharmacodynamic interaction of naproxen with low-dose aspirin in healthy subjects. *J Am Coll Cardiol* 2005; 45:1295–1301.

30.   García Rodríguez LA, Varas-Lorenzo C, Maguire A, Gonzalez-Perez A. Nonsteroidal antiinflammatory drugs and the risk of myocardial infarction in the general population. *Circulation* 2004; 109:3000–3006.

31.   Silverstein FE, Faich G, Goldstein JL *et al*. Gastrointestinal toxicity with celecoxib vs nonsteroidal anti-inflammatory drugs for osteoarthritis and rheumatoid arthritis The CLASS Study: A randomized controlled trial. *JAMA* 2000; 284:1247–1255.

32.   Schnitzer TJ, Burmester DR, Mysler E *et al*; TARGET Study Group. Comparison of lumiracoxib with naproxen and ibuprofen in the Therapeutic Arthritis Research and Gastrointestinal Event Trial (TARGET), reduction in ulcer complications: randomised controlled trial. *Lancet* 2004; 364:664–674.

33.   Patrono C. Aspirin resistance: definition, mechanisms and clinical read-outs. *J Thromb Haemostas* 2003; 1:1710–1713.

34.   Rocca B, Patrono C. Determinants of the interindividual variability in response to antiplatelet drugs. *J Thromb Haemostas* 2005;3:1597–1602.

35.   Cattaneo M. Aspirin and clopidogrel. Efficacy, safety, and the issue of drug resistance. *Arterioscler Thromb Vasc Biol* 2004; 24:1980–1987.

36.   FitzGerald GA, Pedersen AK, Patrono C. Analysis of prostacyclin and thromboxane biosynthesis in cardiovascular disease. *Circulation* 1983; 67:1174–1177.

37.   Cipollone F, Rocca B, Patrono C. Cyclooxygenase-2 expression and inhibition in atherothrombosis. *Arterioscler Thromb Vasc Biol* 2004; 24:246–255.

38.   Gum PA, Kottke-Marchant K, Welsh PA, White J, Topol EJ. A prospective, blinded determination of the natural history of aspirin resistance among stable patients with cardiovascular disease. *J Am Coll Cardiol* 2003; 41:961–965.

39.   Matetzky S, Shenkman B, Guetta V *et al*. Clopidogrel resistance is associated with increased risk of recurrent atherothrombotic events in patients with acute myocardial infarction. *Circulation* 2004; 109:3171–3175.

40.   García Rodríguez LA, Hernández-Díaz S, de Abajo FJ. Association between aspirin and upper gastrointestinal complications: systematic review of epidemiologic studies. *Br J Clin Pharmacol* 2001; 52:563–571.

41.   Patrono C, Bachmann F, Baigent C *et al*. Expert consensus document on the use of antiplatelet agents. *Eur Heart J* 2004; 25:166–181.

42.   Peto R, Gray R, Collins R *et al*. Randomised trial of prophylactic daily aspirin in British male doctors. *BMJ* 1988; 296:313–316.

43.   Steering Committee of the Physicians' Health Study Research Group. Final report on the aspirin component of the ongoing Physicians' Health Study. *N Engl J Med* 1989; 321:129–135.

44.   MRC General Practice Framework. Thrombosis prevention trial: randomised trial of low intensity oral anticoagulation with warfarin and low-dose aspirin in primary prevention of ischaemic heart disease in men at increased risk. *Lancet* 1998; 351:233–241.

45.   Hansson L, Zanchetti A, Carruthers SG *et al*. Effects of intensive blood-pressure lowering and low-dose aspirin in patients with hypertension: principal results of the Hypertension Optimal Treatment (HOT) randomised trial. *Lancet* 1998; 351:1755–1762.

46.   Collaborative Group of the Primary Prevention Project. Low-dose aspirin and vitamin E in people at cardiovascular risk: a randomised trial in general practice. *Lancet* 2001; 357:89–95.

47.   Ridker PM, Cook NR, Lee IM *et al*. A randomized trial of low-dose aspirin in the primary prevention of cardiovascular disease in women. *N Engl J Med* 2005; 352:1293–1304.

48.   ETDRS Investigators. Aspirin effects on mortality and morbidity in patients with diabetes mellitus. Early Treatment Diabetic Retinopathy Study Report 14. *JAMA* 1992; 268:1292–1300.

49.   Barbui T, Finazzi G. When and how to treat essential thrombocythemia. *N Engl J Med* 2005; 353:85–86.

50. Landolfi R, Marchioli R, Kutti J *et al*. Efficacy and safety of low-dose aspirin in polycythemia vera. *N Engl J Med* 2004; 350:114–124.

51. Harrison CN, Campbell PJ, Buck G *et al*. Hydroxyurea compared with anagrelide in high-risk essential thrombocythemia. *N Engl J Med* 2005; 353:33–45.

52. Sanmuganathan PS, Ghahramani P, Jackson PR, Wallis EJ, Ramsay LE. Aspirin for primary prevention of coronary heart disease: safety and absolute benefit related to coronary risk derived from meta-analysis of randomised trials. *Heart* 2001; 85:265–271.

53. Hayden M, Pignone M, Philipps C, Mulrow C. Aspirin for the primary prevention of cardiovascular events: a summary of the evidence for the US Preventive Services Task Force. *Ann Intern Med* 2002; 136:161–171.

54. Wood D, De Backer G, Faergeman O, Graham I, Mancia G, Pyorala K. Prevention of coronary heart disease in clinical practice: recommendations of the Second Joint Force of European and Other Societies on Coronary Prevention. *Atherosclerosis* 1998; 140:199–270.

55. US Preventive Services Task Force. Aspirin for the primary prevention of cardiovascular events: recommendation and rationale. *Ann Intern Med* 2002; 136:157–160.

56. Pearson TA, Blair SN, Daniels SR *et al*. AHA guidelines for primary prevention of cardiovascular disease and stroke: 2002 Update. *Circulation* 2002; 106:388–391.

57. Lauer M. Aspirin for primary prevention of coronary events. *N Engl J Med* 2002; 346:1468–1474.

58. Juul-Moller S, Edvardsson N, Jahnmatz B, Rosen A, Sorensen S, Omblus R. Double-blind trial of aspirin in primary prevention of myocardial infarction in patients with stable chronic angina pectoris. *Lancet* 1992; 340:1421–1425.

3

Clopidogrel and other platelet ADP inhibitors

R. B. Fathi, D. L. Bhatt, E. J. Topol

INTRODUCTION

Atherosclerotic plaque rupture and endothelial denudation expose blood to the subendo-thelial collagen and lipid-rich core that commence the cascade of platelet adhesion, activation, aggregation and thrombin formation, leading to the common pathway of end-organ ischaemia. Platelets and specifically inhibition of their function have emerged on the fore-front of cardiovascular research in the last decade due to the devastating consequences of atherothrombosis. It has long been known that aspirin irreversibly blocks the cyclo-oxygenase pathway and thus prevents the conversion of arachidonic acid to thromboxane A_2. Even though aspirin use has been associated with significant clinical benefits in the secondary prevention of cardiovascular events [1], its relative antiplatelet potency is modest and it has been plagued by adverse side-effects such as gastrointestinal bleeding. Furthermore, many patients continue to have ischaemic events while on aspirin [2], and the concept of 'aspirin resistance' that has been defined as the lack of *in vitro* inhibition of platelet aggregability has been demonstrated in approximately 10% of the population [3]. This effect has not been ameliorated with increasing doses of aspirin and is associated with worst clinical outcomes [4–6]. Thus, newer agents have been developed affecting alternate pathways of platelet biology. Prominent amongst these novel agents are the thienopy-ridines, ticlopidine and clopidogrel, that inhibit adenosine diphosphate (ADP) binding to its platelet receptor, thereby inhibiting platelet aggregation and activation.

ADP RECEPTOR

ADP is a platelet agonist that is secreted from granules in activated platelets and damaged vasculature. After binding to its specific platelet membrane receptor, it leads to activation of a G-protein complex causing the release of cytosolic calcium stores, leading to conformational change of the platelet from a discoid shape to a spiculated one. The platelet glyco-protein IIb/IIIa (GPIIb/IIIa) receptor then becomes activated allowing for fibrinogen binding and promotion of platelet aggregation.

Three major ADP receptors have been described: $P2X_1$, $P2Y_1$ and $P2Y_{12}$. The $P2X_1$ ion channel subtype is associated with platelet shape change and aggregation through calcium influx after activation by ATP. The $P2Y_1$ subtype is a G_q-protein coupled receptor, which also leads to increased calcium influx and platelet shape change through the activation

Robert B. Fathi, Staff, Cardiac, Peripheral and Carotid Intervention, Cleveland Clinic Foundation, Cleveland, Ohio, USA.

Deepak L. Bhatt, Director, Interventional Cardiology Fellowship, Cleveland Clinic Foundation, Cleveland, Ohio, USA.

Eric J. Topol, Chairman, Department of Cardiovascular Medicine and Professor of Medicine and Genetics, Cleveland Clinic Foundation, Cleveland, Ohio, USA.

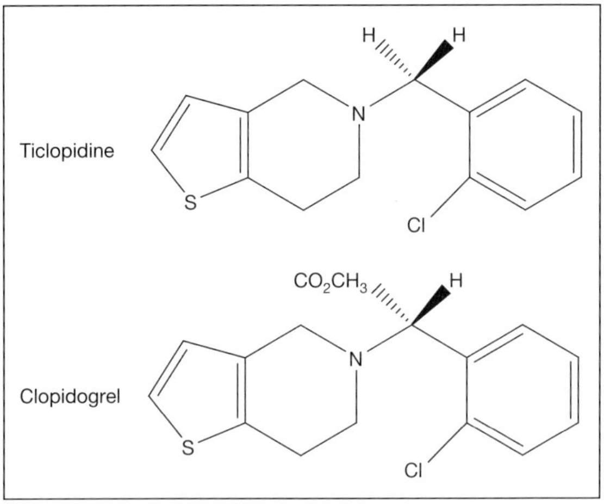

Figure 3.1 The chemical structures of ticlopidine and clopidogrel.

of phospholipase C. The $P2Y_{12}$ receptor is a G_i-protein coupled receptor that decreases cyclic AMP by inhibiting adenylyl cyclase. Its activation is directly associated with platelet aggregation [7].

ADP RECEPTOR ANTAGONISTS

THIENOPYRIDINES

The thienopyridines are irreversible inhibitors of platelet aggregation that act through the adenosine 5'-diphosphate receptor. The two seminal agents in this group are ticlopidine and clopidogrel – two structurally similar agents, differing with an addition of a carboxymethyl group in clopidogrel (Figure 3.1).

TICLOPIDINE

Ticlopidine became available for clinical use in 1978 and was found to be beneficial in patients with established coronary and peripheral vascular disease [8, 9]. Interest in its use though soon turned to the rapidly growing field of percutaneous coronary intervention (PCI). The advent of coronary stenting was embraced as it reduced the rate of restenosis and minimised the incidence of abrupt vessel closure. Its use was initially marred, however, by the high prevalence of acute and subacute stent thrombosis which typically occurred within 30 days [10]. Various antithrombotic strategies including aspirin, heparin, dextran and warfarin were studied, often complicated by extensive bleeding and prolonged hospitalisation. Initial promising attempts at minimising this complication using coumadin and aspirin-based regimens were soon replaced by the dual antiplatelet regimen of aspirin and ticlopidine due to its superior efficacy and lower bleeding risk [11].

The clinical application of ticlopidine was hindered by the development of neutropaenia (2.4%), skin rash, gastrointestinal upset and rarely thrombotic thrombocytopaenic purpura (~0.02%) [12–14]. Furthermore, its use was limited by its delayed onset of action. For these reasons clopidogrel, a structural analogue of ticlopidine, which lacked these adverse haematological side-effects and could be loaded with oral dosing, gained prominence amongst cardiologists even before the first large-scale trials assessing its safety and efficacy were published. Initial studies comparing ticlopidine to clopidogrel were hampered by small sample size and underpowered to show superiority of either agent [15–17], though clopidogrel was better tolerated due to increased discontinuation of ticlopidine because of adverse effects [15]. Despite early concerns of the relative safety of clopidogrel versus ticlopidine [18], a large meta-analysis of all randomised and registry comparisons of clopidogrel and ticlopidine after coronary stenting involving 13 955 patients found that the use of clopidogrel was associated with a decreased 30-day rate of major adverse cardiac events (odds ratio 0.51; $P = 0.001$) [19].

CLOPIDOGREL

Clopidogrel has no significant antiplatelet activity *in vitro*. After oral ingestion it is metabolised by the hepatic cytochrome P450 3A4 enzyme into 2-oxo-clopidogrel, which undergoes hydrolysis before binding to and irreversibly inhibiting the $P2Y_{12}$ receptor [20]. This prevents the coupling of the G_i/adenylyl cyclase system through the formation of a disulfide bridge between the thiol moiety of the active clopidogrel metabolite and a scysteine residue of the $P2Y_{12}$ receptor. It has no direct activity on the platelet GPIIb/IIIa receptor.

The use of a loading dose can substantially decrease the time needed to attain maximal platelet inhibition. This effect can occur within 4–6 h with the use of a loading dose of 300 mg of clopidogrel compared to ticlopidine which can take as long as 5 days. Its absorption and bioavailability is not affected by meals [21]. No dosing adjustment is needed for the elderly, patients with renal or mild to moderate hepatic dysfunction. After discontinuation its effects can persist for up to 10 days.

Clopidogrel also modulates vascular inflammation [22, 23] through decreased production of CD-40 ligand and P-selectin which mediate platelet–leucocyte interactions on the endothelium [24, 25]. Its use has been associated with improved clinical outcomes in patients with elevated levels of C-reactive protein undergoing PCI [26] suggesting its use modulates the vascular inflammatory milieu [27].

Clinical use of clopidogrel

The Clopidogrel vs. Aspirin in Patients at Risk of Ischaemic Events (CAPRIE) study randomised 19 185 patients with symptomatic disease of the coronary, cerebral or peripheral vascular beds to treatment with clopidogrel 75 mg daily or ASA 325 mg daily for an average of 1.6 years. The relative risk of the primary composite endpoint of myocardial infarction (MI), ischaemic stroke or vascular death was 8.7% less in patients treated with clopidogrel ($P = 0.043$) [12]. Clopidogrel was also found to have a lower rate of re-hospitalisation for ischaemic or bleeding events [28]. This benefit was particularly useful in high-risk patients such as those with diabetes, prior ischaemic events or prior coronary bypass grafting [29, 30]. A substudy of 1480 patients in CAPRIE with prior coronary bypass grafting found that the use of clopidogrel was associated with a 31.2% relative risk reduction (RRR) of vascular death, MI, stroke and re-hospitalisation ($P = 0.0003$) [31]. Importantly, unlike ticlopidine, there was no increased incidence of neutropaenia and thrombocytopaenia when compared with aspirin.

Though clopidogrel was found to be modestly superior to aspirin in CAPRIE, combination therapy of aspirin and clopidogrel held significant promise based on the *ex vivo* finding of synergistic platelet inhibition with the combination when compared to aspirin alone [32]. This potential clinical benefit was addressed in the Clopidogrel in Unstable Angina Recurrent Events (CURE) study in which 12 562 patients with unstable angina or non-ST-segment elevation MI were randomised to clopidogrel with aspirin or aspirin alone within 24 h of presentation. Clopidogrel treatment consisted of a loading dose of 300 mg, followed by 75 mg daily. Aspirin therapy was a daily dosing of between 75 and 325 mg as dictated by the treating physician. Dual antiplatelet therapy was associated with a 20% relative risk reduction of the composite endpoint of vascular death, MI, or stroke at a mean follow-up of

Table 3.1 Recent large-scale clinical trials investigating clopidogrel

Study	Number	Group	Therapy	Mean follow-up	Finding
CAPRIE [12]	19 185	Recent, MI, stroke or peripheral vascular disease symptoms	Clopidogrel 75 mg/ day vs. aspirin	1.9 years	8.7% reduction in MI, ischaemic stroke and vascular death
CREDO [46]	2116	Percutaneous coronary intervention (PCI)	Clopidogrel 75 mg/ day + aspirin vs. placebo + aspirin	1.0 year	27% reduction in death, MI, stroke 36% reduction if pre-treated ≥6 h
CURE [36]	12 562	Acute non-ST-segment elevation acute coronary syndrome	Clopidogrel 75 mg/ day + aspirin vs. placebo + aspirin	9.0 months	20% reduction in non-fatal MI, stroke and cardiovascular death
PCI-CURE [45]	2658	Patients within CURE undergoing PCI	Clopidogrel 75 mg/ day + aspirin vs. placebo + aspirin	8.0 months	30% reduction in cardiovascular death, MI, or urgent target vessel revascularisation
ISAR-REACT [39]	2159	Low to intermediate risk PCI	Clopidogrel 75 mg/day + abciximab vs. Clopidogrel 75 mg/day + placebo	30 days	No difference for death, MI or urgent target vessel revascularisation

CAPRIE = Clopidogrel versus Aspirin in Patients at Risk of Ischaemic Events; CREDO = Clopidogrel for the Reduction of Events During Observation; CURE = Clopidogrel in Unstable Angina Recurrent Events; ISAR-REACT = Intracoronary Stenting and Antithrombotic Regimen-Rapid Early Action for Coronary Treatment.

9 months. This beneficial effect on ischaemic events became evident as early as 2 h from randomisation and became statistically significant by 24 h [33–35].

The use of clopidogrel plus aspirin was associated with increased bleeding and requirement of blood transfusions (≥2 units of blood) [36]. Bleeding from clopidogrel associated with coronary bypass grafting has also been a concern – in patients in whom clopidogrel was withheld for a mean of 5 days, no significant difference existed with respect to major bleeding. When clopidogrel was withheld for <5 days, a strong trend towards increased bleeding was evident (9.6 vs. 6.3%; $P = 0.06$). This concern has been reflected and incorporated in the American College of Cardiology/American Heart Association guidelines for patients presenting with non-ST-segment MI undergoing coronary catheterisation within 24–36 h that clopidogrel should be withheld until it is decided that the patient will not undergo coronary bypass surgery in the index admission [37].

Though abciximab has been associated with improved clinical outcomes in patients undergoing high-risk PCI [38], its utility in low- to intermediate-risk PCI in patients pre-treated with clopidogrel is uncertain. Kastrati *et al.* [39] randomised 2159 patients undergoing elective PCI to either abciximab or placebo. All patients received aspirin and a loading dose of clopidogrel 600 mg at least 2 h prior to the intervention. Patients were followed for the composite endpoint of death, MI or urgent target vessel revascularisation. At 30 days there was no significant difference in this composite endpoint (4% in the abciximab group vs. 4% in the placebo group; $P = 0.82$). A summary of these trials is displayed in Table 3.1.

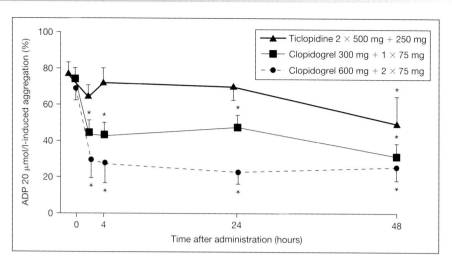

Figure 3.2 The effect on ADP-induced platelet aggregation using 3 different antiplatelet regimens. Near maximal antiplatelet activity can obtained by 4 h using a 600-mg loading dose of clopidogrel. (*$P < 0.05$ from baseline level; modified with permission from [44].

Clopidogrel dosing

Since platelet aggregation after coronary stenting is directly involved with stent thrombosis, clopidogrel has become the primary agent for its prevention. The typical daily dosing regimen for clopidogrel of 75 mg daily was initiated as it provided similar antiplatelet activity to ticlopidine 250 mg twice daily [12]. Prior work has shown that in healthy volunteers, a loading dose of 300 mg of clopidogrel provides near steady-state of ADP-induced platelet aggregation within 6 h; a similar effect with daily dosing of 75 mg requires between 3 and 7 days [40, 41]. Gurbel *et al.* [42] investigated the effect of time dependence of clopidogrel loading on platelet and whole blood aggregation. While no significant difference existed if patients were loaded with 300 mg clopidogrel between 3 and 6 h prior, 12 h prior or 24 h prior to stenting, the use of a loading dose provided increased levels of platelet inhibition compared to 75 mg given at the time of stenting. There is also evidence that 600 mg of clopidogrel exerts both an antiplatelet and an anti-inflammatory effect more rapidly than 300 mg [43]. Loading doses of 600 mg have been shown to more rapidly inhibit platelet aggregability [44] (Figure 3.2), and have been used in recent trials such as ISAR-REACT and the Intracoronary Stenting with Antithrombotic Regimen Cooling-off Trial (ISAR-COOL) with success [39]. There has not been a definitive randomised trial of 600 mg (or higher) compared with 300 mg, for clinical outcomes, but the totality of data strongly favour using a 600 mg loading if vascular intervention is being performed within 24 h of the loading dose.

Duration of treatment post-stenting

Based on data from earlier studies such as the Clopidogrel Aspirin Stent International Cooperative Study (CLASSICS) [15], the arbitrary duration of therapy with clopidogrel after coronary stenting was 28 days, at which time it was felt that the stent had endothelialised and thus risk of stent thrombosis was minimised. The following studies suggest that longer duration of therapy – up to one year – might provide incremental benefit. A substudy termed PCI-CURE evaluated the 2658 patients undergoing PCI within the larger CURE cohort, of whom 2172 (81.7%) received intracoronary stents [45]. Despite the fact that fewer patients in the clopidogrel arm received GPIIb/IIIa inhibitors, this group had a 30% RRR of the primary endpoint of cardiovascular death, MI or urgent target vessel revascularisation at a mean follow-up of 8 months (4.5 vs. 6.4%; $P = 0.03$). This benefit occurred without a significant difference in the rate of major bleeds.

The Clopidogrel for the Reduction of Events During Observation (CREDO) study randomised 2116 patients undergoing elective PCI to 300 mg clopidogrel loading or placebo between 3 and 24 h prior to the procedure, followed by clopidogrel 75 mg/day [46]. After day 28 and up to 12 months, patients who were pre-loaded with clopidogrel continued with 75 mg/day while those with no loading dose received placebo. By 28 days, pre-treatment with clopidogrel was not associated with a reduction of death, MI or urgent target vessel revascularisation, yet a prespecified subgroup analysis suggested that pre-treatment with clopidogrel for ≥6 h had a 38.6% RRR of this primary endpoint ($P = 0.051$) compared to those with pre-treatment of <6 h. At 12 months, patients receiving clopidogrel had a 26.9% RRR in the primary endpoint compared to patients receiving placebo ($P = 0.02$). Similar benefits from dual antiplatelet therapy have been obtained after carotid stenting [47].

Clopidogrel resistance

Though the concept of aspirin resistance is now well accepted, the phenomenon of clopidogrel resistance has only recently been investigated. This interindividual variability may be due in part to inherent variations in the principal metaboliser of clopidogrel, hepatic cytochrome P450 3A4 (CYP 3A4) system. Lau et al. [48] described the incidence of clopidogrel non- and low-responders using the relative inhibition of ADP-induced platelet aggregation. Amongst 32 patients undergoing PCI, 22% were non-responders (<10% inhibition of platelet aggregation) and 32% were low responders (10–29% inhibition of platelet aggregation). This effect was also inversely correlated with the hepatic CYP 3A4 activity ($r = -0.6$; $P = 0.003$). Gurbel et al. [49] investigated the effect of clopidogrel on ADP-induced platelet aggregation in 92 patients undergoing PCI. All patients received 300 mg clopidogrel in the catheterisation laboratory, followed by 75 mg daily. Clopidogrel resistance was defined as a change in ADP-induced (5 µmol/l) platelet aggregation from baseline to post-treatment of ≤10%. Resistance was prominent and gradually decreased over time with 63, 31, 31 and 15% exhibiting resistance at 2 h, 24 h, 5 days and 30 days, respectively.

This effect appears to be associated with worse clinical outcomes. In a small study of 60 patients undergoing PCI for ST-elevation MI, patients were stratified into quartiles of percent reduction of ADP-induced platelet aggregation at day 6 from presentation. Compared to baseline levels, by day 6, variable response was evident with patients from the 1st to 4th quartiles having $103 \pm 8\%$, $69 \pm 3\%$, $58 \pm 7\%$ and $33 \pm 12\%$ reduction of their baseline ADP-induced platelet aggregation levels (P trend 0.007). Over a 6-month duration of follow-up 40% of patients in the 1st and 6.7% of patients in the 2nd quartile had sustained a recurrent cardiovascular event with none in the 3rd or 4th quartiles [50].

Clopidogrel interaction with statins

Patients with coronary artery disease will frequently be co-administered both clopidogrel and an HMG-CoA reductase inhibitor ('statin'). Some statins such as atorvastatin, lovastatin and simvastatin are metabolised by the CYP 3A4 system and others, such as pravastatin, are not. Recently concerns were raised about the possibility that atorvastatin may attenuate the antiplatelet effects of clopidogrel through their competition for activation in the CYP 3A4 system [51]. This effect has been refuted though in a number of studies. Müller et al. [52] randomised 77 patients with stable coronary disease undergoing PCI to atorvastatin, fluvastatin, lovastatin, pravastatin, simvastatin or cerivastatin. All patients were treated with a loading dose of clopidogrel 600 mg and had their ADP-induced platelet aggregation assessed at baseline, 2 h and 4 h. Platelet inhibition after clopidogrel loading was not different by any of the statins tested. Mitsios et al. [53] randomised 45 patients with an acute coronary syndrome to either atorvastatin 10 mg/day or pravastatin 40 mg/day.

Table 3.2 Ongoing trials of clopidogrel

Trial	Patient number	Study group	Study design
ACTIVE	14 000	Atrial fibrillation	Clopidogrel + aspirin vs. warfarin
ARCH	1500	Aortic arch atheroma	Clopidogrel + aspirin vs. warfarin
CASPAR	1460	Peripheral arterial surgery	Clopidogrel + aspirin vs. aspirin
CHARISMA	15 600	Secondary and high-risk primary intervention	Clopidogrel + aspirin vs. aspirin
CLARITY	3000	Acute ST-elevation MI	Clopidogrel + aspirin vs. aspirin
COMMIT	40 000	Acute ST-elevation MI	Clopidogrel + aspirin vs. aspirin
MATCH	7600	Recent transient ischaemic attack or stroke	Clopidogrel + aspirin vs. clopidogrel
WATCH	1600	Heart failure	Clopidogrel vs. aspirin or warfarin

ACTIVE = Atrial fibrillation Clopidogrel Trials with Irbesartan for prevention of Vascular Events; ARCH = Aortic Arch Related Cerebral Hazard; CASPAR = Clopidogrel and Aspirin in Surgery for Peripheral Arterial Disease; CHARISMA = Clopidogrel for High Atherothrombotic Risk and Ischaemic Stabilisation, Management and Avoidance; CLARITY = Clopidogrel as Adjunctive Reperfusion Therapy; COMMIT = Clopidogrel Metoprolol in Myocardia Infarction Trial; MATCH = Management of Atherothrombosis with Clopidogrel in High-risk patients with recent transient ischaemic attack or ischaemic stroke; WATCH = Warfarin and Antiplatelet Therapy in Chronic Heart Failure.

Of these patients 30 underwent PCI and received clopidogrel loading 375 mg/day and then 75 mg/day. After 5 weeks of therapy there was no significant difference in ADP-induced platelet aggregation or soluble levels of CD40L between these two groups. Also a substudy of the CREDO trial found that the benefit obtained from clopidogrel was independent of the type of statin (metabolised by CYP 3A4 or not) and specifically that the 1-year event rates of death, MI or stroke were similar in patients treated with atorvastatin or pravastatin [54].

Pharmaco-economic considerations
If one excludes the need of a thienopyridine for the prevention of stent thrombosis and examines the efficacy of clopidogrel over aspirin – the benefit is modest. The CAPRIE trial [12] demonstrated that treatment with clopidogrel reduced the occurrence of adverse cardiovascular outcomes by 5 events for every 1000 patients treated (8.7% RRR; $P = 0.043$). Gorelick *et al.* [55] performed a cost analysis based on medication cost, cost of likely encountered adverse effects and estimated that the cost to prevent one death would be $8559 for aspirin and $43 843 for clopidogrel. A recent analysis by Gaspoz *et al.* [56] attempted to define and cost-analyse the potential benefit of four antiplatelet models for secondary prevention in all patients with coronary heart disease over a 25-year period: (1) aspirin for all eligible patients (excluding aspirin allergy), (2) aspirin for all eligible patients, clopidogrel if aspirin ineligible, (3) clopidogrel for all patients and (4) aspirin and clopidogrel for all patients (if no aspirin allergy). While aspirin alone was the least efficacious strategy and the combination of aspirin and clopidogrel the most efficacious, this increment comes at a significant price premium. Widespread aspirin use for all eligible patients was estimated to cost $11 000 per quality-adjusted year of life (QAYL) gained, for the second strategy the cost being $31 000 per QAYL and for dual antiplatelet therapy the cost was significantly higher at an extra $130 000 per QAYL.

Future trials of clopidogrel
A number of ongoing clinical trials are due for completion over the next few years (Table 3.2). The Clopidogrel for High Atherothrombotic Risk and Ischaemic Stabilisation (CHARISMA) trial will follow-up 15 603 patients at risk of cardiac events for up to 42 months. Patients will

be randomised to clopidogrel and aspirin or aspirin alone. This study should conclusively address the ideal length of duration of clopidogrel therapy (in addition to aspirin) in a population at risk of events, including those with coronary artery disease, cerebrovascular disease, peripheral arterial disease or multiple risk factors [57].

Though the CURE study showed a reduced incidence of the primary endpoint of non-fatal MI, stroke and vascular death in patients on dual antiplatelet therapy, as opposed to aspirin alone, the absolute numbers of strokes in the study were small (75 with dual therapy, 87 in the aspirin group) [36]. The CURE study was not designed to directly address the question of whether the combination of aspirin and clopidogrel is beneficial in patients with cerebrovascular disease. This question will be addressed in the near future when the results of trials, such as MATCH (clopidogrel and aspirin vs. clopidogrel in recent transient ischaemic attack or stroke patients), ACTIVE (clopidogrel and aspirin vs. warfarin in patients with atrial fibrillation), ARCH (clopidogrel and aspirin vs. warfarin in patients with symptomatic aortic arch atheroma) and CHARISMA (clopidogrel and aspirin vs. aspirin in secondary and high-risk primary prevention), are published.

FUTURE AGENTS

AR-C69931MX (Cangrelor®)
Despite the significant clinical benefits of the thienopyridines, intravenous agents, which act rapidly and have reversible ADP receptor antagonism, have been eagerly investigated. The most promising of this class of agent is AR-C69931MX (Cangrelor®, The Medicines Company), a non-thienopyridine ATP analogue with potent, selective $P2Y_{12}$ receptor antagonism [58], which exhibits greater platelet aggregation inhibition than clopidogrel [59]. Unlike clopidogrel, this agent does not require hepatic conversion to an active metabolite and has a half-life of 3–5 min. After intravenous infusion it provides rapid dose-dependent inhibition of ADP-induced platelet aggregation, and with cessation of infusion its effect is rapidly diminished with platelet function recovery within 50 min.

In a canine model of acute infarction, the use of AR-C69931MX has been associated with improved myocardial perfusion when used adjunctively with tissue-type plasminogen activator [60]. Phase II trials have found that it is safe when administered to patients with unstable angina pectoris [61] and that when compared to abciximab in the setting of PCI it had a similar rate of death, MI or revascularisation with a trend towards decreased major bleeding (using the Thrombosis in Myocardial Infarction [TIMI] criteria). It is expected to undergo Phase III trials in 2005.

AZD6140
An orally active variant of AR-C69931MX has been recently developed by AstraZeneca and is undergoing Phase II investigation. Modifications from the parent compound included the removal of the triphosphate side arm, conversion of the ribose unit to a carbocycle and the purine to a triazolopyridine (Figure 3.3) [62]. It is a nucleotide analogue, has no prodrug activity and provides rapid reversible ADP receptor inhibition ($P2Y_{12}$), with no need for loading.

CS-747
After oral intake CS-747 is converted to its active metabolite, R-99224, that inactivates the $P2Y_{12}$ receptor through the formation of a disulfide bridge with extracellular cysteine residues [63]. The prodrug itself has no activity *in vitro*. It is a potent antiplatelet and -thrombotic agent with a rapid onset and a long duration of action (>3 days). Early studies suggest that this agent may have a role in the future management of atherothrombosis as it is more potent than clopidogrel and ticlopidine [64]. Its clinical safety will be investigated in the upcoming Joint Utilisation of Medications to Block Platelets Optimally (JUMBO-TIMI

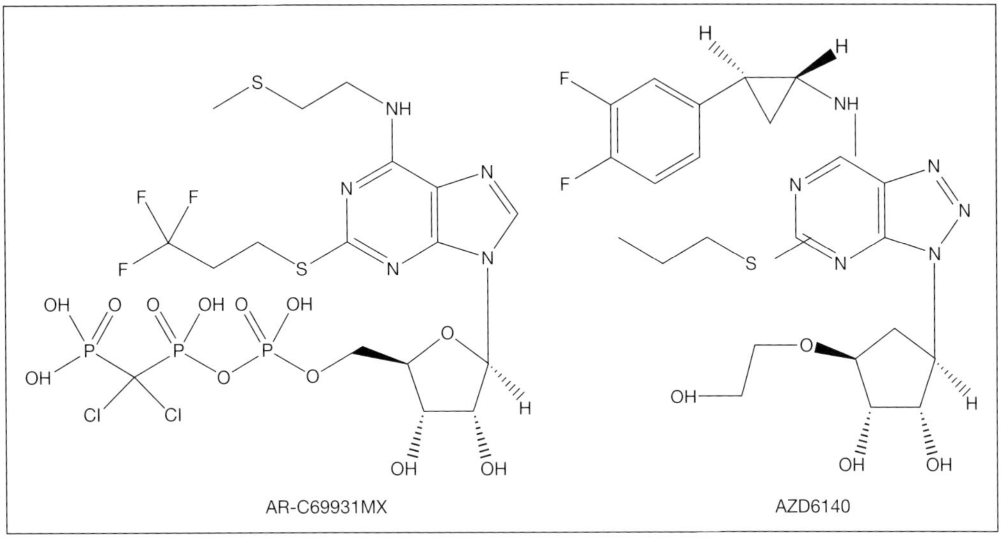

Figure 3.3 The chemical structures of the novel P2Y$_{12}$ inhibitors: AR-C69931MX and AZD6140.

26) study. Patients undergoing elective or urgent PCI will be randomised to receive one of four study arms prior to PCI. These will include low-, intermediate- or high-dose CS-747 (loading and maintenance), or alternatively clopidogrel (300 mg loading, followed by 75 mg daily). The primary endpoint will be significant bleeding by 30 days with secondary endpoints assessing cardiovascular adverse events by 30 days.

MRS-2179

Though agents such as clopidogrel inhibit the function of the P2Y$_{12}$ receptor, it does not adequately inhibit platelet shape change and calcium influx, which are activated *via* the P2Y$_1$ receptor. To address this a selective P2Y$_1$ receptor antagonist, MRS-2179, has recently been described [65]. Theoretically, its use with a selective P2Y$_{12}$ receptor antagonist will provide significant incremental antiplatelet activity, though this will need clinical assessment.

CONCLUSION

Blockade of the ADP receptor has emerged as a potent antiplatelet therapy. Clinical use of clopidogrel been validated in stenting and the treatment of acute coronary syndromes. Several studies are assessing the value of clopidogrel in other settings. Ongoing investigation into other oral and intravenous ADP receptor blockers will likely lead to further clinically useful therapies.

REFERENCES

1.   Collaborative meta-analysis of randomised trials of antiplatelet therapy for prevention of death, myocardial infarction, and stroke in high risk patients. *Br Med J* 2002; 324:71–86.
2.   Alexander JH, Harrington RA, Tuttle RH *et al*. Prior aspirin use predicts worse outcomes in patients with non-ST-elevation acute coronary syndromes. PURSUIT Investigators. Platelet IIb/IIIa in Unstable Angina: Receptor Suppression Using Integrilin Therapy. *Am J Cardiol* 1999; 83:1147–1151.

3.   Gum PA, Kottke-Marchant K, Poggio ED *et al*. Profile and prevalence of aspirin resistance in patients with cardiovascular disease. *Am J Cardiol* 2001; 88:230–235.

4.   Weiss EJ, Bray PF, Tayback M *et al*. A polymorphism of a platelet glycoprotein receptor as an inherited risk factor for coronary thrombosis. *N Engl J Med* 1996; 334:1090–1094.

5.   Chen WH, Lee PY, Ng W, Tse HF, Lau CP. Aspirin resistance is associated with a high incidence of myonecrosis after non-urgent percutaneous coronary intervention despite clopidogrel pretreatment. *J Am Coll Cardiol* 2004; 43:1122–1126.

6.   Bhatt DL. Aspirin resistance: more than just a laboratory curiosity. *J Am Coll Cardiol* 2004; 43:1127–1129.

7.   Bhatt DL, Topol EJ. Scientific and therapeutic advances in antiplatelet therapy. *Nat Rev Drug Discov* 2003; 2:15–28.

8.   Hass WK, Easton JD, Adams HP, Jr *et al*. A randomized trial comparing ticlopidine hydrochloride with aspirin for the prevention of stroke in high-risk patients. Ticlopidine Aspirin Stroke Study Group. *N Engl J Med* 1989; 321:501–507.

9.   Janzon L. The STIMS trial: the ticlopidine experience and its clinical applications. Swedish Ticlopidine Multicenter Study. *Vasc Med* 1996; 1:141–143.

10. Serruys PW, Strauss BH, Beatt KJ *et al*. Angiographic follow-up after placement of a self-expanding coronary-artery stent. *N Engl J Med* 1991; 324:13–17.

11. Leon MB, Baim DS, Popma JJ *et al*. A clinical trial comparing three antithrombotic-drug regimens after coronary-artery stenting. Stent Anticoagulation Restenosis Study Investigators. *N Engl J Med* 1998; 339:1665–1671.

12. A randomised, blinded, trial of clopidogrel versus aspirin in patients at risk of ischaemic events (CAPRIE). CAPRIE Steering Committee. *Lancet* 1996; 348:1329–1339.

13. Bennett CL, Connors JM, Carwile JM *et al*. Thrombotic thrombocytopenic purpura associated with clopidogrel. *N Engl J Med* 2000; 342:1773–1777.

14. Steinhubl SR, Tan WA, Foody JM, Topol EJ. Incidence and clinical course of thrombotic thrombocytopenic purpura due to ticlopidine following coronary stenting. EPISTENT Investigators. Evaluation of Platelet IIb/IIIa Inhibitor for Stenting. *JAMA* 1999; 281:806–810.

15. Bertrand ME, Rupprecht HJ, Urban P, Gershlick AH, Investigators FT. Double-blind study of the safety of clopidogrel with and without a loading dose in combination with aspirin compared with ticlopidine in combination with aspirin after coronary stenting: the clopidogrel aspirin stent international cooperative study (CLASSICS). *Circulation* 2000; 102:624–629.

16. Taniuchi M, Kurz HI, Lasala JM. Randomized comparison of ticlopidine and clopidogrel after intracoronary stent implantation in a broad patient population. *Circulation* 2001; 104:539–543.

17. Muller C, Buttner HJ, Petersen J, Roskamm H. A randomized comparison of clopidogrel and aspirin versus ticlopidine and aspirin after the placement of coronary-artery stents. *Circulation* 2000; 101:590–593.

18. Mueller C, Roskamm H, Neumann FJ *et al*. A randomized comparison of clopidogrel and aspirin versus ticlopidine and aspirin after the placement of coronary artery stents. *J Am Coll Cardiol* 2003; 41:969–973.

19. Bhatt DL, Bertrand ME, Berger PB *et al*. Meta-analysis of randomized and registry comparisons of ticlopidine with clopidogrel after stenting. *J Am Coll Cardiol* 2002; 39:9–14.

20. Savi P, Pereillo JM, Uzabiaga MF *et al*. Identification and biological activity of the active metabolite of clopidogrel. *Thromb Haemost* 2000; 84:891–896.

21. McEwen J, Strauch G, Perles P *et al*. Clopidogrel bioavailability: absence of influence of food or antacids. *Semin Thromb Hemost* 1999; 25(suppl 2):47–50.

22. Bhatt DL, Topol EJ. Need to test the arterial inflammation hypothesis. *Circulation* 2002; 106:136–140.

23. Quinn MJ, Bhatt DL, Zidar F *et al*. Effect of clopidogrel pretreatment on inflammatory marker expression in patients undergoing percutaneous coronary intervention. *Am J Cardiol* 2004; 93:679–684.

24. Xiao Z, Theroux P. Clopidogrel inhibits platelet-leukocyte interactions and thrombin receptor agonist peptide-induced platelet activation in patients with an acute coronary syndrome. *J Am Coll Cardiol* 2004; 43:1982–1988.

25. Hermann A, Rauch BH, Braun M, Schror K, Weber AA. Platelet CD40 ligand (CD40L)—subcellular localization, regulation of expression, and inhibition by clopidogrel. *Platelets* 2001; 12:74–82.

26. Chew DP, Bhatt DL, Robbins MA *et al*. Effect of clopidogrel added to aspirin before percutaneous coronary intervention on the risk associated with C-reactive protein. *Am J Cardiol* 2001; 88:672–674.

27. Vivekananthan D, Bhatt DL, Chew DP *et al*. Clopidogrel pretreatment prior to percutaneous coronary intervention markedly attenuates periprocedural rise in C-reactive protein. *Am J Cardiol* 2004; 94:358–360.

28. Bhatt DL, Hirsch AT, Ringleb PA, Hacke W, Topol EJ. Reduction in the need for hospitalization for recurrent ischemic events and bleeding with clopidogrel instead of aspirin. CAPRIE investigators. *Am Heart J* 2000; 140:67–73.

29. Bhatt DL, Marso SP, Hirsch AT, Ringleb PA, Hacke W, Topol EJ. Amplified benefit of clopidogrel versus aspirin in patients with diabetes mellitus. *Am J Cardiol* 2002; 90:625–628.

30. Ringleb PA, Bhatt DL, Hirsch AT, Topol EJ, Hacke W. Benefit of clopidogrel over aspirin is amplified in patients with a history of ischemic events. *Stroke* 2004; 35:528–532.

31. Bhatt DL, Chew DP, Hirsch AT, Ringleb PA, Hacke W, Topol EJ. Superiority of clopidogrel versus aspirin in patients with prior cardiac surgery. *Circulation* 2001; 103:363–368.

32. Moshfegh K, Redondo M, Julmy F *et al.* Antiplatelet effects of clopidogrel compared with aspirin after myocardial infarction: enhanced inhibitory effects of combination therapy. *J Am Coll Cardiol* 2000; 36:699–705.

33. Yusuf S, Mehta SR, Zhao F *et al.* Early and late effects of clopidogrel in patients with acute coronary syndromes. *Circulation* 2003; 107:966–972.

34. Gerschutz GP, Bhatt DL. The Clopidogrel in Unstable Angina to Prevent Recurrent Events (CURE) study: to what extent should the results be generalizable? *Am Heart J* 2003; 145:595–601.

35. Jneid H, Bhatt DL, Corti R, Badimon JJ, Fuster V, Francis GS. Aspirin and clopidogrel in acute coronary syndromes: therapeutic insights from the CURE study. *Arch Intern Med* 2003; 163:1145–1153.

36. Yusuf S, Zhao F, Mehta SR, Chrolavicius S, Tognoni G, Fox KK. Effects of clopidogrel in addition to aspirin in patients with acute coronary syndromes without ST-segment elevation. *N Engl J Med* 2001; 345:494–502.

37. Braunwald E, Antman EM, Beasley JW *et al.* ACC/AHA guideline update for the management of patients with unstable angina and non-ST-segment elevation myocardial infarction—2002: summary article: a report of the American College of Cardiology/American Heart Association Task Force on Practice Guidelines (Committee on the Management of Patients With Unstable Angina). *Circulation* 2002; 106:1893–1900.

38. Use of a monoclonal antibody directed against the platelet glycoprotein IIb/IIIa receptor in high-risk coronary angioplasty. The EPIC Investigation. *N Engl J Med* 1994; 330:956–961.

39. Kastrati A, Mehilli J, Schuhlen H *et al.* A clinical trial of abciximab in elective percutaneous coronary intervention after pretreatment with clopidogrel. *N Engl J Med* 2004; 350:232–238.

40. Savcic M, Hauert J, Bachmann F, Wyld PJ, Geudelin B, Cariou R. Clopidogrel loading dose regimens: kinetic profile of pharmacodynamic response in healthy subjects. *Semin Thromb Hemost* 1999; 25(suppl 2):15–19.

41. Thebault JJ, Kieffer G, Cariou R. Single-dose pharmacodynamics of clopidogrel. *Semin Thromb Hemost* 1999; 25(suppl 2):3–8.

42. Gurbel PA, Cummings CC, Bell CR, Alford AB, Meister AF, Serebruany VL. Onset and extent of platelet inhibition by clopidogrel loading in patients undergoing elective coronary stenting: the Plavix Reduction Of New Thrombus Occurrence (PRONTO) trial. *Am Heart J* 2003; 145:239–247.

43. Zidar FJ, Moliterno DJ, Bhatt DL *et al.* High-dose clopidogrel loading rapidly reduces both platelet inflammatory marker expression and aggregation. *J Am Coll Cardiol* 2004; 43:64A.

44. Muller I, Seyfarth M, Rudiger S *et al.* Effect of a high loading dose of clopidogrel on platelet function in patients undergoing coronary stent placement. *Heart* 2001; 85:92–93.

45. Mehta SR, Yusuf S, Peters RJ *et al.* Effects of pretreatment with clopidogrel and aspirin followed by long-term therapy in patients undergoing percutaneous coronary intervention: the PCI-CURE study. *Lancet* 2001; 358:527–533.

46. Steinhubl SR, Berger PB, Mann JT, III *et al.* Early and sustained dual oral antiplatelet therapy following percutaneous coronary intervention: a randomized controlled trial. *JAMA* 2002; 288:2411–2420.

47. Bhatt DL, Kapadia SR, Bajzer CT *et al.* Dual antiplatelet therapy with clopidogrel and aspirin after carotid artery stenting. *J Invasive Cardiol* 2001; 13:767–771.

48. Lau WC, Gurbel PA, Watkins PB *et al.* Contribution of hepatic cytochrome P450 3A4 metabolic activity to the phenomenon of clopidogrel resistance. *Circulation* 2004; 109:166–171.

49. Gurbel PA, Bliden KP, Hiatt BL, O'Connor CM. Clopidogrel for coronary stenting: response variability, drug resistance, and the effect of pretreatment platelet reactivity. *Circulation* 2003; 107:2908–2913.

50. Matetzky S, Shenkman B, Guetta V *et al.* Clopidogrel resistance is associated with increased risk of recurrent atherothrombotic events in patients with acute myocardial infarction. *Circulation* 2004; 109:3171–3175.

51. Lau WC, Waskell LA, Watkins PB *et al*. Atorvastatin reduces the ability of clopidogrel to inhibit platelet aggregation: a new drug–drug interaction. *Circulation* 2003; 107:32–37.
52. Muller I, Besta F, Schulz C, Li Z, Massberg S, Gawaz M. Effects of statins on platelet inhibition by a high loading dose of clopidogrel. *Circulation* 2003; 108:2195–2197.
53. Mitsios JV, Papathanasiou AI, Rodis FI, Elisaf M, Goudevenos JA, Tselepis AD. Atorvastatin does not affect the antiplatelet potency of clopidogrel when it is administered concomitantly for 5 weeks in patients with acute coronary syndromes. *Circulation* 2004; 109:1335–1338.
54. Saw J, Steinhubl SR, Berger PB, *et al*. Lack of adverse clopidogrel-atorvastatin clinical interaction from secondary analysis of a randomized, placebo-controlled clopidogrel trial. *Circulation* 2003; 108:921–924.
55. Gorelick PB, Born GV, D'Agostino RB, Hanley DF, Jr, Moye L, Pepine CJ. Therapeutic benefit. Aspirin revisited in light of the introduction of clopidogrel. *Stroke* 1999; 30:1716–1721.
56. Gaspoz JM, Coxson PG, Goldman PA *et al*. Cost effectiveness of aspirin, clopidogrel, or both for secondary prevention of coronary heart disease. *N Engl J Med* 2002; 346:1800–1806.
57. Bhatt DL, Topol EJ, on behalf of the CHARISMA Executive Committee. Clopidogrel added to aspirin versus aspirin alone in secondary prevention and high-risk primary prevention: rationale and design of the clopidogrel for high atherothrombotic risk and ischemic stabilization, management, and avoidance (CHARISMA) trial. *Am Heart J* 2004; 148:263–268.
58. Ingall AH, Dixon J, Bailey A *et al*. Antagonists of the platelet P2T receptor: a novel approach to antithrombotic therapy. *J Med Chem* 1999; 42:213–220.
59. Storey RF, Wilcox RG, Heptinstall S. Comparison of the pharmacodynamic effects of the platelet ADP receptor antagonists clopidogrel and AR-C69931MX in patients with ischaemic heart disease. *Platelets* 2002; 13:407–413.
60. Wang K, Zhou X, Zhou Z *et al*. Blockade of the platelet P2Y12 receptor by AR-C69931MX sustains coronary artery recanalization and improves the myocardial tissue perfusion in a canine thrombosis model. *Arterioscler Thromb Vasc Biol* 2003; 23:357–362.
61. Storey RF, Oldroyd KG, Wilcox RG. Open multicentre study of the P2T receptor antagonist AR-C69931MX assessing safety, tolerability and activity in patients with acute coronary syndromes. *Thromb Haemost* 2001; 85:401–407.
62. Chattaraj SC. Cangrelor AstraZeneca. *Curr Opin Investig Drugs* 2001; 2:250–255.
63. Sugidachi A, Asai F, Yoneda K *et al*. Antiplatelet action of R-99224, an active metabolite of a novel thienopyridine-type G(i)-linked P2T antagonist, CS-747. *Br J Pharmacol* 2001; 132:47–54.
64. Sugidachi A, Asai F, Ogawa T, Inoue T, Koike H. The *in vivo* pharmacological profile of CS-747, a novel antiplatelet agent with platelet ADP receptor antagonist properties. *Br J Pharmacol* 2000; 129:1439–1446.
65. Baurand A, Gachet C. The P2Y(1) receptor as a target for new antithrombotic drugs: a review of the P2Y(1) antagonist MRS-2179. *Cardiovasc Drug Rev* 2003; 21:67–76.

4

Glycoprotein IIb/IIIa inhibitors

B. Brown, D. J. Moliterno

INTRODUCTION

THROMBOSIS IN ACS AND PCI – ROLE OF THE GPIIb/IIIa RECEPTOR

The role of platelets in acute coronary syndromes (ACS) and percutaneous coronary intervention (PCI) has been recognised for years, but recently medicine has seen a dramatic increase in the understanding, development, and clinical application of antiplatelet therapies. The glycoprotein IIb/IIIa (GPIIb/IIIa) inhibitors were introduced to clinical practice in the late 1990s. Currently, three agents are commercially available: abciximab (Reopro, Centocor, Malvern, PA), eptifibatide (Integrillin, COR Therapeutics, San Francisco, CA), and tirofiban (Aggrastat, Guilford Pharmaceuticals, Baltimore, MD). Over 100 000 patients have been studied in randomised controlled trials involving GPIIb/IIIa inhibitors demonstrating their effectiveness in reducing adverse clinical outcomes. While most clinical investigations involving this novel class of antiplatelet medications occurred during the 1990s, recent years have seen continued understanding of the clinical application of GPIIb/IIIa antagonism.

Disruption of an atherosclerotic plaque, which either occurs spontaneously in the setting of an ACS or mechanically during PCI, results in exposure of the coronary arterial subendothelial components with subsequent platelet activation, and thrombus formation. The subendothelial components exposed during plaque rupture such as collagen, von Willebrand factor, fibronectin, etc., are recognised by receptors on the platelet surface. This results in platelet adhesion and subsequent activation. Once activated, platelets release various substances from alpha granules that lead to vasoconstriction, chemotaxis, mitogenesis, and activation of nearby platelets.

Platelet activation then results in recruitment of glycoprotein IIb/IIIa integrins that mediate aggregation. Platelet aggregation promotes production of thrombin by providing the surface for binding of cofactors that are required for conversion of prothrombin to thrombin. Thrombin, in turn, is a potent agonist for further platelet activation and stabilises the developing thrombus by converting fibrinogen to fibrin. Thus, the final common pathway leading to platelet aggregation is binding of fibrinogen to adjacent platelet GPIIb/IIIa receptors. Blocking these receptors would then represent an ideal means of reducing ischaemic complications associated with PCI and ACS.

Despite increased use of aspirin, an effective but weak antiplatelet agent, the rate of admission for unstable angina continues to rise. Furthermore, the rate of percutaneous

Brandon E. Brown, Fellow in Cardiovascular Medicine, Gill Heart Institute, University of Kentucky, Lexington, Kentucky, USA**.**

David J. Moliterno, Chief of Cardiovascular Medicine, Professor and Vice Chair of Medicine, Gill Heart Institute, University of Kentucky, Lexington, Kentucky, USA.

Table 4.1 Characteristics of GPIIb/IIIa inhibitors. Adapted with permission from Topol EJ. *Textbook of Interventional Cardiology*, 2003, p. 19.

	Abciximab	*Eptifibatide*	*Tirofiban*
Type	Monoclonal antibody fragment	Small molecule (KGD sequence)	Small molecule (RGD sequence)
Platelet-bound half-life	Long (h)	Short (sec)	Short (sec)
Plasma half-life	Short (Min)	Long (2.5 h)	Long (1.8 h)
Drug-to-receptor ratio	1.5–2.0	250–2500	>250
Percent of dose in bolus	~75%	<2–5%	<2–5%
Dosage adjustment in renal insufficiency	None	Yes	Yes
Cost	$$$$	$$	$
Specificity/Selectivity			
IIb/IIIa	xxx	xxx	xxx
$\alpha_v\beta_3$	xxx	x	
Mac-1	x		
Anticoagulant properties			
Decreased thrombin generation	++	+	+
Increased activated clotting time	+ 30 sec	+ 20 sec	0
Reversibility without platelets	24–48 h	~4 h	~4 h
Reversibility with platelets	Yes	No	No

interventions in the world also continues to rise at an astonishing rate. Thus, given the prominent role of the platelet in these clinical environments, the development and testing of further antiplatelet therapies is particularly relevant. With an emphasis on knowledge accumulated over the last five years, this chapter seeks to review the basic pharmacology of the available GPIIb/IIIa inhibitors as well as the evidence supporting their use in PCI and ACS. The evidence available for the use of these agents in acute myocardial infarction (both as adjunctive therapy to PCI and fibrinolysis) and the evidence limiting use of oral GPIIb/IIIa agents will be reviewed. Lastly, recent studies evaluating GPIIb/IIIa inhibition in association with newer direct thrombin inhibitors and clopidogrel will be reviewed.

PHARMACOLOGY OF THREE CLINICALLY AVAILABLE DRUGS

GPIIb/IIIa inhibitors have become the most widely studied antiplatelet agents. The three available agents are all potent inhibitors of platelet aggregation, but differ in their pharmacologic and pharmacokinetic profiles (Table 4.1). Pre-clinical studies have established effective antiplatelet activity at greater than 80% inhibition of adenosine diphosphate (ADP)-induced platelet aggregation [1]. While this figure is arbitrary in some respects, it has been validated in clinical trials which have demonstrated efficacy and safety with this level of platelet inhibition [2]. Abciximab was the first GPIIb/IIIa inhibitor to be used clinically and is a humanised murine monoclonal antibody fragment directed against the GPIIb/IIIa integrin [3]. Unlike the small molecule agents tirofiban, lamifiban, and eptifibatide, abciximab is less specific for the $\alpha_{IIb}\beta_3$ receptor and also binds to $\alpha_V\beta_3$ and the activated white blood cell integrin $\alpha_M\beta_3$ (CD11/CD18 or Mac-1 receptor) [4]. In addition, abciximab has unique pharmacokinetic properties in that it possesses a short plasma half-life, but long platelet-bound half-life. Bleeding time returns to normal within 12 h after the end of the standard 12 h infusion in most patients [5]. Platelet aggregation as assessed with 20 μM ADP returns to baseline within 24 h in most patients and within 48 h in all patients. Another unique feature of abciximab is the ability to reverse its antiplatelet effects with platelet transfusion [6].

The small molecule agents were developed because of concerns of potential immuno-genicity, lack of reversibility, and high cost of producing monoclonal antibody agents. These molecules contain the RGD sequence and occupy the RGD binding site of the GPIIb/IIIa receptor. Unlike abciximab, the small molecule agents are specific for the GPIIb/IIIa receptor and do not bind the other integrins. Furthermore, their small molecular size renders them less likely to induce an antibody response. They have a high affinity for the GPIIb/IIIa receptor, but less so than abciximab. However, their effects on platelet aggregation rapidly dissipate once the infusion is terminated [1]. Another important difference between the agents is stoichiometry. The small molecule drugs require 100 molecules of drug per receptor to achieve full platelet inhibition compared to 1.5 molecules of abciximab per receptor. Lastly, since the main route of excretion with tirofiban and eptifibatide is through the kidneys, doses of these drugs should be adjusted in patients with reduced creatinine clearance.

GPIIb/IIIa INHIBITORS IN PCI

BRIEF OVERVIEW OF THE TRIALS

The role of GPIIb/IIIa inhibitors in PCI has been assessed in twelve large-scale, placebo-controlled, randomised trials that enrolled over 20 000 patients. The seven trials introduced below specifically examined the use of GPIIb/IIIa inhibitors in PCI. While most studies were similar in their design, important differences exist with regard to study patient population, drug regimen, adjunctive medical therapies, and endpoint assessment.

Abciximab is the most widely studied of the three agents and its clinical benefits have been studied in a wide range of patients. Since investigational therapies often produce the most clinical efficacy in patients likely to experience a benefit, the first trial published, Evaluation of C7E3 Fab for Prevention of Ischemic Complications (EPIC), investigated the role of abciximab in patients considered high risk for thrombotic complications [7]. A total of 2099 patients who were felt to be high risk for ischaemic complications were enrolled between 1992 and 1993. One focus of the study was to determine whether a single bolus would be sufficient due to the prolonged duration of binding to the GPIIb/IIIa receptor. Thus, patients were randomised to placebo, abciximab 0.25 mg/kg bolus alone, or an abciximab bolus followed by a 10 μg/min infusion for 12 h. All patients received aspirin and heparin to maintain an activated clotting time (ACT) of 300–500 seconds with a heparin infusion continued for the duration of the abciximab infusion. In addition, vascular access sheaths remained in place during the heparin infusion. The primary endpoint of death, myocardial infarction (MI), urgent repeat revascularisation, or stent or balloon pump placement was assessed at 30 days.

The Evaluation in PTCA to Improve Long-term Outcome with abciximab GPII/IIIa blockade (EPILOG) trial was designed to extend the findings of EPIC in two ways [8]. The first objective was to determine if the benefits of abciximab seen in high-risk PCI patients in EPIC could be extrapolated to all patients undergoing PCI. Therefore, patients with acute MI or unstable angina with associated electrocardiographic changes were excluded. The second objective was to determine if the high bleeding rates seen in EPIC could be reduced by modification of the heparin dosing. This was based on results of the Precursor to EPILOG study (PROLOG) [9] study which suggested that the bleeding complications of abciximab could be reduced without affecting clinical efficacy with weight-adjusted heparin and early sheath removal eliminating the need for post-procedure heparin. A total of 2792 patients were randomised. Post-procedure heparin was not given and access sheaths were removed 2–6 h post-procedure. Based on a demonstration of reduced bleeding events in this study, subsequent studies recommended that little or no heparin be administered after the intervention and that vascular access sheaths be removed early. The primary endpoint of death, MI, or urgent repeat revascularisation was assessed at 30 days. Six-month and one-year follow-up of some patients is also available.

The Evaluation of Platelet Inhibition in STENTing (EPISTENT) trial investigated the benefits of abciximab with stent deployment [10]. The trial enrolled 2399 patients undergoing elective or urgent PCI suitable for percutaneous coronary angioplasty (PCA) or stenting during 1996. Patients were randomised to stent plus placebo, stent plus abciximab (bolus followed by 12 h infusion), or PCA plus abciximab. It is noted that all patients in the trial were to receive ticlopidine after stent deployment, but the study protocol allowed one or more doses to be given prior to abciximab. In fact, subsequent analysis determined that early treatment with ticlopidine reduced the risk of periprocedural ischaemic events [11]. The primary endpoint of death, MI, or urgent revascularisation was assessed at 30 days. Follow-up through 6 months and 1 year is also available.

Integrilin to Minimise Platelet Aggregation and Coronary Thrombosis-II (IMPACT-II) tested the efficacy of eptifibatide in 4010 patients undergoing PCI for any indication from 1993 to 1994 [12]. The study randomised 4010 patients to placebo or one of two doses of study drug: 135 µg/kg bolus followed by an infusion of 0.5 µg/kg/min for 20–24 h or a bolus of 135 µg/kg followed by an infusion of 0.75 µg/kg/min for 20–24 h. The primary endpoint of death, MI, or urgent revascularisation was assessed at 30 days.

Subsequently, the European Study Programme for the Relevance of Immunology in liver Transplantation (ESPRIT) trial sought to examine the disappointing effects of eptifibatide seen in IMPACT-II [13]. It was felt that drug under-dosing explained these results and it was later demonstrated that a higher dose of eptifibatide (double bolus of 180 µg/kg followed by an infusion of 2.0 µg/kg/min) resulted in >80% blockade of GPIIb/IIIa receptors [14]. The rationale for a higher dose was based on the discovery that the calcium-chelating anticoagulant citrate used during the dose-finding studies actually exaggerated the binding of eptifibatide to the GPIIb/IIIa receptor because of chelation of calcium [15]. The study sought to evaluate efficacy in non-urgent PCI in patients receiving second and third generation stents using high pressure deployment and concomitant thienopyridine therapy. Therefore, 2064 patients from 92 centres in the United States and Canada were randomised to receive the higher dose of eptifibatide plus heparin vs. placebo. Since patients in the ESPRIT trial were enrolled during 1999–2000, an era when efficacy of GPIIb/IIIa inhibitor therapy in PCI had already been demonstrated, patients were eligible for enrollment if ' . . . in the opinion of the treating physician the patient would not routinely be treated with a glycoprotein IIb/IIIa inhibitor therapy during PCI . . . ' [13]. The study was terminated early as clinical efficacy was demonstrated before all planned 2400 patients could be enrolled. The primary endpoint of death, MI, urgent revascularisation or bailout GPIIb/IIIa inhibitor therapy was assessed at 30 days and up to one year.

Tirofiban was assessed in the Randomised Efficacy Study of Tirofiban for Outcomes and Restenosis (RESTORE) trial in which 2139 patients considered high risk for coronary angioplasty due to unstable angina or MI were randomised to tirofiban given as a bolus of 10 µg/kg followed by an infusion of 0.15 µg/kg/min for 36 h or placebo [16]. The study, which enrolled patients in 1995, assessed a primary endpoint of death, MI, or target vessel revascularisation by 30 days. A unique feature of RESTORE is that myocardial enzyme levels were not routinely obtained as in the other trials. Thus, MI event rates were lower in RESTORE than in other trials.

The Chimeric 7E3 Antiplatelet Therapy in Unstable angina REfractory to standard treatment (CAPTURE) trial differed from the other interventional GPIIb/IIIa trials in that it studied the effects of *pre-treatment* with abciximab prior to angioplasty on patients with unstable angina [17]. To be eligible for enrolment, patients had to have unstable angina with electrocardiographic changes despite medical therapy with heparin and intravenous nitroglycerin. Furthermore, patients were required to have a lesion on angiography suitable for coronary angioplasty. All patients received aspirin and were randomised to placebo or abciximab for 18–24 h prior to the procedure and only 1 h post-procedure as the full benefits of post-procedure abciximab demonstrated in EPIC had yet to be fully appreciated. The trial enrolled 1265

Trial	Number	Agent	IIb/IIIa inhibitor	Control	Odds ratio	Approx. 95% CI	IIb/IIIa better	Placebo better
EPIC	2099	Abciximab	8.3	12.8	0.65	0.45–0.90		
IMPACT-II	4010	Eptifibatide	9.5	11.4	0.83	0.65–1.50		
EPILOG	2792	Abciximab	5.3	11.7	0.45	0.35–0.60		
RESTORE	2141	Tirofiban	8.0	10.5	0.76	0.55–1.00		
EPISTENT[†]	1603	Abciximab	5.3	10.8	0.49	0.35–0.75		
ESPRIT	2064	Eptifibatide	6.8	10.4	0.65	0.40–0.90		

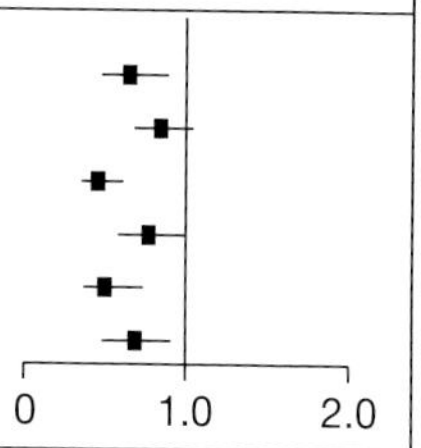

Figure 4.1 Event rates and odds ratio compilation for the 30-day composite endpoint of death, myocardial infarction, or urgent revascularization in GPIIb/IIIa PCI Trials. [†]Stent arms only. Adapted with permission from Topol EJ. *Textbook of Interventional Cardiology*, 2003, p. 19.

patients and was terminated early on the basis of efficacy of the pre-specified primary endpoint of death, MI, or urgent revascularisation at 30 days.

30-DAY EFFICACY

Event rates for the composite 30-day endpoint in the various treatment arms of the above-described studies (excluding CAPTURE and TARGET) are summarised in Figure 4.1 The beneficial effects of GPIIb/IIIa inhibitors are seen across all trials yet the magnitude of benefit is greatest in trials that investigated abciximab, from a 35% relative risk reduction (RRR) in EPIC to a 56% RRR in EPILOG. This benefit is independent of the interventional device used, directional atherectomy or stenting [10, 18], or baseline demographics. It has been shown that no clinical or angiographic parameters identify patients that do not benefit from GPIIb/IIIa inhibition [19]. While IMPACT-II provided evidence that eptifibatide reduces periprocedural events, the magnitude of benefit was less than that seen in the abciximab trials. A 16% RRR ($P = 0.063$) was seen in the higher dose eptifibatide group. The RESTORE trial demonstrated a 16% RRR which also was less than anticipated based on the results of EPIC. A still higher dose of eptifibatide including a double bolus was used in the ESPRIT trial resulting in a greater treatment effect that approximated the degree of benefit seen with abciximab. Perhaps the most significant conclusion drawn from ESPRIT is that small molecule agents such as eptifibatide, when used in appropriate doses, may result in clinical benefits similar to abciximab. While a trend towards a reduction in mortality was seen in most studies, most of the benefit of GPIIb/IIIa inhibition in PCI at 30 days was related to a reduction in MI. The clinical importance of a reduction in MI has been illustrated by studies that have shown that patients who suffer MI during or after PCI are more likely to suffer late cardiac death than those who do not.

LONG-TERM EFFICACY

In all the randomised trials involving GPIIb/IIIa inhibitors, follow-up was obtained through 6 months and even to 1 year in most trials. In general, the benefit in reduction of acute ischaemic events seen at 30 days is extended to 6 months without attenuation (Figure 4.2). For example, in EPILOG, the composite endpoint of death, MI, or target revascularisation was reduced with abciximab compared with placebo from 11.7 to 5.3% at 30 days, 14.7 to 8.4% at 6 months, and from 16.1 to 9.6% at one year. Trends toward a reduction of mortality have been demonstrated with follow-up to one year and longer. EPISTENT provided strong evidence of a complementary benefit of stenting and abciximab as the combination reduced mortality more than either therapy alone (abcixmab plus stent 1.0%, placebo plus stent 2.4%). An analysis of long-term mortality in the three abciximab trials has been reported [20]. For all studies that used the abciximab bolus plus 12 h infusion, mortality rates were reduced 25–30% for as long as 3 years. A significant reduction in mortality has not been demonstrated in the small molecule agents.

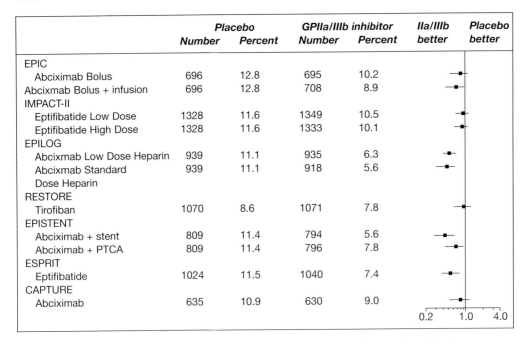

	Placebo		GPIIa/IIIb inhibitor		IIa/IIIb better	Placebo better
	Number	Percent	Number	Percent		
EPIC						
Abciximab Bolus	696	12.8	695	10.2		
Abcixmab Bolus + infusion	696	12.8	708	8.9		
IMPACT-II						
Eptifibatide Low Dose	1328	11.6	1349	10.5		
Eptifibatide High Dose	1328	11.6	1333	10.1		
EPILOG						
Abcixmab Low Dose Heparin	939	11.1	935	6.3		
Abcixmab Standard Dose Heparin	939	11.1	918	5.6		
RESTORE						
Tirofiban	1070	8.6	1071	7.8		
EPISTENT						
Abciximab + stent	809	11.4	794	5.6		
Abciximab + PTCA	809	11.4	796	7.8		
ESPRIT						
Eptifibatide	1024	11.5	1040	7.4		
CAPTURE						
Abciximab	635	10.9	630	9.0		

Figure 4.2 Event rates and odds ratio compilation for the 6-month composite endpoint of death or myocardial infarction in GPIIb/IIIa PCI trials. Adapted with permission from Topol EJ. *Textbook of Interventional Cardiology*, 2003, p. 19.

ABCIXIMAB VS. TIROFIBAN IN TARGET

The only trial to directly compare two GPIIb/IIIa inhibitors was the TARGET trial which was performed to demonstrate the non-inferiority of tirofiban to abciximab in patients expected to undergo stenting [21]. Since all patients in the trial received GPIIb/IIIa inhibition, patients undergoing urgent or elective procedures were eligible for enrolment. A total of 5308 patients were enrolled and 4809 patients were randomised to receive either abciximab 0.25 mg/kg bolus and 0.125 µg/kg/min infusion for 12 h or tirofiban 10 µg/kg bolus and 0.15 µg/kg/min infusion for 18–24 h. Pre-treatment with aspirin and clopidogrel was encouraged and weight-adjusted heparin was given with a target ACT of 250 seconds. A primary composite endpoint of death, MI, or urgent target revascularisation at 30 days was assessed. The primary endpoint occurred in 7.6% of patients in the tirofiban group compared to 6.0% in the abciximab group, a 27% difference (Figure 4.3). The upper bound of the 95% confidence interval (CI) was 1.51 which failed to demonstrate the non-inferiority of tirofiban. The researchers were then able to evaluate the superiority of abciximab. The hazard ratio comparing tirofiban to abciximab revealed a statistically significant difference at 1.26 (95% CI 1.01–1.57; $P = 0.038$). The majority of this difference was derived from the difference of non–fatal MI rates (6.9 vs. 5.4%; $P = 0.04$). At 6 months, the difference between the primary endpoint between the two drugs was attenuated (14.3 vs. 14.8%; $P = 0.591$) and no longer statistically significant [22]. Interestingly, there was no difference in event rates or 1-year mortality among diabetic patients treated with abciximab and tirofiban in TARGET [23]. This suggests that the long-term mortality benefits among diabetic patients treated with abciximab during PCI may not be due to properties unique to abciximab.

Several theories exist to explain the superiority of abciximab over tirofiban observed in TARGET. As discussed earlier, tirofiban and abciximab have different mechanisms of action.

Endpoint	P-value	Odds ratio	Hazard ratio		Tirofiban %	Abciximab %
			Tirofiban better	Abciximab better		
Composite	0.038	1.26			7.6	6.0
Death	0.66	1.21		2.8	0.5	0.4
Non–fatal MI	0.04	1.27			6.9	5.4
Death or non–fatal MI	0.04	1.26			7.2	5.7
Urgent TVR	0.49	1.26		2.43	0.8	0.7
			0.0 1.0 2.0			

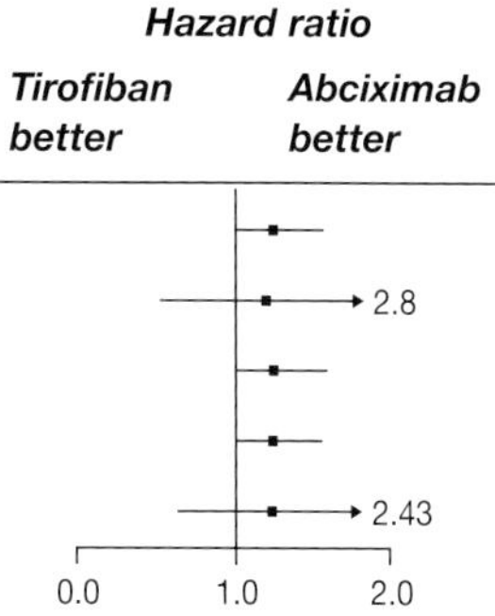

Figure 4.3   Hazard ratios for the individual endpoints in the TARGET trial.
Adapted with permission from Topol EJ *et al. N Engl J Med* 2001; 334(25):1888–1894.
© Massachusetts Medical Society, 2001. All rights reserved.

Whereas tirofiban has a short half-life and marked specificity for the GPIIb/IIIa receptor, abciximab has a prolonged half-life and also binds to the $\alpha_V\beta_3$ integrin receptor and white blood cell $\alpha_M\beta_3$ integrin receptors. Thus, only abciximab has the ability to modify the interaction of platelets with endothelial cells and white cells. Perhaps this ability to attenuate the inflammatory response may help stabilise a ruptured plaque or reduce the degree of platelet activation in PCI. In addition, it is felt that the dose of tirofiban used in TARGET – the same dose used in RESTORE may not have been comparable to the dose of abciximab with regard to platelet inhibition. Herrmann *et al.* conducted a study where patients with ACS in whom PCI was planned were randomised to tirofiban or abciximab at doses used in TARGET [24]. The rapid inhibition of platelet aggregation (IPA) to 20 μM ADP at baseline, 5, 15, 30, 45, and 60 min was measured and demonstrated that the IPA with tirofiban was less than that of abciximab at all time-points. The mean time-to-balloon inflation coincided with the maximum difference in IPA between the two drugs, which supports the notion that tirofiban less potently inhibits platelet activation at the critical moment of balloon inflation. Danzi and colleagues conducted an observational study involving 554 patients that compared the safety and efficacy of a high bolus dose tirofiban vs. abciximab in patients undergoing PCI. There was no statistically significant difference with regard to bleeding or 30-day MACE suggesting that high bolus dosing of tirofiban is safe and efficacious.

ISAR-REACT AND ISAR-SWEET

A subanalysis of EPISTENT demonstrated a reduction of major adverse cardiac events in the first year among patients treated with ticlopidine [25]. However, this benefit was only evident in patients randomised to placebo, not to abciximab. A substudy of the Clopidogrel in Unstable Angina to Prevent Recurrent Events Trial (CURE), PCI-CURE, demonstrated improved outcomes in patients treated with clopidogrel prior to PCI [26], though only a minority of patients were treated with GPIIb/IIIa inhibitors. Therefore it was uncertain if GPIIb/IIIa inhibitors provide additional benefit in PCI for patients pretreated with a thienopyridine. This question was addressed in a recent study, Intracoronary Stenting and Antithrombotic Regimen Trial-Rapid Early Action for Coronary Treatment (ISAR-REACT) [27], in which 2159 patients scheduled to undergo PCI were treated with 600 mg clopidogrel at least 2 h prior to the procedure and randomised to receive abciximab or placebo. The primary composite endpoint of death, MI, or urgent target revascularisation was reached in approximately 4% of patients in each group (relative risk 1.05; 95% CI 0.69–1.59; $P = 0.82$) (Figure 4.4). These findings suggested that abciximab provides no additional benefit in patients treated with

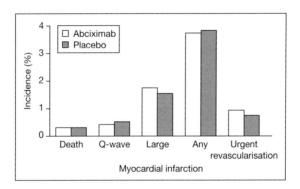

Figure 4.4 The 30-day incidence of adverse events in the abciximab and placebo groups in ISAR-REACT. Reproduced with permission from Kastrati A *et al. N Engl J Med* 2004; 350(3):232–238. © Massachusetts Medical Society, 2004. All rights reserved.

clopidogrel greater than 2 h prior to elective PCI. However, ISAR-REACT enrolled a low-risk study population which is reflected in the low event rate when compared to other PCI trials.

As abciximab had been demonstrated to reduce mortality in diabetics following PCI [28], the ISAR group than conducted the Intracoronary Stenting and Antithrombic Regimen-Is Abciximab a Superior Way to Eliminate Elevated Thrombotic Risk in Diabetes (ISAR-SWEET) study to specifically determine whether the benefits of Clopidogrel in ISAR-REACT could be extended to diabetic patients [29]. A total of 701 diabetic patients undergoing PCI were given a loading dose of clopidogrel and randomized to abciximab or placebo. The primary endpoint death, or MI at one year of $P = 0.01$). Therefore, patients with diabetes otherwise considered low-risk that undergo elective PCI do not seem to benefit from GPIIb/IIIa therapy when high-dose clopidogrel is administered at least 2 hours prior to PCI.

REPLACE-2

Considering the central role of thrombin in platelet activation and thrombosis, its inhibition with heparin has been instrumental in reducing events in PCI. However, heparin is subject to practical limitations such as variable pharmacokinetics and a potential to activate platelets. Bivalirudin, a direct inhibitor of thrombin, was approved for clinical use in 2000 as an alternative to heparin for patients with unstable angina during PCI. The Randomised Evaluation in PCI Linking Angiomax to Reduced Clinical Events (REPLACE-1) trial was an open-labelled pilot trial of bivalirudin compared with heparin in 1056 patients undergoing PCI [30]. Treatment with a thienopyridine was encouraged, but use of GPIIb/IIIa antagonists was on a provisional basis. Although there was a trend in the reduction of a composite endpoint of death, MI, urgent revascularisation, and bleeding in the GPIIb/IIIa treated and untreated arms, there was no statistically significant difference between the two arms.

REPLACE-2, which followed in 2003, involved 6010 patients to answer more definitively the question of whether bivalirudin with GPIIb/IIIa inhibitors used on a provisional basis, could provide comparable protection from ischaemic complications of PCI as compared to the standard of unfractionated heparin (UFH) and GPIIb/IIIa inhibition [31]. The primary composite endpoint of death, MI, urgent repeat revascularisation, or in-hospital major bleeding was assessed at 30 days. Suggested indications for provisional use of GPIIb/IIIa inhibitors included: abrupt or side-branch closure, dissection, new or sustained thrombus, impaired or slow flow, distal embolisation, persistent residual stenosis, and prolonged ischaemia. As a result provisional GPIIb/IIIa inhibitor use was 7.2% in the bivalirudin group (3.7% eptifibatide, 3.5% abciximab). At 30 days, the primary endpoint occurred in 9.2% of the bivalirudin group compared to 10% of the heparin group (OR 0.92; 95% CI 0.77–1.09;

$P = 0.32$). In-hospital bleeding rates were significantly reduced with bivalirudin (2.4 vs. 4.1%, $P < 0.001$). It should be noted that the majority of benefit of bivalirudin in the primary efficacy endpoint was derived from a reduction in bleeding events, while there was a statistically insignificant increase in MI in the bivalirudin group. However, this did not affect one-year mortality rates in long-term follow-up [32].

CONCLUSIONS

Platelet GPIIb/IIIa receptor blockade represents one of the most significant breakthroughs in the pharmacotherapy of interventional cardiology. Large-scale clinical trials have unequivocally demonstrated that these agents reduce the risk of periprocedural complications as much as 50–60% in a broad range of patients without increasing the major bleeding risk so long as appropriate heparin dosing and early vascular sheath removal is employed. While GPIIb/IIIa inhibitor therapy possesses a role with intermediate- and high-risk PCI procedures, it does not improve outcomes in PCI of coronary artery bypass grafts [23]. Also, among lower-risk patients in whom pre-treatment with 600 mg clopidogrel several hours before PCI is possible, use of GPIIb/IIIa inhibitors confers no additional benefit. Abciximab, given as a bolus and 12-h infusion appears to be the gold standard in PCI, but small molecule agents are more frequently utilised in clinical practice given their lower cost. It may be reasonable to withhold use of abciximab except for patients at higher risk of ischaemic events. For example, patients with unstable ischaemic syndromes in TARGET derived particular benefit with abciximab. Furthermore, diabetic patients seem to derive greater benefit with abciximab, a finding initially observed in a substudy of EPISTENT [33], but challenged in TARGET and ISAR-SWEET. As discussed in subsequent sections, abciximab has not been demonstrated to be of benefit in the medical management of ACS, but it is the only agent well studied during primary PCI for acute MI.

GPIIb/IIIa INHIBITORS IN UNSTABLE ANGINA

While the benefit of GPIIb/IIIa receptor inhibition in planned PCI is well-established, the role of these agents in the medical therapy of ACS has been less clear. This may result from the inherent heterogeneity of patients who present with ACS. The diversity of symptoms upon presentation and the diversity of conditions that lead to unstable angina have made the definition of unstable angina difficult. For example, as opposed to a relatively predictable and 'planned' vessel injury in patients undergoing PCI, patients with unstable angina or non-ST-elevation myocardial infarction (NSTEMI) present with ongoing platelet-mediated thrombosis over a ruptured plaque. Thus, maximal platelet inhibition with GPIIb/IIIa receptor blockade cannot be attained at the time of vessel injury in ACS as in planned PCI. Despite these circumstances, the benefits of these agents in ACS have been demonstrated in six large-scale clinical trials enrolling over 30 000 patients.

CLINICAL TRIAL DESIGNS

The six trials examining the role of GPIIb/IIIa inhibitors in unstable angina and non-ST-elevation myocardial infarction (NSTEMI) include the '4 P's' (PRISM, PRISM-PLUS, PURSUIT, PARAGON) and the more recent abciximab trial, GUSTO IV-ACS. Most of these trials aimed to enrol high-risk patients with true unstable coronary artery disease requiring treatment for chest pain within 12 to 24 h and either ischaemic ECG changes or elevated cardiac enzymes. The Platelet IIb/IIIa Antagonism for the Reduction of Acute Coronary Syndrome Events in a Global Organisation Network (PARAGON)-B [34] and The Global Use of Strategies to Open Occluded Arteries (GUSTO-IV) [35] were the first to include troponin positive as an enrolment criterion as this group of patients seemed to derive greater benefit in earlier studies. The Platelet Receptor Inhibition in Ischaemic Syndrome Management (PRISM) Study [36] enrolled lower-risk patients due to the inclusion of patients without ischaemic ECG changes or elevated cardiac enzymes.

In the PURSUIT [37], PARAGON-B, and GUSTO IV-ACS trials GPIIb/IIIa inhibition was compared to placebo and all patients received aspirin and heparin. However, PRISM-PLUS [38] and PARAGON-A [39] included arms which compared GPIIb/IIIa receptor blockade with heparin. In PRISM-PLUS, the tirofiban-only arm was terminated early due to an unexpected increase in mortality in this arm. While this may have been due to chance, it raised the possibility of a pro-thrombotic effect of GPIIb/IIIa antagonism without adjunctive heparin use. However, this was not repeated in the subsequent larger PRISM trial which compared tirofiban to heparin. In all studies, the study drug was continued for 24–48 h at least, or until hospital discharge, whichever came first. In PRISM, PRISM-PLUS, and PARAGON-A coronary angiography was discouraged in the first 48 h and for the first 60 h in GUSTO IV-ACS. The primary endpoint in PARAGON-A, PURSUIT, and GUSTO IV-ACS was the composite of death and MI at 30 days. In the other trials, refractory ischaemia was included in the primary composite endpoint and was assessed at 48 h in PRISM, 7 days in PRISM-PLUS, and 30 days in PARAGON-B. Event rates were higher in PURSUIT due to a definition of non-procedure-related MI as any increase in CK-MB. In GUSTO IV-ACS, MI was defined as an increase in CK-MB greater than 3 times the upper limit of normal while in the remaining trials MI was defined as an increase in CK-MB greater than 2 times the upper limit of normal.

CLINICAL TRIAL OUTCOMES

The benefit of GP IIb/IIIa inhibitors in the treatment of ACS has been demonstrated in many trials, but the results are inconsistent and the degree of benefit has fallen short of expectations. In PRISM, patients who received tirofiban compared to heparin alone had a reduced rate of the composite endpoint of death, MI, or refractory ischaemic during the 48-h drug infusion (3.8 vs. 5.6%; RR 0.67; $P = 0.01$), mostly due to a reduction in refractory ischaemia. However, at 30 days this difference was no longer significant. PRISM-PLUS observed a significant reduction in 30-day death or MI in patients receiving tirofiban and heparin vs. heparin alone (8.7 vs. 11.9%; $P = 0.03$) which was extended to 6 months. The large, international trial PURSUIT observed a significant absolute risk reduction of 1.5% as early as 96 h after drug infusion. This benefit was also seen in higher-risk patients at 7 days, 30 days, and 6 months of follow-up suggesting that the benefits are durable. In contrast to the clinical benefit seen in the other trials, PARAGON-A did not show a benefit of lamifiban for a reduction of the composite endpoint of 30-day death, MI, or recurrent ischaemia. Retrospective analyses of PARAGON-A showed that optimal outcomes were obtained when drug levels were maintained at 18 and 42 ng/ml [40]. Therefore, PARAGON-B examined the effects of an optimal dose of lamifiban based on renal function. Patients assigned to the active therapy group did not experience a reduction in the 30-day death or MI despite the change in dosing guidelines. GUSTO IV-ACS was designed on the basis of benefit in reduction of death, MI, or urgent revascularisation seen in patients with refractory angina given abciximab for 18–24 h prior to planned angioplasty in the CAPTURE trial [17]. In contrast to other trials, abciximab actually increased the risk of death at 30 days (3.9 vs. 4.3%; $P = 0.66$). The precise mechanisms responsible for these findings are unclear, but several theories exist. First, in GUSTO IV-ACS discouragement of early revascularisation may have led investigators to select a lower-risk population as early revascularisation which is closely linked to the beneficial effects of GPIIb/IIIa inhibitor therapy was discouraged. Next, the trial raises questions about potential paradoxical toxic properties of prolonged abciximab infusions [41] due to significant peak–trough variations in platelet inhibition.

A meta-analysis by Boersma et al. published in 2002 [42] sought to better understand the treatment benefits of GPIIb/IIIa inhibitors in patients with ACS 'not routinely scheduled for early revascularisation'. A total of 31 402 patients from the '5 P's' and GUSTO IV-ACS met the inclusion criteria for the study. At 30 days, a 9% reduction in the odds of death or MI was seen with GPIIb/IIIa inhibitors compared with control (10.8 vs. 11.8%; odds ratio [OR] 0.91; 95% CI 0.84–0.98; $P = 0.15$).

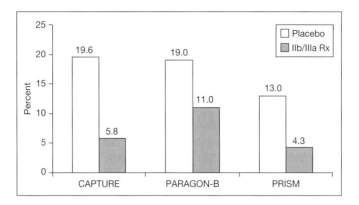

Figure 4.5 30-day death or myocardial infarction with troponin (+) in CAPTURE, PARAGON-B, and PRISM.

TROPONIN POSITIVE

The overwhelming finding from the unstable angina trials is that the greatest clinical benefit is seen in patients at highest risk for ischaemic complications. Patients with elevated troponin have a 3–8 fold increase in the risk of death in non-ST-segment elevation ACS [43]. Such patients derived particular benefit for GP IIb/IIIa inhibition in CAPTURE [44], PARAGON B [45], and PRISM [46] with reductions in 30-day death or MI of 42–74% (Figure 4.5). Such preferential benefit was also demonstrated in the meta-analysis by Boersma *et al*. In the 45% of patients with elevated troponins, therapy with GPIIb/IIIa inhibitors was associated with a 15% reduction in the odds of death or MI at 30 days compared to placebo (10.3 vs. 12.0%). In those patients with negative troponin, no treatment benefit was seen.

PERCUTANEOUS CORONARY INTERVENTION

Another important observation from the Boersma *et al*. meta-analysis was the 23% reduction in the combined endpoint of 30-day death or MI (OR 0.77; 95% CI 0.64–0.92) in patients that underwent PCI within 5 days of randomisation. Similar findings were noted in a post-randomisation meta-analysis from CAPTURE, PURSUIT, and PRISM-PLUS. An overall 34% reduction in death or MI was noted during medical management with GPIIb/IIIa inhibition preceding PCI (2.5 vs. 3.8%; OR 0.66) and an additional 41% reduction in PCI-related ischaemic complications in patients that received GPIIb/IIIa inhibitor therapy and subsequently underwent PCI [47]. Thus, a clear complementary relationship exists between benefit of GPIIb/IIIa inhibitor therapy and PCI.

TACTICS-TIMI 18

Further evidence supporting the role of GPIIb/IIIa inhibition in ACS and its complementary benefits with PCI came from the TACTICS-TIMI 18 trial [48] which sought to determine whether a routine early invasive strategy was superior to a conservative strategy. In this study, patients with high-risk unstable angina were treated with aspirin, heparin, and tirofiban for 48 h including ≥12 h prior to PCI. Angiography was performed in the conservative arm only for patients with rest ischaemic or a positive stress test. Overall, there was a significant reduction in the primary endpoint of death, MI, or re-hospitalisation for ACS at 6 months: 15.9% in the early invasive strategy vs. 19.4% in the conservative strategy (OR 0.78; $P = 0.025$) (Figure 4.6). Similar benefits were also seen at 30 days. Interestingly, a reduction in death or MI was seen as early as the first week in contrast to earlier conservative vs. invasive trials where the rate of MI in the first few weeks tended to be greater in the invasive group consistent with

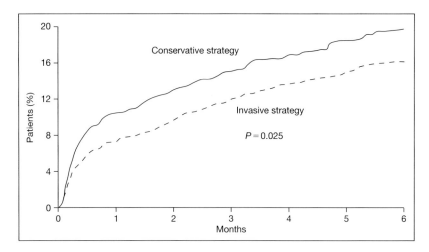

Figure 4.6 Cumulative incidence of the primary endpoint of death, non-fatal myocardial infarction, or rehospitalisation for an acute coronary syndrome during the 6-month follow-up period in TACTICS-TIMI 18. Reproduced with permission from Cannon CP *et al. N Engl J Med* 2001; 344(25):1879–1887. © Massachusetts Medical Society, 2001. All rights reserved.

an early hazard of PCI. Such findings reflect the benefits of GPIIb/IIIa inhibition in reduction of periprocedural ischaemic events with PCI. The role of troponin levels to predict patients likely to benefit from an invasive strategy was once again demonstrated in this study. In patients with a troponin T > 0.1 ng/ml, there was a relative risk reduction of 39% in the primary endpoint with the invasive strategy compared to the conservative strategy ($P < 0.001$) [49]. This study demonstrated improved outcomes of an invasive strategy when combined with new advances in cardiology of stenting and GPIIb/IIIa inhibition.

ISAR-COOL

Unlike ST-elevation MI where time-to-reperfusion is clearly linked with improved survival, optimal timing of revascularisation for NSTEMI remains controversial. Therefore, the ISAR-COOL trial tested the hypothesis that there would be an incremental benefit of prolonged antiplatelet and antithrombotic therapy before revascularisation in high-risk ACS patients [50]. Therefore, 410 patients with angina pectoris and myocardial ischemia confirmed by ST-segment depression or elevated troponin T levels from two centres in Germany were randomised to pre-treatment with UFH, aspirin, clopidogrel, and tirofiban for 3 to 5 days or ≤6 h. The primary endpoint was the composite of incidence of large MI (new Q waves on ECG, new left bundle branch block, or elevation of CK-MB five times the upper limit of normal) or death from any cause during 30 days of follow-up. The primary endpoint was reached in 11.6% of patients in the pre-treatment group and 5.9% in the early intervention group (RR 1.96; $P = 0.04$). The majority of this difference was due to a reduction in non-fatal MI. Interestingly, subgroup analysis, although underpowered, failed to demonstrate a significant benefit of either strategy in patients with elevated troponin T or in patients undergoing PCI. While ISAR-COOL has limited applicability due to small sample size and a limited number of endpoints, it strongly suggests that delaying angiography and PCI in patients with ACS in order to allow more time for potent antithrombotic therapies may be harmful.

RECOMMENDATIONS

Overall, GPIIb/IIIa inhibitors confer a 9% reduction in the combined endpoint of 30-day death or MI in patients with unstable angina or NSTEMI. Subgroup analyses indicate

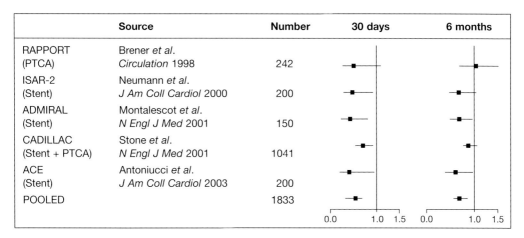

	Source	Number	30 days	6 months
RAPPORT (PTCA)	Brener *et al.* *Circulation* 1998	242		
ISAR-2 (Stent)	Neumann *et al.* *J Am Coll Cardiol* 2000	200		
ADMIRAL (Stent)	Montalescot *et al.* *N Engl J Med* 2001	150		
CADILLAC (Stent + PTCA)	Stone *et al.* *N Engl J Med* 2001	1041		
ACE (Stent)	Antoniucci *et al.* *J Am Coll Cardiol* 2003	200		
POOLED		1833		

Figure 4.7 Relative risk of death, MI, or target vessel revascularisation from meta-analysis of trials of abciximab during percutaneous coronary intervention for acute myocardial infarction.
Adapted with permission from Topol EJ. *Textbook of Interventional Cardiology*, 2003; p. 752.

that troponin positive patients or those who undergo PCI derive the greatest benefit. Thus, when taken in conjunction with the TACTICS-TIMI 18 data which have helped make early PCI the treatment of choice in ACS, patients with planned PCI and/or positive troponin should receive GPIIb/IIIa inhibitor therapy. As a result, the 2002 joint American Heart Association/American College of Cardiology Guidelines on the Management of Non-ST-segment Elevation ACS Glycoprotein IIb/IIIa Inhibitor Therapy was given a class IA recommendation in patients treated with heparin and aspirin and in whom percutaneous revascularisation is planned [51]. Abciximab, however, on the basis of GUSTO IV-ACS, was given a class III indication for patients in whom PCI is not planned.

ADJUNCTIVE THERAPY TO PCI IN ACUTE MYOCARDIAL INFARCTION

The primary goal of reperfusion therapy in acute MI is the preservation of myocardial function. It has been demonstrated that only patients in whom Thrombolysis in Myocardial Infarction (TIMI) grade 3 flow is achieved can reperfusion of epicardial coronary arteries improve regional ejection fraction and clinical outcomes [52]. However, positron emission tomography and myocardial contrast echocardiography studies have demonstrated that despite large vessel TIMI 3 flow, microvascular perfusion may remain impaired. It is logical to consider GPIIb/IIIa inhibition as a pharmacologic adjunct to mechanical reperfusion as platelets are known to interfere with both large vessel and microvascular flow via occlusive thrombus formation and distal embolisation of small aggregates and release of vasoconstrictive mediators [53].

Subgroup analysis from EPIC demonstrated that patients with ST-elevation MI (STEMI) who received abciximab experienced a benefit in clinical outcomes [54]. Of the three agents approved for clinical use, abciximab is the only agent well studied in clinical trials of primary PCI. The first of these studies, ReoPro in Acute myocardial infarction and Primary PCTA Organization Randomized Trial (RAPPORT) [55], enrolled 483 patients with acute STEMI-deemed candidates for primary percutaneous transluminal coronary angioplasty (PTCA) and randomised them to abciximab or placebo. Treatment with abciximab was associated with a 48% reduction in the primary composite endpoint of death, re-infarction, or need for urgent revascularisation by 30 days ($P = 0.03$). While this benefit was maintained at 6 months, the majority of benefit in the composite end point was due to a reduction in the need for urgent revascularisation (Figure 4.7). However, bleeding in the abciximab arm occurred significantly more often and the trial was limited by a low utilisation of stents

(<20%) which was appropriate at the time of the study. ISAR-2 [56] and Abciximab Before Direct Angioplasty and Stenting in Myocardial Infarction Regarding Acute and Long-term Follow-up (ADMIRAL) [57] assessed the effect of abciximab with stenting in acute MI. ISAR-2 randomised 401 patients undergoing primary stenting for acute STEMI to abciximab plus reduced-dose heparin or high-dose heparin. At 30 days, the primary composite endpoint of death, re-infarction, or target lesion revascularisation was reached in 5.0% of the abciximab group and 10.5% in the control group resulting in a RRR of 53% (P = 0.038). At one year, the absolute risk reduction was still 5.7%, but had lost its statistical significance. ADMIRAL randomised 300 patients with STEMI within 24 h of onset of pain to abciximab or placebo. Angiographic data demonstrated more complete reperfusion in the abciximab group (TIMI grade 3 flow: 95.1 in the abciximab group and 86.7% in the placebo group; P = 0.04) and left ventricular function was better preserved. The 30-day rate of death, re-infarction, or target vessel revascularisation (TVR) was 6.0% in the abciximab group and 14.6% in the placebo group resulting in a RRR of 59% (P = 0.01). The magnitude of clinical benefit persisted to 6 months without attenuation. An important feature of ADMIRAL compared to the other trials is that patients received the study drug immediately after the decision to proceed with catheter-based intervention. Thus, 26% of patients received the study drug in the emergency department or mobile intensive care unit. These patients had substantially better 30-day and 6-month outcomes adding weight to the notion that abciximab, when administered upstream, improves outcomes in patients who undergo stenting in acute MI.

In contrast to ADMIRAL and RAPPORT, Controlled Abciximab and Device Investigation to Lower Late Angioplasty Complications (CADILLAC) [58] suggested that abciximab may not be required for all patients undergoing PCI for acute MI. This was a much larger trial, enrolling 2082 patients in a 2-by-2 factorial design into four groups: primary angioplasty with or without abciximab, and primary stenting with or without abciximab. When compared to placebo, abciximab reduced the primary composite end point of death, MI, and TVR by 30% (5.0 vs. 7.1%; P = 0.04) at 30 days and by 14%; (13.0 vs. 15.1%; P = 0.17) at 6 months. A subsequent analysis revealed that abciximab did not affect the composite endpoint at one year [59]. While the effect of abciximab was consistent with the other trials, the magnitude of benefit was lower than expected. This may be due to enrolment of lower-risk patients in CADILLAC as overall mortality was remarkably low (3.3%). Of 2681 patients screened for enrolment, 599 (22.3%) were excluded ' . . . if the angiographic findings indicated that non-interventional management was the proper approach . . . ' Furthermore, this study demonstrated a marked benefit in clinical outcomes at 6 months with stenting as compared to angioplasty, but no incremental benefit with use of abciximab.

The most recent study published, ACE (Abciximab and Carbostent Evaluation) trial sought to clarify the conflicting results of the earlier studies [60]. Four hundred patients with STEMI were randomised to infarct-related artery stenting alone or with abciximab. The primary composite endpoint of death, re-infarction, TVR, and stroke at 30 days occurred in 4.5% of the abciximab group compared with 10.5% of the stenting alone group (P = 0.023). At 6 months the composite of death and re-infarction was lower in the abciximab group (5.5 vs. 13.5%; P = 0.006). Although it was not a prespecified endpoint, 1-year survival was greater in the abciximab group (95 ± 2 vs. 88 ± 2%; P = 0.017) [61].

The only head-to-head comparison GPIIb/IIIa inhibitors in STEMI is High-dose Bolus TiRofibAn and Sirolimus Eluting STEnt vs. Abciximab and Bare Metal Stent in Acute Myocardial Infarction study (STRATEGY) whose primary aim was to assess whether high-dose tirofiban with a drug-eluting stent (DES) vs. abciximab with a bare metal stent would result in a similar incidence of major adverse cardiovascular events (MACE) but a lower binary rate of restenosis at six months [62]. The results, presented at the 2004 sessions of the American Heart Association, revealed that the tirofiban–DES combination resulted in a lower incidence of the primary composite endpoint of death, MI, stroke, and binary restenosis (23 vs. 48%; P = 0.003). While the small sample size limits the study's conclusions, it still adds evidence to the notion that a higher dose of tirofiban may result in clinical benefits similar to those seen with abciximab. It also hints to a cost-reduction potential of small molecule GPIIb/IIIa inhibition and DES.

Despite differences among the trials, abciximab has a clear adjunctive role to mechanical reperfusion in acute MI. Although it may not be required in all cases, it should be strongly considered in higher-risk patients such as those with a large thrombus burden and upstream administration should be achieved when possible. The recent update to the ACC/AHA Guidelines for the Management of Patients with ST-Elevation Myocardial Infarction issued a class IIa indication for starting abciximab as early as possible before primary PCI with or without stenting [63]. The small molecule agents were given a class IIb indication for administration before primary PCI.

GLYCOPROTEIN IIb/IIIa THERAPY IN ACUTE MYOCARDIAL INFARCTION

ADJUNCTIVE THERAPY TO FIBRINOLYSIS

Fibrinolytic therapy in acute STEMI clearly improves survival when administered within 12 h of symptom onset [64–66]. Despite this marked clinical benefit, tissue-level perfusion may be achieved in as few as 25% of patients [67]. As platelets are a key component of coronary thrombosis and predispose to distal microembolisation, it is logical to consider GPIIb/IIIa inhibitors, the most potent inhibitors of platelets available, as adjunctive therapy for acute MI. Pilot angiographic studies of patients with acute MI demonstrated a benefit of platelet GPIIb/IIIa inhibition in combination with reduced doses of fibrinolytic agents in improvement in infarct artery patency as well as tissue-level perfusion relative to plasminogen activator therapy [68–70]. Two recent large-scale clinical trials, GUSTO [71] and The Assessment of Safety and Efficacy of a New Thrombolytic Regimen (ASSENT-3) Trial [72] have examined the role of GPIIb/IIIa inhibitors as an adjunct to fibrinolytic therapy in acute MI (Figure 4.8).

GUSTO V enrolled 16 588 patients with acute MI within 6 h of symptom onset to either full-dose reteplase (two 10-U boluses, 30 min apart) or half-dose reteplase (two 5-U boluses, 30 min apart) and abciximab (0.25 mg/kg bolus and 0.125 μg/kg/min infusion for 12 h). The primary endpoint of all-cause death at 30 days was 5.9% in the reteplase group compared to 5.6% in the combination therapy group (RR 0.95; 95% CI 0.84–1.08; $P = 0.43$). However, a significant reduction in recurrent MI and a reduction in need for urgent revascularisation occurred in the combination arm. The importance of this result is illustrated by the association of a reduction in re-infarction rates and reduced mortality at one year [73]. Nevertheless, follow-up at one year also demonstrated no difference in overall mortality [74]. One issue that must be considered in evaluating these results is the reasonably low mortality rates in the control group (5.9%) compared to GUSTO III (7.5%), which could diminish the power of the study to detect a mortality difference. This low mortality rate may be due to selection bias in which higher-risk patients were treated with primary PCI rather than fibrinolysis, enrolment of lower-risk patients, and/or improvement in other aspects of medical treatment of acute MI. Patients enrolled in GUSTO V were lower risk: 90% were Killip class I, a minority was diabetic, and two-thirds of patients were enrolled with inferior wall infarctions.

ASSENT-3 examined a composite efficacy endpoint of 30-day death, in-hospital re-infarction, or in-hospital refractory ischaemia. In this trial 6095 patients were randomised to full-dose tenecteplase (TNK) with enoxaparin (continued up to 7 days), half-dose TNK with abciximab and low-dose UFH, or full-dose TNK with weight-adjusted UFH. The activated partial thromboplastin time was maintained at 50–70 seconds. The primary composite endpoint was reduced in the combination regimens compared to standard TNK therapy at 30 days (UFH 15.4%, abciximab 11.1%, enoxaparin 11.4%; $P = 0.0001$). The difference in

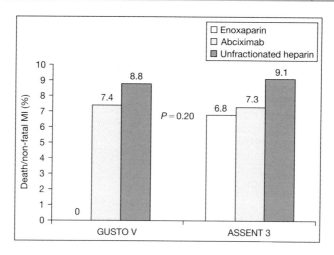

Figure 4.8 30-day combined death and non-fatal/MI rates from GUSTO V and ASSENT-3.
Adapted with kind permission of Springer Science and Business Media from DP Vivekananthan, DJ Moliterno, *et al. J Throm and Throm* 2002; 13(1):35–39.

efficacy was evident at 48 h, the time of discontinuation of heparin. While the study was not powered to detect a difference in mortality, rates of death were similar in all groups. However, in-hospital re-infarction (UFH 4.2%, abciximab 2.2%, enoxaparin 2.7%; $P = 0.0009$) and refractory ischaemia (UFH 6.5%, abciximab 3.2%, enoxaparin 4.6%; $P < 0.0001$) occurred significantly less frequently in the combination therapy arms. No difference in mortality was discerned at 1-year follow-up. [75].

While a reduction in ischaemic complications is important, it is difficult to advocate use of combination fibrinolytic and GP IIb/IIIa inhibition for all STEMI patients. The increased incidence of bleeding complications and a fearful trend toward an increase in intracranial haemorrhage (ICH) in patients older than 75 years in GUSTO V (2.1 vs. 1.1%; RR 1.91; 95% CI 0.95–3.84; $P = 0.069$) renders this strategy relatively contraindicated in a growing elderly population. Furthermore, the efficacy of a combination strategy in a higher-risk patient population is unknown. Likewise, early percutaneous revascularisation is the treatment of choice in patients with cardiogenic shock. The recent update of the ACC/AHA Guidelines for the Management of Patients with ST-Elevation Myocardial Infarction gave combination reperfusion with abciximab and half-dose TNK or reteplase a class IIb indication when used for prevention of re-infarction or other complications of MI. It is only recommended for use in selected patients: anterior MI, age less than 75 years, and no risk factors for bleeding. Likewise, a class III recommendation was given for combined therapy in patients greater than 75 years of age due to an increased risk of ICH [63].

FACILITATED PCI WITH GPIIb/IIIa RECEPTOR INHIBITION

In hospitals with cardiac catheterisation facilities, primary PCI is better than fibrinolysis in patients presenting with STEMI [76]. Furthermore, patients with STEMI that present to hospitals without catheterisation facilities benefit more from PCI performed after transport to facilities with catheterisation laboratories than from fibrinolysis [77–79]. However, a criticism of these trials is the low number of patients that underwent rescue PCI if there was no ECG evidence of reperfusion (as a greater use of this strategy may have improved the outcomes in patients receiving fibrinolysis). However, bleeding complications may occur more frequently with full-dose fibrinolysis, GPIIb/IIIa inhibition, aspirin, and heparin, particularly if streptokinase were used. With equivalence in outcomes using a combination of reduced-dose fibrinolytics and GPIIb/IIIa inhibitors compared to full-dose fibrinolysis [71], it may be rational to employ this strategy when PCI is planned. The administration of pharmacologic therapies to bridge the delay between presentation and PCI has been termed 'facilitated PCI.'

Two small trials recently published have examined the benefit of GPIIb/IIIa therapy when employed as part of a facilitated PCI strategy. The Bavarian Reperfusion Alternatives Evaluation (BRAVE) trial involved 253 STEMI patients who were randomised to facilitated PCI with half-dose reteplase plus abciximab or abciximab alone [80]. The primary endpoint, infarct size by technetium (Tc)-sestamibi, was similar between the two groups. Major bleeding was higher in the facilitated group (5.6% vs. 1.6%, $P = 0.16$) and MACE at 6 months was similar. The ongoing Tirofiban in Myocardial Infarction Evaluation (ON-TIME) study randomised 507 patients with STEMI to receive tirofiban or placebo prior to transfer for PCI [81]. Post-PCI perfusion was unchanged as assessed by TIMI flow grade, blush score, or corrected TIMI frame counts. The facilitated strategy also exhibited a trend toward an increase in MACE at 30 days (8.6% vs. 4.4%, $P = 0.06$). Therefore, no trial has yet to demonstrate a benefit of facilitated PCI compared to primary PCI alone. Three new trials, Addressing the Value of Facilitated Angioplasty after Combination Therapy or Eptifibatide Monotherapy in Acute Myocardial Infarction (ADVANCE-MI), Facilitated Intervention with Enhanced Reperfusion Speed to Stop Events (FINESSE), and Trial of Inhibitors of Glycoprotein IIb/IIIa with Enoxaparin for Reperfusion (TIGER), seek to address the role of such a strategy of facilitated reperfusion for STEMI. ADVANCE-MI randomises patients to either therapy with eptifibatide or a combination of reduced-dose tenecteplase and eptifibatide while FINESSE includes a third arm that has neither upstream drug strategy, but uses abciximab in the catheterisation laboratory [82]. Both TIGER and ADVANCE-MI test the role of enoxaparin compared to UFH. Collectively, these three trials should add greatly to our understanding of how to employ such pharmacologic therapies in the management of STEMI.

ORAL GPIIb/IIIa INHIBITORS

Orally administered GPIIb/IIIa inhibitors were developed following the remarkable efficacy demonstrated with the intravenous agents in the setting of PCI and ACS. Their structure is based on the RGD motif to compete with fibrinogen for the RGD sequence on the GPIIb/IIIa integrin. Orally active drugs that have been examined in large-scale phase III studies include xemilofiban (Searle, Skokie, IL), orbofiban (Searle), sibrafiban (Hoffman-LaRoche, Basel, Switzerland), and lotrafiban (Smith-Kline Beecham, Middlesex, England). As with the intravenous drugs, oral agents must maintain a steady level of 80% platelet inhibition in response to 20-μM ADP agonist to achieve therapeutic efficacy. However, due to their pharmacokinetic properties, there are inevitable fluctuations in their degree of platelet inhibition as a result of serum peak and trough levels. A total of 42 636 patients have been enrolled in phase III studies. Evaluation of oral Xemilofiban in Controlling Thrombotic Events (EXCITE) [83] was the only trial specifically investigating the role of oral GPIIb/IIIa inhibitors in PCI and studied xemilofiban. Orbofiban in Patients with Unstable coronary Syndromes-TIMI 16 (OPUS-TIMI 16) [84] enrolled 10 232 patients within 72 h of presentation with ACS to either aspirin or one of two doses of orbofibran. Sibrafiban cespirin to yield maximum protection from ischaemic heart events post acute coronary syndromes (SYMPHONY) [85] and 2nd SYMPHONY [86] were designed to test the hypothesis that long-term therapy with a more potent inhibitor of platelet aggregation with an oral GPIIb/IIIa inhibitor would be more effective and better tolerated than aspirin in secondary prevention. Blockade of the GPIIb/IIIa Receptor to Avoid Vascular Occlusion (BRAVO) [87] was unique in that it was a true secondary prevention trial examining lotrafiban in patients with either cerebrovascular disease, cardiovascular disease, or peripheral vascular disease. Overall, the results of all phase 3 trials were disappointing and failed to demonstrate a benefit of oral GPIIb/IIIa inhibitors. The odds ratio for mortality for patients treated with oral GPIIb/IIIa inhibitor relative to aspirin control from the individual trials

	Number	Event rate Treatment	Event rate Control	Odds ratio	95% CI
EXCITE					
Xemilofiban	7232	1.4	1.0	1.40	0.88–2.24
OPUS					
Orbofiban	10 288	4.8	3.7	1.31	1.06–1.61
SYMPHONY					
Sibrafiban	9169	2.0	1.8	1.14	0.83–1.58
2nd SYMPHONY					
Sibrafiban	6637	2.1	1.3	1.55	1.02–2.35
BRAVO					
Lotrafiban	9200	1.6	1.7	0.94	0.85–1.03
POOLED	42 526	0.1	0.1	1.21	0.96–1.52

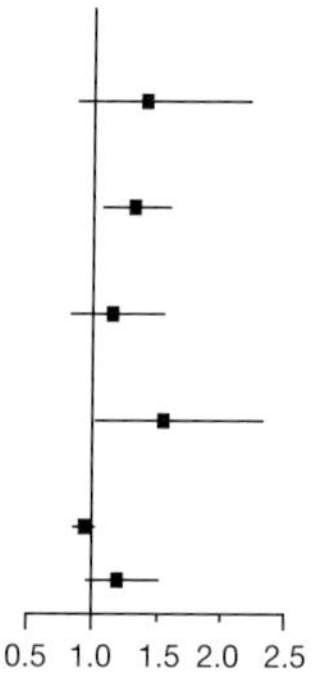

0.5 1.0 1.5 2.0 2.5

Figure 4.9 Odds ratios for mortality in published studies of oral GPIIb/IIIa inhibitors. Adapted with permission from Lincoff AM, *Contemporary Cardiology: Platelet Glycoprotein IIb/IIIa Inhibitors in Cardiovascular Disease*. Humana Press, Inc., 2003, p. 379.

(except BRAVO) when pooled was 1.31 (1.12–1.53; $P = 0.0001$) [88] (Figure 4.9). Furthermore, bleeding events were increased with oral GPIIb/IIIa inhibitors in a dose-dependent fashion. No one single clear explanation for the failure of oral GPIIb/IIIa inhibitors exists, though theories abound. As mentioned earlier, both intravenous and oral agents have demonstrated potential proinflammatory and prothrombotic properties. Perhaps these factors, on a background of fluctuating plasma levels, variability in patient response, and rapid receptor reversibility may explain these disappointing results. Whether long-acting agents may avoid these problems is yet to be determined.

SAFETY

The large number of clinical trials involving intravenous GPIIb/IIIa inhibitors have enrolled well over 100 000 patients and demonstrated an acceptable bleeding safety profile; the rate of transfusion, an endpoint examined in most studies, is summaried in Figure 4.10. However, the bleeding risk is increased in the setting of fibrinolytic therapy. In TIMI-14, the study group that included abciximab and full-dose streptokinase had to be discontinued due to excessive bleeding. In GUSTO V, rates of severe bleeding were roughly doubled in the reteplase plus abciximab group compared to the reteplase only group. Nevertheless, there appears to be no increased risk of ICH [89] except for the trend toward an increased risk in patients older than 75 treated with combination therapy.

As mentioned in early PCI trials, the risk of bleeding in EPIC was largely due to inappropriate heparin dosing and indwelling vascular access sheaths. With appropriate heparin dosing and monitoring, bleeding risk remains at acceptable levels. GPIIb/IIIa inhibitors have been used in combination with low-molecular-weight heparin and have also demonstrated an acceptable safety profile.

A lingering concern with GPIIb/IIIa inhibitors is their use in patients that require urgent coronary artery bypass grafting (CABG). Due to their short duration of action and rapid reversibility, the small-molecule agents likely do not confer any significant perioperative bleeding risk [35, 90]. In addition, pooled analysis from the abciximab trials, EPILOG and EPISTENT, demonstrated that CABG may be performed without an incremental bleeding risk [91]. Nevertheless, a small-molecule agent should be used preferentially if there exists a high suspicion that CABG may be required.

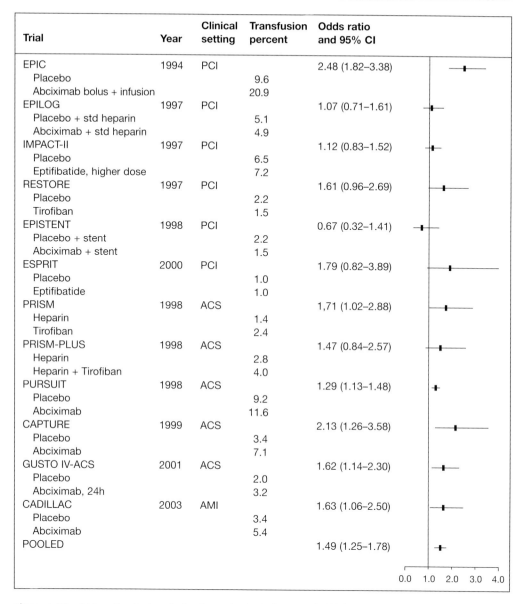

Trial	Year	Clinical setting	Transfusion percent	Odds ratio and 95% CI
EPIC	1994	PCI		2.48 (1.82–3.38)
Placebo			9.6	
Abciximab bolus + infusion			20.9	
EPILOG	1997	PCI		1.07 (0.71–1.61)
Placebo + std heparin			5.1	
Abciximab + std heparin			4.9	
IMPACT-II	1997	PCI		1.12 (0.83–1.52)
Placebo			6.5	
Eptifibatide, higher dose			7.2	
RESTORE	1997	PCI		1.61 (0.96–2.69)
Placebo			2.2	
Tirofiban			1.5	
EPISTENT	1998	PCI		0.67 (0.32–1.41)
Placebo + stent			2.2	
Abciximab + stent			1.5	
ESPRIT	2000	PCI		1.79 (0.82–3.89)
Placebo			1.0	
Eptifibatide			1.0	
PRISM	1998	ACS		1,71 (1.02–2.88)
Heparin			1.4	
Tirofiban			2.4	
PRISM-PLUS	1998	ACS		1.47 (0.84–2.57)
Heparin			2.8	
Heparin + Tirofiban			4.0	
PURSUIT	1998	ACS		1.29 (1.13–1.48)
Placebo			9.2	
Abciximab			11.6	
CAPTURE	1999	ACS		2.13 (1.26–3.58)
Placebo			3.4	
Abciximab			7.1	
GUSTO IV-ACS	2001	ACS		1.62 (1.14–2.30)
Placebo			2.0	
Abciximab, 24h			3.2	
CADILLAC	2003	AMI		1.63 (1.06–2.50)
Placebo			3.4	
Abciximab			5.4	
POOLED				1.49 (1.25–1.78)

0.0 1.0 2.0 3.0 4.0

Figure 4.10 Odds ratios for transfusion in randomised glycoprotein IIb/IIIa trials. Std = Standard dose.

Thrombocytopaenia is a rare complication of GPIIb/IIIa inhibitor administration, but when it occurs it has a deleterious effect on clinical outcomes and bleeding risk. Overall, it occurs in approximately 1–2% of patients and severe thrombocytopaenia ($<20 \times 10^7/l$) occurs in 0.4 to 1.0% of cases [92]. A retrospective review of the TARGET trial revealed that development of thrombocytopaenia led to more severe bleeding (5.1 vs. 0.7%; $P = 0.001$), blood transfusions (6.1 vs. 1.4%, $P = 0.001$), and a higher risk of mortality (2.0 vs. 0.4%; $P = 0.022$). Furthermore, there was a higher rate of TVR [93]. It is recommended that platelet levels should be checked within 2–4 h of starting abciximab and within 24 h of starting small-molecule agents.

CONCLUSIONS

As the important role of arterial thrombosis in ACS and PCI was better recognised, glycoprotein IIb/IIIa inhibitors were developed for the purpose of overcoming the limitations of aspirin, an effective but weak inhibitor of platelets. Platelets are activated by many mechanisms involving multiple different agonists, but all converge on the GPIIb/IIIa receptor, the final common pathway to thrombosis. Over 100 000 patients have been enrolled in randomised clinical trials that have paved the way for approval of three parenteral agents available for clinical use. While the results of clinical trials have been inconsistent, the role of this novel class of drugs in the modern day management of high-risk ACS and PCI is firmly established. This benefit is most firmly established in the subgroup of ACS patients that are troponin positive or who undergo early PCI. Likewise, highly significant reductions in ischaemic complications of PCI have been demonstrated with abciximab and to a lesser extent, the small-molecule agents, tirofiban and eptifibatide. In STEMI, abcixmab appears to be the drug of choice as an adjunct to primary PCI, but its use as adjunctive therapy to fibrinolysis has been hampered by increased bleeding. However, in low-risk PCI patients that have been given upfront dosing of clopidogrel, it seems that GPIIb/IIIa inhibition is unnecessary. Likewise, the use of bivalirudin in lower-risk patients may preclude the need for GPIIb/IIIa inhibitors, which again emphasises the particular benefit of GPIIb/IIIa inhibition in high-risk patients [31].

The questions that remain have to do with explaining the marked heterogeneity of clinical trial results and exploring the possibility of paradoxical prothrombotic or toxic mechanisms which may clarify such differences and shed light on the failure of oral GPIIb/IIIa inhibitors. It is likely that point-of-care platelet activation testing will allow more insight into safer and more effective patient-specific dosing regimens. In the era of drug-eluting stents, one wonders about the incremental benefit of GPIIb/IIIa inhibition in prevention of restenosis. Currently enrolling trials will help define the role of GPIIb/IIIa inhibition for facilitated PCI. Lastly, further head-to-head trials should help determine the extent of class effects and the relevance of other non-platelet actions of GPIIb/IIIa inhibitors.

ACKNOWLEDGEMENT

Donna Gilbreath for editorial assistance.

REFERENCES

1. Kleiman NS. Pharmacokinetics and pharmacodynamics of glycoprotein IIb–IIIa inhibitors. *Am Heart J* 1999; 138(4 Pt 2):263–275.
2. Neumann FJ *et al.* Anti-platelet effects of abciximab, tirofiban and eptifibatide in patients undergoing coronary stenting. *J Am Coll Cardiol* 2001; 37:1323–1328.
3. Coller BS. Binding of abciximab to alpha V beta 3 and activated alpha M beta 2 receptors: with a review of platelet-leukocyte interactions. *Thromb Haemost* 1999; 82:326–336.
4. Coller BS. A new murine monoclonal antibody reports an activation-dependent change in the conformation and/or microenvironment of the platelet glycoprotein IIb/IIIa complex. *J Clin Invest* 1985; 76:101–108.
5. Tcheng JE *et al.* Pharmacodynamics of chimeric glycoprotein IIb/IIIa integrin antiplatelet antibody Fab 7E3 in high-risk coronary angioplasty. *Circulation* 1994; 90:1757–1764.
6. Wagner C *et al.* Reversal of the anti-platelet effects of 7E3 Fab treatment by platelet transfusion in cynomolgus monkeys. *Thromb Haemost* 1995; 73:1313.
7. Use of a monoclonal antibody directed against the platelet glycoprotein IIb/IIIa receptor in high-risk coronary angioplasty. The EPIC Investigation. *N Engl J Med* 1994; 330:956–961.
8. Platelet glycoprotein IIb/IIIa receptor blockade and low-dose heparin during percutaneous coronary revascularization. The EPILOG Investigators. *N Engl J Med* 1997; 336:1689–1696.
9. Lincoff A *et al.* A multicenter, randomised, double-blind pilot trial of standard versus low dose weight-adjusted heparin in patients treated with the platelet glycoprotein IIb/IIIa receptor antibody 7E3 during percutaneous coronary revascularization. *J Am Coll Cardiol* 1995; 25:80A (Abstract).

10. Randomized placebo-controlled and balloon-angioplasty-controlled trial to assess safety of coronary stenting with use of platelet glycoprotein-IIb/IIIa blockade. The EPISTENT Investigators. Evaluation of Platelet IIb/IIIa Inhibitor for Stenting. *Lancet* 1998; 352:87–92.

11. Steinhubl SR *et al*. The duration of pretreatment with ticlopidine prior to stenting is associated with the risk of procedure-related non-Q-wave myocardial infarctions. *J Am Coll Cardiol* 1998; 32:1366–1370.

12. Randomized placebo-controlled trial of effect of eptifibatide on complications of percutaneous coronary intervention: IMPACT-II. Integrilin to Minimise Platelet Aggregation and Coronary Thrombosis-II. *Lancet* 1997; 349:1422–1428.

13. Novel dosing regimen of eptifibatide in planned coronary stent implantation (ESPRIT): a randomized, placebo-controlled trial. *Lancet* 2000; 356:2037–2044.

14. Tcheng JE *et al*. Clinical pharmacology of higher dose eptifibatide in percutaneous coronary intervention (the PRIDE study). *Am J Cardiol* 2001; 88:1097–1102.

15. Phillips DR *et al*. Effect of Ca2+ on GP IIb-IIIa interactions with integrilin: enhanced GP IIb-IIIa binding and inhibition of platelet aggregation by reductions in the concentration of ionized calcium in plasma anticoagulated with citrate. *Circulation* 1997; 96:1488–1494.

16. Effects of platelet glycoprotein IIb/IIIa blockade with tirofiban on adverse cardiac events in patients with unstable angina or acute myocardial infarction undergoing coronary angioplasty. The RESTORE Investigators. Randomized Efficacy Study of Tirofiban for Outcomes and REstenosis. *Circulation* 1997; 96:1445–1453.

17. Randomized placebo-controlled trial of abciximab before and during coronary intervention in refractory unstable angina: the CAPTURE Study. *Lancet* 1997; 349:1429–1435.

18. Ghaffari S *et al*. Platelet glycoprotein IIb/IIIa receptor blockade with abciximab reduces ischemic complications in patients undergoing directional coronary atherectomy. EPILOG Investigators. Evaluation of PTCA to Improve Long-term Outcome by c7E3 GP IIb/IIIa Receptor Blockade. *Am J Cardiol* 1998; 82:7–12.

19. Ellis SG *et al*. Reduction in complications of angioplasty with abciximab occurs largely independently of baseline lesion morphology. EPIC and EPILOG Investigators. Evaluation of 7E3 for the Prevention of Ischemic Complications. Evaluation of PTCA To Improve Long-term Outcome with abciximab GPIIb/IIIa Receptor Blockade. *J Am Coll Cardiol* 1998; 32:1619–1623.

20. Anderson KM *et al*. Long-term mortality benefit with abciximab in patients undergoing percutaneous coronary intervention. *J Am Coll Cardiol* 2001; 37:2059–2065.

21. Topol EJ *et al*. Comparison of two platelet glycoprotein IIb/IIIa inhibitors, tirofiban and abciximab, for the prevention of ischemic events with percutaneous coronary revascularization. *N Engl J Med* 2001; 344:1888–1894.

22. Moliterno DJ *et al*. Outcomes at 6 months for the direct comparison of tirofiban and abciximab during percutaneous coronary revascularisation with stent placement: the TARGET follow-up study. *Lancet* 2002; 360:355–360.

23. Roffi M *et al*. Lack of benefit from intravenous platelet glycoprotein IIb/IIIa receptor inhibition as adjunctive treatment for percutaneous interventions of aortocoronary bypass grafts: a pooled analysis of five randomized clinical trials. *Circulation* 2002; 106:3063–3067.

24. Herrmann HC *et al*. Comparison of degree of platelet inhibition by abciximab versus tirofiban in patients with unstable angina pectoris and non-Q-wave myocardial infarction undergoing percutaneous coronary intervention. *Am J Cardiol* 2002; 89:1293–1297.

25. Steinhubl SR *et al*. Ticlopidine pretreatment before coronary stenting is associated with sustained decrease in adverse cardiac events: data from the Evaluation of Platelet IIb/IIIa Inhibitor for Stenting (EPISTENT) Trial. *Circulation* 2001; 103:1403–1409.

26. Mehta SR *et al*. Effects of pretreatment with clopidogrel and aspirin followed by long-term therapy in patients undergoing percutaneous coronary intervention: the PCI-CURE study. *Lancet* 2001; 358:527–533.

27. Kastrati A *et al*. A clinical trial of abciximab in elective percutaneous coronary intervention after pretreatment with clopidogrel. *N Engl J Med* 2004; 350:232–238.

28. Bhatt DL *et al*. Abciximab reduces mortality in diabetics following percutaneous coronary intervention. *J Am Coll Cardiol* 2003; 35:922–928.

29. Mehilli J *et al*. Randomized clinical trial of abciximab in diabetic patients undergoing elective percutaneous coronary interventions after pretreatment with a high loading dose of Clopidogrel. *Circulation* 2004; 110:3627–3625.

30. Lincoff AM *et al*. The REPLACE 1 Trial: a pilot study of bivalirudin vs. heparin during percutaneous coronary intervention with stenting and GP IIb/IIIa blockade. *J Am Coll Cardiol* 2002; 39:16A (Abstract).

31. Lincoff AM *et al.* Bivalirudin and provisional glycoprotein IIb/IIIa blockade compared with heparin and planned glycoprotein IIb/IIIa blockade during percutaneous coronary intervention: REPLACE-2 randomized trial. *JAMA* 2003; 289:853–863.

32. Lincoff AM *et al.* Long-term efficacy of bivalirudin and provisional glycoprotein IIb/IIIa blockade vs. heparin and planned glycoprotein IIb/IIIa blockade during percutaneous coronary revascularization: REPLACE-2 randomized trial. *JAMA* 2004; 292:696–703.

33. Marso SP *et al.* Optimizing the percutaneous interventional outcomes for patients with diabetes mellitus: results of the EPISTENT (Evaluation of platelet IIb/IIIa inhibitor for stenting trial) diabetic substudy. *Circulation* 1999; 100:2477–2484.

34. Randomized, placebo-controlled trial of titrated intravenous lamifiban for acute coronary syndromes. The PARAGON-B Investigators. *Circulation* 2002; 105:316–321.

35. Cohen M. Glycoprotein IIb/IIIa receptor blockers in acute coronary syndromes: Gusto IV-ACS. *Lancet* 2001; 357:1899–1900.

36. A comparison of aspirin plus tirofiban with aspirin plus heparin for unstable angina. Platelet Receptor Inhibition in Ischemic Syndrome Management (PRISM) Study Investigators. *N Engl J Med* 1998; 338:1498–1505.

37. Inhibition of platelet glycoprotein IIb/IIIa with eptifibatide in patients with acute coronary syndromes. The PURSUIT Trial Investigators. Platelet Glycoprotein IIb/IIIa in Unstable Angina: Receptor Suppression Using Integrilin Therapy. *N Engl J Med* 1998; 339:436–443.

38. Inhibition of the platelet glycoprotein IIb/IIIa receptor with tirofiban in unstable angina and non-Q-wave myocardial infarction. Platelet Receptor Inhibition in Ischemic Syndrome Management in Patients Limited by Unstable Signs and Symptoms (PRISM-PLUS) Study Investigators. *N Engl J Med* 1998; 338:1488–1497.

39. International, randomized, controlled trial of lamifiban (a platelet glycoprotein IIb/IIIa inhibitor), heparin, or both in unstable angina. The PARAGON Investigators. Platelet IIb/IIIa Antagonism for the Reduction of Acute coronary syndrome events in a Global Organization Network. *Circulation* 1998; 97:2386–2395.

40. Moliterno DJ. Patient-specific dosing of IIb/IIIa antagonists during acute coronary syndromes: rationale and design of the PARAGON B study. The PARAGON B International Steering Committee. *Am Heart J* 2000; 139:563–566.

41. Peter K *et al.* Induction of fibrinogen binding and platelet aggregation as a potential intrinsic property of various glycoprotein IIb/IIIa (alphaIIbbeta3) inhibitors. *Blood* 1998; 92:3240–3249.

42. Boersma E *et al.* Platelet glycoprotein IIb/IIIa inhibitors in acute coronary syndromes: a meta-analysis of all major randomized clinical trials. *Lancet* 2002; 359:189–198.

43. Heidenreich PA *et al.* The prognostic value of troponin in patients with non-ST elevation acute coronary syndromes: a meta-analysis. *J Am Coll Cardiol* 2001; 38:478–485.

44. Hamm CW *et al.* Benefit of abciximab in patients with refractory unstable angina in relation to serum troponin T levels. c7E3 Fab Antiplatelet Therapy in Unstable Refractory Angina (CAPTURE) Study Investigators. *N Engl J Med* 1999; 340:1623–1629.

45. Newby LK *et al.* Benefit of glycoprotein IIb/IIIa inhibition in patients with acute coronary syndromes and troponin t-positive status: the paragon-B troponin T substudy. *Circulation* 2001; 103:2891–2896.

46. Heeschen C *et al.* Troponin concentrations for stratification of patients with acute coronary syndromes in relation to therapeutic efficacy of tirofiban. PRISM Study Investigators. Platelet Receptor Inhibition in Ischemic Syndrome Management. *Lancet* 1999; 354:1757–1762.

47. Boersma E *et al.* Platelet glycoprotein IIb/IIIa receptor inhibition in non-ST-elevation acute coronary syndromes: early benefit during medical treatment only, with additional protection during percutaneous coronary intervention. *Circulation* 1999; 100:2045–2048.

48. Cannon CP *et al.* Comparison of early invasive and conservative strategies in patients with unstable coronary syndromes treated with the glycoprotein IIb/IIIa inhibitor tirofiban. *N Engl J Med* 2001; 344:1879–1887.

49. Morrow DA *et al.* Ability of minor elevations of troponins I and T to predict benefit from an early invasive strategy in patients with unstable angina and non-ST elevation myocardial infarction: results from a randomized trial. *JAMA* 2001; 286:2405–2412.

50. Neumann FJ *et al.* Evaluation of prolonged antithrombotic pretreatment ('cooling-off' strategy) before intervention in patients with unstable coronary syndromes: a randomized controlled trial. *JAMA* 2003; 290:1593–1599.

51. Braunwald E *et al.* ACC/AHA 2002 guideline update for the management of patients with unstable angina and non-ST-segment elevation myocardial infarction summary article: a report of the American

College of Cardiology/American Heart Association task force on practice guidelines (Committee on the Management of Patients With Unstable Angina). *J Am Coll Cardiol* 2002; 40:1366–1374.

52. Simes RJ *et al.* Link between the angiographic substudy and mortality outcomes in a large randomized trial of myocardial reperfusion. Importance of early and complete infarct artery reperfusion. GUSTO-I Investigators. *Circulation* 1995; 91:1923–1928.

53. Topol EJ. Toward a new frontier in myocardial reperfusion therapy: emerging platelet preeminence. *Circulation* 1998; 97:211–218.

54. Lefkovits J *et al.* Effects of platelet glycoprotein IIb/IIIa receptor blockade by a chimeric monoclonal antibody (abciximab) on acute and six-month outcomes after percutaneous transluminal coronary angioplasty for acute myocardial infarction. EPIC investigators. *Am J Cardiol* 1996; 77:1045–1051.

55. Brener SJ *et al.* Randomized, placebo-controlled trial of platelet glycoprotein IIb/IIIa blockade with primary angioplasty for acute myocardial infarction. ReoPro and Primary PTCA Organization and Randomized Trial (RAPPORT) Investigators. *Circulation* 1998; 98:734–741.

56. Neumann FJ *et al.* Effect of glycoprotein IIb/IIIa receptor blockade with abciximab on clinical and angiographic restenosis rate after the placement of coronary stents following acute myocardial infarction. *J Am Coll Cardiol* 2000; 35:915–921.

57. Montalescot G *et al.* Platelet glycoprotein IIb/IIIa inhibition with coronary stenting for acute myocardial infarction. *N Engl J Med* 2001; 344:1895–1903.

58. Stone GW *et al.* Comparison of angioplasty with stenting, with or without abciximab, in acute myocardial infarction. *N Engl J Med* 2002; 346:957–966.

59. Tcheng JE *et al.* Benefits and risks of abciximab use in primary angioplasty for acute myocardial infarction: the Controlled Abciximab and Device Investigation to Lower Late Angioplasty Complications (CADILLAC) trial. *Circulation* 2003; 108:1316–1323.

60. Antoniucci D *et al.* A randomized trial comparing primary infarct artery stenting with or without abciximab in acute myocardial infarction. *J Am Coll Cardiol* 2003; 42:1879–1885.

61. Antoniucci D *et al.* Abciximab-supported infarct artery stent implantation for acute myocardial infarction and long-term survival: a prospective, multicenter, randomized trial comparing infarct artery stenting plus abciximab with stenting alone. *Circulation* 2004; 109:1704–1706.

62. Valgimigli M *et al.* High-dose bolus tirofiban and sirolimus eluting stent versus abiciximab and bare metal stent in acute myocardial infarction (STRATEGY) study – protocol design and demography of the first 100 patients. *Cardiovasc Drugs Ther* 2004; 18:225–230.

63. Antman EM *et al.* ACC/AHA guidelines for the management of patients with ST-elevation myocardial infarction – executive summary. A report of the American College of Cardiology/American Heart Association Task Force on Practice Guidelines (Writing Committee to revise the 1999 guidelines for the management of patients with acute myocardial infarction). *J Am Coll Cardiol* 2004; 44:671–719.

64. Effectiveness of intravenous thrombolytic treatment in acute myocardial infarction. Gruppo Italiano per lo Studio della Streptochinasi nell'Infarto Miocardico (GISSI). *Lancet* 1986; 1:397–402.

65. Randomized trial of intravenous streptokinase, oral aspirin, both, or neither among 17,187 cases of suspected acute myocardial infarction: ISIS-2. ISIS-2 (Second International Study of Infarct Survival) Collaborative Group. *Lancet* 1988; 2:349–360.

66. An international randomized trial comparing four thrombolytic strategies for acute myocardial infarction. The GUSTO investigators. *N Engl J Med* 1993; 329:673–82.

67. Lincoff AM, Topol EJ. Illusion of reperfusion. Does anyone achieve optimal reperfusion during acute myocardial infarction? *Circulation* 1993; 88:1361–1374.

68. Antman EM *et al.* Abciximab facilitates the rate and extent of thrombolysis: results of the thrombolysis in myocardial infarction (TIMI) 14 trial. The TIMI 14 Investigators. *Circulation* 1999; 99:2720–2732.

69. Trial of abciximab with and without low-dose reteplase for acute myocardial infarction. Strategies for Patency Enhancement in the Emergency Department (SPEED) Group. *Circulation* 2000; 101:2788–2794.

70. de Lemos JA *et al.* Abciximab improves both epicardial flow and myocardial reperfusion in ST-elevation myocardial infarction. Observations from the TIMI 14 trial. *Circulation* 2000; 101:239–243.

71. Topol EJ. Reperfusion therapy for acute myocardial infarction with fibrinolytic therapy or combination reduced fibrinolytic therapy and platelet glycoprotein IIb/IIIa inhibition: the GUSTO V randomized trial. *Lancet* 2001; 357:1905–14.

72. Efficacy and safety of tenecteplase in combination with enoxaparin, abciximab, or unfractionated heparin: the ASSENT-3 randomized trial in acute myocardial infarction. *Lancet* 2001; 358:605–613.

73. Hudson MP *et al.* Early reinfarction after fibrinolysis: experience from the global utilization of streptokinase and tissue plasminogen activator (alteplase) for occluded coronary arteries (GUSTO I)

and global use of strategies to open occluded coronary arteries (GUSTO III) trials. *Circulation* 2001; 104:1229–1235.

74. Lincoff AM *et al*. Mortality at 1 year with combination platelet glycoprotein IIb/IIIa inhibition and reduced-dose fibrinolytic therapy vs. conventional fibrinolytic therapy for acute myocardial infarction: GUSTO V randomized trial. *JAMA* 2002; 288:2130–2135.

75. Sinnaeve PR *et al*. Efficacy of tenecteplase in combination with enoxaparin, abciximab, or unfractionated heparin: one-year follow-up results of the Assessment of the Safety of a New Thrombolytic-3 (ASSENT-3) randomized trial in acute myocardial infarction. *Am Heart J* 2004; 147:993–998.

76. Keeley EC, Boura JA, Grines CL. Primary angioplasty versus intravenous thrombolytic therapy for acute myocardial infarction: a quantitative review of 23 randomized trials. *Lancet* 2003; 361:13–20.

77. Widimsky P *et al*. Long distance transport for primary angioplasty vs. immediate thrombolysis in acute myocardial infarction. Final results of the randomized national multicentre trial – PRAGUE-2. *Eur Heart J* 2003; 24:94–104.

78. Grines CL *et al*. A randomized trial of transfer for primary angioplasty versus on-site thrombolysis in patients with high-risk myocardial infarction: the Air Primary Angioplasty in Myocardial Infarction study. *J Am Coll Cardiol* 2002; 39:1713–1719.

79. Andersen HR *et al*. A comparison of coronary angioplasty with fibrinolytic therapy in acute myocardial infarction. *N Engl J Med* 2003; 349:733–742.

80. Kastrati A *et al*. Early administration of reteplase plus abciximab vs abciximab alone in patients with acute myocardial infarction referred to percutaneous coronary intervention *JAMA* 2004; 291:947–954.

81. van't Hof AWJ *et al*. Facilitation of primary coronary angioplasty by early start of a glycoprotein IIb/IIIa inhibitor: results of the Ongoing Tirofiban In Myocardial Infarction (ON-TIME) trial. *Eur Heart J* 2004; 25:837–846.

82. Ellis SG *et al*. Facilitated percutaneous coronary intervention versus primary percutaneous coronary intervention: design and rationale of the Facilitated Intervention with Enhanced Reperfusion Speed to Stop Events (FINESSE) trial. *Am Heart J* 2004; 147:E16.

83. O'Neill WW *et al*. Long-term treatment with a platelet glycoprotein-receptor antagonist after percutaneous coronary revascularization. EXCITE Trial Investigators. Evaluation of Oral Xemilofiban in Controlling Thrombotic Events. *N Engl J Med* 2000; 342:1316–1324.

84. Cannon CP *et al*. Oral glycoprotein IIb/IIIa inhibition with orbofiban in patients with unstable coronary syndromes (OPUS-TIMI 16) trial. *Circulation* 2000; 102:149–156.

85. Comparison of sibrafiban with aspirin for prevention of cardiovascular events after acute coronary syndromes: a randomized trial. The SYMPHONY Investigators. Sibrafiban versus Aspirin to Yield Maximum Protection from Ischemic Heart Events Post-acute Coronary Syndromes. *Lancet* 2000; 355:337–345.

86. Randomized trial of aspirin, sibrafiban, or both for secondary prevention after acute coronary syndromes. *Circulation* 2001; 103:1727–1733.

87. Topol EJ *et al*. Randomized, double-blind, placebo-controlled, international trial of the oral IIb/IIIa antagonist lotrafiban in coronary and cerebrovascular disease. *Circulation* 2003; 108:399–406.

88. Newby LK *et al*. The failure of orally administered glycoprotein IIb/IIIa inhibitors to prevent recurrent cardiac events. *Am J Med* 2002; 112:647–658.

89. Blankenship JC. Bleeding complications of glycoprotein IIb-IIIa receptor inhibitors. *Am Heart J* 1999; 138(4 Pt 2):287–296.

90. Marso SP *et al*. Enhanced efficacy of eptifibatide administration in patients with acute coronary syndrome requiring in-hospital coronary artery bypass grafting. PURSUIT Investigators. *Circulation* 2000; 102:2952–2958.

91. Lincoff AM *et al*. Abciximab and bleeding during coronary surgery: results from the EPILOG and EPISTENT trials. Improve Long-term Outcome with abciximab GP IIb/IIIa blockade. Evaluation of Platelet IIb/IIIa Inhibition in STENTing. *Ann Thorac Surg* 2000; 70:516–526.

92. Madan M *et al*. Efficacy of abciximab readministration in coronary intervention. *Am J Cardiol* 2000; 85:435–440.

93. Merlini PA *et al*. Thrombocytopenia caused by abciximab or tirofiban and its association with clinical outcome in patients undergoing coronary stenting. *Circulation* 2004; 109:2203–2226.

5

Unfractionated heparin and low-molecular-weight heparin in coronary heart disease

M. Cohen

INTRODUCTION

Unfractionated heparin (UFH) and low-molecular-weight heparins (LMWHs) can be used as prophylaxis to prevent thromboembolism and are also used to treat patients with acute coronary syndromes (ACS). In this chapter, the pharmacology and mode of action of both UFH and LMWH are outlined and the evidence supporting their use in ACS, including unstable angina (UA), non-ST-segment elevation myocardial infarction (NSTEMI) and ST-segment elevation myocardial infarction (STEMI), is summarised.

PHARMACOLOGY AND MODE OF ACTION OF HEPARINS

- UFH and LMWHs mediate the majority of their anticoagulant effect through binding to antithrombin and inhibition of enzymes in the coagulation cascade, particularly thrombin (IIa) and factor Xa.
- LMWH has a more predictable anticoagulation response than UFH, eliminating the need for response monitoring.

Heparin consists of a heterogeneous group of negatively charged, highly sulfated glycosaminoglycan molecules. The majority of its anticoagulant activity is mediated through binding to antithrombin and subsequent inactivation of a number of enzymes in the coagulation cascade, including thrombin (IIa) and factors Xa, IXa, XIa and XIIa (Figure 5.1) [1]. Thrombin (IIa) and factor Xa are the most sensitive to binding and inactivation [1]. Inactivation of thrombin prevents fibrin formation and inhibits thrombin-induced activation of factors V and VIII. Heparin can also increase vessel wall permeability and can inhibit platelet activation through binding to von Willebrand factor (vWF) [1].

LMWHs are derivatives of heparin produced by enzymatic or chemical depolymerisation methods. Like other types of heparin, including UFH, LMWHs mediate their major anticoagulant activity through binding to antithrombin, leading to inactivation of IIa and factor Xa. LMWHs bind less to IIa and therefore have a reduced antifactor IIa to antifactor Xa (anti-IIa/anti-Xa) ratio relative to UFH [1]. Additional actions of LMWHs are outlined in Table 5.1 [2]. The major advantage of LMWH over UFH is its reduced propensity to bind to proteins and cells, leading to a more predictable anticoagulant response and eliminating the

Marc Cohen, Professor of Medicine, Mount Sinai School of Medicine, Chief of Cardiology, Newark Beth Israel Medical Center, Newark, New Jersey, USA.

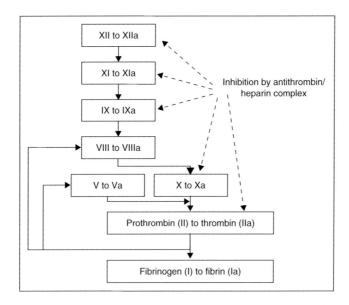

Figure 5.1　Points of inhibition by heparin, including low-molecular-weight heparin, in the coagulation cascade. The heparin/antithrombin complex inhibits factors XIIa, XIa, IXa, Xa and thrombin (IIa). Factor Xa and IIa are the most sensitive to inhibition.

Table 5.1　Non-antithrombin-mediated actions of low-molecular-weight heparins

Release of tissue factor pathway inhibitor
Interaction with heparin co-factor II
Inhibition of pro-coagulant actions of leucocytes
Promotion of fibrinolysis
Protein binding
Modulation of vascular endothelium (receptor- and non-receptor-mediated)
Reproduced with permission from [2].

need to monitor its anticoagulant effect [1]. Further research into the mechanisms of action of LMWH is ongoing. Heparin, including LMWH, has been shown to release a Kunitz-type inhibitor, tissue factor pathway inhibitor (TFPI), the effects of which may contribute to heparin- or LMWH-mediated anticoagulation [2, 3]. The antithrombotic effects of TFPI are summarised in Table 5.2 [2]. LMWHs have been shown to have a more consistent effect on TFPI than UFH [3]. Individual LMWHs differ with respect to manufacturing method (e.g., chemical vs. enzymatic digestion), average molecular weight and molecular weight profile, binding to antithrombin, anti-IIa/anti-Xa ratio, TFPI release, and vWF-mediated platelet function [2, 4, 5]. Table 5.3 summarises the biological heterogeneity of LMWHs [4].

The anticoagulant actions of UFH and LMWH have been exploited to treat ACS, including UA, NSTEMI and STEMI (Figure 5.2). UA and NSTEMI are characterised by an insufficient supply of oxygen to the heart as a result of narrowing of the coronary arteries, which in turn is caused by non-occlusive thrombus formation after rupture of an atherosclerotic plaque. STEMI occurs when thrombus formation completely occludes the blood vessel, blocking blood flow to the heart. UA and NSTEMI can progress to STEMI [6].

Table 5.2 Antithrombotic properties of tissue factor pathway inhibitor

Multi-domain inhibition of protease generation
Direct inhibition of factor Xa and elastase
Inhibition of tissue-factor-mediated activation of platelets and macrophages
Interaction with low-density lipoproteins, altering their pathological role
Interaction with vascular endothelium
Modulation of endogenous glycosaminoglycans
Neutralisation of endogenously formed tissue factor
Regulatory functions?
Reproduced with permission from [2].

Table 5.3 Biological heterogeneity of low-molecular-weight heparins

Wide variations in the affinity profile to the proteins:	
Antithrombin	Platelet factor 4
Heparin co-factor II	Protamine
Histidine-rich glycoprotein	Fibronectin
Albumin	Factor VIII
Fibrinogen	
Differential binding to endothelial cell lining and other cellular components of blood	
Variation in protease-inhibition profile	
Differential bioavailability and pharmacokinetics	
From Fareed J *et al.*, with permission [4].	

UFH TREATMENT OF UA AND NSTEMI

- ▪ UFH alone or in combination with aspirin is more effective than aspirin alone for treating UA and NSTEMI.
- ▪ The anticoagulation response must be monitored and the dose of UFH adjusted to maintain an activated partial thromboplastin time (aPTT) within the therapeutic range (1.5–2 times the control or 50–70 seconds).

Anticoagulation with UFH has been a cornerstone of treatment for patients with UA and NSTEMI for over a decade, on the basis of several randomised trials that found lower rates of death or myocardial infarction (MI) with UFH either alone or in combination with aspirin compared with aspirin alone [7–11]. A meta-analysis of 6 randomised trials, comparing treatment with aspirin plus UFH vs. aspirin alone in patients with UA, showed that combination treatment led to a relative reduction in the risk of death or MI of 33% compared with aspirin alone (risk ratio [RR] 0.67; 95% confidence interval [CI] 0.44–1.02) [10].

The anticoagulant effect of UFH is monitored by measuring aPTT, usually 6 h after the initial bolus dose. The subsequent continuous intravenous (IV) dose is adjusted accordingly to maintain the aPTT within a therapeutic range (1.5–2 times control or 50–70 seconds) [11]. Some patients require higher doses of heparin (UFH) to prolong the aPTT and are described as heparin-resistant [1]. A number of mechanisms have been proposed to account for this phenomenon, including antithrombin deficiency, increased heparin clearance, elevation of heparin-binding proteins, and elevation of factor VIII and fibrinogen [1].

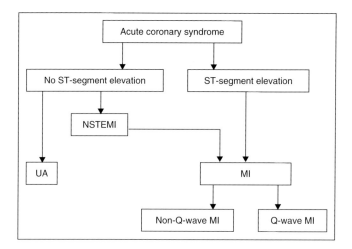

Figure 5.2   Summary of acute coronary syndromes.
MI = Myocardial infarction; NSTEMI = non-ST-segment elevation myocardial infarction; UA = unstable
angina. From Braunwald E *et al.*, 2002 [41].

   Monitoring of aPTT varies widely among different laboratories, and nomograms are recommended to standardise dose-adjustment methods [1, 12]. Several studies have investigated the relationship between aPTT and recurrent cardiovascular events and bleeding in patients with ACS treated with UFH [13–15]. In the Organisation to Assess Strategies for Ischaemic Syndromes 2 (OASIS-2) trial, subtherapeutic aPTT values below 60 seconds were associated with an increased risk of recurrent cardiovascular events compared with aPTT values greater than or equal to 60 seconds [13]. Higher aPTT values were associated with an increased risk of major bleeding, with a 7% increase in risk for every 10-second increase in aPTT [13]. Furthermore, the Global Utilization of Streptokinase and t-PA for Occluded Coronary Arteries I (GUSTO-I) study, which was actually conducted in STEMI patients, showed that aPTT values greater than 70 seconds were associated with an increased likelihood of death, bleeding, stroke or re-infarction [14]. An aPTT at 12 h of between 50 and 70 seconds was associated with the lowest rate of bleeding and death [14]. Becker *et al.* [15] also found that higher levels of anticoagulation, as indicated by increased aPTT, were not associated with a reduction in ischaemic events (from a substudy analysis of the Thrombolysis In Myocardial Infarction IIIB [TIMI-IIIB] study).
   Low body weight has been shown to be related to high aPTT levels [14]. On the basis of available data, the current optimal dosing regimen is, therefore, weight-adjusted. For patients weighing less than 70 kg, the recommended dose of UFH is a 60 IU/kg bolus followed by an IV infusion of 12 IU/kg/h [16]. The aPTT should be monitored frequently (every 6 h until the target range is reached and every 12–24 h thereafter) and the UFH dose adjusted according to a standardised nomogram to ensure a therapeutic range of 1.5–2 times the control or 50–70 seconds [16].

LMWH TREATMENT OF UA AND NSTEMI

■ Treatment of UA and NSTEMI with LMWH can reduce the rate of death or MI relative to placebo.
■ Enoxaparin alone or in combination with a glycoprotein (GP) IIb/IIIa receptor antagonist is superior to UFH for the treatment of UA and NSTEMI.

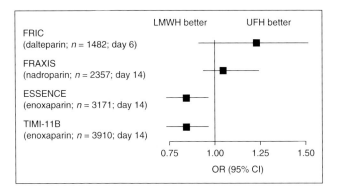

Figure 5.3 Efficacy of LMWH vs. UFH in patients with unstable angina and non-ST-segment elevation myocardial infarction. Plot of odds ratios (ORs) and 95% confidence intervals (CIs), with LMWH and UFH, for the triple efficacy endpoint of death, myocardial infarction and recurrent ischaemia and/or urgent revascularisation from the FRIC, FRAX.I.S, ESSENCE and TIMI-11B studies. From Braunwald *et al.*, 2002 [41].

■ The recommended dose of enoxaparin (1 mg/kg twice daily) does not require adjustment in obese patients, but should be reduced in patients with severe renal impairment (creatinine clearance less than 30 ml/min).

The potential advantages of LMWH over UFH prompted many studies investigating the efficacy and safety of LMWH in the treatment of patients with ACS. An overview of the results from some of these studies is presented in Figure 5.3.

EFFICACY OF LMWH VERSUS PLACEBO

Two multicentre, randomised, double-blind trials, FRagmin during InStability in Coronary Artery Disease (FRISC) and Fragmin and Fast Revascularisation during InStability in Coronary Artery Disease (FRISC II), have shown that LMWH (dalteparin) treatment of patients with unstable coronary artery disease can reduce the risk of coronary events within the first month of therapy, although these benefits are lost after 1 year [17, 18].

LMWH VS. UFH

A number of studies have compared the efficacy of LMWH vs. UFH in patients with either UA or non-Q-wave MI receiving aspirin therapy, with mixed results [19–24]. Gurfinkel *et al.* [19] conducted a small randomised, single-blind study comparing the efficacy and safety of subcutaneous (SC) nadroparin and aspirin vs. either aspirin alone or aspirin and IV UFH for up to 7 days. Treatment with aspirin and nadroparin was more effective than aspirin alone or aspirin plus UFH, with a significantly greater reduction in the risk of major cardiovascular events (odds ratio [OR] 5.06; 95% CI 2.28–11.39; $P = 0.00001$ and OR 5.63; 95% CI 2.50–12.81; $P = 0.00001$, respectively). A significant reduction in the rate of recurrent angina compared with the other treatment regimens and reductions in the rates of non-fatal MI and urgent revascularisation compared with aspirin alone were also seen. However, the results from this study should be interpreted with caution, owing to its single-blind nature and its failure to demonstrate superiority of aspirin plus UFH over aspirin alone [19]. In contrast, the randomised, double-blind, parallel-controlled FRagmin In Unstable Coronary Artery Disease (FRIC) study showed that the rate of the composite endpoint of death, MI or recurrent angina was comparable after acute treatment (days 1–6; open-label phase) between SC dalteparin and IV UFH (9.3 vs. 7.6%, respectively; RR 1.18; 95% CI 0.84–1.66). Rates of the composite endpoint were also similar after prolonged treatment (days 6–45; double-blind) with either dalteparin or placebo [20]. Similarly, the FRAXiparine in Ischaemic Syndrome (FRAX.I.S.) trial showed that the efficacy of nadroparin treatment for up to 8 days was comparable to that of UFH [21].

Some of the most convincing evidence comes from two randomised, double-blind trials of SC enoxaparin vs. IV UFH treatment for up to 8 days in patients with unstable coronary artery disease: the Efficacy and Safety of Subcutaneous Enoxaparin in Non-Q-Wave Coronary Events (ESSENCE) and TIMI-11B trials [22–24]. In the ESSENCE trial, treatment with enoxaparin was associated with a significantly lower risk of the composite endpoint of death, MI or recurrent angina at 14 days (16.6 vs. 19.8%, respectively; OR 0.80; 95% CI 0.67–0.96; $P = 0.02$) and also at 30 days (19.8 vs. 23.3%, respectively; OR 0.81; 95% CI 0.68–0.96; $P = 0.02$). Enoxaparin treatment was also associated with a reduction in the need for urgent revascularisation compared with UFH treatment [22]. Furthermore, the benefits with enoxaparin treatment were also evident at 1-year follow-up [23]. In agreement with the results of the ESSENCE trial, the TIMI 11B trial also showed a significantly lower rate of death, MI or urgent revascularisation at 48 h with enoxaparin treatment compared with UFH (5.5 vs. 7.3%, respectively; OR 0.75; 95% CI 0.58–0.97; $P = 0.026$), and also at 8 days (12.4 vs. 14.5%, respectively; OR 0.83; 95% CI 0.69–1.00; $P = 0.048$). The treatment effect was sustained during an additional 35 days of outpatient therapy with either enoxaparin or placebo, although there was no further additional treatment benefit of administering enoxaparin long-term over 35 days [24]. From a safety point of view, both trials showed that enoxaparin treatment did not lead to an increase in the rate of major bleeding during hospitalisation, although the rate of minor bleeding was increased [22, 24]. Enoxaparin in the outpatient treatment phase did, however, lead to increased bleeding, and this treatment course is thus not recommended. Meta-analyses of the results from these two trials indicated that the demonstrated efficacy of enoxaparin treatment was comparable between the two trials [25, 26]. Overall, treatment with enoxaparin led to a 20% relative reduction in the incidence of death and serious cardiac ischaemic events during the initial few days of treatment that was sustained through 43 days [25]. Furthermore, at one year there was a significant absolute reduction in the rate of death, non-fatal MI or urgent revascularisation of 2.5% [26].

TRIALS OF LMWH IN THE ERA OF GLYCOPROTEIN IIb/IIIa RECEPTOR ANTAGONISTS

A number of clinical trials have investigated the feasibility, efficacy and safety of LMWH in combination with a GPIIb/IIIa receptor antagonist as treatment for patients with UA or non-Q-wave MI. The Antithrombotic Combination Using Tirofiban and Enoxaparin (ACUTE) pilot study ($n = 55$) compared the pharmacokinetics and pharmacodynamics of randomised, blinded treatment with a combination of tirofiban (0.1 µg/kg/min IV) and either enoxaparin (1 mg/kg SC every 12 h) or UFH (adjusted according to aPTT) [27]. Enoxaparin treatment did not affect plasma clearance of tirofiban. In addition, there was a non-significant trend toward a greater and less variable inhibition of platelet aggregation and significantly lower adjusted bleeding times with enoxaparin and tirofiban compared with UFH and tirofiban (19.6 vs. 24.9 min, respectively; $P = 0.02$) [27]. As an extension of the ACUTE study, the larger randomised, double-blind ACUTE-II study investigated the effects of these two treatment regimens on clinical outcomes and safety [28]. Although both treatments led to comparable rates of death and MI at 30 days, the rates of major and minor bleeding at 24 h were slightly lower with enoxaparin and tirofiban compared with UFH and tirofiban. Furthermore, although not a primary endpoint of the study, treatment with tirofiban and enoxaparin led to greater reductions in the incidence of refractory ischaemia requiring urgent intervention and re-hospitalisation for UA [28].

In two randomised, double-blind trials, Platelet IIb/IIIa Antagonist for the Reduction of Acute Coronary Syndrome Events in a Global Organisation Network B (PARAGON B) and Global Utilization of Strategies To Open Occluded Coronary Arteries Trial IV in Acute Coronary Syndromes (GUSTO IV-ACS), designed to assess the efficacy of the GPIIb/IIIa receptor antagonists lamifiban and abciximab in patients receiving UFH or LMWH (enoxaparin or dalteparin), both treatment combinations led to comparable clinical and major-bleeding event rates [29, 30].

Similar results were obtained in two observational studies, National Investigators Collaborating on Enoxaparin (NICE)-3 ($n = 671$) and NICE-4 ($n = 818$), designed to assess the safety profile of enoxaparin plus either abciximab, eptifibatide or tirofiban in patients who may undergo percutaneous coronary intervention (PCI) [31, 32]. Clinical and major bleeding event rates were similar to those from previous studies where GPIIb/IIIa receptor antagonists were given alone [31]. In a further small study by Kereiakes *et al.* [33] ($n = 56$) comparing 2 doses of dalteparin (40 or 60 IU/kg IV) in combination with abciximab, patients undergoing PCI who received the higher dose of dalteparin had less procedural thrombosis, a more consistent anti-Xa effect, and a lower incidence of major bleeding compared with patients receiving the lower dose.

In the Coronary Revascularisation Using Integrilin and Single Bolus Enoxaparin (CRUISE) study, treatment of patients undergoing PCI with a combination of enoxaparin and eptifibatide did not increase the incidence of bleeding or vascular complications relative to concomitant treatment with UFH and eptifibatide [34].

A number of randomised, open-label studies have compared the efficacy of enoxaparin and UFH in combination with a GPIIb/IIIa receptor antagonist [35–37]. In the Integrilin and Enoxaparin Randomised Assessment of Acute Coronary Syndrome Treatment (INTERACT) study, treatment with enoxaparin in combination with a GPIIb/IIIa receptor antagonist for 48 h before any necessary revascularisation led to lower rates of recurrent ischaemia at 96 h (12.7 vs. 25.9%, respectively; $P < 0.0001$), the composite endpoint of death or MI at 30 days (5 vs. 9%, respectively; $P = 0.031$), and major bleeding at both 96 h and 30 days (2.1 vs. 5.5% for 96 h, respectively; $P = 0.016$; and 5.3 vs. 8.7% for 30 days, respectively; $P = 0.062$) compared with UFH plus a GPIIb/IIIa receptor antagonist [35]. Similarly, in the A to Z trial, treatment with enoxaparin and tirofiban was shown not to be inferior to treatment with UFH and tirofiban, with a trend in favour of the enoxaparin combination with respect to the incidence of the composite endpoint of death, MI or refractory ischaemia at 7 days (8.4 vs. 9.4%, respectively; hazard ratio [HR] 0.88; 95% CI 0.71–1.08) [36].

In contrast, in the Superior Yield of the New Strategy of Enoxaparin, Revascularization and Glycoprotein IIb/IIIa Receptor Antagonists (SYNERGY) trial (approximately 10 000 patients), similar rates of death or non-fatal MI at 30 days were seen after treatment with either enoxaparin or UFH in combination with a GPIIb/IIIa receptor antagonist (14 vs. 14.5%, respectively; HR 0.96; 95% CI 0.86–1.06), and there was no difference in the incidence of ischaemic events during PCI between treatments [37]. On the other hand, the enoxaparin combination significantly increased the incidence of major bleeding, according to the TIMI definition, relative to treatment with the UFH combination (9.1 vs. 7.6%, respectively; $P = 0.008$). However, when using the GUSTO definition for severe bleeding, the increase was not significantly different (2.7 vs. 2.2%, respectively; $P = 0.08$) [37]. The SYNERGY study was complicated by pre-randomisation treatment and post-randomisation treatment crossovers. In patients treated consistently, there was a significant 18% relative reduction in the composite endpoint of death or non-fatal MI with the enoxaparin combination compared with the UFH combination, with no excess of bleeding (Figure 5.4) [37].

The benefit with enoxaparin has been confirmed by a meta-analysis of the six major trials comparing enoxaparin and UFH with or without additional GPIIb/IIIa receptor antagonist therapy in ACS patients (ESSENCE, TIMI-11B, ACUTE-II, INTERACT, A to Z and SYNERGY) [38]. Overall, there was a significant decrease in the composite endpoint of

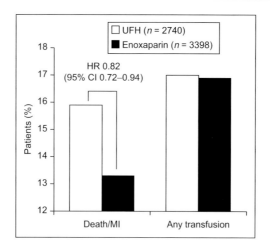

Figure 5.4 Efficacy and safety of enoxaparin vs. unfractionated heparin (UFH) in patients with unstable angina and non-ST-segment elevation myocardial infarction: results from a subgroup analysis of the SYNERGY study. Rates of death or myocardial infarction (MI) and any transfusion among patients randomised to a combination of a glycoprotein IIb/IIIa receptor antagonist and either enoxaparin or UFH. Patients in the subgroup analysis either received no pre-study antithrombin treatment or received pre-study treatment that was the same as the study-allocated treatment [37]. CI = Confidence interval; HR = hazard ratio.

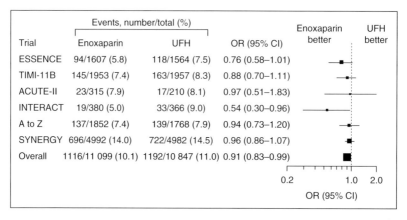

Figure 5.5 Efficacy of enoxaparin versus unfractionated heparin (UFH) in patients with unstable angina and non-ST-segment elevation myocardial infarction: death or myocardial infarction at 30 days. Plot of overall and individual study odds ratio (OR) with 95% confidence interval (CI) for the efficacy endpoint of death or myocardial infarction at 30 days. The size of each square reflects the statistical weight of a trial in calculating the OR. From Peterson JL *et al.*, 2004 [38].

death or MI at 30 days with enoxaparin compared with UFH (10.1 vs. 11.0%, respectively; OR 0.91; 95% CI 0.83–0.99). This was also true in the subgroup of patients who did not receive treatment pre-randomisation (8 vs. 9.4%, respectively; OR 0.81; 95% CI 0.70–0.94) [38]. An overview of the results for the composite endpoint of death or MI at 30 days is presented for each study in Figure 5.5. In the Enoxaparin VErsus Tinzaparin in Non-ST-Segment Elevation Acute Coronary Syndromes (EVET) trial, the efficacy of up to 7 days of treatment with two LMWHs, enoxaparin and tinzaparin, in patients with non-ST-segment ACS was directly compared. Enoxaparin led to a significantly lower incidence of the composite endpoint of recurrent angina, MI or death at 7 days compared with tinzaparin (12.3 vs. 21.1%, respectively; $P = 0.015$) [39], and this effect was maintained at 6 months (25.5 vs. 44.0%, respectively; $P < 0.001$) [40].

In conclusion, enoxaparin is the only LMWH to have shown superiority over UFH in combination with a GPIIb/IIIa receptor antagonist and is, therefore, the LMWH of choice in the treatment of UA or NSTEMI.

ACC/AHA GUIDELINES FOR UA/NSTEMI: HEPARIN THERAPY [41]

Class I indications (evidence or general agreement that the treatment or procedure is useful and effective)

■ 'Anticoagulation with subcutaneous LMWH or intravenous unfractionated heparin should be added to antiplatelet therapy with ASA (aspirin) and/or clopidogrel' (level of evidence: A)

Class IIa indications (weight of evidence or opinion in favor of usefulness and efficacy of treatment or procedure)

■ 'Enoxaparin is preferable to UFH as an anticoagulant in patients with UA/NSTEMI, unless CABG (coronary artery bypass grafting) is planned within 24 h' (level of evidence: A)

LMWH DOSING ISSUES

For treatment of UA or NSTEMI, the recommended dose of enoxaparin is 1 mg/kg twice daily, which gives predictable anti-Xa levels within the target therapeutic range in most patients [42]. A low anti-Xa activity of below 0.5 IU/ml in enoxaparin-treated patients has been shown to be associated with a significant increase in death at 30 days, with a greater than 3-fold increase, compared with an anti-Xa activity of over 0.5 IU/ml [43]. For this reason, it is important to achieve the minimum prescribed anti-Xa level with enoxaparin (0.5 IU/ml) when possible.

Studies have shown that the recommended dose of LMWH does not need to be adjusted for obese patients [44–46]. Total plasma clearance and anti-Xa and -IIa activity are not affected by body weight or body mass index [44–46]. Furthermore, a retrospective combination analysis of patient subgroups in the ESSENCE and TIMI 11B trials showed that obesity had no impact on clinical outcomes after treatment with enoxaparin [47].

In contrast, studies have shown that the dose of LMWH should be reduced in patients with severe renal impairment (creatinine clearance of less than 30 ml/min) [48, 49]. Studies comparing the pharmacokinetics of LMWH in patients with renal impairment and healthy volunteers have shown that severe renal impairment reduces LMWH clearance [48, 49]. A combined analysis of the ESSENCE and TIMI 11B trials also showed that renal impairment was associated with an increased risk of clinical events and major or any bleeding after either UFH or enoxaparin treatment [47].

LMWH TREATMENT OF STEMI

■ The addition of LMWH to fibrinolytic therapy can reduce ischaemic events and improve coronary reperfusion in patients with STEMI.

■ Enoxaparin has been shown to be superior to UFH as adjunctive therapy to fibrino-lysis in patients with STEMI.

■ Full-dose LMWH should not be used to treat patients aged over 75 years because it increases the rate of stroke and intracranial bleeding in this patient population.

Prompt coronary reperfusion with either thrombolysis or PCI is the recommended treatment strategy for patients presenting with STEMI within 12 h of symptom onset [50]. An overview of these initial treatment options is given in Figure 5.6. A number of studies have investigated the benefits of anticoagulation with UFH and LMWH as adjunctive therapy to fibrinolysis, or as treatment in patients ineligible for any kind of reperfusion therapy, and these are discussed in the following text.

LMWH VS. PLACEBO

A number of randomised, placebo-controlled studies have shown that LMWH can be used effectively to treat patients with STEMI in combination with fibrinolytic therapy and/or aspirin [51–54]. In a study by Glick et al. [51], LMWH (enoxaparin) use 5 days after treatment with streptokinase and heparin significantly reduced the re-infarction rate during the first 6 months (4.6 vs. 21.6%, respectively; $P = 0.01$) and also led to a non-significant reduction in the incidence of angina pectoris at 6 months (9.3 vs. 21.6%, respectively; $P = 0.078$), compared with placebo. The Fragmin in Acute Myocardial Infarction (FRAMI) study showed that treatment of patients with dalteparin and oral aspirin after an acute MI significantly reduced the risk of left ventricular thrombus formation compared with placebo and aspirin treatment (13.8 vs. 21.9%, respectively; RR 0.63; 95% CI 0.43–0.92; $P = 0.02$) [52]. Furthermore, in the BIOchemical Markers in Acute Coronary Syndromes II (BIOMACS II) study, dalteparin treatment of patients with acute MI undergoing fibrinolytic therapy with streptokinase led to a higher rate of TIMI grade 3 flow in the infarct-related arteries (68% for dalteparin vs. 51% with placebo; $P = 0.10$) and significantly fewer ischaemic episodes 6–24 h after the start of treatment compared with placebo (16% for dalteparin vs. 38% for placebo; $P = 0.04$) [53].

More recently, the Acute Myocardial Infarction – StreptoKinase (AMI–SK) study documented improved coronary reperfusion with the addition of a LMWH to fibrinolytic therapy with streptokinase [54]. Patients with acute MI ($n = 496$) were randomised to treatment with either enoxaparin or placebo in combination with streptokinase and aspirin for 3–8 days. Significantly more enoxaparin-treated patients had TIMI grade 3 flow at 5–10 days (70.3 vs. 57.8%, respectively; $P = 0.01$) and achieved complete resolution of the ST segment at 90 min compared with placebo (15.7 vs. 11.2%, respectively; $P = 0.012$) [54]. Coronary patency, defined as TIMI flow grades of 2 or 3, at 5–10 days was significantly better (87.6 vs. 71.7%, respectively; $P < 0.001$) and the incidence of the triple endpoint of death, MI, or recurrent angina was significantly lower after enoxaparin treatment (13.4 vs. 21.0%, respectively; $P = 0.03$) [54].

LMWH VS. UFH

Four randomised, open-label studies have compared the efficacy and safety of LMWH and UFH as adjunctive therapy to fibrinolysis in patients with STEMI [55–58]. In the Heparin and Aspirin Reperfusion Therapy (HART) II study, enoxaparin was shown to be non-inferior to UFH with respect to coronary patency (TIMI 2 and 3 reperfusion rates at 90 min.), with a trend in favour of enoxaparin that approached superiority (80.1 vs. 75.1%) [55]. There was also a non-significant trend toward lower rates of reocclusion, defined as deterioration from TIMI grade 2 or 3 at 90 min to grade 0 or 1 at follow-up, with enoxaparin

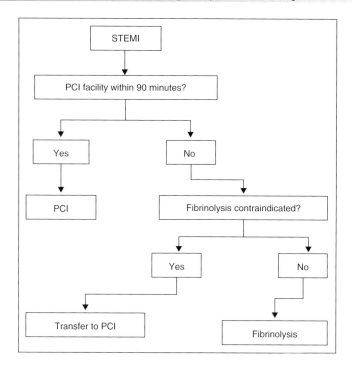

Figure 5.6 Early treatment options in patients with ST-segment elevation myocardial infarction (STEMI). Reproduced with permission from [50]. PCI = percutaneous coronary intervention.

compared with UFH (5.9 vs. 9.8%, respectively) [55]. In the ENTIRE-TIMI 23 trial, comparable TIMI 3 flow rates were seen with enoxaparin and UFH when used as adjunctive therapy to tenecteplase (TNK) [56]. On the other hand, enoxaparin significantly reduced the composite endpoint of death or MI at 30 days (4.4 vs. 15.9%, respectively; $P = 0.005$) and the rate of non-fatal re-infarction at 30 days (1.9 vs. 12.2%, respectively; $P = 0.003$) compared with UFH, with no increase in major bleeding [56]. Similarly, in the Assessment of the Safety and Efficacy of a New Thrombolytic Regimen 3 (ASSENT-3) study, the addition of enoxaparin for up to 7 days to lytic therapy significantly reduced the rate of the composite endpoint of 30-day death, in-hospital re-infarction, or in-hospital refractory ischaemia compared with UFH (11.4 vs. 15.4%, respectively; $P = 0.0002$) due mainly to reductions in both in-hospital re-infarction and refractory ischaemia, but not 30-day death [57]. More major bleeding complications were seen with enoxaparin than UFH, although the difference between treatments was not significant [57].

In an open-label extension of the ASSENT-3 study (ASSENT-3 PLUS), the addition of either enoxaparin or UFH to fibrinolytic therapy with TNK was compared in approximately 1600 patients in a pre-hospital setting [58]. There was a significant reduction in the incidence of in-hospital re-infarction (3.5 vs. 5.8%, respectively; RR 1.65; 95% CI 1.05–2.59; $P = 0.028$), and a trend toward a reduction in the incidence of in-hospital refractory ischaemia (4.4 vs. 6.5%; RR 1.47; 95% CI 0.97–2.22; $P = 0.067$) with enoxaparin compared with UFH [58]. Significant efficacy benefits with enoxaparin were seen in the subgroup of patients aged under 75 years [58]. Enoxaparin was associated with a significant increase in the incidence of total stroke (2.9 vs. 1.3%, respectively; RR 0.46; 95% CI 0.23–0.93; $P = 0.026$) and intracranial bleeding (2.2 vs. 0.97%, respectively; RR 0.44; 95% CI 0.19–1.01; $P = 0.047$) compared with UFH; this was due to high rates in patients aged over 75 years [58]. In a multivariate analysis, both age and age-by-treatment interaction were shown to significantly influence the risk of intracranial bleeding. The results from this study highlighted the need to test lower doses of LMWH in the elderly.

A large randomised, double-blind, phase III study is currently under way, which has been designed to compare the efficacy and safety of enoxaparin (30 mg IV bolus followed by 1 mg/kg SC twice daily) with UFH as adjunctive therapy to lysis in approximately 21 000 patients with STEMI (Enoxaparin and Thrombolysis Reperfusion for Acute Myocardial Infarction – Study 25 [ExTRACT TIMI 25]). In patients over 75 years, the initial bolus injection of enoxaparin has been eliminated and the twice-daily dose has been reduced to 75% of that used for younger patients (i.e., 0.75 mg/kg).

Most recently, the randomised, double-blind Clinical Trial of REviparin and Metabolic Modulation in Acute Myocardial Infarction Treatment Evaluation (CREATE) trial has shown that treatment with the LMWH reviparin, in patients on standard therapy (79% received a lytic or PCI), significantly reduces the incidence of death at both 7 days (8 vs. 8.9%, respectively; HR 0.89; 95% CI 0.80–0.99; $P = 0.04$) and 30 days (9.8 vs. 11.3%, respectively; HR 0.87; 95% CI 0.79–0.96; $P = 0.005$) compared with placebo [59]. The incidence of re-infarction was also significantly lower with reviparin at both 7 days (1.6 vs. 2.1%, respectively; HR 0.75; 95% CI 0.60–0.95; $P = 0.02$) and 30 days (2 vs. 2.6%, respectively; HR 0.77; 95% CI 0.62–0.95; $P = 0.01$), although there was no difference in the incidence of stroke compared with placebo. There was an increased bleeding risk with reviparin relative to UFH, but this was outweighed by the benefits of treatment [59].

ACC/AHA GUIDELINES FOR STEMI: USE OF UFH AND LMWH [50]

Class I indications (evidence or general agreement that the treatment or procedure is useful and effective)

- ■ 'Patients undergoing percutaneous or surgical revascularisation should be given UFH' (level of evidence: C)
- ■ 'UFH should be given intravenously to patients undergoing reperfusion therapy with alteplase, reteplase, or tenecteplase . . .' (level of evidence: C)
- ■ 'UFH should be given intravenously to patients treated with non-selective fibrinolytic agents . . . who are at high risk for systemic emboli . . .' (level of evidence: B)
- ■ 'Platelet counts should be monitored daily in patients given UFH' (level of evidence: C)

Class IIb indications (usefulness and efficacy of treatment is less well established by evidence or opinion)

- ■ 'LMWH might be considered an acceptable alternative to UFH as ancillary therapy for patients less than 75 years of age who are receiving fibrinolytic therapy provided that renal dysfunction . . . is not present' (level of evidence: B). Enoxaparin 30 mg IV bolus followed by 1.0 mg/kg SC q12h is the most comprehensively studied regimen in patients less than 75 years.

Class III indications (evidence or general agreement that the treatment or procedure is not useful or effective and may be harmful)

- ■ 'LMWH should not be used as an alternative to UFH as ancillary therapy in patients over 75 years of age who are receiving fibrinolytic therapy' (level of evidence: B)
- ■ 'LMWH should not be used as an alternative to UFH as ancillary therapy in patients less than 75 years of age who are receiving fibrinolytic therapy but have significant renal dysfunction (serum creatinine greater than 2.5 mg/dl in men, or 2.0 mg/dl in women).' (level of evidence: B)

IN PATIENTS INELIGIBLE FOR REPERFUSION

The randomised, double-blind Treatment with Enoxaparin and Tirofiban in Acute Myocardial Infarction (TETAMI) study compared treatment with enoxaparin vs. UFH in 1216 patients with STEMI who were ineligible for reperfusion [60]. This study did not show a significant difference between the efficacy of treatments, with a comparable incidence of the composite endpoint of death, re-infarction or recurrent ischaemia at 30 days with enoxaparin and UFH (15.7 vs. 17.3%, respectively; OR 0.89; 95% CI 0.66–1.21) and a comparable safety profile [60].

SUMMARY

LMWH offers many benefits over UFH and, for most patients with ACS, appears to be the best treatment option when an antithrombin is required. Of the LMWHs, enoxaparin has been the most extensively studied and has the most favourable efficacy profile in ACS; it is therefore the drug of choice. However, the use of LMWHs to treat STEMI is not currently recommended in patients receiving fibrinolytic therapy and who are older than 75 years of age or have renal dysfunction. The results of the ExTRACT TIMI 25 study will hopefully establish whether lower doses of enoxaparin can be safely used to treat patients over the age of 75.

REFERENCES

1. Hirsh J, Raschke R. Heparin and low-molecular-weight heparin: the Seventh ACCP Conference on Antithrombotic and Thrombolytic Therapy. *Chest* 2004; 126(3 suppl):188S–203S.
2. Fareed J, Jeske W, Hoppensteadt D, Clarizio R, Walenga JM. Low-molecular-weight heparins: pharmacologic profile and product differentiation. *Am J Cardiol* 1998; 82(5B):3L-10L.
3. Fareed J, Hoppensteadt D, Walenga J *et al*. Pharmacodynamic and pharmacokinetic properties of enoxaparin: implications for clinical practice. *Clin Pharmacokinet* 2003; 42:1043–1057.
4. Fareed J, Walenga JM, Hoppensteadt D, Racanelli A, Coyne E. Chemical and biological heterogeneity in low molecular weight heparins: implications for clinical use and standardisation. *Semin Thromb Hemost* 1989; 15(4):440–463.
5. Montalescot G, Bal-dit-Sollier C, Chibedi D *et al*; ARMADA Investigators. Comparison of effects on markers of blood cell activation of enoxaparin, dalteparin, and unfractionated heparin in patients with unstable angina pectoris or non-ST-segment elevation acute myocardial infarction (the ARMADA study). *Am J Cardiol* 2003; 91(8):925–930.
6. Wiviott SD, Braunwald E. Unstable angina and non-ST-segment elevation myocardial infarction: part I. Initial evaluation and management, and hospital care. *Am Fam Physician* 2004; 70(3):525–532.
7. Theroux P, Ouimet H, McCans J *et al*. Aspirin, heparin, or both to treat acute unstable angina. *N Engl J Med* 1988; 319(17):1105–1111.
8. Theroux P, Waters D, Qiu S, McCans J, de Guise P, Juneau M. Aspirin versus heparin to prevent myocardial infarction during the acute phase of unstable angina. *Circulation* 1993; 88(5 Pt 1):2045–2048.
9. Cohen M, Adams PC, Parry G *et al*. Combination antithrombotic therapy in unstable rest angina and non-Q-wave infarction in nonprior aspirin users. Primary end points analysis from the ATACS trial. *Circulation* 1994; 89(1):81–88.
10. Oler A, Whooley MA, Oler J, Grady D. Adding heparin to aspirin reduces the incidence of myocardial infarction and death in patients with unstable angina. A meta-analysis. *JAMA* 1996; 276(10):811–815.
11. Braunwald E, Jones RH, Mark DB *et al*. Diagnosing and managing unstable angina. Agency for Health Care Policy and Research. *Circulation* 1994; 90(1):613–622.
12. Flaker GC, Bartolozzi J, Davis V, McCabe C, Cannon CP. Use of a standardised nomogram to achieve therapeutic anticoagulation after thrombolytic therapy in myocardial infarction. *Arch Intern Med* 1994; 154(13):1492–1496.

13. Anand SS, Yusuf S, Pogue J, Ginsberg JS, Hirsh J; Organization to Assess Strategies for Ischemic Syndromes Investigators. Relationship of activated partial thromboplastin time to coronary events and bleeding in patients with acute coronary syndromes who receive heparin. *Circulation* 2003; 107(23):2884–2888.

14. Granger CB, Hirsch J, Califf RM *et al*. Activated partial thromboplastin time and outcome after thrombolytic therapy for acute myocardial infarction: results from the GUSTO-I Trial. *Circulation* 1996; 93(5):870–878.

15. Becker RC, Cannon CP, Tracy RP *et al*. Relationship between systemic anticoagulation as determined by activated partial thromboplastin time and heparin measurements and in-hospital clinical events in unstable angina and non-Q wave myocardial infarction. *Am Heart J* 1996; 131(3):421–433.

16. Hochman JS, Wali AU, Gavrila D *et al*. A new regimen for heparin use in acute coronary syndromes. *Am Heart J* 1999; 138(2 Pt 1):313–318.

17. Fragmin during Instability in Coronary Artery Disease (FRISC) study group. Low-molecular-weight heparin during instability in coronary artery disease. *Lancet* 1996; 347(9001):561–568.

18. Fragmin and Fast Revascularisation during Instability in Coronary artery disease (FRISC II) Investigators. Long-term low-molecular-mass heparin in unstable coronary-artery disease: FRISC II prospective randomised multicentre study. *Lancet* 1999; 354(9180):701–707.

19. Gurfinkel EP, Manos EJ, Mejail RI *et al*. Low molecular weight heparin versus regular heparin or aspirin in the treatment of unstable angina and silent ischemia. *J Am Coll Cardiol* 1995; 26(2):313–318.

20. Klein W, Buchwald A, Hillis WS *et al*. Comparison of low-molecular-weight heparin with unfractionated heparin acutely and with placebo for 6 weeks in the management of unstable coronary artery disease. Fragmin in unstable coronary artery disease study (FRIC). *Circulation* 1997; 96(1):61–68.

21. The FRAX.I.S. Study Group. Comparison of two treatment durations (6 days and 14 days) of a low molecular weight heparin with a 6-day treatment of unfractionated heparin in the initial management of unstable angina or non-Q wave myocardial infarction: FRAX.I.S. (FRAxiparine in Ischaemic Syndrome). *Eur Heart J* 1999; 20(21):1553–1562.

22. Cohen M, Demers C, Gurfinkel EP *et al*. A comparison of low-molecular weight heparin with unfractionated heparin for unstable coronary artery disease. Efficacy and Safety of Subcutaneous Enoxaparin in Non-Q-Wave Coronary Events Study Group. *N Engl J Med* 1997; 337(7):447–452.

23. Goodman SG, Cohen M, Bigonzi F *et al*. Randomized trial of low molecular weight heparin (enoxaparin) versus unfractionated heparin for unstable coronary artery disease: one-year results of the ESSENCE Study. Efficacy and Safety of Subcutaneous Enoxaparin in Non-Q-Wave Coronary Events. *J Am Coll Cardiol* 2000; 36(3):693–698.

24. Antman EM, McCabe CH, Gurfinkel EP *et al*. Enoxaparin prevents death and cardiac ischemic events in unstable angina/non-Q-wave myocardial infarction. Results of the thrombolysis in myocardial infarction (TIMI) 11B trial. *Circulation* 1999; 100(15):1593–1601.

25. Antman EM, Cohen M, Radley D *et al*. Assessment of the treatment effect of enoxaparin for unstable angina/non-Q-wave myocardial infarction. TIMI 11B/ESSENCE meta-analysis. *Circulation* 1999; 100(15):1602–1608.

26. Antman EM, Cohen M, McCabe C, Goodman SG, Murphy SA, Braunwald E; TIMI 11B and ESSENCE Investigators. Enoxaparin is superior to unfractionated heparin for preventing clinical events at 1-year follow-up of TIMI 11B and ESSENCE. *Eur Heart J* 2002; 23(4):308–314.

27. Cohen M, Theroux P, Weber S *et al*. Combination therapy with tirofiban and enoxaparin in acute coronary syndromes. *Int J Cardiol* 1999; 71(3):273–281.

28. Cohen M, Theroux P, Borzak S *et al*; ACUTE II Investigators. Randomized double-blind safety study of enoxaparin versus unfractionated heparin in patients with non-ST-segment elevation acute coronary syndromes treated with tirofiban and aspirin: the ACUTE II study. The Antithrombotic Combination Using Tirofiban and Enoxaparin. *Am Heart J* 2002; 144(3):470–477.

29. Mukherjee D, Mahaffey KW, Moliterno DJ *et al*. Promise of combined low-molecular-weight heparin and platelet glycoprotein IIb/IIIa inhibition: results from Platelet IIb/IIIa Antagonist for the Reduction of Acute coronary syndrome events in a Global Organization Network B (PARAGON B). *Am Heart J* 2002; 144(6):995–1002.

30. Simoons ML; GUSTO IV-ACS Investigators. Effect of glycoprotein IIb/IIIa receptor blocker abciximab on outcome in patients with acute coronary syndromes without early coronary revascularisation: the GUSTO IV-ACS randomised trial. *Lancet* 2001; 357(9272):1915–1924.

31. Ferguson JJ, Antman EM, Bates ER *et al*; NICE-3 Investigators. Combining enoxaparin and glycoprotein IIb/IIIa antagonists for the treatment of acute coronary syndromes: final results of

the National Investigators Collaborating on Enoxaparin-3 (NICE-3) study. *Am Heart J* 2003; 146(4):628–634.

32. Kereiakes DJ, Grines C, Fry E *et al*; NICE 1 and NICE 4 Investigators. National Investigators Collaborating on Enoxaparin. Enoxaparin and abciximab adjunctive pharmacotherapy during percutaneous coronary intervention. *J Invasive Cardiol* 2001; 13(4):272–278.

33. Kereiakes DJ, Kleiman NS, Fry E *et al*. Dalteparin in combination with abciximab during percutaneous coronary intervention. *Am Heart J* 2001; 141(3):348–352.

34. Bhatt DL, Lee BI, Casterella PJ *et al*; Coronary Revascularisation Using Integrilin and Single bolus Enoxaparin Study. Safety of concomitant therapy with eptifibatide and enoxaparin in patients undergoing percutaneous coronary intervention: results of the Coronary Revascularisation Using Integrilin and Single bolus Enoxaparin Study. *J Am Coll Cardiol* 2003; 41(1):20–25.

35. Goodman SG, Fitchett D, Armstrong PW, Tan M, Langer A; Integrilin and Enoxaparin Randomised Assessment of Acute Coronary Syndrome Treatment (INTERACT) Trial Investigators. Randomised evaluation of the safety and efficacy of enoxaparin versus unfractionated heparin in high-risk patients with non-ST-segment elevation acute coronary syndromes receiving the glycoprotein IIb/IIIa inhibitor eptifibatide. *Circulation* 2003; 107(2):238–244.

36. Blazing MA, de Lemos JA, White HD *et al*; A to Z Investigators. Safety and efficacy of enoxaparin vs unfractionated heparin in patients with non-ST-segment elevation acute coronary syndromes who receive tirofiban and aspirin: a randomised controlled trial. *JAMA* 2004; 292(1):55–64. Erratum in: *JAMA* 2004; 292(10):1178.

37. Ferguson JJ, Califf RM, Antman EM *et al*. SYNERGY Trial Investigators. Enoxaparin vs unfractionated heparin in high-risk patients with non-ST-segment elevation acute coronary syndromes managed with an intended early invasive strategy: primary results of the SYNERGY randomized trial. *JAMA* 2004; 292(1):45–54.

38. Petersen JL, Mahaffey KW, Hasselblad V *et al*. Efficacy and bleeding complications among patients randomised to enoxaparin or unfractionated heparin for antithrombin therapy in non-ST-Segment elevation acute coronary syndromes: a systematic overview. *JAMA* 2004; 292(1):89–96.

39. Michalis LK, Katsouras CS, Papamichael N *et al*. Enoxaparin versus tinzaparin in non-ST-segment elevation acute coronary syndromes: the EVET trial. *Am Heart J* 2003; 146(2):304–310.

40. Katsouras CS, Michalis LK, Papamichael N *et al*. Enoxaparin versus tinzaparin in non-ST-segment elevation acute coronary syndromes: results of the EVET trial at 6 months. *Am Heart J* 2005; in press.

41. Braunwald E, Antman EM, Beasley JW *et al*; American College of Cardiology; American Heart Association. Committee on the Management of Patients With Unstable Angina. ACC/AHA 2002 guideline update for the management of patients with unstable angina and non-ST-segment elevation myocardial infarction—summary article: a report of the American College of Cardiology/American Heart Association task force on practice guidelines (Committee on the Management of Patients With Unstable Angina). *J Am Coll Cardiol* 2002; 40(7):1366–1374.

42. Martin JL, Fry ET, Sanderink GJ *et al*. Reliable anticoagulation with enoxaparin in patients undergoing percutaneous coronary intervention: The pharmacokinetics of enoxaparin in PCI (PEPCI) study. *Catheter Cardiovasc Interv* 2004; 61(2):163–170.

43. Montalescot G, Collet JP, Tanguy ML *et al*. Anti-Xa activity relates to survival and efficacy in unselected acute coronary syndrome patients treated with enoxaparin. *Circulation* 2004; 110(4): 392–398.

44. Becker RC, Spencer FA, Bruno R *et al*. Excess body weight does not adversely influence either bioavailability or anticoagulant activity of enoxaparin administered subcutaneously in acute coronary syndromes. *Circulation* 2000; 102(18):II-427–8 (Abstract 2080).

45. Hainer JW, Barrett JS, Assaid CA *et al*. Dosing in heavy-weight/obese patients with the LMWH, tinzaparin: a pharmacodynamic study. *Thromb Haemost* 2002; 87(5):817–823.

46. Sanderink GJ, Le Liboux A, Jariwala N *et al*. The pharmacokinetics and pharmacodynamics of enoxaparin in obese volunteers. *Clin Pharmacol Ther* 2002; 72(3):308–318.

47. Spinler SA, Inverso SM, Cohen M, Goodman SG, Stringer KA, Antman EM; ESSENCE and TIMI 11B Investigators. Safety and efficacy of unfractionated heparin versus enoxaparin in patients who are obese and patients with severe renal impairment: analysis from the ESSENCE and TIMI 11B studies. *Am Heart J* 2003; 146(1):33–41.

48. Sanderink GJ, Guimart CG, Ozoux ML, Jariwala NU, Shukla UA, Boutouyrie BX. Pharmacokinetics and pharmacodynamics of the prophylactic dose of enoxaparin once daily over 4 days in patients with renal impairment. *Thromb Res* 2002; 105(3):225–231.

49. Hulot JS, Vantelon C, Urien S et al. Effect of renal function on the pharmacokinetics of enoxaparin and consequences on dose adjustment. *Ther Drug Monit* 2004; 26(3):305–310.
50. Antman EM, Anbe DT, Armstrong PW et al; American College of Cardiology; American Heart Association; Canadian Cardiovascular Society. ACC/AHA guidelines for the management of patients with ST-elevation myocardial infarction—executive summary. A report of the American College of Cardiology/American Heart Association Task Force on Practice Guidelines (Writing Committee to revise the 1999 guidelines for the management of patients with acute myocardial infarction). *J Am Coll Cardiol* 2004; 44(3):671–719.
51. Glick A, Kornowski R, Michowich Y et al. Reduction of reinfarction and angina with use of low-molecular-weight heparin therapy after streptokinase (and heparin) in acute myocardial infarction. *Am J Cardiol* 1996; 77(14):1145–1148.
52. Kontny F, Dale J, Abildgaard U, Pedersen TR. Randomized trial of low molecular weight heparin (dalteparin) in prevention of left ventricular thrombus formation and arterial embolism after acute anterior myocardial infarction: the Fragmin in Acute Myocardial Infarction (FRAMI) Study. *J Am Coll Cardiol* 1997; 30(4):962–969.
53. Frostfeldt G, Ahlberg G, Gustafsson G et al. Low molecular weight heparin (dalteparin) as adjuvant treatment of thrombolysis in acute myocardial infarction—a pilot study: biochemical markers in acute coronary syndromes (BIOMACS II). *J Am Coll Cardiol* 1999; 33(3):627–633.
54. Simoons ML, Krzeminska-Pakula M, Alonso A et al; AMI-SK Investigators. Improved reperfusion and clinical outcome with enoxaparin as an adjunct to streptokinase thrombolysis in acute myocardial infarction. The AMI–SK study. *Eur Heart J* 2002; 23:1282–1290.
55. Ross AM, Molhoek P, Lundergan C et al; HART II Investigators. Randomized comparison of enoxaparin, a low-molecular-weight heparin, with unfractionated heparin adjunctive to recombinant tissue plasminogen activator thrombolysis and aspirin: second trial of Heparin and Aspirin Reperfusion Therapy (HART II). *Circulation* 2001; 104(6):648–652.
56. Antman EM, Louwerenburg HW, Baars HF et al. Enoxaparin as adjunctive antithrombin therapy for ST-elevation myocardial infarction: results of the ENTIRE-Thrombolysis in Myocardial Infarction (TIMI) 23 Trial. *Circulation* 2002; 105(14):1642–1649. Erratum in: *Circulation* 2002; 105(23):2799.
57. Assessment of the Safety and Efficacy of a New Thrombolytic Regimen (ASSENT)-3 Investigators. Efficacy and safety of tenecteplase in combination with enoxaparin, abciximab, or unfractionated heparin: the ASSENT-3 randomised trial in acute myocardial infarction. *Lancet* 2001; 358(9282):605–613.
58. Wallentin L, Goldstein P, Armstrong PW et al. Efficacy and safety of tenecteplase in combination with the low-molecular-weight heparin enoxaparin or unfractionated heparin in the prehospital setting: the Assessment of the Safety and Efficacy of a New Thrombolytic Regimen (ASSENT)-3 PLUS randomized trial in acute myocardial infarction. *Circulation* 2003; 108(2):135–142.
59. Yusuf S, Mehta SR, Xie C et al; CREATE Trial Group Investigators. Effects of reviparin, a low-molecular-weight heparin, on mortality, reinfarction, and strokes in patients with acute myocardial infarction presenting with ST-segment elevation. *JAMA* 2005; 293(4):427–435.
60. Cohen M, Gensini GF, Maritz F et al; TETAMI Investigators. The safety and efficacy of subcutaneous enoxaparin versus intravenous unfractionated heparin and tirofiban versus placebo in the treatment of acute ST-segment elevation myocardial infarction patients ineligible for reperfusion (TETAMI): a randomized trial. *J Am Coll Cardiol* 2003; 42(8):1348–1356.

6

Intravenous direct thrombin inhibition: acute coronary syndromes and heparin-induced thrombocytopaenia

E. D. Crouch, V. Menon, E. M. Ohman, G. W. Stone

INTRODUCTION

Anticoagulation therapy with indirect thrombin inhibitors, such as unfractionated heparin (UFH) and low-molecular-weight heparin (LMWH), has been a cornerstone of therapy for acute coronary syndromes (ACS) and has been shown to reduce the risk of recurrent myocardial infarction (MI) and cardiovascular death by up to 50% when used in combination with aspirin [1]. Nevertheless, UFH and LMWH carry the risk of heparin-induced thrombocytopaenia (HIT) and have several mechanistic and pharmacokinetic limitations, which have led to an increased interest in alternative anticoagulants. There is established evidence that direct thrombin inhibitors (DTIs) are effective anticoagulants in patients with HIT and HIT with thrombotic complications (HITT) [2]. There is also emerging evidence to suggest that some DTIs are at least as safe and effective as heparin in the treatment of many patients with ACS [3], but without the risk of developing HIT or HITT.

This chapter will:

(i)   summarise the mechanism of action and limitations of indirect thrombin inhibitors;
(ii)   highlight the potential benefits of DTIs as alternative anticoagulants;
(iii) review the key pharmacological features of the different DTIs and the major clinical trials evaluating their efficacy and safety in ACS and HIT; and,
(iv) discuss the clinical role of DTIs in the management of ACS and HIT.

MECHANISMS OF ACTION OF DIRECT AND INDIRECT THROMBIN INHIBITORS

Thrombin cleaves fibrinogen into fibrin, which serves to stabilise aggregated platelets (Figure 6.1). In addition, thrombin activates and recruits platelets to the site of coronary vascular injury [4] and amplifies its own generation by activating factors V, VIII and XI [5].

Eron D. Crouch, Cardiology Fellow, University of North Carolina at Chapel Hill, Chapel Hill, North Carolina, USA.

Venugopal Menon, Director, Coronary Care Unit, Assistant Professor of Medicine and Emergency Medicine, University of North Carolina at Chapel Hill, Chapel Hill, North Carolina, USA.

E. Magnus Ohman, Ernest and Hazel Craige Professor of Cardiovascular Medicine, Chief, Division of Cardiology and Director, University of North Carolina Heart Center, Chapel Hill, North Carolina, USA.

Gregg W. Stone, Professor of Medicine, Columbia University Medical Center, Director of Cardiovascular Research and Education, Center for Interventional Vascular Therapy, Columbia University Medical Center, Vice-chairman, The Cardiovascular Research Foundation, New York, USA.

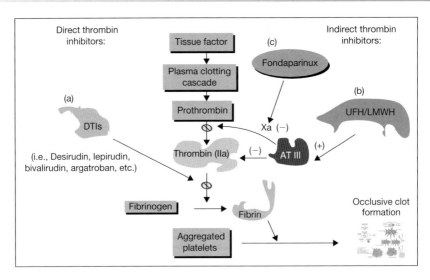

Figure 6.1 Mechanisms of action of thrombin inhibitors. (a) DTIs directly inhibit the activation of thrombin, which prevents thrombin-dependent cleavage of fibrinogen to fibrin. (b) UFH primarily catalyses antithrombin III (ATIII) to inhibit the activation of thrombin. LMWH primarily inhibits factor Xa-mediated cleavage of prothrombin to thrombin. (c) fondaparinux, an novel indirect thrombin inhibitor, directly inhibits factor Xa-mediated cleavage of prothrombin into thrombin.

Thrombin has three key binding sites: the active site, the fibrin-binding site, and the heparin-binding site (Figure 6.2A). *In vivo*, antithrombin III (ATIII) inhibits the active site, thus inactivating thrombin. This is part of the autoregulation of the coagulation cascade.

Indirect thrombin inhibitors, such as UFH and LMWH (i.e., enoxaparin and dalteparin), utilise the heparin-binding site to bridge antithrombin III (ATIII) to thrombin (Figure 6.2A). This process catalyses the ATIII inhibition of thrombin. These agents also inhibit the production of thrombin by catalysing the ATIII-mediated inhibition of factor Xa cleavage of prothrombin into thrombin (Figure 6.1). LMWHs are far more potent inhibitors of factor Xa and far less potent catalysts of ATIII than UFHs [6].

Indirect thrombin inhibitors have several limitations which have led to an increased interest in alternative anticoagulants. One limitation of UFH is its large molecular size, which leads to a propensity to non-specifically bind to numerous plasma proteins and factors released by platelets and endothelial cells at the site of vascular injury [4]. This causes unpredictable plasma bioavailability and efficacy at the site of vascular injury, necessitating frequent activated clotting time (ACT) or activated partial thromboplastin time (aPTT) monitoring to ensure a therapeutic anticoagulant response [7]. Since the affinity of heparins for plasma proteins is chain-length dependent, LMWH has less affinity for plasma proteins. Subsequently, LMWH has a more predictable bioavailability and therapeutic effect at the site of vascular injury [4]. Typically, dosing of LMWH is weight-adjusted with little need for laboratory monitoring. Bioavailability may become less predictable in patients with renal insufficiency [8] and morbid obesity. If needed, monitoring can be accomplished via a quantitative factor Xa assay [8]; however, enoxaparin is typically avoided in patients with significant renal insufficiency. Rebound ischaemia after the discontinuation of anticoagulation has been reported with UFH and dalteparin [9]. Enoxaparin has not been associated with rebound ischaemia [10].

Although LMWHs have overcome some pharmacokinetic limitations of UFH, mechanistically, both UFH and LMWH depend on ATIII to inhibit thrombin and have limited activity against thrombin with fibrin bound to its fibrin-binding site [4, 11, 12]. When UFH or LMWH

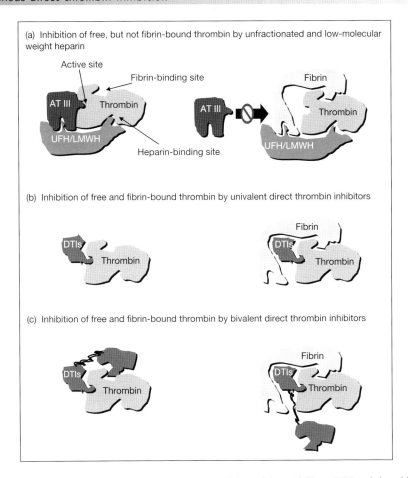

(a) Inhibition of free, but not fibrin-bound thrombin by unfractionated and low-molecular weight heparin

Active site

Fibrin-binding site

Fibrin

AT III   Thrombin

AT III

Thrombin

UFH/LMWH

Heparin-binding site

UFH/LMWH

(b) Inhibition of free and fibrin-bound thrombin by univalent direct thrombin inhibitors

Fibrin

DTIs

Thrombin

DTIs

Thrombin

(c) Inhibition of free and fibrin-bound thrombin by bivalent direct thrombin inhibitors

Fibrin

DTIs

Thrombin

DTIs

Thrombin

Figure 6.2 Binding sites of direct and indirect thrombin inhibitors. (a) UFH bridges ATIII and thrombin through the heparin binding site. LMWH also bridges ATIII and thrombin, but to a lesser extent (primarily inhibits factor Xa.) (left). When heparin binds fibrin-bound thrombin, it forms a very stable, active tertiary complex, which can not be deactivated by ATII, because of conformational changes which obscure the active site of thrombin (right). (b) Univalent DTIs can bind the active site of both free and fibrin-bound thrombin, thus inactivating the thrombin complex. (c) Bivalent DTIs can also bind the active site of both free and fibrin-bound thrombin, thus inactivating the thrombin complex. In the case of free thrombin, bivalent DTIs also bind the fibrin binding site.

binds to the heparin-binding site of a fibrin-bound thrombin molecule, it forms a very stable, highly active, ternary thrombin/fibrin/heparin complex that changes the conformation of the thrombin active site, limiting its availability for inhibition by ATII (Figure 6.2(a), right) [13, 14]. In addition, since the heparin-binding site on a ternary thrombin/fibrin/heparin complex is occupied, other heparin molecules cannot bridge ATII to the thrombin active site [4]. As a result, thrombin molecules in these ternary complexes remain active, cleaving fibrinogen into fibrin, which stabilises aggregated platelets into occlusive clots. The thrombin molecule in these complexes also continue to activate platelets at the site of vascular injury [15]. For reasons that are not completely understood, platelet-bound factor Xa also appears to be protected from inhibition by UFH and LMWH [4].

Finally, UFH and LMWH can lead to intense, autoantibody-mediated thrombin activation and potentially life-threatening venous and arterial thrombosis (i.e., HITT) [16–18]. In the past, HIT has been defined as a drop in platelet count to less than 100×10^9/l; however, more recent definitions have emphasised a drop of ≥50%, typically beginning between days 5 and 10 of UFH or LMWH therapy [19]. Even in the absence of a thrombotic syndrome, suspicion of HIT mandates prompt discontinuation of all UFH and LMWH [20]. In addition to discontinuing all heparins, using an alternative anticoagulant in patients with HIT is also suggested, because of the relatively high risk for progression to HITT, which is associated with significant morbidity and mortality [20].

BENEFITS OF DIRECT THROMBIN INHIBITORS AS ALTERNATIVE ANTICOAGULANTS

Several factors make DTIs a very attractive alternative to indirect thrombin inhibition. DTIs independently bind and inhibit thrombin and do not require the inhibitory actions of ATIII [13]. Consequently, they inactivate both freely circulating and fibrin-bound thrombin by directly inhibiting the active site (Figure 6.2(b) and (c)). Univalent DTIs, such as argatroban and efegatran, block only the active site of thrombin, preventing the enzyme from cleaving fibrinogen into fibrin (Figure 6.2(b), Table 6.1). Bivalent DTIs, such as hirudin and bivalirudin, also block the active site of thrombin; but in the absence of fibrin, they simultaneously bind to the fibrin-binding site, forming a more stable inhibitory complex (Figure 6.2(c), Table 6.1).

DTIs also have a very low affinity for plasma proteins. In addition, since DTIs do not interact with the heparin-binding site on thrombin, they do not form ternary thrombin/fibrin/heparin complexes [13]. Both of these features lead to a more predictable bioavailability and effect at the site of vascular injury and ultimately a decreased need for laboratory monitoring (Table 6.1).

Finally, and possibly most importantly, DTIs have not been shown to cause HIT or HITT. Conversely, in patients with HITT some DTIs have been shown to be effective alternative anticoagulants as well as effective therapy to prevent additional thrombotic complications [2].

BIVALENT DIRECT THROMBIN INHIBITORS

HIRUDIN

Key pharmacological features of hirudin

Hirudin, the prototypical DTI, is a 65- or 66-amino acid polypeptide first isolated from the salivary glands of the medicinal leech, *Hirudo medicinalis* [21]. There are two commercially available recombinant hirudin preparations, desirudin and lepirudin. These hirudin preparations are known as desulphatohirudins, because they lack a sulpha group that is present on position 63 of native hirudin [4]. Hirudins are bivalent inhibitors that typically bind both the active site and the fibrin-binding site of thrombin (Figure 6.2(c)). Consequently, they have high affinity for thrombin, forming an essentially irreversible 1:1 hirudin/thrombin complex [4]. The normal half-life of the hirudin is approximately 90–120 min when given intravenously [22, 23] and 120–180 min by subcutaneous injection [22, 23]. They are cleared *via* the kidney and can accumulate to dangerously high levels in patients with significant renal insufficiency. The manufacturers of both lepirudin [22] and desirudin [23] recommend renal dose adjustments in this patient population (Table 6.1). There is no selective antagonist that can reverse over-anticoagulation with hirudin; however, it can be managed with dialysis using high- or low-flux polysulfondialysers [24]. The anticoagulant effect of the hirudin can be monitored using the aPTT (Table 6.1) [25]; however, this assay is unreliable at higher hirudin concentrations [25]. The ecarin clotting time (ECT) assay demonstrates a linear relationship, even at higher hirudin concentrations, but it is not widely available [26] and is seldom utilised due to lack of clinical familiarity.

Table 6.1 Prescribing information for current direct thrombin inhibitors

Drug (Trade)	FDA-approved indications(s)	Label-recommended dosing	Label-recommended monitoring	Metabolism	Half-life (min)	Major clinical trials
Bivalent direct thrombin inhibitors						
Desirudin (Revasc™, Iprivask™)	APR 2003: Prophylaxis of deep vein thrombosis in patients undergoing elective hip replacement surgery.	15 mg subcutaneously every 12 h, beginning 5–15 min prior to surgery.	Normally none. Check aPTT and creatinine at least once daily in renal insufficiency; target aPTT 1.5–2.0x normal.	Kidney	60	**ACS:** GUSTO-IIa, GUSTO-IIb, TIMI-9A, TIMI-9B, HELVETICA.
Lepirudin (Refludan™)	MAR 1998: Anticoagulant in patients with HIT and associated thromboembolic disease.	0.4 mg/kg bolus, then 0.15 mg/kg infusion for 2–10 days (up to 110 kg).	Check first aPTT 4 h after drug initiation, then at least once daily; target aPTT 1.5–2.5x normal.	Kidney	90	**ACS:** HIT-3, HIT-4, OASIS, OASIS-2. **HIT:** HAT-1, HAT-2, HAT-3.
Bivalirudin (Angiomax™, Hirulog™)	DEC 2000 and JUNE 2005: Anticoagulant in conjunction with aspirin in patients with unstable angina undergoing PCI and with provisional glycoprotein IIb/IIIa inhibitor use in patients with stable and unstable angina undergoing PCI.	1.0 mg/kg bolus, then mg/kg/h infusion for 4 h, then 0.2 mg/kg/h for up to 20 h.	Check initial ACT after 5 min, again at 45 min, and 5 min after any; target ACT >350.	Plasma, liver and kidney	25	**ACS:** HERO, HERO-2, BAT, CACHET, REPLACE-2, PROTECT-TIMI 30♦, ACUITY♦, HORIZONS*. **HIT:** ATBAT.
Univalent direct thrombin inhibitors						
Argatroban (Acova™, Novastan™)	APR 2002: Anticoagulant in patients undergoing PCI who have or are at risk for HIT.	350 μ/kg bolus over 3–5 min, then 25 mg/kg/min infusion.	Check initial ACT 5–10 min after the initial bolus and after each dose adjustment; target ACT 300–450.	Liver	45	**ACS:** ARGAMI-2, MINT, ARG 216/310/311▲ **HIT:** ARG 911, ARG 915.
Efegatran	None	–	–	–	–	**ACS:** ESCALAT, PRIME, Klootwijk et al.
Inogatran	None	–	–	–	–	**ACS:** TRIM.

ACS = acute coronary syndrome; HIT = heparin-induced thrombocytopaenia; PCI = percutaneous coronary intervention; aPTT = activated partial thromboplastin time; ACT = activated clotting time.
♦In renal insufficient patients, renal adjustment is recommended and outlined in packet insert.
*Currently enrolling.
▲Trials enrolled 91 patients with HIT undergoing PCI for UA.

Table 6.2 Clinical trials evaluating direct thrombin inhibitors vs. unfractionated heparin as adjunct to thrombolysis in acute ST-segment elevation myocardial infarction

Trial	Patients	Treatment regimen	Control regimen	Clinical outcome
Bivalent direct thrombin inhibitors				
TIMI-9A (1994)[28]	757	Desirudin 0.6 mg/kg bolus, then 0.2 mg/kg/h then 1000 or 1300 infusion × 96 h; (ASA + SK or tPA)	UFH 5000 IU bolus, then 1000 or 1300 IU/h infusion × 96 h, target aPTT 60–90 seconds; (ASA + SK or tPA)	Stopped early due to ↑ rate of intracranial haemorrhage with both regimens and ↑ rate of major non-intra-cranial haemorrhage with desirudin.
GUSTO-IIa (1994)[27]	2564	Desirudin 0.6 mg/kg bolus, then 0.2 mg/kg/h infusion × 72 to 120 h; (SK or tPA)	UFH 5000 IU bolus, then 1000–1300 IU/h infusion × 72 to 120 h, target aPTT 60–90 sec; (SK or tPA)	Stopped early due to ↑ rate of haemorrhagic stroke with desirudin.
TIMI-9B (1996)*[30]	3002	Desirudin 0.1 mg/kg bolus, then 0.1 mg/kg/h infusion × 96 h; (ASA + SK or tPA)	UFH 5000 IU bolus, then 1000 IU h infusion × 96 h, target aPTT 55–85 sec; (ASA + SK or tPA)	No difference in death, MI, CHF, shock, intracranial haemorrhage or major non-intracranial haemorrhage at 30 days.
GUSTO-IIb (1998†)*[33]	3289	Desirudin 0.1 mg/kg bolus, then 0.1 mg/kg/h infusion × 72 h; (ASA + SK or tPA)	UFH 5000 IU bolus, then 1000 IU/h infusion × 72 h, target aPTT 60–85 sec; (SK or tPA)	No difference in death, MI, intracranial or major non-intracranial haemorrhage at 30 days with tPA, but ↓ death and MI with desirudin over UFH when used as adjunct to SK.
HIT-3 (1994)[29]	302	Lepirudin 0.4 mg/kg bolus, then 0.15 mg/kg/h infusion × 48 to 72 h; (SK or tPA)	UFH 70 IU/kg bolus, then 15 IU/kg/h infusion × 48 to 72 h; (SK or tPA)	Stopped early due to ↑ rate of major haemorrhage with lepirudin.
HIT-4 (1999)*[32]	1208	Lepirudin 0.2 mg/kg bolus, then 0.5 mg/kg subcutaneously twice daily × 5 to 7 days; (ASA + SK)	Placebo bolus, then UFH 12 500 IU subcutaneously twice daily × 5 to 7 days; (ASA + SK)	No difference in death, MI, CVA, PCI, recurrent angina, intracranial haemorrhage, or major non-intracranial haemorrhage at 30 days.
HERO (1997)*[50]	412	Bivalirudin 0.125 or 0.250 mg/kg bolus, then 0.125 or 0.500 mg/kg/min infusion × up to 60 h; (given after SK + ASA)	UFH 5000 IU bolus, then 1000–1200 IU/h infusion × up to 69 h; (SK + ASA)	↑ incidence of TIMI 3 flow at 90–120 minutes and ↓ incidence of major haemorrhage at 35 days with low-dose bivalirudin; no difference in death, MI, or shock.
HERO-2 (2001)[52]	17 073	Bivalirudin 0.250 mg/kg bolus, then 0.250–0.500 mg/kg/h infusion × 48 h; (given before SK + ASA)	UFH 5000 IU bolus, then 800–1000 IU/h infusion × 48 h, target aPTT 50–75 sec; (SK + ASA)	↓ incidence of MI at 96 hours –30 days; ↑ incidence of moderate haemorrhage with bivalirudin, but no difference in the rate of intracranial haemorrhage.

Table 6.2 (Continued)

Trial	Patients	Treatment regimen	Control regimen	Clinical outcome
Univalent direct thrombin inhibitors				
ARGAMI-2 (1998)*∞ [59]	1201	Argatroban 60 or 120 mcg/kg bolus, then 2 or 4 mcg/kg/min infusion × 72 h; (ASA + SK or tPA)	UFH 5000 IU bolus, then 1000 IU/h infusion × 72 h; (ASA + SK or tPA)	No difference in death, MI, CHF, PCI, or CVA at 30 days.
MINT (1999) [61]	125	Argatroban 100 mcg/kg bolus, then 1 or 3 mcg/kg/min infusion × 48 to 72 h; (ASA + tPA)	UFH 70 IU/kg bolus, then 15 IU/kg/h infusion up to 1500 IU/h × 72 h, target aPTT 50–70 seconds; (ASA + tPA)	No difference in <TIMI 3 flow at 90 min or composite of death, MI, CHF, shock, PCI, CABG, recurrent angina, or major haemorrhage at 30 days.
ESCALAT (1999) [66]	245	Efegatran 0.05–0.2 mg/kg bolus, then 1 mg/kg/h infusion × 72 to 96 h; (SK)	UFH 5000 IU bolus, then 1000 IU/h infusion × 72 to 96 h; (tPA)	Trend, but no significant ↑ in the incidence of death, MI, <TIMI 3 flow or major haemorrhage with efegatran.
PRIME (2002) [67]	336	Efegatran 0.05–0.3 mg/kg bolus, then 0.3–1.2 mg/kg/h infusion × 72 to 96 h; (ASA + tPA)	UFH 5000 IU bolus, then 1000 IU/h infusion × 72 to 96 h; (ASA + tPA), target aPTT 60–85 sec	No difference in <TIMI 3 flow, death, MI at 96 h – discharge or 30 days; no difference in intracranial haemorrhage or major non-intracranial haemorrhage.

SK = streptokinase; tPA = tissue plasminogen activator; ASA = aspirin; MI = myocardial infarction; CHF = congestive heart failure; PCI = percutaneous coronary intervention; CVA = cerebral vascular accident; CABG = coronary artery bypass graft.
†Enrolled 12 142 patients with STEMI, NSTEMI, or UA; Subgroup analysis of 3289 STEMI patients shown above.
*Included in The Direct Thrombin Inhibitor Trialists' Collaborative Group meta-analysis.
∞Unpublished trial.

Clinical trials evaluating hirudin in ST-segment elevation myocardial infarction (STEMI)

Several clinical trials have evaluated hirudin as adjunct to thrombolysis in the setting of acute STEMI (Table 6.2). The Global Use of Strategies to Open Occluded Coronary Arteries (GUSTO-IIa) [27], Thrombolysis in Myocardial Infarction (TIMI-9A) [28], and Hirudin for Improvement of Thrombolysis (HIT-3) [29] trials randomised patients with acute ST-elevation myocardial infarction (STEMI) to hirudin or UFH as an adjunct to streptokinase (SK) or tissue-type plasminogen activator (tPA) therapy (Table 6.2). All three randomised, double-blind, phase II trials were stopped prematurely due to an unacceptably high rate of major bleeding in patients treated with hirudin [25]. GUSTO-IIa and HIT-3 also showed a trend toward more intracranial bleeding with hirudin [25]. The median aPTT was higher in patients with major bleeding complications than in those without major bleeding (106 vs. 76 seconds) [25]; therefore, the GUSTO-IIb [30], TIMI-9B [31], and HIT-4 [32] trials were re-started with lower doses of hirudin (Table 6.2). A lower dose of UFH was used as well, because more major bleeding was also seen in the UFH arm than in contemporary trials [25].

The GUSTO-IIb trial randomised 12 142 patients presenting within 12 h of STEMI, non-ST-segment elevation myocardial infarction (NSTEMI) or unstable angina (UA) to receive either desirudin or UFH (Table 6.2). Patients with STEMI also received thrombolytic therapy (SK or tPA) and aspirin. When compared to UFH, desirudin significantly reduced the overall risk of death or MI during the initial 24 h of treatment (1.3 and 2.1%; $P = 0.001$) [30]. This reduction became insignificant at 30 days (8.9 and 9.8%; odds ratio [OR] 0.89; 95% confidence interval [CI] 0.79–1.00; $P = 0.06$) [30]. The overall benefit of desirudin was not influenced by ST-segment status [30]. A retrospective subgroup analysis of 3289 patients with STEMI (2 274 receiving tPA and 1015 receiving SK) suggested that when used as adjunct to SK, desirudin significantly reduced the risk of death or MI at 30 days compared to UFH (9.1 and 14.9%; OR 0.57; 95% CI 0.38–0.87; $P = 0.009$) [33]. In contrast, desirudin was not superior to UFH in patients given tPA (10.3 and 10.5%; OR 0.98; 95% CI 0.74–1.30; $P = 0.91$) [33]. Overall, there was no significant difference in serious or life-threatening bleeding, including intracranial haemorrhage; however, desirudin was associated with a higher incidence of moderate bleeding compared with UFH (8.8 and 7.7%; $P = 0.03$) [30].

The TIMI-9B trial randomised 3002 patients presenting within 12 h of onset of STEMI, to lepirudin or UFH plus aspirin and either SK or tPA. There was no difference in the primary endpoint of death, recurrent MI, severe heart failure, or cardiogenic shock at 30 days between lepirudin and UFH (11.9 and 12.9%, respectively; OR 1.09; 95% CI 0.88–1.36; $P = \text{NS}$) [31]. Likewise, subgroup analyses revealed no significant differences between any patient populations [31]. These results were confounded by the fact that patients randomised to lepirudin were significantly more likely, at all charted time intervals, to have a therapeutic aPTT (cumulatively, $P = 0.0001$) [31]. Lepirudin and UFH had a similar rate of major haemorrhage (4.6 and 5.3%, respectively; $P = \text{NS}$), including intracranial haemorrhage (0.4 and 0.9%, respectively; $P = \text{NS}$) [31].

The HIT-4 trial randomised 1208 patients presenting within 6 h of STEMI to lepirudin or UFH bolus followed by subcutaneous injection as adjunct to aspirin and SK. This double-blind study resulted in no significant difference between the two groups in the composite endpoint of death, MI, CVA, rescue percutaneous transluminal colonary angioplasty (PTCA) or recurrent angina at 30 days (22.7 vs. 24.3%; $P = \text{NS}$) [32]. An angiographic substudy of 447 patients found TIMI 3 flow of the infarct-related artery in 40.7% of the lepirudin and in 33.5% of the heparin group ($P = 0.16$). There was also no significant difference in the incidence of intracranial haemorrhage (0.2 vs. 0.3%) or major non-intracranial haemorrhage (3.3 vs. 3.5%) [32].

Clinical trials evaluating hirudin in NSTEMI and UA

The GUSTO-IIb trial randomised 8011 patients with NSTEMI or UA to receive either desirudin (3994 patients) or standard-dose UFH (4017 patients). In this subgroup, there was no significant difference in the incidence of the primary endpoint of death or MI between desirudin and standard-dose UFH at 30 days (8.3 vs. 9.1% respectively; OR 0.90; 95% CI 0.78–1.06; $P = 0.22$). However, the patients treated with desirudin did show a trend towards increased severe haemorrhage (1.3 vs. 0.9% respectively; $P = 0.06$), including intracranial haemorrhage (0.2 vs. 0.02% respectively; $P = 0.06$) (Table 6.3) [30].

The Organisation to Assess Strategies for Ischaemic Syndromes (OASIS) trial was a pilot study that randomised 909 conservatively managed patients with NSTEMI or UA to a 72-h infusion of either low- or intermediate-dose lepirudin vs. standard-dose UFH (Table 6.3). Compared with UFH, intermediate-dose lepirudin produced a significant reduction in the primary endpoint of cardiovascular death, MI, or refractory angina at 7 days

Table 6.3 Clinical trials evaluating non-STEMI on unstable angina with direct thrombin inhibitors vs. unfractionated heparin therapy in non ST-segment elevation myocardial infarction and unstable angina

Trial (Date) Patients		Treatment regimen	Control regimen	Clinical outcome
Bivalent direct thrombin inhibitors				
GUSTO-IIb[†] (1996)* [30]	8011	Desirudin 0.1 mg/kg bolus, then 0.1 mg/kg/h infusion × 72 h.	UFH 5000 IU bolus, then 1000 IU/h infusion × 72 h, target aPTT 60–85 sec.	No difference in death or MI at 30 days; trend toward ↑ severe haemorrhage, including intracranial haemorrhage.
OASIS (1997)* [34]	909	Lepirudin 0.2–0.6 mg/kg bolus, then 0.1–0.2 mg/kg/h infusion × 72 h.	UFH 5000 IU bolus, then 1000–1200 IU/h infusion, target aPTT 60–100 sec	↓ death, MI, angina at 7 days with intermediate-dose lepirudin; no difference in major haemorrhage; ↑ minor bleeding with intermediate-dose hirudin.
OASIS-2 (1999)* [35]	10 141	Lepirudin 0.4 mg/kg bolus, then 0.15 mg/kg/h infusion × 72 h.	UFH 5000 IU bolus, then 15 IU/kg/h infusion, target aPTT 60–100 sec.	↓ cardiovascular death, new MI, or angina at 7 days, but ↑ major non-intracranial haemorrhage in the first 72 h with lepirudin.
Univalent direct thrombin inhibitors				
TRIM (1997)* [69]	1209	Inogatran 1.1–5.5 mg bolus, then 2.0–10.0 mg/h infusion × 72 h.	UFH 5000 IU bolus, then 1200 IU/h infusion.	↑ death, MI, refractory or recurrent angina with inogatran after 3-day infusion, which became insignificant at 7 days; no difference in major haemorrhage at 7 days.
Klootwijk *et al.* (1999)* [68]	432	Efegatran 0.1 or 0.3 mg/kg bolus, then 0.105–0.840 mg/kg/h infusion × 48 h.	UFH 5000 IU bolus, then 1000 IU/h infusion.	↑ minor haemorrhage and thrombophlebitis with efegatran; no difference in death, MI, angina, or revascularisation.

SK = streptokinase; tPA = tissue plasminogen activator, MI = myocardial infarction.
*Included in the Direct Thrombin Inhibitor Trialists' Collaborative Group meta-analysis.
[†]Enrolled 12 142 patients with STEMI, NSTEMI, or UA; Subgroup analysis of 8011 NSTEMI and UA patients shown above.

(6.5 vs. 3.0%; OR 0.57; 95% CI 0.32–1.02; $P = 0.047$) [34]. In addition, compared with standard-dose UFH, intermediate-dose lepirudin produced a significant reduction in the secondary composite endpoint of death, MI, or refractory/severe angina requiring revascularisation at 7 days (7.3 vs. 3.4%; OR 0.49; 95% CI 0.27–0.86; $P = 0.035$) [34]. There was no significant difference in major bleeding between low-dose lepirudin (0.7%) or intermediate-dose lepirudin (1.1%) and standard-dose UFH (1.1%); however, compared with UFH (10.5%), minor bleeding was significantly more frequent in patients treated with intermediate-dose (21.3%; $P = 0.001$) or low-dose lepirudin (16.2%; $P = 0.033$) [34].

The OASIS-2 trial randomised 10 141 patients with NSTEMI or UA to a 72-h infusion of either intermediate-dose lepirudin or standard-dose UFH (Table 6.3). There was a trend, but not statistically significant reduction in the primary composite endpoint of death or MI at 7 days favouring lepirudin over UFH (3.6 and 4.2%; OR 0.84; 95% CI 0.69–1.02; $P = 0.077$) and at 35 days (6.8 and 7.7%; OR 0.87; 95% CI 0.75–1.01; $P = 0.06$) [35]. Lepirudin produced a significant reduction in the secondary composite endpoint of cardiovascular death, new MI, or refractory angina at 7 days, compared with UFH (5.6 vs. 6.7%; OR 0.82; 95% CI 0.70–0.96; $P = 0.0125$) [35]. Major bleeding occurred more frequently with lepirudin than with heparin (1.2 and 0.7%; OR 1.73; 95% CI 1.13–2.63; $P = 0.01$), but the rate of life-threatening bleeding was 0.4% in both groups [35].

When the results of the OASIS and OASIS-2 trials are combined, lepirudin showed a significant reduction in the composite endpoint of cardiovascular death or MI at 7 days (3.5 vs. 4.3%; $P = 0.039$) and all-cause death or MI at 35 days when compared with heparin (6.7 vs. 7.7%; OR 0.86; 95% CI 0.74–0.99; $P = 0.04$) [35]. The results of these trials also show a significantly increased bleeding risk with lepirudin when compared to UFH.

Clinical trials evaluating hirudin as adjunct to percutaneous intervention

The Hirudin in a European Restenosis Prevention Trial vs. Heparin Treatment in PTCA (HELVETICA) trial randomised in a double-blind fashion 1141 patients scheduled for coronary angioplasty in the UA, to receive either desirudin or UFH given as a bolus, followed by infusion for 24 h (Table 6.3) [36]. This was followed by either subcutaneous desirudin or placebo for an additional 72 h in the desirudin group or by subcutaneous placebo injections for 72 h in the UFH group (Table 6.3) [36]. An additional bolus of placebo (in the desirudin group) or UFH (in the UFH group) could be given if the procedure lasted longer than 1 h [36]. At 30 weeks, there was no significant difference in the primary endpoint of death, non-fatal MI, coronary artery bypass grafting, bailout angioplasty with or without coronary stenting, or repeat PCI at the previous angioplasty site among the three groups (intravenous UFH group, 67.3%; intravenous desirudin group, 63.5% and intravenous desirudin followed by subcutaneous desirudin group, 68.0%; $P = $ NS) [36]. Compared with UFH, however, desirudin produced a significant reduction in recurrent cardiac events within 96 h of angioplasty (OR 0.61 in combined desirudin groups 95% CI 0.41–0.90; $P = 0.023$) [36]. The time-to-event curves converged thereafter, reflecting the development of restenosis for both groups [36]. On repeat angiography at 6 months, the mean change in luminal diameter of the dilated vessel was similar among the three groups [36]. There was no excess in major or minor bleeding seen with desirudin compared to UFH [36].

The GUSTO-IIb Angioplasty Substudy investigators randomised 1138 patients in the setting of acute STEMI to primary angioplasty or accelerated thrombolytic therapy. Compared with accelerated thrombolytic therapy, primary angioplasty was associated with a decreased occurrence of the primary endpoint of death, re-infarction or disabling stroke at 30 days (13.6 vs. 9.6%; OR 0.67; 95% CI 0.47–0.97; $P = 0.033$). Of the 565 patients randomised to primary angioplasty, there was a trend favouring desirudin, but no significant difference in the occurrence of the primary endpoint at 30 days between the 256 patients who received desirudin and the 247 patients who received standard-dose UFH (8.2 vs. 10.6% respectively; OR 0.76; 95% CI 0.42–1.39; $P = 0.37$) (Table 6.4) [71].

In the OASIS-2 trial, PCI was performed at the discretion of the investigator. Of the 117 patients who underwent PCI within the first 72 h, lepirudin was associated with a significantly lower incidence of death or MI at 96 h (6.4 vs. 21.4%, respectively; OR 0.30; 95% CI 0.10–0.88) and 35 days (6.4 vs. 22.9%; OR 0.25; 95% CI 0.07–0.86) when compared with UFH. In the UFH group, death or MI was significantly higher at 35 days in patients

Table 6.4 Clinical trials evaluating percutaneous intervention with adjunctive bivalent direct thrombin inhibitor vs. unfractionated heparin therapy

Name	Patients	Clinical setting	Treatment regimen	Control regimen	Clinical outcomes
Desirudin					
HELVETICA (1995)* [36]	1141	UA	Desirudin 40 mg bolus, then 0.2 mg/kg/h infusion for 24 h, then 40 mg or placebo twice daily (ASA)	UFH 10 000 IU bolus, then 15 IU/kg/h infusion for 24 h, then placebo twice daily (ASA).	↓ early cardiac events at 96 h with hirudin; no difference in event-free survival, major or minor haemorrhage at 30 weeks.
GUSTO-IIb (1997)[71]	565	STEMI	Desirudin 30 mg bolus; repeat to ACT of >350 sec (ASA)	UFH 3000 IU bolus; repeat to ACT of >350 sec (ASA)	Trend in death, re-infarction, or disabling stroke favouring desirudin at 30 days.
Lepirudin					
OASIS-2 (2002)[72]	117	NSTEMI and UA	Lepirudin 0.4 gm/kg bolus, then 0.15 mg/kg/h infusion (ASA).	UFH 5000 IU bolus, then 15 IU/kg/h infusion; to aPTT of 60–100 (ASA)	↓ death or MI at 96 h and 35 days with lepirudin; all 3 PCI-related major haemorrhages with lepirudin.
Bivalirudin					
BAT (1995)* [53]	4098	UA or post-infarction angina	Bivalirudin 1.0 mg/kg bolus, then 2.5 mg/kg/h for 4 h , then 2.0 mg/kg/h infusion (ASA).	UFH 175 IU/kg bolus, then 15 IU/kg/h infusion (ASA)	↓ major haemorrhage with bivalirudin; ↓ death, MI, vessel occlusion, or rapid deterioration in post-infarction subgroup, but not in total population.
CACHET (2000)[54]	268	UA	Bivalirudin 0.5–1.0 mg/kg bolus, then 1.75–2.5 mg/kg/h infusion with planned OR provisional abciximab therapy (ASA + clopidogrel).	UFH 70 IU/kg bolus, then repeat bolus to maintain ACT >200 and planned abciximab therapy (ASA + clopidogrel).	No difference in death, MI, revascularisation, or rate of major haemorrhage at 7 days.
REPLACE-1 (2001)[73]	1056	Urgent or elective PCI	Bivalirudin 0.75 mg/kg bolus, then 1.75 mg/kg/h infusion during procedure and provisional GPIIb/IIIa inhibition (ASA + clopidogrel).	UFH 70 IU/kg bolus, then repeat bolus to maintain ACT 200–300 and provisional GPIIb/IIIa inhibition (ASA + clopidogrel).	No difference in death, MI, or repeat revascularisation at 48 h; overall, no significant difference in the rate of major bleeding; ↓ major bleeding events with bivalirudin compared to UFH in patients not receiving GPIIb/IIIa inhibition.

Table 6.4 (continued)

REPLACE-2 (2003)[55]	6010	Urgent or elective PCI	Bivalirudin 0.75 mg/kg bolus, then 1.75 mg/kg/h infusion; use of provisional GPIIb/IIIa inhibitor (ASA + clopidogrel).	UFH 65 IU/kg bolus, then planned abciximab or eptifibatide therapy (ASA + clopidogrel).	Currently enrolling Bivalirudin non-inferior in terms of death, MI, urgent repeat revascularisation, or in-hospital major bleeding at 30 days; ↓ in-hospital major bleeding with bivalirudin; trend towards ↓ one-year, all-cause mortality with bivalirudin.
PROTECT-TIMI 30 (2004)[75]	857	NSTEMI and UA	Planned eptifibatide therapy, plus UFH 50 IU/kg bolus; target ACT >200 OR enoxaparin 0.5 mg/kg IV bolus (ASA + clopidogrel).	Bivalirudin 0.75 mg/kg bolus, then 1.75 mg/kg/h (ASA + clopidogrel).	Change in coronary flow reserve of open arteries after PCI favoured bivalirudin; TIMI minor bleeding and need for transfusion significantly ↓ with bivalirudin. Currently enrolling.
ACUITY[76]♦		NSTEMI and UA	Bivalirudin IV 0.1 mg/kg bolus followed by 0.25 mg/kg/h through angiography with increase in dose for PCI to 0.5 mg/kg bolus and increased infusion to 1.75 mg/kg/h for duration of PCI plus planned eptifibatide OR bivalirudin alone. (ASA + clopidogrel).	Enoxaparin 1 mg/kg SC given every 12 h, through angiography with adjustments for PCI (0.3 mg/kg IV bolus if last SC dose given ≥ 8 h) plus planned eptifibatide. (ASA + clopidogrel).	
HORIZONS*	3400	STEMI	Bivalirudin 0.75 mg/kg bolus, then 1.75 mg/kg/h infusion; use of provisional GPIIb/IIIa inhibitor (ASA + clopidogrel).	UFH 60 IU/kg bolus, then planned abciximab or eptifibatide therapy (ASA + clopidogrel).	Currently enrolling.

MI = myocardial infarction; UFH = unfractionated heparin; GPIIb/IIIa inhibitors = glycoprotein IIb-IIIa inhibitors; ASA = aspirin; PCI = percutaneous coronary intervention; SC = subcutaneous.
*Included in The Direct Thrombin Inhibitor Trialists' Collaborative Group meta-analysis.
†Enrolled patients with STEMI and NSTEMI.
♦Currently enrolling.

undergoing PCI compared with those managed conservatively (22.9 vs. 7.3% respectively; OR 3.14; $P < 0.001$). This PCI-related hazard was not observed in lepirudin-treated patients (6.4 vs. 6.8%; OR 0.94; $P = 1.0$); however, all three PCI-related major haemorrhages were in patients randomised to lepirudin (Table 6.4) [72].

Clinical trials evaluating hirudin in HIT and HITT

The Heparin-Associated Thrombocytopenia (HAT)-1 trial was a prospective, multicentre, historical control study of 82 HIT antibody-positive patients who received one of four intravenous lepirudin regimens based on diagnosis (HIT, $n = 18$; HITT, $n = 51$; HITT with thrombolysis, $n = 5$; HIT with cardiopulmonary bypass surgery, $n = 8$) [37]. The platelet counts rapidly increased by ≥30% or $>10^9/l$ in 88.7% of lepirudin-treated patients with HIT or HITT [37]. The overall incidence of the combined endpoint of death, amputation, or new thromboembolic complications was significantly reduced in lepirudin-treated patients compared with historical control patients by day 14 (9.1 vs. 32.8%, respectively; $P = 0.001$) [37]. The rate of major bleeding was similar in both groups [37].

In the HAT-2 trial, 112 HIT antibody-positive patients received one of three different lepirudin regimens, based on diagnosis (HIT, $n = 43$; HITT, $n = 65$; HITT with thrombolysis, $n = 4$). The platelet count normalised by day 10 in 69.1% of lepirudin-treated patients. At 5 weeks, the combined incidence of death, limb amputation, and/or new thromboembolic complications was lower in the lepirudin-treated group (30.9%; 95% CI 0.21–0.41) vs. the historical control group (52.1%; 95% CI 0.40–0.64). Bleeding occurred significantly more frequently, in the lepirudin group vs. the historical control group (44.6 vs. 27.2%, respectively; $P = 0.0001$). There was no difference in bleeding requiring transfusion (12.9 vs. 9.1%, respectively; $P = 0.23$). No intracranial bleeding was observed in the lepirudin group [38].

The HAT-3 trial was a prospective study of 98 HIT antibody-positive patients who received lepirudin therapy for a median of 14 days [39]. There was a relatively low incidence of new thrombosis in the lepirudin-treated group, when compared to the 75 historical controls from the HAT-1 and HAT-2 trial meta-analysis (6.1 vs. 27.2%, respectively). Likewise, the incidence of the composite endpoint of all-cause mortality, limb amputation or new thromboembolic event was lower in patients treated with lepirudin vs. historical controls (21.5 vs. 47.8%, respectively). The incidence of major bleeding, however, was relatively high in the lepirudin group vs. the control group (20.4 vs. 7.1%, respectively).

Current clinical role of hirudin in ACS and HIT

The TIMI-9B, HIT-4 and GUSTO-IIb trials suggest that hirudin provided no definite added benefit, but was probably at least as safe and effective as UFH when used as an adjunct to thrombolytic therapy in patients with acute STEMI (Table 6.2). The HELVETICA, GUSTO-IIb and OASIS-2 trials, however, suggest that hirudin, especially lepirudin, offers modest benefit over UFH as an adjunct to PCI in patients not receiving glycoprotein IIb/IIIa (GPIIb/IIIa) inhibitors (Table 6.4). In patients managed conservatively, the OASIS and OASIS-2 trials showed a significant reduction in cardiovascular death or MI as well, but also showed an increased bleeding risk with lepirudin when compared to UFH (Table 6.3).

As a result, lepirudin is not routinely used for ACS, but is approved by the Food and Drug Administration (FDA) as an anticoagulant in patients with HITT, in order to prevent further thromboembolic events (Table 6.1) [40, 41]. The American College of Cardiology/American Heart Association (ACC/AHA) clinical guidelines recommend the use of lepirudin as an alternative to UFH or LMWH in patients with HIT or HITT [42]. This recommendation is supported by the HAT-1 [37], HAT-2 [38] and HAT-3 [2] trials and post-marketing data which suggest that lepirudin therapy is safe and effective in the prevention

Table 6.5 Treatment of isolated HIT with lepirudin and argatroban

Study description	HIT-Ab Pos (%)[a]	Treatment duration (mean days)	New thrombosis[b]				Composite endpoint[b]				Major bleeding[c]		
			DTI (%)[c]	Control (%)[c]	RRR	P (%)	DTI (%)	Control (%)	RRR	P	DTI (%)	Control (%)	P
Lepirudin													
Meta-analysis, n = 111[d]	100	13.5	2.7	–	–	–	9.0	–	–	–	14.4	–	–
Post-marketing, n = 612	66	11.1	2.1	–	–	–	15.7[e]	–	–	–	5.9	–	–
Argatroban (139 controls)													
ARG-911 study, n = 160	50	5.3	8.1	23.0[f]	0.65	<0.001	25.6	38.8	0.34[g]	0.014	3.1	8.2	0.078
ARG-915, n = 189	–	5.1	5.8	23.0	0.75	<0.001	28.0	38.8	0.28[g]	0.04	5.3	8.6	0.27

DTI = direct thrombin inhibitor; HIT-Ab Pos (%) = percent testing positive for HIT antibodies; RRR = relative risk reduction.
[a]The heparin-induced platelet activation test was used in the lepirudin trials; for the argatroban studies, either the platelet aggregation test (using platelet aggregometry) or the serotonin release assay or no assay was performed.
[b]Composite endpoint defined as all-cause mortality, limb amputation, or new thrombosis (each patient could contribute only one event).
[c]Major bleeding defined as bleeding requiring transfusion (lepirudin meta-analysis) or as 'major bleeding likely caused by lepirudin' (lepirudin post-marketing study); or as overt bleeding associated with haemoglobin fall >2 g/l that led to transfusion of >2 units of blood or bleeding that was intracranial, retroperitoneal, or into a prosthetic joint (argatroban studies).
[d]Meta-analysis of patients with isolated HIT identified in three trials (HAT-1, HAT-2, and HAT-3); control group data not reported; although n = 111 is indicated, 17 of these patients had a history of HIT and had normal platelet counts when treated.
[e]Value may overestimate composite endpoint (not reported), as 15.7% represents the sum of the individual efficacy endpoints reported.
[f]Control group data from the ARG-915 study report is shown (the control groups were identical in the two argatroban studies, except that 8 of 147 controls from the ARG-911 study were not included in the ARG-915 study, as they had a history of HIT, rather than acute HIT).
[g]The RRR values shown were determined from the categorical analysis; using time-to-event analysis, somewhat greater RRR values (determined from the hazard ratios) were obtained: ARG-911, 0.40 (P = 0.01) and ARG-915, 0.36) (P = 0.018).

Reproduced with modifications and permission of Wakentin TE. *Thrombosis Research* 2003;110:76 [2].

Table 6.6   Treatment of HIIT by analysis of new thrombosis and major bleeding

Study description (n = number of patients receving DTI)	HIT-Ab Pos (%)[a]	Treatment duration (days)	New thrombosis DTI (%)[c]	New thrombosis Control (%)[c]	RRR	P (%)	Major bleeding[b] DTI (%)	Major bleeding[b] Control	P
Lepirudin (75 controls)									
Meta-analysis (HAT-1,2 studies), n = 113	100	13.3	10.1	27.2	0.63	0.005[d]	18.8	7.1	0.02
Third study (HAT-3), n = 98	100	14.0	6.1	–	0.78	<0.05[f]	20.4	–	<0.05[f]
Post-marketing, n = 496	77	12.1	5.2	–	0.81	<0.05[f]	5.4	–	NA
Argatroban (46 controls)									
First study (Arg-911), n = 144	65	5.9	19.4	34.8	0.44	0.044	11.1	2.2	0.077
Second study (Arg-915)[c], n = 229	NA	7.1	13.1	–	0.62	<0.001	6.1	–	0.48

DTI = direct thrombin inhibitor; HAT = heparin-associated thrombocytopaenia; NA = not applicable; RRR = relative risk reduction.

[a] The heparin-induced platelet activation test was used in the lepirudin trials; for the argatroban studies, either the platelet aggregation test (using platelet aggregometry) or the serotonin release assay or no assay was performed.

[b] Major bleeding defined in the lepirudin studies as that requiring blood transfusion and/or 'likely caused by lepirudin', and defined in the argatroban studies as overt bleeding associated with haemoglobin fall >2 g/l or transfusion of >2 units of blood or that was intracranial, retroperitoneal, or into a prosthetic joint.

[c] Categorical values and analysis shown for argatroban studies; in contrast, for lepirudin studies, values shown represent day 35 endpoints using time-to-event analysis.

[d] P-value determined by log-rank test (time-to-event analysis).

[e] RRR calculation performed using the control group data shown above.

[f] Statistical analysis not provided in the study abstract report, although it is apparent that the P-value would be significant.

Reproduced with modifications and permission of Wakentin TE. *Thrombosis Research* 2003;110:76 [2].

and treatment of thrombosis in patients with HIT or HITT (Tables 6.5 and 6.6) [39]. Currently, desirudin has no FDA-approved indications in ACS or HIT, but is approved as prophylaxis for deep venous thrombosis in patients undergoing elective hip replacement surgery (Table 6.1) [43–45]. Thus lepirudin is accepted as the preferred alternative anticoagulant among ACS patients with suspected HIT or HITT.

BIVALIRUDIN

Key pharmacological features of bivalirudin
Bivalirudin is a 20-amino acid, synthetic version of hirudin [25]. Like hirudin, it is a bivalent inhibitor, binding both the active and fibrin-binding sites of thrombin (Figure 6.2C). In contrast to hirudin, bivalirudin is slowly cleaved by thrombin, restoring active site function to the enzyme [25]. The cleaved molecule of bivalirudin remains bound to the fibrin-binding site; however, this is with a greatly reduced affinity for thrombin [4]. As a result, other substrates, such as fibrin, can compete for access to this cleaved bivalirudin-bound exosite [4]. Bivalirudin is degraded primarily by a combination of hepatic metabolism and proteolytic cleavage, with a small proportion being eliminated by renal mechanisms [46]. It has a half-life of 25 min in patients with normal renal function [25]. It can be used safely in patients with significant renal insufficiency [47]; however, the manufacturers of bivalirudin recommend renal dose adjustment based on creatinine clearance [48]. Bivalirudin is cleared approximately 25% by standard haemodialysis [48]. The anticoagulant effect of bivalirudin can be effectively monitored using the aPTT or ACT; both of which exhibit a dose-dependent linear prolongation (Table 6.1) [49].

Clinical trials evaluating bivalirudin in STEMI
The Hirulog Early Reperfusion/Occlusion (HERO) trial, a phase II, double-blind study, randomised 412 patients to either standard-dose UFH, low-dose bivalirudin, or high-dose bivalirudin administered after SK and aspirin (Table 6.2). The primary endpoint of TIMI 3 flow of the infarct-related artery at 90–120 min was achieved significantly less frequently in patients treated with heparin (35%; 95% CI 28–44%) when compared to patients treated with either low-dose bivalirudin (46%; 95% CI 38–55%; $P = 0.023$) or high-dose bivalirudin (48%; 95% CI 40–57%; $P = 0.03$) [50]. There was no significant difference in the incidence of death, cardiogenic shock or re-infarction between patients treated with UFH (17.9%), low-dose bivalirudin (14.7%) and high-dose bivalirudin (12.5%) at 35 days [50]. It was hypothesised that bivalirudin administered before thrombolytic therapy may have had greater efficacy, since thrombolysis is known to result in the exposure of tissue-bound thrombin, which could lead to further clot formation [51]. Major bleeding occurred significantly less often with low-dose bivalirudin vs. standard-dose UFH (14 vs. 27%; $P < 0.01$) [50], with a trend towards less bleeding with high-dose bivalirudin as well (19 vs. 27%; $P = 0.12$) [50].

The HERO-2 trial enrolled 17 073 patients in a randomised, double-blind fashion to evaluate whether high-dose bivalirudin was more effective when administered before SK (Table 6.2) [51]. The study demonstrated no difference between high-dose bivalirudin and standard-dose UFH in the primary endpoint of mortality at 30 days (10.8 vs. 10.9%; OR 0.99; CI 95% 0.90–1.09; $P = 0.85$) [52]; however, high-dose bivalirudin produced a significant reduction in the rate of re-infarction at 96 h (1.6 vs. 2.3%; OR 0.70; 95% CI 0.56–0.87; $P = 0.001$) [52]. In addition, reduction of the composite endpoint of death, re-infarction and disabling stroke favoured bivalirudin over UFH (12.7 vs. 13.8%; OR 0.91; 95% CI 0.83–1.00; $P = 0.049$) [52]. Furthermore, there was no significant difference in the incidence of intracranial haemorrhage between bivalirudin and UFH (0.6 vs. 0.4%; OR 1.48; 95% CI 0.94–2.32;

$P = 0.09$), but overall the incidence was substantially lower than that seen in contemporary trials of UFH used as adjunct to thrombolytic therapy [52]. Unfortunately, there was a significant increase in moderate bleeding with bivalirudin compared with UFH (1.4 vs. 1.1%; OR 1.32; 95% CI 1.0–1.74; $P = 0.05$) and a trend toward excessive severe bleeding (0.7 vs. 0.5%; OR 1.46; 95% CI 0.98–2.19; $P = 0.07$) [50]. This increase in bleeding rate was unexpected, since the first HERO trial suggested a trend toward a reduced risk of bleeding with high-dose bivalirudin [50] and may have resulted from higher aPTT levels at 12 and 24 h in patients receiving high-dose bivalirudin compared with standard-dose UFH [52].

Clinical trials evaluating bivalirudin as adjunct to percutaneous intervention

The Bivalirudin Angioplasty Trial (BAT) investigators randomised, in a double-blind fashion, 4098 patients undergoing coronary angioplasty for unstable angina or post-infarction angina to adjunctive bivalirudin vs. high-dose UFH (Table 6.3). There was no significant difference in the primary endpoint of in-hospital death, MI, abrupt vessel closure, or clinical deterioration of cardiac origin necessitating coronary intervention, intra-aortic balloon pump, or coronary artery bypass graft (CABG) between the total bivalirudin and UFH populations (11.8 vs. 12.9%, respectively; $P = 0.26$) [53]. However, in the prospectively stratified subgroup of 704 patients with post-infarction angina, bivalirudin produced a significantly decreased incidence of the primary endpoint (9.1 vs. 14.2%; $P = 0.04$) and bleeding rate (3.0 and 11.1%; $P < 0.001$) [53] compared to UFH. Moreover, in a re-analysis of the data designed to reflect more contemporary clinical endpoints, bivalirudin compared to UFH resulted in a significant reduction in the composite endpoint of death, myocardial infarction, or repeat revascularization 7 days (6.2% vs. 7.9% respectively; $P = 0.039$) and at 90 days (15.7% vs. 18.5%; $P = 0.01$) [78]. In the total study population there was also significantly less major bleeding in patients randomised to bivalirudin compared with UFH (3.8 and 9.8%; $P < 0.001$) [53].

The promising results of the BAT trial led to the Comparison of Abciximab Complications with Hirulog for Ischemic Events (CACHET) [54], the Randomised Evaluation in PCI Linking Bivalirudin to Reduced Clinical Events (REPLACE-1 & 2) [55], and the Randomized Trial To Evaluate the Relative Protection Against Post-PCI Microvascular Dysfunction and Post-PCI Ischaemia Among Anti-platelet and Anti-Thrombotic Agents (PROTECT-TIMI 30) trials to evaluate the use of bivalirudin in the modern era of percutaneous intervention with adjunctive GPIIb/IIIa inhibitors and stenting.

The CACHET trial was the first study to evaluate the feasibility of administering a DTI in conjunction with a GPIIb/IIIa inhibitor. The trial randomised 268 patients with UA, undergoing PCI with stenting to treatment with either one of three doses of bivalirudin or standard-dose UFH (Table 6.3). Clopidogrel was administered 2 or more hours before PCI and continued for at least 30 days thereafter. The first 60 patients enrolled in the trial were used to establish the safety of bivalirudin when administered with abciximab [54]. The remaining 208 patients were randomised to UFH with abciximab or to bivalirudin with or without abciximab [54]. The primary composite endpoint of death, MI or revascularisation at 7 days occurred infrequently among both the UFH and the three bivalirudin groups, with no suggestion of increased risk among patients receiving bivalirudin (0 vs. 4.7% vs. 0 vs. 6.4%; $P = $ NS) [54]. There was, however, a significant reduction in the composite endpoint of death, MI, revascularisation, or clinically important bleeding in bivalirudin and planned or provisional use of abciximab compared to UFH and abciximab at 7 days (3.3 vs. 10.6%; $P = 0.018$) [54].

The REPLACE-1 trial was a pilot study for REPLACE-2 and randomised 1056 patients undergoing elective or urgent PCI in an open-label fashion to bivalirudin (532 patients) or standard-dose UFH (524 patients). A GPIIb/IIIa inhibitor was used at the discretion of the investigator. Clopidogrel was encouraged to be given before the procedure. Stents were used in 85% of patients. The primary endpoint of death, MI or repeat revascularisation at

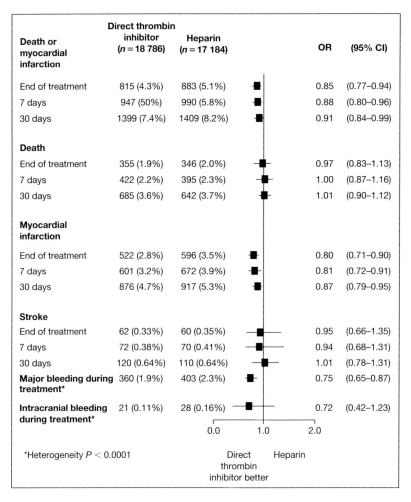

Figure 6.3 Meta-analysis of efficacy and safety of direct thrombin inhibitors relative to heparin. Horizontal lines represent 95% CI. Reproduced with modifications and permission of *Lancet* 2002; 359:296 [3].

48 h occurred in 5.6% of patients receiving bivalirudin, compared to 6.9% of patients receiving UFH (RRR 19%; $P = 0.40$). Overall, there was no significant difference in the rate of major bleeding between patients randomised to bivalirudin compared to those randomised to UFH (2.1 vs. 2.7%, respectively; $P = 0.52$). In the subset of 304 patients not receiving adjunctive GPIIb/IIIa inhibition, bivalirudin was associated with no major bleeding events compared to a 2.0% event rate in those receiving UFH (Table 6.4) [73].

REPLACE-2 was a phase III, randomised, double-blind, international trial of 6010 patients with UA undergoing angioplasty with stenting and compared bivalirudin plus provisional GPIIb/IIIa inhibitors with UFH plus planned GPIIb/IIIa inhibitors (Table 6.3). All patients received ASA, and more than 85% received clopidogrel. Patients with unprotected left main disease, those undergoing staged or repeated PCI within the month and those undergoing emergent PCI for acute MI were excluded from the trial [55]. There was no significant difference in the primary composite endpoint of death, MI, urgent repeat revascularisation or in-hospital major bleeding with bivalirudin plus provisional GPIIb/IIIa inhibitors

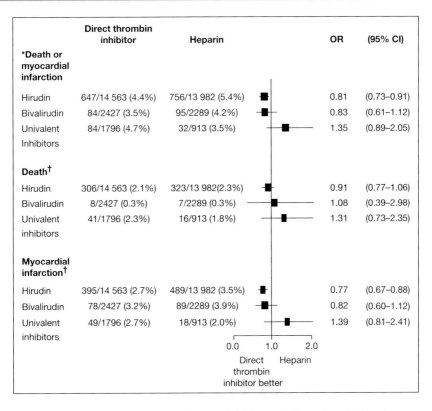

Figure 6.4 Meta-analysis of efficacy of direct thrombin inhibitors relative to heparin by subgroup according to agent. Horizontal lines represent 95% CI. Reproduced with modifications and permission of *Lancet* 2002; 359:299 [3].

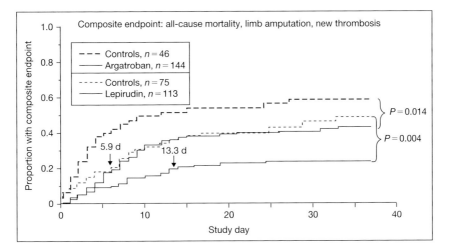

Figure 6.5 Therapeutic efficacy of lepirudin and argatroban (Arg-911 trial) compared with their respective historical controls. Therapeutic efficacy of lepirudin (meta-analysis of HAT1 and HAT2 studies) and argatroban (Arg-911 trial), compared with their respective historical controls, in patients with thrombosis complicating HIT. Reproduced with modifications and permission of Wakentin TE. *Thrombosis Research* 2003;110:78 [2].

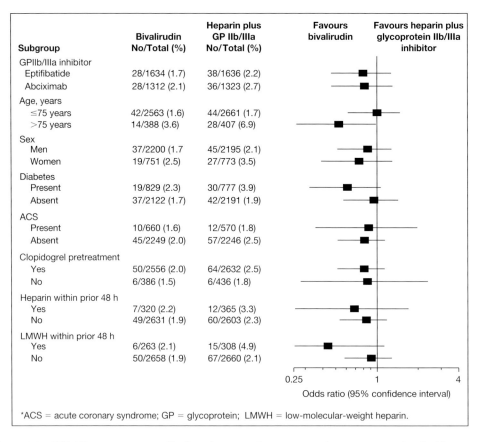

Subgroup	Bivalirudin No/Total (%)	Heparin plus GP IIb/IIIa No/Total (%)		
GPIIb/IIIa inhibitor				
Eptifibatide	28/1634 (1.7)	38/1636 (2.2)		
Abciximab	28/1312 (2.1)	36/1323 (2.7)		
Age, years				
≤75 years	42/2563 (1.6)	44/2661 (1.7)		
>75 years	14/388 (3.6)	28/407 (6.9)		
Sex				
Men	37/2200 (1.7	45/2195 (2.1)		
Women	19/751 (2.5)	27/773 (3.5)		
Diabetes				
Present	19/829 (2.3)	30/777 (3.9)		
Absent	37/2122 (1.7)	42/2191 (1.9)		
ACS				
Present	10/660 (1.6)	12/570 (1.8)		
Absent	45/2249 (2.0)	57/2246 (2.5)		
Clopidogrel pretreatment				
Yes	50/2556 (2.0)	64/2632 (2.5)		
No	6/386 (1.5)	6/436 (1.8)		
Heparin within prior 48 h				
Yes	7/320 (2.2)	12/365 (3.3)		
No	49/2631 (1.9)	60/2603 (2.3)		
LMWH within prior 48 h				
Yes	6/263 (2.1)	15/308 (4.9)		
No	50/2658 (1.9)	67/2660 (2.1)		

Odds ratio (95% confidence interval)

*ACS = acute coronary syndrome; GP = glycoprotein; LMWH = low-molecular-weight heparin.

Figure 6.6   REPLACE-2 one-year mortality by subgroup and treatment assignment*. Reproduced with modifications and permission of *JAMA* 2004; 292:696–703 [74].

compared with UFH plus planned GPIIb/IIIa inhibitors at 30 days (9.2 vs. 10.0%; OR 0.92; 95% CI 0.77–1.09; $P = 0.32$) [55]. Likewise, there was no significant difference in secondary composite endpoint of death, MI or urgent repeat revascularisation (7.6 vs. 7.1%; OR 0.92; 95% CI 0.90–1.32; $P = 0.40$) [55]. Prespecified statistical criteria for non-inferiority to UFH and a planned GPIIb/IIIa inhibitor were satisfied for both endpoints. In addition, there was a significant reduction of in-hospital major bleeding in the bivalirudin group compared with UFH plus a GPIIb/IIIa inhibitor (2.4 vs. 4.1%; $P < 0.001$) [55]. Furthermore, one-year, all-cause mortality consistently trended toward bivalirudin over UFH plus a GPIIb/IIIa inhibitor on the whole and in all prespecified subgroups (Figure 6.6) [74].

The PROTECT-TIMI 30 trial was an open-label, randomised trial to evaluate the efficacy of eptifibatide for 18–24 h in combination with either standard-dose UFH or LMWH, vs. bivalirudin (REPLACE-2 dosing) in patients undergoing PCI for NSTEMI or UA (Table 6.3). The prespecified primary endpoint of change in coronary flow reserve of open arteries after PCI favoured bivalirudin over eptifibatide plus either adjunctive UFH or LMWH (1.43 vs. 1.33; $P = 0.036$). The primary safety endpoint of TIMI major bleeding was low for both groups, but there was a trend toward less bleeding with bivalirudin (0.0 vs. 0.7%, respectively; $P = 0.308$). TIMI minor bleeding (0.4 vs. 2.5%, respectively; $P = 0.027$) and need for transfusion (0.4 vs. 4.4%, respectively; $P < 0.001$) were significantly less with bivalirudin [75].

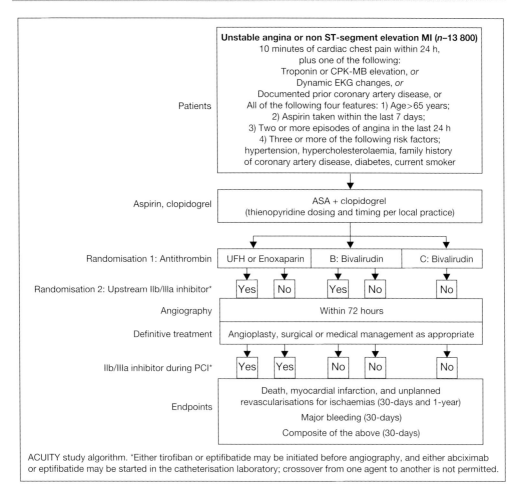

ACUITY study algorithm. *Either tirofiban or eptifibatide may be initiated before angiography, and either abciximab or eptifibatide may be started in the catheterisation laboratory; crossover from one agent to another is not permitted.

Figure 6.7 ACUITY study algorithm. Reproduced with modifications and permission of *AHJ* 2004; 148:764–775 [76].

The Randomised Comparison of Angiomax (bivalirudin) vs. Lovenox/Clexane (enoxaparin) in Patients Undergoing Early Invasive Management for Acute Coronary Syndromes Without ST-segment Elevation (ACUITY) trial is an ongoing, open-label, parallel group study projected to randomise 13 800 patients within 24 h of NSTEMI or UA to either (i) standard-dose UFH or LMWH plus planned GPIIb/IIIa inhibition *(upstream and/or during PCI)*, (ii) bivalirudin plus planned GPIIb/IIIa inhibition *(upstream and/or during PCI)* or (iii) bivalirudin alone (Table 6.3, Figure 6.7). The primary study endpoint is a composite of death, MI, unplanned revascularisation for ischaemia or major bleeding using the ACUITY scale at 30 days (Figure 6.7) [76].

The Harmonizing Outcomes with Revascularization and Stents in Acute Myocardial Infarction (HORIZONS AMI) trial is an ongoing 200 centre international trial in which 3400 patients with STEMI within 12 hours onset undergoing a primary angioplasty revascularization strategy are randomized to either (i) standard dose UFH plus planned GPIIb/IIIa inhibition with either abciximab or eptifibatide, or (ii) bivalirudin alone. The primary study end point is a composite of death, MI, unplanned revascularisation for ischaemia or major bleeding at 30 days. Patients are also randomized to drug-eluting stent implantation using the paclitaxel-eluting stent vs. bare metal stenting.

Clinical trials evaluating bivalirudin in HIT and HITT

The Anticoagulant Therapy with Bivalirudin to Assist in the Performance of PCI in Patients with Heparin-Induced Thrombocytopenia (ATBAT) trial was a prospective, multicentre, open-label study to evaluate the efficacy and safety of bivalirudin in 52 patients with HIT or HITT undergoing PCI [56]. High- or low-dose bivalirudin was given 5 min before PCI and continued for a median of 4 h. TIMI grade 3 flow and <50% stenosis was achieved in 98% of patients, and absence of death, emergency bypass surgery or Q-wave infarction was achieved in 96%. The primary endpoint of major bleeding within 48 h of discontinuation or until discharge occurred in only one patient who was on high-dose bivalirudin and underwent elective bypass surgery [56].

Current clinical role of bivalirudin in ACS and HIT

Taken together, the HERO and HERO-2 trials suggest that bivalirudin is at least as effective as UFH when used as an adjunct to thrombolytic therapy within 12 h of STEMI (Table 6.2); however, optimal dosing and the true risk of haemorrhage are unclear. Consequently, bivalirudin is not routinely used in this patient population. In addition, there is limited experience with bivalirudin as an anticoagulant in patients with HIT. Currently, bivalirudin has no FDA-approved or AHA/ACC-recommended indication for the treatment of HIT or HITT; although, limited experience from the ATBAT trial suggests that it is safe and effective in patients with HIT or HITT who are undergoing PCI.

There is a growing body of evidence from the BAT, CACHET, REPLACE- 1 & 2 and PROTECT-TIMI 30 trials that bivalirudin is more effective than UFH in patients with UA undergoing PCI and probably as effective as UFH plus GPIIb/IIIa inhibition, and carries a significantly decreased risk of bleeding complications (Table 6.4) [57]. As a result, bivalirudin in conjunction with aspirin is FDA-approved in patients with stable and unstable angina undergoing PCI (Table 6.1) [49] and is used routinely in some interventionalists' practices. Although the updated AHA/ACC guidelines are not currently available, the American College of Chest Physicians (ACCP) practice guidelines recommend bivalirudin over UFH in patients undergoing PCI who are not treated with a GPIIb/IIIa inhibitor (Grade 1A). In addition, ACCP guidelines recommend bivalirudin as an alternative to UFH as an adjunct to GPIIb/IIIa inhibitors during PCI in patients who are at low risk for complications (Grade 1B). Finally, in PCI patients who are at high risk for bleeding, bivalirudin is recommended over UFH as an adjunct to GPIIb/IIIa antagonists (Grade 1B) [77]. The ongoing ACUITY trial should offer more insight into the emerging role of bivalirudin as adjunct to PCI in ACS patients in the modern era of drug-eluting stents, clopidogrel and GPIIb/IIIa inhibition (Figure 6.7) [76]. Finally, the HORIZONS trial will determine if bivalirudin is as effective as UFH plus GPIIb/IIIa inhibition while also reducing major bleeding complications in patients with STEMI.

UNIVALENT DIRECT THROMBIN INHIBITORS

ARGATROBAN

Key pharmacological features of argatroban

Argatroban is a small, synthetic, univalent molecule that competitively and reversibly inhibits the active site of free and fibrin-bound thrombin (Figure 6.2B). It is metabolised in the liver via a process that generates three active intermediates [4]. As a result, the normal half-life of argatroban is 45 min [4], but may be prolonged in patients with significant hepatic dysfunction. No dose adjustment is needed for patients with renal insufficiency [25]. The anticoagulant effect of argatroban can be effectively monitored using aPTT [25]; however, the packet insert suggests monitoring the ACT. Both methods demonstrate dose-dependent linear prolongation [58]. Argatroban is the only univalent DTI approved for clinical use [25].

Clinical trials evaluating argatroban in STEMI

The Argatroban in Acute Myocardial Infarction (ARGAMI)-2 [59] trial was an unpublished [60], phase II, double-blind, randomised study of low- or high-dose argatroban vs. standard-dose UFH as an adjunct to either tPA or SK in acute STEMI (Table 6.2). The trial was originally designed to enrol 1200 patients; however, after enrolling 600 patients, the low-dose argatroban arm was terminated due to lack of efficacy [59]. Therefore, 1001 patients were randomised to receive either high-dose argatroban or standard-dose UFH, which resulted in no significant difference in the separate or combined clinical endpoints of total mortality, recurrent MI, pump failure, interventions for ischaemia or ischaemic stroke at 30 days [59]. There were trends toward a decreased incidence of major and minor bleeding, including intracranial haemorrhage with argatroban vs. UFH; however, it was not statistically significant [59].

The Myocardial Infarction with Novastan and tPA (MINT) trial was a single-blinded pilot study of 125 patients randomised to receive a 100 μg/kg bolus of argatroban, followed by low- or high-dose argatroban infusion vs. standard-dose UFH as an adjunct to tPA in the setting of acute STEMI (Table 6.2). There was a trend toward a decreased incidence of patients achieving the primary endpoint of TIMI 3 flow at 90 min with UFH (42.1%) vs. low-dose argatroban (56.8%; $P = 0.20$) or high-dose argatroban (58.7%; $P = 0.13$) [61]. There was also a trend towards a decreased incidence of minor and major haemorrhage in the high-dose argatroban group when compared to UFH (59 vs. 77.5%; $P = 0.07$) [61]. There was also no difference in the composite endpoint of death, MI, CHF, shock, PTCA, CABG or recurrent angina at 30 days between UFH, low-dose argatroban and high-dose argatroban (37.5 vs. 31.6 and 25.5%, respectively; $P = 0.23$); however, this should be interpreted with caution, because the study was not powered to demonstrate a clinical benefit [61].

Clinical trials evaluating argatroban as adjunct to percutaneous intervention

The ARG 216/310/311 Study investigators enrolled 91 patients with HIT and UA undergoing PCI while on argatroban [62]. The primary endpoints of satisfactory procedural outcome and adequate anticoagulation were achieved in 94.5 and 97.8%, respectively [63]. Only one patient experienced periprocedural major bleeding (1.1%) [62]. These rates were comparable to historical control patients on UFH undergoing PCI [62].

Clinical trials evaluating argatroban in HIT and HITT

The ARG 911 trial was a prospective study of 304 patients evaluating the efficacy and safety of argatroban as anticoagulant therapy in patients with HIT ($n = 160$) or HITT ($n = 144$) when compared with 193 historical control patients with HIT ($n = 147$) or HITT ($n = 46$) [64]. Argatroban was administered for an average of 6 days. Compared with control subjects, argatroban-treated patients had a significantly more rapid rise in platelet counts [64]. The incidence of the primary composite endpoint of all-cause death, all-cause amputation or new thrombosis was reduced significantly in argatroban-treated patients vs. historical control patients with HIT (25.6 vs. 38.8%, respectively; $P = 0.014$) and HITT (OR 0.57; 95% CI 0.36–0.90; $P = 0.014$ by time-to-event analysis) (Figure 6.5) [64]. Bleeding events were similar between groups [64].

The ARG 915 trial was a multicentre, non-randomised, prospective study of 418 patients with HIT ($n = 189$) or HITT ($n = 229$) that were administered intravenous argatroban for a mean of 5–7 days [65]. Comparisons were made with a historical control cohort of 185 patients (HIT, $n = 139$; HITT, $n = 46$). Platelet counts recovered more rapidly in argatroban-treated patients than in controls [65]. The primary composite endpoint of all-cause death, all-cause amputation or new thrombosis was significantly reduced in argatroban-treated patients with HIT vs. controls (28.0 vs. 38.8%; $P = 0.04$) and in argatroban-treated patients with HITT vs. controls (OR 0.56; 95% CI 0.36–0.87; $P = 0.008$ by time-to-event analysis) [65]. Argatroban therapy also significantly reduced new thrombosis in HIT (Table 6.5), HITT (Table 6.6), and death due to thrombosis in HITT [65]. Bleeding rates were similar between groups [65].

Clinical role of argatroban in ACS and HIT

The ARGAMI-2 [59] and MINT [61] trials suggest that argatroban has no benefit over, but is probably as safe as UFH when used as an adjunct to thrombolytic therapy in the setting of STEMI; however, these results should be interpreted with caution because the ARGAMI-2 trial was unpublished and the MINT trial was under-powered to show clinical benefit. The ARG 911 [64] and ARG 915 [65] trials found that, in patients with HIT or HITT, a combination of discontinuation of heparin and argatroban therapy significantly reduced the incidence of adverse outcomes in this high-risk population. Furthermore, the ARG 216/310/311 Study investigators found argatroban to be safe and effective in patients with HIT and UA undergoing PCI [62]. Currently, argatroban is not routinely used as an adjunct to thrombolytic therapy, but is FDA-approved as an anticoagulant in patients undergoing PCI who have or are at high risk for HIT (Table 6.1) [40, 41].

EFEGATRAN AND INOGATRAN

Key pharmacological features of efegatran and inogatran

Efegatran and inogatran are both synthetic, univalent, reversible inhibitors of the thrombin active site that have been evaluated in patients with ACS.

Clinical trials evaluating efegatran and inogatran in STEMI

The Efegatran Sulfate as an Adjunct to Streptokinase vs. Heparin as an Adjunct to Tissue Plasminogen Activator in Patients with Acute Myocardial Infarction (ESCALAT) trial [66] was a phase II, double-blind study of 245 patients with acute STEMI randomised within 12 h of onset of symptoms to either SK with one of four different doses of efegatran or tPA with standard-dose UFH (Table 6.2). The regimen of SK and efegatran was no more effective than the regimen of tPA and UFH in achieving TIMI 2 or 3 flow of the infarct-related artery at 90 min (73 vs. 79%, respectively; $P = $ NS) [66]. There was a trend toward an increased incidence of the composite endpoint of death, re-infarction or <TIMI 3 flow (47 vs. 32%, respectively; $P = 0.07$), as well as the composite endpoint of death, myocardial re-infarction, stroke or refractory angina (15 vs. 7%, respectively; $P = 0.14$) in the SK and efegatran group vs. the tPA and UFH group [66]. There was also a trend toward increased major bleeding with efegatran (23 vs. 11%, respectively; $P = 0.07$); although there were no intracranial haemorrhages [66].

The Promotion of Reperfusion in Myocardial Infarction Evolution (PRIME) trial was a single-blind study that randomised 336 patients receiving tPA within 12 h of an acute STEMI to one of five doses of efegatran vs. standard-dose UFH (Table 6.2). The lowest dose of efegatran was terminated early because of an unacceptably low incidence of TIMI 3 flow at 90 min (27%) and a high rate of rescue PCI (40%) [67]. In the remaining population, there was no significant difference between the combined efegatran group and the UFH group in the primary endpoint of death, re-infarction or <TIMI 3 flow by the time of discharge or at 30 days (53.8 vs. 53.0%; $P = 0.74$) [67]. However, the efegatran group did show a shorter time to recovery of the ST segments compared with the UFH group (107 vs. 154 min, respectively; $P = 0.025$) [67]. Additionally, there was no significant difference in the composite endpoint of death, stroke, re-infarction, new congestive heart failure or refractory ischaemia between groups (34%

intermediate-dose efagatran, 30% high-dose efegatran and 23% standard-dose UFH; $P = 0.231$ [67]. Furthermore, there was no significant difference in the combined incidence of intracranial haemorrhage, >5 g/dl decrease in haemoglobin or 15% decrease in haematocrit between the combined efegatran and UFH-treated groups (26 vs. 22%; $P = 0.72$) [67].

Clinical trials evaluating efegatran and inogatran in NSTEMI and UA

Klootwijk *et al.* [68] evaluated efegatran in the conservative management of NSTEMI and UA. The trial randomised 432 patients with NSTEMI or UA, in a single-blind fashion, to one of five different doses of efegatran or standard-dose UFH therapy for 48 h (Table 6.3). There was no significant difference in the composite endpoint of death, MI, recurrent angina, or ischaemia-driven revascularisation between any one of the five efegatran-treated groups and the UFH-treated group at 7 days (ranged from 52% to 71% with efegatran vs. 71% with UFH) or at 30 days (ranged from 73% to 81% with efegatran vs. 81% with UFH). The high incidence of patients reaching the composite endpoint was driven by recurrent angina, which was very frequent in all groups [68]. Patients receiving efegatran also experienced a significantly increased incidence of minor haemorrhage (ranged from 17 to 32% with efegatran vs. 11% with UFH; $P = 0.001$) and thrombophlebitis (ranged from 7.7 to 20% with efegatran; $P = 0.0001$) [68].

The Thrombin Inhibition in Myocardial Infarction (TRIM) trial evaluated inogatran in the conservative management of NSTEMI and UA (Table 6.3) [69]. The TRIM trial was a phase II study of 1209 patients with NSTEMI or UA that were randomised, in a double-blind fashion, to receive either low-, intermediate- or high-dose inogatran vs. standard-dose UFH therapy for 72 h (Table 6.3). There was a significant increase in the composite endpoint of death, MI, refractory angina or recurrence of angina at 3 days in the combined inogatran groups (39.4% with low-dose, 37.6% with intermediate-dose and 36.1% with high-dose inogatran vs. 29.5% with UFH; OR 1.48; 95% CI 1.12–1.96; $P = 0.01$), which became insignificant by the pre-determined primary endpoint of 7 days (45.7, 45.9, and 45.5 vs. 41.0%, respectively; OR 1.23; 95% CI 0.95–1.61; $P = NS$) [69]. In addition, the secondary endpoint of death or myocardial (re)infarction occurred in 3.6% of the low-dose, 2.0% of the intermediate-dose and 4.0% of the high-dose inogatran group vs. only 0.7% of the UFH group at 3 days (OR 5.02; 95% CI 1.19–21.17; $P < 0.05$) [69]. This difference became insignificant at 7 days (4.0, 4.3, and 6.7 vs. 2.6%, respectively; OR 1.99; 95% CI 0.93–4.27; $P = 0.10$) [69]. There was no significant difference in major bleeding at 7 days between the groups [69]. There were no intracerebral haemorrhages in this study [69]. Overall, the results of this study suggested that inogatran was inferior to UFH in the conservative management of NSTEMI and UA.

Clinical roles of efegatran and inogatran in ACS and HIT

Based on the ESCALAT [66] and PRIME [67] trials, the efficacy and safety of efegatran as an adjunct to thrombolytic therapy is questionable. In addition, the results of Klootwijk *et al.* [68] and TRIM suggested that the efficacy and safety of efegatran and inogatran are suboptimal in the conservative management of patients with NSTEMI or UA. Currently, neither agent is approved for clinical use [25].

THE DIRECT THROMBIN INHIBITOR TRIALISTS' COLLABORATIVE GROUP META-ANALYSIS

In 1999, the Direct Thrombin Inhibitor Trialists' Collaborative Group published a meta-analysis of TIMI-9B, GUSTO-IIb, HIT-4, HERO, ARGAMI-2, OASIS, OASIS-2, TRIM, Klootwijk *et. al.*, HELVETICA and BAT comparing lepirudin, desirudin, bivalirudin, argatroban, inogatran and efegatran with UFH in the treatment of ACS (Tables 6.2–6.4) [70]. These eleven randomised trials represented over 30 000 patients [3]. The meta-analysis excluded trials with less than 200 patients, those improperly randomised, uncontrolled, those with no data for death and MI or those using clinically irrelevant dose DTIs or UFH [3]. They found that the use of DTIs was associated with a lower risk of death and MI at the end of treatment (4.3 vs. 5.1%; OR 0.85; 95% CI 0.77–0.94; $P = 0.001$) and at 30 days (7.4 vs. 8.2%; OR 0.91; 95% CI 0.84–0.99; $P = 0.02$) (Figure 6.3) [3]. This was primarily due to a reduction in the incidence of recurrent MI, (2.8 vs. 3.5%; OR 0.80; 95% CI 0.71–0.90; $P = 0.001$), with no reduction in death (1.9 vs. 2.0%; OR 0.97; 95% CI 0.83–1.13; $P = 0.69$) (Figure 6.3) [3]. Subgroup analysis revealed that these benefits were seen with hirudin and bivalirudin, but not with the univalent DTIs (Figure 6.4) [3]. Overall, there was an increased risk of major bleeding with hirudin compared to UFH (2.3 vs. 1.9%; OR 0.75; 95% CI 0.65–0.87), but a decreased risk of major bleeding with bivalirudin compared to UFH (4.2 vs. 9.0%; OR 0.44; 95% CI 0.34–0.56) [3]. There was no excess in intracranial haemorrhage with the use of DTIs (0.11 vs. 0.16%; OR 0.72; 95% CI 0.42–1.23; $P = 0.27$) [3].

It is worth mentioning that this meta-analysis was done prior to the release of the HERO-2 trial (over 17 000 patients), which showed an increased risk of moderate bleeding and a trend toward excessive severe bleeding with bivalirudin compared with UFH [52]. Additionally, the meta-analysis represents patients treated prior to the modern era of PCI with adjunctive GPIIb/IIIa inhibitor and clopidogrel therapy, including the REPLACE-2 study that demonstrates reduced bleeding complications when bivalirudin is used as a procedural anticoagulant for PCI rather than UFH and GPIIb/IIIa inhibition.

SUMMARY

Direct thrombin inhibitors (DTI) have been extensively studied in cardiovascular diseases. They offer some unique properties that make them an attractive alternative to either UFH or LMWH. The initial studies with hirudin were somewhat tainted by (probably) too high dosages and their use in combination with fibrinolytic therapy. These early studies showed a consistent reduction in reinfarction both in the STEMI and non-STEMI populations. Furthermore, when PCI was applied, the benefit appeared to be exaggerated. These benefits were offset by higher major bleeding rates, although the absolute rates were low. Uniquely, bivalirudin has been shown to have a similar reduction in reinfarction, but at a cost of less major bleeding. This has been most pronounced in the PCI population, but on the other hand, when combined with streptokinase, higher bleeding rates were observed. The recent focus on prevention of bleeding in ACS and PCI has led to a resurgence of interest and use of DTIs. In particular, the use of bivalirudin has grown in the PCI population and the ACUITY trial will add considerably to our knowledge base with DTI.

One of the most important and frequently unrecognized side-effects of UFH and LMWH remains HIT with the associated risk of thrombosis and death. DTIs remain the first line therapy for this devastating condition. While DTIs are frequently under-used in this setting, lepirudin remains the first choice for patients with ACS. The overall benefits in reduction in death and non-fatal MI in ACS, coupled with the elegant studies in HIT, provide a solid foundation for its use. On the other hand, bivalirudin is an attractive approach for patients with suspected HIT who are planned to undergo elective PCI.

Anticoagulant therapy is a key component for reduction of re-thrombosis among patients with ACS. DTI offer some very important characteristics that may, ultimately, replace UFH or LMWH as better alternatives with comparable efficacy and fewer side-effects, including the feared consequences of HIT.

REFERENCES

1. Eikelboom JW, Anand SS, Malmberg K, Weitz JI, Ginsberg JS, Yusuf S. Unfractionated heparin and low-molecular-weight heparin in acute coronary syndrome without ST elevation: a meta-analysis. *Lancet* 2000; 355:1936–1942.
2. Warkentin TE. Management of heparin-induced thrombocytopenia: a critical comparison of lepirudin and argatroban. *Thromb Res* 2003; 110:73–82.
3. Direct thrombin inhibitors in acute coronary syndromes: principal results of a meta-analysis based on individual patients' data. *Lancet* 2002; 359:294–302.
4. Weitz JI, Crowther M. Direct thrombin inhibitors. *Thromb Res* 2002; 106:V275-V284.
5. Kumar R, Beguin S, Hemker HC. The effect of fibrin clots and clot-bound thrombin on the development of platelet procoagulant activity. *Thromb Haemost* 1995; 74:962–968.
6. Fareed J, Hoppensteadt D, Walenga J et al. Pharmacodynamic and pharmacokinetic properties of enoxaparin: implications for clinical practice. *Clin Pharmacokinet* 2003; 42:1043–1057.
7. Hirsh J. Heparin. *N Engl J Med* 1991; 324:1565–1574.
8. Spinler SA, Inverso SM, Cohen M, Goodman SG, Stringer KA, Antman EM. Safety and efficacy of unfractionated heparin versus enoxaparin in patients who are obese and patients with severe renal impairment: analysis from the ESSENCE and TIMI 11B studies. *Am Heart J* 2003; 146:33–41.
9. Bijsterveld NR, Moons AH, Meijers JC et al. Rebound thrombin generation after heparin therapy in unstable angina. A randomized comparison between unfractionated and low-molecular-weight heparin. *J Am Coll Cardiol* 2002; 39:811–817.
10. Bijsterveld NR, Peters RJ, Murphy SA, Bernink PJ, Tijssen JG, Cohen M. Recurrent cardiac ischemic events early after discontinuation of short-term heparin treatment in acute coronary syndromes: results from the Thrombolysis in Myocardial Infarction (TIMI) 11B and Efficacy and Safety of Subcutaneous Enoxaparin in Non-Q-Wave Coronary Events (ESSENCE) studies. *J Am Coll Cardiol* 2003; 42:2083–2089.
11. Liaw PC, Becker DL, Stafford AR, Fredenburgh JC, Weitz JI. Molecular basis for the susceptibility of fibrin-bound thrombin to inactivation by heparin cofactor ii in the presence of dermatan sulfate but not heparin. *J Biol Chem* 2001; 276:20959–20965.
12. Hogg PJ, Bock PE. Modulation of thrombin and heparin activities by fibrin. *Thromb Haemost* 1997; 77:424–433.
13. Weitz JI, Hudoba M, Massel D, Maraganore J, Hirsh J. Clot-bound thrombin is protected from inhibition by heparin-antithrombin III but is susceptible to inactivation by antithrombin III-independent inhibitors. *J Clin Invest* 1990; 86:385–391.
14. Weitz JI, Leslie B, Hudoba M. Thrombin binds to soluble fibrin degradation products where it is protected from inhibition by heparin-antithrombin but susceptible to inactivation by antithrombin-independent inhibitors. *Circulation* 1998; 97:544–552.
15. Bates SM, Weitz JI. Direct thrombin inhibitors for treatment of arterial thrombosis: potential differences between bivalirudin and hirudin. *Am J Cardiol* 1998; 82:12P-18P.
16. King DJ, Kelton JG. Heparin-associated thrombocytopenia. *Ann Intern Med* 1984; 100:535–540.
17. Laster J, Cikrit D, Walker N, Silver D. The heparin-induced thrombocytopenia syndrome: an update. *Surgery* 1987; 102:763–770.
18. Boshkov LK, Warkentin TE, Hayward CP, Andrew M, Kelton JG. Heparin-induced thrombocytopenia and thrombosis: clinical and laboratory studies. *Br J Haematol* 1993; 84:322–328.
19. Warkentin TE, Roberts RS, Hirsh J, Kelton JG. An improved definition of immune heparin-induced thrombocytopenia in postoperative orthopedic patients. *Arch Intern Med* 2003; 163:2518–2524.
20. Hirsh J, Heddle N, Kelton JG. Treatment of heparin-induced thrombocytopenia: a critical review. *Arch Intern Med* 2004; 164:361–369.
21. Markwardt F. The development of hirudin as an antithrombotic drug. *Thromb Res* 1994; 74:1–23.
22. Laboratories. B. RefludanTM [lepirduin (rDNA) for injection] prescribing information as of 10/2002.
23. Inc. AP. IprivaskTM [desirudin for injection] prescribing information.
24. Greinacher A, Lubenow N. Recombinant hirudin in clinical practice: focus on lepirudin. *Circulation* 2001; 103:1479–1484.
25. Eikelboom JW, French J. Management of patients with acute coronary syndromes: what is the clinical role of direct thrombin inhibitors? *Drugs* 2002; 62:1839–1852.
26. Toschi V, Lettino M, Gallo R, Badimon JJ, Chesebro JH. Biochemistry and biology of hirudin. *Coron Artery Dis* 1996; 7:420–428.

27.   Randomized trial of intravenous heparin versus recombinant hirudin for acute coronary syndromes. The Global Use of Strategies to Open Occluded Coronary Arteries (GUSTO) IIa Investigators. *Circulation* 1994; 90:1631–1637.

28.   Antman EM. Hirudin in acute myocardial infarction. Safety report from the Thrombolysis and Thrombin Inhibition in Myocardial Infarction (TIMI) 9A Trial. *Circulation* 1994; 90:1624–1630.

29.   Neuhaus KL, von Essen R, Tebbe U *et al*. Safety observations from the pilot phase of the randomized r-Hirudin for Improvement of Thrombolysis (HIT-III) study. A study of the Arbeitsgemeinschaft Leitender Kardiologischer Krankenhausarzte (ALKK). *Circulation* 1994; 90:1638–1642.

30.   A comparison of recombinant hirudin with heparin for the treatment of acute coronary syndromes. The Global Use of Strategies to Open Occluded Coronary Arteries (GUSTO) IIb investigators. *N Engl J Med* 1996; 335:775–782.

31.   Antman EM. Hirudin in acute myocardial infarction. Thrombolysis and Thrombin Inhibition in Myocardial Infarction (TIMI) 9B trial. *Circulation* 1996; 94:911–921.

32.   Neuhaus KL, Molhoek GP, Zeymer U *et al*. Recombinant hirudin (lepirudin) for the improvement of thrombolysis with streptokinase in patients with acute myocardial infarction: results of the HIT-4 trial. *J Am Coll Cardiol* 1999; 34:966–973.

33.   Metz BK, White HD, Granger CB *et al*. Randomized comparison of direct thrombin inhibition versus heparin in conjunction with fibrinolytic therapy for acute myocardial infarction: results from the GUSTO-IIb Trial. Global Use of Strategies to Open Occluded Coronary Arteries in Acute Coronary Syndromes (GUSTO-IIb) Investigators. *J Am Coll Cardiol* 1998; 31:1493–1498.

34.   Comparison of the effects of two doses of recombinant hirudin compared with heparin in patients with acute myocardial ischemia without ST elevation: a pilot study. Organization to Assess Strategies for Ischemic Syndromes (OASIS) Investigators. *Circulation* 1997; 96:769–777.

35.   Effects of recombinant hirudin (lepirudin) compared with heparin on death, myocardial infarction, refractory angina, and revascularisation procedures in patients with acute myocardial ischaemia without ST elevation: a randomized trial. Organisation to Assess Strategies for Ischemic Syndromes (OASIS-2) Investigators. *Lancet* 1999; 353:429–438.

36.   Serruys PW, Herrman JP, Simon R *et al*. A comparison of hirudin with heparin in the prevention of restenosis after coronary angioplasty. Helvetica Investigators. *N Engl J Med* 1995; 333:757–763.

37.   A clinical trial comparing primary coronary angioplasty with tissue plasminogen activator for acute myocardial infarction. GUSTO-IIb Angioplasty Substudy Investigators. *N Engl J Med* 1997; 336:1621–1628.

38.   Mehta SR, Eikelboom JW, Rupprecht HJ *et al*. Efficacy of hirudin in reducing cardiovascular events in patients with acute coronary syndrome undergoing early percutaneous coronary intervention. *Eur Heart J* 2002; 23:117–123.

39.   Greinacher A, Janssens U, Berg G *et al*. Lepirudin (recombinant hirudin) for parenteral anticoagulation in patients with heparin-induced thrombocytopenia. Heparin-Associated Thrombocytopenia Study (HAT) investigators. *Circulation* 1999; 100:587–593.

40.   Greinacher A, Volpel H, Janssens U *et al*. Recombinant hirudin (lepirudin) provides safe and effective anticoagulation in patients with heparin-induced thrombocytopenia: a prospective study. *Circulation* 1999; 99:73–80.

41.   Greinacher A. Lepirudin: a bivalent direct thrombin inhibitor for anticoagulation therapy. *Expert Rev Cardiovasc Ther* 2004; 2:339–357.

42.   McCrae KR, Bussel JB, Mannucci PM, Remuzzi G, Cines DB. Platelets: an update on diagnosis and management of thrombocytopenic disorders. *Hematology (Am Soc Hematol Educ Program)* 2001:282–305.

43.   Greinacher A. Treatment options for heparin-induced thrombocytopenia. *Am J Health Syst Pharm* 2003; 60(suppl 5):S12–S18.

44.   Brogan GX. Update on acute coronary syndromes and implications for therapy. *Expert Opin Investig Drugs* 2003; 12:1971–1983.

45.   Heiz-Valle C, de Maistre E, Commun N, Heck M, Lecompte T, Hoffman M. [Desirudin (Revasc) to prevent thromboembolic complications after hip or knee replacement surgery]. *Therapie* 2002; 57:34–38.

46.   Matheson AJ, Goa KL. Desirudin: a review of its use in the management of thrombotic disorders. *Drugs* 2000; 60:679–700.

47.   Eriksson BI, Dahl OE. Prevention of venous thromboembolism following orthopaedic surgery: clinical potential of direct thrombin inhibitors. *Drugs* 2004; 64:577–595.

48. Lincoff AM. Direct thrombin inhibitors for non-ST-segment elevation acute coronary syndromes: what, when, and where? *Am Heart J* 2003; 146:S23–S30.

49. Chew DP, Bhatt DL, Kimball W *et al.* Bivalirudin provides increasing benefit with decreasing renal function: a meta-analysis of randomized trials. *Am J Cardiol* 2003; 92:919–923.

50. Laboratories. BV. Angiomax® [bivalirudin for injection] prescribing information as of 11/2003. 2003.

51. Gladwell TD. Bivalirudin: a direct thrombin inhibitor. *Clin Ther* 2002; 24:38–58.

52. White HD, Aylward PE, Frey MJ *et al.* Randomized, double-blind comparison of hirulog versus heparin in patients receiving streptokinase and aspirin for acute myocardial infarction (HERO). Hirulog Early Reperfusion/Occlusion (HERO) Trial Investigators. *Circulation* 1997; 96:2155–2161.

53. White HD. Direct thrombin inhibition and thrombolytic therapy: rationale for the Hirulog and Early Reperfusion/Occlusion (HERO-2) trial. *Am J Cardiol* 1998; 82:57P–62P.

54. White H. Thrombin-specific anticoagulation with bivalirudin versus heparin in patients receiving fibrinolytic therapy for acute myocardial infarction: the HERO-2 randomised trial. *Lancet* 2001; 358:1855–1863.

55. Bittl JA, Strony J, Brinker JA *et al.* Treatment with bivalirudin (Hirulog) as compared with heparin during coronary angioplasty for unstable or postinfarction angina. Hirulog Angioplasty Study Investigators. *N Engl J Med* 1995; 333:764–769.

56. Lincoff AM, Kleiman NS, Kottke-Marchant K *et al.* Bivalirudin with planned or provisional abciximab versus low-dose heparin and abciximab during percutaneous coronary revascularization: results of the Comparison of Abciximab Complications with Hirulog for Ischemic Events Trial (CACHET). *Am Heart J* 2002; 143:847–853.

57. Comparison of bivalirudin versus heparin during percutaneous coronary intervention (the randomized evaluation of PCI linking angiomax to reduced clinical events trial). REPLACE-1 Investigators. *AJC* 2004; 93:1092–1096.

58. Lincoff AM, Bittl JA, Harrington RA *et al.* Bivalirudin and provisional glycoprotein IIb/IIIa blockade compared with heparin and planned glycoprotein IIb/IIIa blockade during percutaneous coronary intervention: REPLACE-2 randomized trial. *JAMA* 2003; 289:853–863.

59. Lincoff AM, Kleiman N, Kereiakes D *et al.* Long-term efficacy of bivalirudin and provisional glycoprotein IIb/IIIa blockade vs. heparin and planned glycoprotein IIb/IIIa blockade during percutaneous coronary revascularization. *JAMA* 2004; 292:696–703.

60. Gibson, presented at AHA Annual Scientific Sessions 2004.

61. Stone G, Bertrand M, Colombo A *et al.* Acute catheterization and urgent intervention triage strategy (ACUITY) trial: study design and rationale. *Am Heart J* 2004; 148:764–775.

62. Mahaffey KW, Lewis BE, Wildermann NM *et al.* The anticoagulant therapy with bivalirudin to assist in the performance of percutaneous coronary intervention in patients with heparin-induced thrombocytopenia (ATBAT) study: main results. *J Invasive Cardiol* 2003; 15:611–616.

63. Wittkowsky AK. The role of thrombin inhibition during percutaneous coronary intervention. *Pharmacotherapy* 2002; 22:97S-104S.

64. Popma JJ, Berger P, Ohman EM *et al.* Antithrombotic therapy during percutaneous coronary intervention. The seventh ACCP conference on antithrombotic and thrombolytic therapy. *Chest* 2004; 126:576S–599S.

65. Laboratories. A. Argatroban [argatroban injection] prescribing information as of 04/2002. 2002.

66. Alderman EL. Results from late-breaking clinical trials sessions at ACC '98. American College of Cardiology. *J Am Coll Cardiol* 1998; 32:1–7.

67. Jang IK. Direct thrombin inhibitors in acute coronary syndromes. *Lancet* 2002; 360:491–492; author reply 492.

68. Jang IK, Brown DF, Giugliano RP *et al.* A multicenter, randomized study of argatroban versus heparin as adjunct to tissue plasminogen activator (TPA) in acute myocardial infarction: myocardial infarction with novastan and TPA (MINT) study. *J Am Coll Cardiol* 1999; 33:1879–1885.

69. Lewis BE, Matthai WH, Jr, Cohen M, Moses JW, Hursting MJ, Leya F. Argatroban anticoagulation during percutaneous coronary intervention in patients with heparin-induced thrombocytopenia. *Catheter Cardiovasc Interv* 2002; 57:177–184.

70. Wykrzykowska JJ, Kathiresan S, Jang IK. Clinician update: direct thrombin inhibitors in acute coronary syndromes. *J Thromb Thrombolysis* 2003; 15:47–57.

71. Lewis BE, Wallis DE, Berkowitz SD *et al.* Argatroban anticoagulant therapy in patients with heparin-induced thrombocytopenia. *Circulation* 2001; 103:1838–1843.

72. Lewis BE, Wallis DE, Leya F, Hursting MJ, Kelton JG. Argatroban anticoagulation in patients with heparin-induced thrombocytopenia. *Arch Intern Med* 2003; 163:1849–1856.

73. Fung AY, Lorch G, Cambier PA *et al*. Efegatran sulfate as an adjunct to streptokinase versus heparin as an adjunct to tissue plasminogen activator in patients with acute myocardial infarction. ESCALAT Investigators. *Am Heart J* 1999; 138:696–704.

74. Multicenter, dose-ranging study of efegatran sulfate versus heparin with thrombolysis for acute myocardial infarction: The Promotion of Reperfusion in Myocardial Infarction Evolution (PRIME) trial. *Am Heart J* 2002; 143:95–105.

75. Klootwijk P, Lenderink T, Meij S *et al*. Anticoagulant properties, clinical efficacy and safety of efegatran, a direct thrombin inhibitor, in patients with unstable angina. *Eur Heart* J 1999; 20:1101–1111.

76. A low molecular weight, selective thrombin inhibitor, inogatran, vs heparin, in unstable coronary artery disease in 1209 patients. A double-blind, randomized, dose-finding study. Thrombin inhibition in Myocardial Ischaemia (TRIM) study group. *Eur Heart J* 1997; 18:1416–1425.

77. Direct thrombin inhibitors in acute coronary syndromes and during percutaneous coronary intervention: design of a meta-analysis based on individual patient data. Direct Thrombin Inhibitor Trialists' Collaborative Group. *Am Heart J* 2001; 141:E2.

78. Bittl JA, Chaitman BR, Feit F, Kimball W, Topol EJ, on behalf of the Bivalirudin Angioplasty Study Investigators. Bivalirudin versus heparin during coronary angioplasty for unstable or post-infarction angina: final report reanalysis of the Bivalirudin Angioplasty Study. *Am Heart J* 2001;142:952–959.

7

Direct thrombin inhibition during percutaneous coronary interventions

V. Kalahasti, A. M. Lincoff

INTRODUCTION

Antithrombin treatment is an important adjunct to oral and intravenous platelet inhibitors, during and after percutaneous coronary intervention (PCI) to prevent complications due to arterial thrombosis at the site of vessel injury. Unfractionated heparin (UFH) has been the principal anticoagulant used in unstable angina and PCI for more than two decades [1, 2]. UFH has significant limitations including the requirement of antithrombin as a cofactor, inability to bind to clot-bound thrombin [3–9], inhibition by plasma proteins and platelet factors resulting in unpredictable pharmacokinetics [10, 11]. Moreover, UFH has the potential to activate platelets, inducing thrombocytopaenia and leading to a thrombotic syndrome [12, 13]. The lack of predictable response to UFH may lead to excessive bleeding due to increased anticoagulation or to ischaemic complications secondary to inadequate anticoagulation[14, 15]. Direct thrombin inhibitors (DTI) have been developed to overcome these deficiencies associated with the use of UFH [16–19]. DTIs were initially studied in the early 1990s in the setting of acute coronary syndrome (ACS) and PCI. These earlier trials suggested that any advantage of DTIs over UFH with regard to suppression of ischaemic events was offset by increased bleeding complications. Those early data, however, were dominated by trials using hirudin, an irreversible DTI. More recent studies of bivalirudin, a synthetic reversible DTI, have shown more encouraging results and contemporary large randomised controlled trials have established the safety of DTIs in PCI. This chapter will briefly review indirect thrombin inhibitors and then examine the pharmacology, clinical trials of DTIs in PCI and the therapeutic applications of DTIs in PCI.

THROMBIN AND THROMBIN INHIBITORS

THROMBIN

Thrombin generation and degradation
Thrombin plays a pivotal role in thrombosis at sites of arterial injury through activation of platelets and fibrin generation. Thrombin has multiple actions that directly and indirectly influence clot formation [20, 21]. In addition to cleaving fibrinogen to fibrin, thrombin

Vidyasagar Kalahasti, Staff, Department of Cardiovascular Medicine, Cleveland Clinic Foundation, Cleveland, Ohio, USA.

A. Michael Lincoff, Professor of Medicine, Cleveland Clinic Lerner College of Medicine of Case Western Reserve University, Cleveland, Ohio, USA.

activates factor XIII, which leads to increased fibrin strand cross-linking and enhanced integrity of the fibrin clot. Thrombin activates factors V and VIII which amplify the coagulation cascade, leading to further thrombin generation [22]. Thrombin also stimulates platelet activation and aggregation which helps in the formation of a platelet-rich thrombus [23].

The mechanisms that limit thrombin generation and thereby restrict fibrin production are the two naturally occurring inhibitors of coagulation, antithrombin system and thrombomodulin–protein C–protein S system. Antithrombin binds to circulating thrombin and inactivates this molecule until the complex is subsequently cleared by the reticulo-endothelial system [24]. Thrombin also binds to thrombomodulin, which is found on intact endothelium. The thrombin–thrombomodulin complex activates protein C, a plasma protein which in conjunction with protein S, a cofactor, inhibits activated factor V and VIII and rapidly slows arterial clotting [25].

Thrombin structure
Thrombin has three distinct enzymatic sites, an active site, exosite 1 and exosite 2 (Figure 7.1) [26, 27] . The active site is the primary binding site and is responsible for most of the proteolytic activity of thrombin. Exosite 1 is responsible for the binding of substrates in proper orientation. Thrombin binds to fibrin *via* exosite 1 [28, 29]. Exosite 2 is the binding site for heparin. DTIs bind to either or both the active site or exosite 1.

Indirect thrombin inhibitors
UFH and low-molecular-weight heparins (LMWH) are indirect thrombin inhibitors, in that they require the presence of antithrombin. UFH forms a complex with antithrombin and rapidly inactivates thrombin and factor Xa [30]. This activity is primarily mediated by a unique pentasaccharide sequence with a high affinity for antithrombin and is randomly distributed along approximately one-third of the molecules present in pharmaceutical preparations of UFH [31]. This interaction between heparin and antithrombin induces a conformational change in antithrombin, which enhances the rate at which it inhibits thrombin and factor Xa by 1000-fold. Heparin must bind to both antithrombin and its substrate (thrombin or factor Xa) in order to inactivate these enzymes by forming a ternary complex. In order to anchor to thrombin, pentasaccharide-containing heparin chains of 18 or more saccharide units in length are required to form the ternary complex; factor Xa may be inhibited by heparin molecules of any length bound to antithrombin. Since most of the UFH chains are at least 18 saccharide units long, UFH preparations have similar activity against factor Xa and thrombin [31].

LMWHs are fragments of UFH and are produced by depolymerisation, whereby many of the higher weight molecular chains are eliminated. LMWHs retain the 'essential pentasaccharide' sequence, which is required for the binding to antithrombin. LMWHs produce their anticoagulant effect in a fashion similar to UFH by binding to antithrombin, but the increased proportion of molecules with chain lengths less than 18 saccharide units in LMWH leads to preferential inhibition of factor Xa over thrombin. Potential advantages of LMWH include ease of administration, improved bioavailability after subcutaneous injection, less binding to plasma proteins, greater Xa/IIa inhibition, and more predictable anticoagulant response [32]. Both UFH and LMWH lack the ability to inhibit thrombin bound to fibrin and fibrin degradation products. This is due to the fact that fibrin-bound thrombin is relatively protected from heparin–antithrombin complex because UFH binds concurrently to fibrin and to exosite 2 on thrombin, thereby bridging thrombin onto fibrin [28]. This ternary heparin–thrombin–fibrin complex increases the affinity of the thrombin–fibrin interaction. Allosteric modulation of thrombin's active site impairs the reactivity of antithrombin with thrombin [33, 34]. In addition, factor Xa bound to the surface of activated platelets is

Table 7.1 Mechanistic and pharmacokinetic comparison of different antithrombins

	UFH	LMWH	Lepirudin	Argatroban	Bivalirudin
Direct bivalent binding	No	No	Yes	No	Yes
Clearance mechanism	Both renal and non-renal	Mostly renal	Renal	Hepatic	Hepatic, renal and proteolysis
Inhibition of clot-bound thrombin	No	No	Yes	Yes	Yes
Half-life (min)	30–60 (dose-dependent)	270	60	53	25
Clinically relevant antibody formation	Yes	Possible	Yes	No	No

UFH = Unfractionated heparin; LMWH = low-molecular-weight heparin.
Adapted from Lincoff A. Direct thrombin inhibitors for non-ST-segment elevation acute coronary syndromes: What, when, and where? *Am Heart J* 2003;146:S23–S30.

also resistant to inactivation by heparin–antithrombin complex, and this protected factor Xa enhances the conversion of prothrombin to thrombin. Similar to UFH, longer chains of LMWH will also bridge thrombin to fibrin and heighten the thrombin–fibrin interaction. Thus, LMWHs are also relatively ineffective in inhibiting clot-bound thrombin.

Direct thrombin inhibitors
The principal DTIs include hirudin (or its recombinant forms lepirudin or desirudin), bivalirudin (known previously as hirulog) and argatroban. The US Food and Drug Administration (FDA) has approved hirudin and argatroban for use in patients with heparin-induced thrombocytopaenia (HIT), and bivalirudin for use in PCI. Other DTIs, like efegatran and inogatran have been studied in patients with acute coronary syndromes, but not in the setting of PCI [35, 36].

DTIs inhibit thrombin by blocking its active site and by preventing thrombin from interacting with its substrates [37]. They antagonise both clot-bound thrombin as well as fluid phase thrombin and are not affected by plasma proteins or platelet factor 4. They therefore theoretically have a more predictable anticoagulant response than UFH. DTIs can be classified according to structure and nature of their interaction with thrombin [38–40]. Hirudin and bivalirudin are bivalent inhibitors of thrombin, as they bind to both the active site and exosite 1. Univalent DTIs, such as argatroban and ximlegatran, target only the active catalytic site of thrombin.

The various properties of indirect and direct thrombin inhibitors are summarised in Table 7.1 and the binding properties are shown in Figure 7.1.

Hirudin
Hirudin is the prototypical direct thrombin inhibitor and is a 65-amino acid polypeptide. It was originally isolated from the salivary glands of the medicinal leech *Hirudo medicinalis* [41]. Hirudin is a bivalent inhibitor with the amino-terminal domain interacting with the active site of thrombin, and the acidic carboxy-terminal domain binding to exosite 1. Lepirudin and desirudin are recombinant forms of hirudin. Both the native and recombinant hirudins bind to thrombin with high affinity, forming an essentially irreversible 1:1 stoichiometric complex with thrombin [27]. Although recombinant forms of hirudin bind

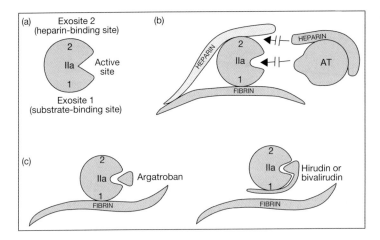

Figure 7.1 Thrombin (IIa) interactions with fibrin. (a) In addition to its active site, thrombin possesses two positively charged exosites; exosite 1 serves as the substrate-binding domain, whereas exosite 2 binds heparin. (b) Thrombin binds to fibrin via exosite 1. By simultaneously binding to fibrin and exosite 2 on thrombin, heparin bridges thrombin to fibrin, thereby heightening the apparent affinity of thrombin for fibrin and inducing conformational changes at the active site of the enzyme. Because exosite 2 is occupied by the heparin molecule bridging thrombin to fibrin, antithrombin (AT)-bound heparin cannot bind to thrombin to form a ternary heparin/thrombin/AT complex. The conformational changes in the active site of thrombin may also limit access of AT to the active site of the enzyme. (c) Active site-directed inhibitors, such as argatroban, inhibit fibrin-bound thrombin without displacing the enzyme from fibrin, whereas bivalent inhibitors, such as hirudin or bivalirudin, displace thrombin from fibrin during the inactivation process. Adapted from: Weitz JI and Buller HR. Direct thrombin inhibitors in acute coronary syndromes. *Circulation* 2002; 105:1004–1011.

thrombin with 10-fold lower affinity than hirudin, they remain potent inhibitors of thrombin. Hirudin has a plasma half-life of 40 min after intravenous administration and is eliminated primarily by renal excretion. Lepirudin and desirudin are also excreted through renal mechanisms and accumulate in patients with renal insufficiency [42].

Bivalirudin
Bivalirudin (originally termed hirulog) is a specific and reversible DTI [43]. It is a synthetic, 20-amino acid polypeptide with a chemical structure similar to hirudin. Its amino-terminal D-Phe-Pro-Arg-Pro domain, which interacts with the active site of thrombin, is linked *via* four glycine residues to a dodecapeptide analogue of the carboxy-terminal of hirudin [44]. Like hirudin, bivalirudin forms a 1:1 stoichiometric complex with thrombin. Once bound, however, the Arg-Pro bond at the amino terminal of bivalirudin is cleaved by thrombin, thereby restoring active site functions of thrombin. Bivalirudin has a half-life of 25 min and in contrast to hirudin, renal excretion is not the major route of bivalirudin clearance [45]. Instead, bivalirudin is mostly cleared by proteolytic cleavage. Accordingly, bivalirudin may be safer than hirudin, particularly in patients with renal impairment. Robson and colleagues described the pharmacokinetics of bivalirudin in patients with normal kidney function and in those with renal insufficiency. Patients with mild renal insufficiency have almost normal clearance of bivalirudin, but in patients with moderate and severe renal insufficiency the clearance is decreased by 45 and 68% respectively [46].

Activated clotting time (ACT), given its use in PCI, has been evaluated to monitor bivalirudin. Bivalirudin increased ACTs in a consistent and dose-dependent fashion [47, 48] but the rates of bleeding noted in clinical trials using bivalirudin showed poor correlation with ACT values. Cho and associates used a thrombin-inhibitor management point-of-care test based upon the ecarin clotting time (TIM-ECT) and compared with two other ACT methods (Hemochron ACT and CoaguChek Pro/DM ACT) to correlate with bivalirudin concentrations [49]. In their study both non-citrated and citrated TIM-ECT provided a more accurate assessment of the anticoagulation effect of bivalirudin ($r = 0.58$; $P < 0.0001$ and $r = 0.72$; $P < 0.0001$ respectively). In contrast, there was no correlation between Hemochron ACT ($r = 0.15$; $P = 0.267$) and bivalirudin concentration and only a weak correlation between the Pro/DM ACT ($r = 0.42$; $P = 0.002$) and bivalirudin concentration. In a related study, Casserly and colleagues found that both TIM-ECT and ACT demonstrated a strong correlation with bivalirudin concentration and TIM-ECT had a higher correlation and also appeared to more consistently reflect bivalirudin concentrations [50]. In another recent study by Cheneau and associates, ACT reflected bivalirudin concentrations consistently, but there was no correlation between ACT and clinical events, both bleeding and ischaemic events [51]. This lack of correlation may explain the poor relation between ACT values and bleeding rates in previous trials with bivalirudin. Therefore, the dose of bivalirudin should not be adjusted solely on the basis of ACT measurements.

Argatroban

Argatroban is a potent and competitive univalent inhibitor of thrombin [52]. It is a synthetically manufactured arginine derivative, which interacts only with the active site of thrombin and reversibly binds soluble and clot-bound thrombin. It is currently approved for use in patients with heparin-induced thrombocytopaenia. Argatroban is primarily metabolised in the liver *via* hydroxylation and aromatisation and the CYP3A4/5 microsomal system plays only a minor role. This may explain the lack of interaction between argatroban and the drugs metabolised by the CYP3A4/5 system. The half-life of argatroban is 45 min, which is prolonged in patients with hepatic dysfunction. Argatroban is primarily eliminated in the faeces [53].

CLINICAL TRIALS OF DIRECT THROMBIN INHIBITORS IN PCI

Hirudin

Hirudin has been compared with UFH in patients undergoing PCI in one dedicated randomised trial as well as in subgroups of patients in acute coronary syndromes studies. The Hirudin in a European Trial vs. Heparin in the Prevention of Restenosis after PTCA (HELVETICA) study randomised a total of 1141 patients with unstable angina undergoing PCI to either hirudin or UFH, [54] with a principal goal of determining if hirudin would decrease restenosis. This study compared three regimens: 1) intravenous UFH given as a bolus plus infusion for 24 h, followed by subcutaneous placebo for 3 days; 2) hirudin given as an intravenous bolus plus infusion for 24 h, followed by subcutaneous placebo for 3 days; and 3) hirudin given as an intravenous bolus plus infusion for 24 h, followed by subcutaneous hirudin for 3 days. The primary outcome was event-free survival at 7 months, defined as absence of death, myocardial infarction (MI), coronary artery bypass grafting (CABG), or repeat revascularisation at the previous angioplasty site. Secondary endpoints included early adverse cardiac events (within 96 h), bleeding, and angiographic measurements of coronary diameter at 6-month follow-up. At 7 months, event-free survival was similar in those given UFH, intravenous hirudin, or intravenous hirudin followed by subcutaneous hirudin (67.3, 63.5, and 68.0%, respectively; $P = $ NS). Likewise, on repeat angiography at 6 months, there was no significant difference in mean luminal diameter of the dilated vessel among the 3 groups. But, the hirudin group experienced a significant reduction in the early adverse ischaemic events at 96 h (OR 0.61; 95% CI 0.41 to 0.90; $P = 0.023$) that was preserved at 30 days. There was a non-significant trend

Table 7.2 Composite endpoints and bleeding complications in the three treatment arms of the HELVETICA study at 96 hours and at 30 weeks

	Heparin IV (n = 382)		Intravenous hirudin (n = 381)		Intravenous and subcutaneous hirudin (n = 378)	
	96 hours	30 weeks	96 hours	30 weeks	96 hours	30 weeks
Death, MI, revascularisation, bailout procedure* (%)	11	32.7	7.9	36.5	5.6	32
Major bleeding (%)		6.2		5.5		7.7
Minor bleeding (%)		11.3		13.1		15.1

*At 96 hours the combined relative risk in the hirudin groups as compared with the heparin group was 0.61 (95% confidence interval 0.41–0.90; $P = 0.023$)
Adapted from: Serruys PW, Herrman JP, Simon R et al. A comparison of hirudin with heparin in the prevention of restenosis after coronary angioplasty (HELVETICA trial). N Engl J Med 1995; 333:757–763.

for increased major bleeding with hirudin, mostly seen in the subcutaneous hirudin treatment arm, and a trend for a higher incidence of minor haemorrhagic events with hirudin compared with heparin (Table 7.2).

The early reduction in ischaemic complications seen in the HELVETICA study is consistent with that in other trials. Among 117 patients with unstable angina who underwent PCI in the OASIS-2 trial [55], hirudin produced a significant reduction in death or MI compared with UFH at 35 days (6.4 and 22.9%, respectively; OR 0.25; 95% CI 0.07 to 0.86). Likewise, in the GUSTO-IIB trial [56] in the patients who underwent early PCI during study drug infusion, the risk of MI was lower in the hirudin group than in those given UFH at 30 days (4.9 and 7.6%, respectively; $P = 0.04$) and 6 months (6.7 and 9.7%, respectively; $P = 0.04$). Censored analysis showed that hirudin was associated with a trend for a reduction in death or MI before PCI and within 48 h from the intervention.

Bivalirudin

Bivalirudin has been the most extensively studied DTI in PCI. The first large trial done in 1993 compared bivalirudin and UFH among 4098 patients undergoing coronary angioplasty for unstable or post-infarction angina. Patients were assigned to receive UFH (bolus of 175 U/kg followed by 15 U/kg/h infusion for 24 h with a goal activated clotting time of 350–400 seconds) or bivalirudin (1 mg/kg bolus followed by 2.5 mg/kg/h infusion for four hours and then 0.2 mg/kg/h infusion for 20 h) immediately before and following angioplasty [57]. In the initial report of that trial using an incomplete database, there was no significant difference in the incidence of primary endpoint of in-hospital death, MI, abrupt vessel closure or cardiac deterioration between the two treatment arms (11.4% for bivalirudin vs. 12.2% for UFH; $P = 0.44$). In a predefined subgroup of patients with post-infarction angina, bivalirudin was associated with a significant reduction in the primary endpoint (9.1 vs. 14.2% for UFH; $P = 0.04$). In the entire cohort, treatment with bivalirudin, as compared with UFH, was associated with marked decrease in major haemorrhage rates (3.8 and 9.8%, respectively; $P < 0.001$) as well as in the need for blood transfusions (3.7 and 8.6% respectively; $P < 0.001$). Bleeding rates in the subgroup with post-infarction angina were also significantly lower with bivalirudin than with heparin (3.0 and 11.1%, respectively; $P < 0.001$).

Table 7.3 Clinical ischaemic endpoints (death, MI, or revascularisation) in the *total cohort* at 7, 90 and 180 days in the final report reanalysis of the Bivalirudin Angioplasty Study

Days	Bivalirudin (n = 2161)	Heparin (n = 2151)	Odds ratio (95% CI)	P-value
7	135 (6.2%)	169 (7.9%)	0.78 (0.62–0.99)	0.039
90	340 (15.7%)	399 (18.5%)	0.82 (0.70–0.96)	0.012
180	496 (23%)	532 (24.7%)	0.90 (0.78–1.04)	0.153

Adapted from Bittl J, Chaitman B, Feit F et al. Bivalirudin vs. heparin during coronary angioplasty for unstable or postinfarction angina: final report reanalysis of the bivalirudin angioplasty study. *Am Heart J* 2001; 142:952–959.

Table 7.4 Clinical ischaemic endpoints (death, MI, or revascularisation) in the *postinfarction angina cohort* at 7, 90 and 180 days in the final report reanalysis of the Bivalirudin Angioplasty Study

Days	Bivalirudin (n = 369)	Heparin (n = 372)	Odds ratio (95% CI)	P-value
7	18 (4.9%)	37 (9.9%)	0.47 (0.26–0.84)	0.009
90	43 (11.7%)	75 (20.2%)	0.54 (0.36–0.81)	0.003
180	69 (18.7%)	94 (25.3%)	0.70 (0.49–1.00)	0.049

Adapted from Bittl J, Chaitman B, Feit F et al. Bivalirudin vs. heparin during coronary angioplasty for unstable or postinfarction angina: final report reanalysis of the bivalirudin angioplasty study. *Am Heart J* 2001; 142:952–959.

Despite these promising results with regard to bleeding, interest in development of bivalirudin waned until a re-analysis was undertaken on an intent-to-treat basis of the entire 4312-patient cohort [58]. In this re-analysis, a more contemporary endpoint of death, MI or revascularisation was used, complete follow-up data were obtained, and Kaplan-Meier time-to-event statistical analyses were performed. Using this more complete and appropriate analysis, bivalirudin was found to significantly reduce the combined endpoint of death, MI, or revascularisation in the entire cohort at 7 days compared to UFH (6.2 vs. 7.9% respectively; $P = 0.039$) an absolute risk reduction that was sustained at 90 days (15.7 vs. 18.5% respectively; $P = 0.012$) and 180 days (23 vs. 24.7% respectively; $P = 0.15$) (Tables 7.3 and 7.4). As with the initial published analysis, the incidence of clinically significant bleeding events was substantially less frequent with bivalirudin than with heparin (3.5% and 9.3%, respectively; $P < 0.001$) (Table 7.5). Based on this trial, bivalirudin appeared to be more effective than heparin in patients undergoing coronary angioplasty while at the same time producing a significant reduction in major bleeding. However, the findings of this trial were of unclear relevance to contemporary clinical practice, given that interventional procedures at that time did not routinely utilise stents nor include the use of thienopyridine and glycoprotein IIb/IIIa (GPIIb/IIIa) platelet inhibitors.

The Comparison of Abciximab Complications with Hirulog for Ischemic Events Trial (CACHET) was the first clinical investigation to use bivalirudin in conjunction with aspirin, clopidogrel, GPIIb/IIIa inhibitors, and stents in patients undergoing elective PCI [59]. CACHET was a single centre, open-label, randomised, controlled, pilot study conducted in three phases. In the initial phase (Phase A) of the study, 60 patients undergoing elective PCI

Table 7.5 Bleeding endpoints (major haemorrhage) in the total cohort by treatment group in the Bivalirudin Angioplasty Study

Days	Bivalirudin (n = 2161)	Heparin (n = 2151)	Odds ratio (95% CI)	P-value
7	76 (3.5%)	199 (9.3%)	0.34 (0.26–0.45)	<0.001
90	79 (3.7%)	199 (9.3%)	0.35 (0.27–0.46)	<0.001
180	79 (3.7%)	199 (9.3%)	0.35 (0.27–0.46)	<0.001

Adapted from Bittl J, Chaitman B, Feit F et al. Bivalirudin vs. heparin during coronary angioplasty for unstable or postinfarction angina: final report reanalysis of the bivalirudin angioplasty study. *Am Heart J* 2001; 142:952–959.

received abciximab and were randomised to receive either a bolus dose of bivalirudin of 1 mg/kg followed by a 2.5 mg/kg/h infusion for 4 h (the bivalirudin dose used in the prior large-scale angioplasty trial) or UFH given as 70 U/kg bolus (maximum 7000 U). After the safety of this regimen of high-dose bivalirudin with abciximab was established, the remaining two phases were carried out in 208 patients using two lower doses of bivalirudin (0.75 mg/kg bolus in Phase B or 0.5 mg/kg bolus in Phase C, with infusion of 1.75 mg/kg/h for the procedure duration) with provisional abciximab, compared again with UFH and planned abciximab. Criteria for provisional use of abciximab in the bivalirudin arms included coronary dissection, new or suspected thrombus formation, impaired or slow coronary flow, or other procedural complications, and this agent was administered provisionally in 24%. The composite clinical endpoint of death, MI, repeat revascularisation, or major bleeding by 7 days occurred in 3.3, 5.9, and 0% of the patients treated with bivalirudin in Phases A, B, and C respectively and in 10.6% of patients receiving UFH and abciximab ($P = 0.018$ for the pooled bivalirudin groups vs. the UFH group) (Figure 7.2). This small pilot trial suggested that bivalirudin could be safely used in conjunction with potent GPIIb/IIIa inhibitors.

Following the initial demonstration of potential safety and efficacy of bivalirudin with provisional GPIIb/IIIa inhibition in the CACHET study, a larger pilot experience with bivalirudin was obtained in the Randomised Evaluation in PCI Linking Angiomax to Reduced Clinical Events (REPLACE)-1 trial [60]. In this trial, 1056 patients undergoing elective or urgent PCI were randomised to receive UFH (70 U/kg) bolus or bivalirudin (0.75 mg/kg bolus, 1.75 mg/kg/h infusion during the procedure). GPIIb/IIIa inhibitor use was at the discretion of the physician and was used in 72% of patients; 85% of the patients received stents. The primary efficacy endpoint, a composite of death, MI, or repeat revascularisation by hospital discharge or within 48 h, occurred in 6.9% of patients in the heparin group and in 5.6% in the bivalirudin group ($P = 0.40$) (Table 7.6). Bivalirudin reduced major bleeding by 22% compared with heparin (2.1 vs. 2.7%, respectively; $P = 0.52$). Thus, CACHET and REPLACE-1 provided substantial preliminary evidence that bivalirudin can be used safely and effectively in the setting of potent antiplatelet agents and contemporary PCI.

The Randomised Evaluation in PCI Linking Angiomax to Reduced Clinical Events (REPLACE)-2 trial was a large, multicentre, double-blind, active-controlled trial [61]. This study was done to determine the efficacy of bivalirudin with GPIIb/IIIa inhibition used only on a provisional basis, compared with heparin plus planned GPIIb/IIIa blockade with regard to protection from periprocedural ischaemic and haemorrhagic complications during urgent or elective PCI. The objective was to determine if bivalirudin with provisional GPIIb/IIIa blockade was not inferior to heparin plus GPIIb/IIIa blockade and was superior to heparin alone.

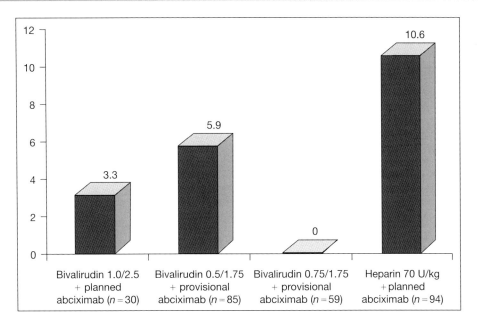

Figure 7.2 Incidence of quadruple endpoint of death, MI, revascularisation or in-hospital major bleeding in the four treatment arms of the CACHET pilot trial. Adapted from Lincoff A. Direct thrombin inhibitors for non-ST-segment elevation acute coronary syndromes: what, when, and where? *Am Heart J* 2003; 146:S23–S30.

Table 7.6   Efficacy endpoints by hospital discharge or at 48 hours in REPLACE–1 trial

	Heparin (n = 524)	*Bivalirudin (n = 532)*
Composite - death, MI, or revascularisation	36 (6.9%)	30 (5.6%)
Death	3 (0.6%)	0 (0%)
MI	27 (5.2%)	26 (4.9%)
Revascularisation	12 (2.3%)	8 (1.5%)

Adapted from: Lincoff A, Bittl J, Kleiman N *et al*: Comparison of bivalirudin vs. heparin during percutaneous coronary intervention (the Randomised Evaluation of PCI Linking Angiomax to Reduced Clinical Events [REPLACE]-1 trial). *Am J Cardiol* 2004; 93:1092–1096.

In this trial, 6010 patients were randomly assigned to receive intravenous bivalirudin (0.75 mg/kg bolus plus 1.75 mg/kg/h for the duration of PCI), with provisional GPIIb/IIIa inhibition vs. heparin (65 U/kg bolus) with planned GPIIb/IIIa inhibition (abciximab or eptifibatide at the operator's discretion). The primary 'quadruple' endpoint was a 30-day composite of death, MI, urgent revascularisation or in-hospital major bleeding. The secondary 'triple' endpoint was 30-day incidence of death, MI or urgent revascularisation. More than 85% of patients received clopidogrel prior to their intervention. Provisional GPIIb/IIIa inhibitor was required due to a procedural complication among 7.2% of patients in the bivalirudin arm; however, provisional drug (placebo) was also administered to 5.2% of patients in the heparin plus planned GPIIb/IIIa arm that were thought by the operator to require provisional

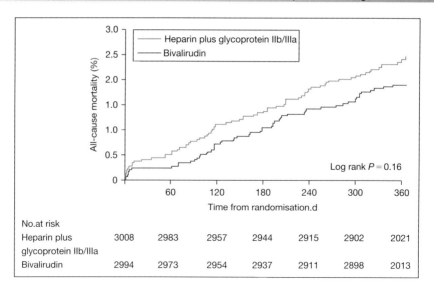

Figure 7.3 Cumulative incidence of one-year all-cause mortality in the REPLACE-2 trial. Adapted from Lincoff A, Kleiman N, Kereiakes D *et al*. Long-term efficacy of bivalirudin and provisional glycoprotein IIb/IIIa blockade vs. heparin and planned glycoprotein IIb/IIIa blockade during percutaneous coronary revascularisation. REPLACE-2 randomised trial. *JAMA* 2004; 292:696–703.

GPIIb/IIIa inhibition despite ongoing (blinded) GPIIb/IIIa therapy. The quadruple composite endpoint occurred in 9.2% of the patients in the bivalirudin group and 10.0% of patients in the heparin plus GPIIb/IIIa group ($P = 0.32$), and the triple composite endpoint occurred in 7.6% of patients in the bivalirudin arm vs. 7.1% of patients in the heparin arm ($P = 0.40$). Both endpoints satisfied formal prespecified statistical criteria for non-inferiority of bivalirudin compared with heparin plus GPIIb/IIIa blockade and superiority compared with heparin alone. In-hospital major bleeding was significantly lower among patients randomised to bivalirudin (2.4 vs. 4.1% with heparin plus GPIIb/IIIa inhibitor $P < 0.001$).

The long-term results of REPLACE-2 trial confirmed the efficacy of bivalirudin compared to UFH plus GPIIb/IIIa inhibition [62]. At 6 months, death occurred in 1.4% of patients in the heparin plus GPIIb/IIIa group and in 1.0% of patients in the bivalirudin group (hazard ratio [HR] 0.70; 95% CI 0.43–1.14; $P = 0.15$). MI occurred in 7.4 and 8.2% of patients, respectively (HR 1.12; 95% CI 0.93–1.34; $P = 0.24$) and repeat revascularisation was required in 11.4 and 12.1% of patients, respectively (HR 1.06; 95% CI 0.91–1.23; $P = 0.45$). At one year, death occurred in 2.46% patients in the heparin plus GPIIb/IIIa group and in 1.89% of patients treated with bivalirudin (HR 0.78; 95% CI 0.55–1.11; $P = 0.16$) (Figure 7.3). This trend toward mortality benefit at one year with bivalirudin, despite a small and non-significant excess risk of non-Q-wave MI at 30 days, was particularly seen in high-risk subgroups, including those older than 75 years, female and those with diabetes, and this effect was independent of GPIIb/IIIa inhibitor (abciximab or eptifibatide) or pre-treatment with a thienopyridine. The patients in this trial were also classified into tertiles of risk based on multivariate modelling by incorporating baseline factors that independently contribute to poor long-term outcome. In the patients in the highest tertile of risk, death occurred significantly less frequently with bivalirudin than with heparin plus GPIIb/IIIa inhibition (6.0 vs 3.9%, respectively; $P = 0.047$). Patients with acute coronary syndromes (ACS; unstable angina/ non-ST-segment elevation myocardial infarction) were largely excluded in the REPLACE-2 trial. This question about use of bivalirudin in patients with ACS undergoing early invasive strategy is currently being studied in ACUITY (Acute Catheterisation and Urgent Intervention Triage strategY), a large, multicentre randomised trial [63]. In ACUITY, approximately 13 800 patients with moderate to high-risk ACS undergoing an early invasive strategy will be enrolled internationally at 600 medical centres. Patients with ACS are randomly assigned to UFH or enoxaparin plus GPIIb/IIIa inhibition vs. bivalirudin plus GPIIb/IIIa inhibition vs. bivalirudin plus provisional GPIIb/IIIa inhibition. All patients undergo cardiac catheterisation within 72 h followed by percutaneous or surgical revascularisation when appropriate. In a second random assignment, patients assigned to receive GPIIb/IIIa inhibitors are subrandomised to upstream drug initiation vs. GPIIb/IIIa administration during angioplasty only. The primary study endpoint is the composite of death, MI, unplanned revascularisation for ischaemia, and major bleeding at 30 days. In a recent substudy of the REPLACE-2 trial, bivalirudin was shown to be safe and efficacious in patients with diabetes. There were no differences in clinical outcomes at 30 days in 1624 diabetic patients when compared to 4368 non-diabetic patients [64]. In fact, the one-year mortality was lower in the bivalirudin arm but did not reach statistical significance (2.3% vs. 3.9%). No differences were noted in the risk of major bleeding (3.0 vs. 3.3%) with less minor bleeding (12.6% vs. 24.4%; $P < 0.001$) in the bivalirudin arm in diabetic patients. Among patients with renal impairment in the REPLACE-2 trial, there was increased risk of ischaemic events (HR 1.45; 95% CI 1.13–1.88; $P = 0.004$), bleeding complications (HR 1.72; 95% CI 1.00–2.80; $P = 0.028$), and mortality at 12 months (HR 3.85; 95% CI 2.67–5.54; $P < 0.001$). Bivalirudin proved protection from ischaemic events that was comparable to–heparin and glycoprotein–inhibition in patients with renal impairment consistent with the results of the overall trial [65].

The combination of bivalirudin and GPIIb/IIIa inhibition was also studied in a non-randomised single centre series by Cho and colleagues [66]. In this study, 162 patients who received bivalirudin were compared to 172 patients who received heparin. At 30 days, the incidence of death, MI or revascularisation was 2.8% in the bivalirudin group compared to 4.2% in the heparin group ($P = 0.5$). In a separate analysis, the 30-day combined endpoint of death, MI and revascularisation was 4.0% in patients receiving heparin and a GPIIb/IIIa inhibitor (155 of 172 patients, 90.1%) compared to 3.7% in patients who received bivalirudin and GPIIb/IIIa inhibitor (132 of 162 patients, 86.8%) ($P = 0.78$). In multivariate analysis, bivalirudin use was associated with improved outcome at 120 days (odds ratio 0.33; 95% CI 0.13–0.85). Bleeding rates were similar between the two groups (4.3% for bivalirudin and 6.4% for heparin) with a trend toward more blood transfusions in the heparin group. This study was one of the first 'real world' experiences using bivalirudin in a contemporary interventional practice incorporating the use of stents, thienopyridines and GPIIb/IIIa inhibitors.

Gurm and colleagues also analysed bivalirudin in the 'real world' setting in a single centre registry study [67]. In this study, 6996 patients who underwent PCI were analysed to compare the outcomes with bivalirudin and heparin. Bivalirudin was used in 1070 patients, heparin alone in 801 patients, and heparin plus GPIIb/IIIa inhibitors in 5125 remaining patients. In this study, the incidence of bleeding (blood transfusion rate 1.7 vs. 4.3%; $P < 0.001$) and periprocedural MI (CK-MB > 5X ULN 2.7 vs. 4.3%; $P = 0.016$) were significantly lower in patients treated with bivalirudin. There was no difference in the unadjusted or propensity-adjusted long-term survival. This is another study that validates the findings of REPLACE-2.

Patients with acute ST-elevation myocardial infarction (STEMI) were also excluded in randomised trials of bivalirudin. In a recent study, 91 consecutive patients with STEMI from a single centre were treated with bivalirudin as a sole anticoagulant [68]. Patients with STEMI <24 h old underwent PCI with or without stent placement and bivalirudin was administered as a bolus dose (0.75 mg/kg) followed by infusion (1.75 mg/kg/h) for the duration of the procedure. The primary endpoints were death, clinical evidence of re-infarction, subacute thrombosis, or disabling stroke at 30 days. This series included a substantial number of patients with high-risk characteristics known to predict adverse outcomes, including female, diabetes or patients with history of prior MI and with cardiogenic shock. More than 60% of patients received balloons and stents with 97.8% of patients achieving

TIMI 3 flow. GPIIb/IIIa inhibitors (abciximab) were used in only two of the patients secondary to poor TIMI flow. Three patients died (3.3%) in this cohort of patients with no reports of recurrent ischaemia, stroke, subacute thrombosis, bleeding and transfusion. This study is not randomised and only a retrospective evaluation without a control group, but suggests that bivalirudin may be an attractive alternative to use of heparin and GPIIb/IIIa inhibitors. Indeed, this issue is currently being studied in a large, phase IIIb study evaluating the safety and efficacy of bivalirudin in patients undergoing primary PCI for STEMI (BIAMI trial). Patients with STEMI <12 h duration will be enrolled and treated with clopidogrel plus bivalirudin 0.75 mg/kg IV bolus followed by 1.75 mg/kg/hr for the duration of the PCI procedure. GPIIb/IIIa inhibitors will be used only for bailout. The primary safety endpoint is the frequency of major and minor bleeding and thrombocytopaenia. The primary efficacy endpoint is the composite of death, re-infarction, ischaemic target vessel revascularisation and stroke at 30 days and 6 months.

Bivalirudin has also been used recently in conjunction with drug-eluting stents (DES) and reported in a series of patients [69]. In this study, 323 patients who received bivalirudin as a single antithrombotic regimen during PCI with DES were compared to 352 patients who received heparin alone. Few patients received GPIIb/IIIa inhibitors and most of these patients were in the heparin group. The major in-hospital clinical outcomes including death, MI, and repeat revascularisation were similar between the two groups as well as the bleeding and vascular complications. This was the first study to show the safety of bivalirudin administration for patients who undergo PCI with DES. Further studies are needed to assess the role of bivalirudin as a sole agent for use with DES.

Bivalirudin thus far is the most extensively studied DTI in PCI. REPLACE-2 is the definitive trial that demonstrated the safety and effectiveness of this agent with provisional GPIIb/IIIa blockade in the era of contemporary interventional cardiology practice. Both the short- and long-term results of bivalirudin favour the usefulness of this agent as a replacement for heparin during PCI. The principal advantages of bivalirudin are decreased rates of bleeding and convenience of short infusions during the procedure. Bivalirudin is also more cost-effective than a combination of heparin plus GPIIb/IIIa inhibition, and would be reasonably cost-effective compared with heparin as well. The cost-effectiveness of bivalirudin with provisional GPIIb/IIIa inhibition compared to heparin plus routine GPIIb/IIIa inhibition was analysed recently [70]. The in-hospital and 30-day costs are reduced by $405 (95% CI $37 to $773) and $374 (95% CI $61 to $688) per patient with bivalirudin as compared to heparin plus routine GPIIb/IIIa administration. The hospital costs were also decreased primarily due to reductions in major bleeding (cost savings = $107/patient), minor bleeding ($52/patient), and thrombocytopaenia ($47/patient). Although bivalirudin is approved by the Food and Drug Administration (FDA) for use in elective PCI, it has not been studied in a systematic fashion in the setting of primary PCI for STEMI and as part of an early invasive strategy in ACS (unstable angina and NSTEMI) and the ongoing trials discussed above should shed more light on the appropriate role of this agent in those situations. These trials may also give us important information about bivalirudin's effectiveness with DES.

Bivalirudin should be the anticoagulant of choice in all low-risk patients undergoing PCI as an alternative to heparin plus GPIIb/IIIa inhibitors. Also, for patients undergoing PCI who are not treated with GPIIb/IIIa inhibitors, bivalirudin is favoured over heparin. Bivalirudin is also particularly useful in certain specific patient groups like the elderly, patients with renal insufficiency and patients with thrombocytopaenia who may be at higher risk for bleeding complications during PCI [71].

Argatroban

There are no large randomised controlled trials assessing the use of argatroban during PCI. There have been case reports, which have shown the feasibility of anticoagulation with argatroban during PCI in patients with heparin-induced thrombocytopaenia (HIT). In a series by

Lewis *et al.* argatroban was used as an anticoagulant in 91 HIT patients who had 112 PCI procedures [72]. Argatroban was given as 350 µg/kg initial bolus followed by 25 mcg/kg/min infusion, adjusted to achieve an ACT of 300–450 sec. Favourable outcomes were observed and most patients achieved adequate anticoagulation with argatroban. There were few adverse events reported with the use of this agent. Further studies are awaited to establish the role of argatroban as an alternative anticoagulant in PCI for patients without HIT.

SUMMARY

Thrombin plays a central role in thrombus formation and activation of platelets. Until recently, UFH has been the gold standard antithrombin used in PCI. DTIs have undergone widespread recent evaluation in the setting of PCI. Bivalirudin, is the most extensively studied and its safety and efficacy has now been very well established in conjunction with potent antiplatelet regimens and contemporary PCI with the use of stents. Bivalirudin should be considered as a very attractive alternative to heparin and routine GPIIb/IIIa blockade. Ongoing randomised controlled trials should clarify the usefulness of bivalirudin in the setting of primary PCI for STEMI and as part of an early invasive strategy in the treatment of ACS. Further studies are also needed to assess the role of new oral DTIs in the setting of PCI.

REFERENCES

1. Theroux P *et al.* Aspirin, heparin, or both to treat acute unstable angina. *N Engl J Med* 1988; 319:1105–1111.
2. Chesebro JH, Badimon L, Fuster V. Importance of antithrombin therapy during coronary angioplasty. *J Am Coll Cardiol* 1991; 17(6 suppl B):96B–100B.
3. Teitel JM, Rosenberg RD. Protection of factor Xa from neutralization by the heparin-antithrombin complex. *J Clin Invest* 1983; 71:1383–1391.
4. Pieters J *et al.* Inhibition of factor IXa and factor Xa by antithrombin III/heparin during factor X activation. *J Biol Chem* 1988; 263:15313–15318.
5. Hogg PJ, Jackson CM. Fibrin monomer protects thrombin from inactivation by heparin-antithrombin III: implications for heparin efficacy. *Proc Natl Acad Sci USA* 1989; 86:3619–3623.
6. Weitz JI *et al.* Clot-bound thrombin is protected from inhibition by heparin-antithrombin III but is susceptible to inactivation by antithrombin III-independent inhibitors. *J Clin Invest* 1990; 86:385–391.
7. Young E *et al.* Heparin binding to plasma proteins, an important mechanism for heparin resistance. *Thromb Haemost* 1992; 67:639–643.
8. Weitz JI, Leslie B, Hudoba M. Thrombin binds to soluble fibrin degradation products where it is protected from inhibition by heparin-antithrombin but susceptible to inactivation by antithrombin-independent inhibitors. *Circulation* 1998; 97:544–552.
9. Bar-Shavit R, Eldor A, Vlodavsky I. Binding of thrombin to subendothelial extracellular matrix. Protection and expression of functional properties. *J Clin Invest* 1989; 84:1096–1104.
10. Hirsh J *et al.* Heparin and low-molecular-weight heparin: mechanisms of action, pharmacokinetics, dosing, monitoring, efficacy, and safety. *Chest* 2001; 119(suppl 1):64S–94S.
11. Hirsh J *et al.* Mechanism of action and pharmacology of unfractionated heparin. *Arterioscler Thromb Vasc Biol* 2001; 21:1094–1096.
12. Warkentin TE *et al.* Heparin-induced thrombocytopenia in patients treated with low-molecular-weight heparin or unfractionated heparin. *N Engl J Med* 1995; 332:1330–1335.
13. Aster RH. Heparin-induced thrombocytopenia and thrombosis. *N Engl J Med* 1995; 332:1374–1376.
14. Morabia A. Heparin doses and major bleedings. *Lancet* 1986; 1:1278–1279.
15. Anand S *et al.* The relation between the activated partial thromboplastin time response and recurrence in patients with venous thrombosis treated with continuous intravenous heparin. *Arch Intern Med* 1996; 156:1677–1681.

16. Lefkovits J, Topol EJ. Direct thrombin inhibitors in cardiovascular medicine. *Circulation* 1994; 90:1522–1536.
17. Hirsh J, Weitz JI. New antithrombotic agents. *Lancet* 1999; 353:1431–1436.
18. Weitz JI, Crowther M. Direct thrombin inhibitors. *Thromb Res* 2002; 106:V275-V284.
19. Kaplan KL, Francis CW. Direct thrombin inhibitors. *Semin Hematol* 2002; 39:187–196.
20. Davie EW. Biochemical and molecular aspects of the coagulation cascade. *Thromb Haemost* 1995; 74:1–6.
21. Chesebro JH *et al*. Role of thrombin in arterial thrombosis: implications for therapy. *Thromb Haemost* 1991; 66:1–5.
22. Kumar R, Beguin S, Hemker HC. The influence of fibrinogen and fibrin on thrombin generation – evidence for feedback activation of the clotting system by clot bound thrombin. *Thromb Haemost* 1994; 72: 713–721.
23. Kumar R, Beguin S, Hemker HC. The effect of fibrin clots and clot-bound thrombin on the development of platelet procoagulant activity. *Thromb Haemost* 1995; 74: 962–968.
24. Fiore LD, Deykin D. Mechanisms of hemostasis and arterial thrombosis. *Cardiol Clin* 1994; 12:399–409.
25. Shah PK. New insights into the pathogenesis and prevention of acute coronary syndromes. *Am J Cardiol* 1997; 79:17–23.
26. Stubbs MT, Bode W. A player of many parts: the spotlight falls on thrombin's structure. *Thromb Res* 1993; 69:1–58.
27. Weitz JI, Buller HR. Direct thrombin inhibitors in acute coronary syndromes: present and future. *Circulation* 2002; 105:1004–1011.
28. Hogg PJ, Bock PE. Modulation of thrombin and heparin activities by fibrin. *Thromb Haemost* 1997; 77:424–433.
29. Liaw PC *et al*. Molecular basis for the susceptibility of fibrin-bound thrombin to inactivation by heparin cofactor ii in the presence of dermatan sulfate but not heparin. *J Biol Chem* 2001; 276:20959–20965.
30. Olson ST, Bjork I. Regulation of thrombin activity by antithrombin and heparin. *Semin Thromb Hemost* 1994; 20:373–409.
31. Hirsh J. Heparin. *N Engl J Med* 1991; 324:1565–1574.
32. Weitz JI. Low-molecular-weight heparins. *N Engl J Med* 1997; 337:688–698.
33. Hogg PJ *et al*. Binding of fibrin monomer and heparin to thrombin in a ternary complex alters the environment of the thrombin catalytic site, reduces affinity for hirudin, and inhibits cleavage of fibrinogen. *J Biol Chem* 1996; 271:26088–26095.
34. Becker DL *et al*. Exosites 1 and 2 are essential for protection of fibrin-bound thrombin from heparin-catalyzed inhibition by antithrombin and heparin cofactor II. *J Biol Chem* 1999; 274:6226–6233.
35. Andersen K, Dellborg M. Heparin is more effective than inogatran, a low-molecular weight thrombin inhibitor in suppressing ischemia and recurrent angina in unstable coronary disease. Thrombin Inhibition in Myocardial Ischemia (TRIM) Study Group. *Am J Cardiol* 1998; 81:939–944.
36. Klootwijk P *et al*. Anticoagulant properties, clinical efficacy and safety of efegatran, a direct thrombin inhibitor, in patients with unstable angina. *Eur Heart J* 1999; 20:1101–1111.
37. Bates SM, Weitz JI. The mechanism of action of thrombin inhibitors. *J Invasive Cardiol* 2000; 12(suppl F): 27F–32F.
38. Das J, Kimball SD. Thrombin active site inhibitors. *Bioorg Med Chem* 1995; 3:999–1007.
39. Weitz JI, Hirsh J. New antithrombotic agents. *Chest* 1998; 114(suppl 5):715S–727S.
40. Hauptmann J. Pharmacokinetics of an emerging new class of anticoagulant/antithrombotic drugs. A review of small-molecule thrombin inhibitors. *Eur J Clin Pharmacol* 2002; 57:751–758.
41. Wallis RB. Hirudins: from leeches to man. *Semin Thromb Hemost* 1996; 22:185–196.
42. Lefevre G *et al*. Effect of renal impairment on the pharmacokinetics and pharmacodynamics of desirudin. *Clin Pharmacol Ther* 1997; 62:50–59.
43. Maraganore JM *et al*. Design and characterization of hirulogs: a novel class of bivalent peptide inhibitors of thrombin. *Biochemistry* 1990; 29:7095–7101.
44. Parry MA, Maraganore JM, Stone SR. Kinetic mechanism for the interaction of Hirulog with thrombin. *Biochemistry*, 1994; 33:14807–14814.
45. Fox I *et al*. Anticoagulant activity of Hirulog, a direct thrombin inhibitor, in humans. *Thromb Haemost* 1993; 69:157–163.
46. Robson R. The use of bivalirudin in patients with renal impairment. *J Invasive Cardiol* 2000; 12(suppl F): 33F–36F.
47. Cannon CP *et al*. Anticoagulant effects of hirulog, a novel thrombin inhibitor, in patients with coronary artery disease. *Am J Cardiol* 1993; 71:778–782.

48. Topol EJ *et al*. Use of a direct antithrombin, hirulog, in place of heparin during coronary angioplasty. *Circulation* 1993; 87:1622–1629.

49. Cho L *et al*. Correlation of point-of-care ecarin clotting time versus activated clotting time with bivalirudin concentrations. *Am J Cardiol* 2003; 91:1110–1113.

50. Casserly IP *et al*. Point-of-care ecarin clotting time versus activated clotting time in correlation with bivalirudin concentration. *Thromb Res* 2004; 113:115–121.

51. Cheneau E *et al*. Value of monitoring activated clotting time when bivalirudin is used as the sole anticoagulation agent for percutaneous coronary intervention. *Am J Cardiol* 2004; 94:789–792.

52. Hursting MJ *et al*. Novastan (brand of argatroban): a small-molecule, direct thrombin inhibitor. *Semin Thromb Hemost* 1997; 23:503–516.

53. Swan SK, Hursting MJ. The pharmacokinetics and pharmacodynamics of argatroban: effects of age, gender, and hepatic or renal dysfunction. *Pharmacotherapy* 2000; 20:318–329.

54. Serruys PW *et al*. A comparison of hirudin with heparin in the prevention of restenosis after coronary angioplasty. Helvetica Investigators. *N Engl J Med* 1995; 333:757–763.

55. Effects of recombinant hirudin (lepirudin) compared with heparin on death, myocardial infarction, refractory angina, and revascularisation procedures in patients with acute myocardial ischaemia without ST elevation: a randomised trial. Organisation to Assess Strategies for Ischemic Syndromes (OASIS-2) Investigators. *Lancet* 1999; 353:429–438.

56. Roe MT *et al*. Comparison of benefits and complications of hirudin versus heparin for patients with acute coronary syndromes undergoing early percutaneous coronary intervention. *Am J Cardiol* 2001; 88:1403–1406, A6.

57. Bittl JA *et al*. Treatment with bivalirudin (Hirulog) as compared with heparin during coronary angioplasty for unstable or postinfarction angina. Hirulog Angioplasty Study Investigators. *N Engl J Med* 1995; 333:764–769.

58. Bittl JA *et al*. Bivalirudin versus heparin during coronary angioplasty for unstable or postinfarction angina: Final report reanalysis of the Bivalirudin Angioplasty Study. *Am Heart J* 2001; 142:952–959.

59. Lincoff AM *et al*. Bivalirudin with planned or provisional abciximab versus low-dose heparin and abciximab during percutaneous coronary revascularization: results of the Comparison of Abciximab Complications with Hirulog for Ischemic Events Trial (CACHET). *Am Heart J* 2002; 143:847–853.

60. Lincoff AM *et al*. Comparison of bivalirudin versus heparin during percutaneous coronary intervention (the Randomized Evaluation of PCI Linking Angiomax to Reduced Clinical Events [REPLACE]-1 trial). *Am J Cardiol* 2004; 93:1092–1096.

61. Lincoff AM *et al*. Bivalirudin and provisional glycoprotein IIb/IIIa blockade compared with heparin and planned glycoprotein IIb/IIIa blockade during percutaneous coronary intervention: REPLACE-2 randomized trial. *JAMA* 2003; 289:853–863.

62. Lincoff AM *et al*. Long-term efficacy of bivalirudin and provisional glycoprotein IIb/IIIa blockade vs heparin and planned glycoprotein IIb/IIIa blockade during percutaneous coronary revascularization: REPLACE-2 randomized trial. *JAMA* 2004; 292:696–703.

63. Stone GW *et al*. Acute Catheterization and Urgent Intervention Triage strategY (ACUITY) trial: study design and rationale. *Am Heart J* 2004; 148:764–775.

64. Gurm HS *et al*. Use of bivalirudin during percutaneous coronary intervention in patients with diabetes mellitus: an analysis from the randomized evaluation in percutaneous coronary intervention linking angiomax to reduced clinical events (REPLACE)-2 trial. *J AM Coll Cardiol* 2005; 45:1932–1938.

65. Chew DP *et al*. Bivalirudin versus heparin and glycoprotein IIb/IIIa inhibition among patients with renal impairment undergoing percutaneous coronary intervention (a subanalysis of the REPLACE-2 trial). *AM J Cardiol* 2005; 95:581–585.

66. Cho L *et al*. Safe and efficacious use of bivalirudin for percutaneous coronary intervention with adjunctive platelet glycoprotein IIb/IIIa receptor inhibition. *Am J Cardiol* 2003; 91:742–743.

67. Gurm HS *et al*. Effectiveness and safety of bivalirudin during percutaneous coronary intervention in a single medical center. *AM J Cardiol* 2005; 95:716–721.

68. Stella JF, *et al*. Anticoagulation with bivalirudin during percutaneous coronary intervention for ST-segment elevation myocardial infarction. *J Invasive Cardiol* 2004; 16:451–454.

69. Rha SW *et al*. Bivalirudin versus heparin as an antithrombotic agent in patients treated with a sirolimus-eluting stent. *Am J Cardiol* 2004; 94:1047–1050.

70. Cohen DJ *et al.* Economic evaluation of bivalirudin with provisional glycoprotein IIB/IIIA inhibition versus heparin with routine glycoprotein IIB/IIIA inhibition for percutaneous coronary intervention: results from the REPLACE-2 trial. *J Am Coll Cardiol* 2004; 44:1792–1800.

71. Popma JJ *et al.* Antithrombotic therapy during percutaneous coronary intervention: the Seventh ACCP Conference on Antithrombotic and Thrombolytic Therapy. *Chest* 2004; 126(suppl 13):576S–599S.

72. Lewis BE *et al.* Argatroban anticoagulation during percutaneous coronary intervention in patients with heparin-induced thrombocytopenia. *Catheter Cardiovasc Interv* 2002; 57:177–184.

8

Pentasaccharide and other factor Xa inhibitors

P. Tricoci, J. H. Alexander, R. A. Harrington

INTRODUCTION

Factor X has been recognised to play an important role in the coagulation system for decades [1]. Deficiency of factor X leads to a haemorrhagic diathesis first described in two families, Stuart and Prower [2, 3]. It has been suggested that only levels of factor X less than 5% of normal lead to a clinically significant bleeding tendency [4].

Factor X is the zymogen of factor Xa (fXa), a serine protease that plays a critical role in the coagulation cascade. Factor Xa activation is located in the common pathway of both intrinsic and extrinsic systems, at an earlier stage than thrombin and can be activated by either factor VIIa–tissue factor complex (extrinsic Xase) or factor VIIIa/IXa complex (intrinsic Xase). Factor Xa combines with factor Va on the activated platelet membrane surface to form the 'prothrombinase' complex that converts prothrombin to thrombin (Figure 8.1). Prothrombinase is 300 000-fold more active than fXa in catalysing prothrombin activation [5]. Effective and selective inhibition of fXa is expected to strongly inhibit the generation of thrombin.

Current approaches to anticoagulant (antithrombin) therapy include unfractionated heparin (UFH), low-molecular-weight heparins (LMWH), vitamin K antagonists (VKA), and recently, direct thrombin inhibitors. These drugs have a number of limitations that make them less than ideal antithrombotic agents. Given the limitations of classic antithrombotic drugs, alternative approaches have been developed, attempting to offer pharmacological and clinical advantages over currently available antithrombotics. The pivotal position of fXa in the coagulation cascade has made its inhibition an attractive target for the development of new antithrombotis. Since the amount of activated serine protease is amplified at each step of the coagulation cascade, the upstream inhibition of fXa may be a more effective way to inhibit coagulation than the downstream inhibition of thrombin. In addition, given the multiple feedback loops in the coagulation cascade and the multiple procoagulant effects of even small amounts of thrombin, preventing thrombin generation may be a more effective strategy than inhibiting its activity after the fact. Factor Xa does not have anticoagulant properties. Additionally, fXa has slower activation kinetics than thrombin, thus making it a more attractive target for pharmacologic inhibition. Finally, the potential clinical advantage of selective inhibition of fXa has been underlined by the results of clinical trials with LMWH. Those LMWHs that have a higher anti-Xa activity than antithrombin

Peirluigi Trioci, Cardiology Fellow, Duke Clinical Research Institute, Durham, North Carolina, USA.

John H. Alexander, Assistant Professor of Medicine in Cardiovascular Medicine, Duke Clinical Research Institute, Durham, North Carolina, USA.

Robert A. Harrington, Professor of Medicine, Director, Cardiovascular Clinical Trials, Duke Clinical Research Institute, Durham, North Carolina, USA.

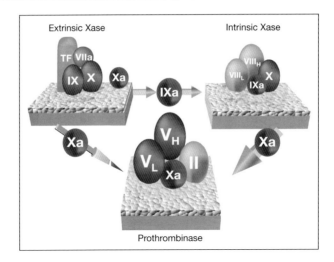

Figure 8.1 Extrinsic and intrinsic Xase generate factor Xa, which combines with factor Va on platelet's surface to form the 'prothrombinase complex'. With permission from Mann KG. *Coagulation Explosion*. Vermont Business Graphics, Burlington, 1997.

activity, have tended to show greater superiority over UFH in both vein and arterial thrombosis [6, 7].

CLASSIFICATION

There are a number of fXa inhibitors that are in various stages of development, and one, fondaparinux, that is commercially available. These agents are a heterogeneous group of compounds, ranging from non-peptidic molecules to peptidic or saccharidic sequences. The pharmacodynamic and pharmacokinetic properties of these drugs differ. A proposed classification scheme based on their specificity for fXa and on their mechanism of action divides these drugs into four categories: indirect selective, indirect non-selective, direct selective, and direct non-selective fXa inhibitors. Direct inhibitors act directly by binding to fXa while indirect inhibitors catalyse or facilitate the interaction between antithrombin (AT) and fXa. Both direct and indirect inhibitors may act selectively on fXa or may have other targets in the coagulation cascade as well (Table 8.1).

FONDAPARINUX

Fondaparinux, an indirect fXa inhibitor, is the first and, currently, the only commercially available fXa inhibitor. It is synthetically derived from the pentasaccharidic sequence of heparin [8]. The pentasaccharidic sequence of heparin is the minimal sequence of heparin-binding AT that produces a high fXa activity without having any antithrombin property [9, 10]. The natural pentasaccharide sequence was identified using fractionation methods, and was subsequently synthesised [8].

Structural analyses showed that four specific sulphate groups are critical in the interaction between the pentasaccharide of heparin and AT [11, 12].

The α-methyl glycoside derivative of original pentasaccharide was first synthesised by Petitou and colleagues [13]. The compound was subsequently known as SR 90107A/Org 31540 (fondaparinux) and was developed by Sanofi-Synthelabo and Organon (Figure 8.2).

Table 8.1 Classification of factor Xa inhibitors

	Target	AT dependent	Route of administration
Indirect-selective			
Fondaparinux	Factor Xa	Yes	Parenteral
Idraparinux	Factor Xa	Yes	Parenteral
Indirect-non-selective			
Unfractionated Heparin	Factors IIa, Xa, IX, XI, XII	Yes	Parenteral
Low-molecular-weight heparins	Factors Xa, IIa	Yes	Parenteral
Direct-selective			
DX-9065a	Factor Xa	No	Parenteral
Razaxaban (DPC 906)	Factor Xa	No	Oral
Direct-non-selective			
Tifacogin (rTFPI)	Factor Xa, complex inhibits fVIIa	No	Parenteral
NAPc	Factor Xa, complex inhibits fVIIa	No	Parenteral

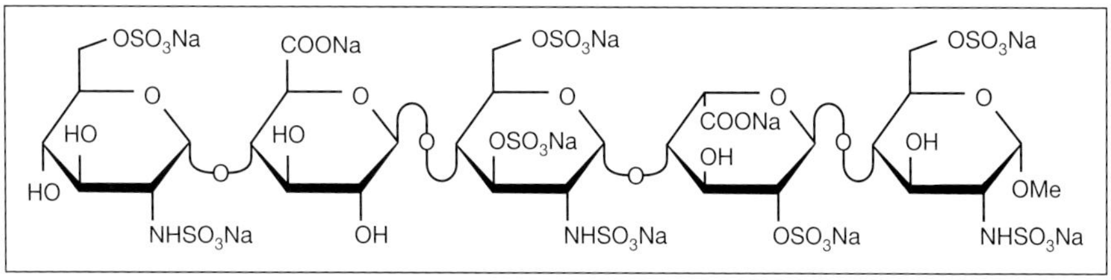

Figure 8.2 Chemical structure of fondaparinux.

PHARMACODYNAMICS

Fondaparinux has a highly specific binding capacity toward AT. At clinically relevant concentrations, more than 95% of the drug is bound to AT, with a stoichiometric ratio of 1:1 [8, 14]. The binding site is specific and possesses high affinity. Binding capacity (B_{max}) and dissociation constant (K_D) are similar for human plasma ($B_{max} = 2072\,nmol/l$; $K_D = 28\,nmol/l$) and purified AT ($B_{max} = 1627\,nmol/l$; $K_D = 32\,nmol/l$), suggesting that at clinically relevant concentration interactions with other plasma proteins, such as albumin and α1-acid glycoprotein are unlikely. This may reduce the potential interactions with other drugs by the competition for protein binding. Fondaparinux and heparins have a similar affinity for AT, but fondaparinux does not inhibit thrombin because thrombin inhibition requires sequences longer than 18 saccharides [15]. The lack of antithrombin effects of fondaparinux has been confirmed *in vivo* [16].

The bond between fondaparinux and AT is non-covalent and reversible. After the binding, AT undergoes conformational changes leading to the exposure of an arginine containing loop. The exposure of this loop greatly increases the affinity of AT for fXa (approximately 300-fold) without increasing the antithrombin activity [17, 18]. After AT binds fXa, further conformational changes lead to the release of unmodified fondaparinux from AT. This means that one molecule of fondaparinux can activate several molecules of AT [19].

The bond between AT and fXa is covalent and irreversible. AT–Xa complexes are then eventually cleared from plasma.

As the drug concentration increases there is a concentration-dependent decrease in the fraction of fondaparinux bound to AT. This suggests that the chemical interaction between fondaparinux and AT is saturable, and the concentration of AT is the limiting factor in fondaparinux's anticoagulant effect. [14, 20]. Since the fondaparinux is pharmacologically active only in its AT-bound fraction, once there is no free AT the antithrombotic effect of the drug reaches a plateau [21].

The inhibition of the fXa, caused by the fondaparinux–AT interaction, results in the impairment of thrombin generation. A dose-dependent inhibition of thrombin generation caused by fondaparinux has been demonstrated in several models using either extrinsic or intrinsic pathway activation [22–25]. Fondaparinux showed a greater effect when the coagulation was triggered by the tissue-factor pathway compared to the intrinsic pathway. Fondaparinux, unlike heparin, effectively inhibits thrombin generation in platelet-rich plasma. This is probably due to the absence of interaction between fondaparinux and platelet proteins, such as platelet factor 4.

At clinically relevant doses, fondaparinux has a minimal effect on the standard tests for monitoring antithrombotic therapy. A subcutaneous dose of 10 mg of fondaparinux did, however, result in an average increase in activated partial thromboplastin time (aPTT) from 33.5 ± 4.1 to 38.8 ± 5.3 seconds and in an average increase of prothombin time (PT) from 13.2 ± 0.6 to 14.3 ± 0.9 seconds, 1.5 h after the administration [26]. The modest effect of fondaparinux on the aPTT recalls the similar finding observed with therapeutic doses of LMWH. Although fondaparinux can inhibit fXa bound to a clot it is unable to inhibit fXa already included in the pro-thrombinase complex [27]. This is thought to be due to its relatively large size, and is a limitation that fondaparinux shares with both UFH and LMWH. Whether the inability of fondaparinux to act on fXa bound in the pro-thrombinase complex is a significant limitation is unknown and will require further investigations comparing fondaparinux with other direct, small-molecule fXa inhibitors that are active within the pro-thrombinase complex.

The antithrombotic effect of fondaparinux has been demonstrated in several animal models. The first demonstration of its antithrombotic effect *in vivo* was made by Walenga and colleagues in 1985 [28]. Subsequently venous thrombosis models showed that fondaparinux inhibits clot formation in a dose-dependent fashion, and that the antithrombotic effect is closely related to the *ex vivo* anti-Xa activity [29–32]. The antithrombotic properties of fondaparinux were also demonstrated in arterial thrombosis models and in arterovenous shunt models [33–35]. Although fondaparinux does not possess fibrinolytic activity, it was effective to enhance lysis induced by tPA and to prevent re-occlusion in a rabbit artery thrombosis model, suggesting a possible role as adjunctive therapy during fibrinolysis [36].

PHARMACOKINETICS

The pharmacokinetics of fondaparinux have been studied in healthy volunteers [37]. Fondaparinux sodium is completely and rapidly absorbed after subcutaneous administration. After a single 2.5 mg subcutaneous injection the time to reach C_{max} is 1.7 ± 0.4 h. The bioavailability is complete. Plasma half-life after a subcutaneous dose of 2.5 mg is 17 h in young individuals and 21 h in elderly. Then, the steady-state is reached after 3 to 4 days. For concentrations less than 2 mg/dl, fondaparinux is highly bound to plasma proteins (>97%), predominantly AT. The pharmacokinetic profile of fondaparinux is linear in the range from 2 to 8 mg single subcutaneous doses. For clinically relevant doses, 64 to 77% of fondaparinux is excreted unmodified in urine up to 72 h. The total clearance of fondaparinux is reduced by 25% in patients with mild renal impairment (CrCl > 50–80 ml/min), by 40% in patients with moderate renal impairment (CrCl > 30–50 ml/min) and by 55% in patients with severe renal impairment (CrCl < 30ml/min). The renal clearance of fondaparinux is also 25% lower in patients older than 75 years and 30% lower in patients weighing less than 50 kg [38]. Data from patients on chronic dialysis suggest that fondaparinux is dialysable [39]. Although *in vivo* metabolism of fondaparinux has not been studied, there is no evidence that fondaparinux is bio-transformed. In clinical studies, fondaparinux has been shown not to have pharmacokinetic interactions with aspirin, piroxicam, digoxin or warfarin [40–43]. In particular fondaparinux does not influence the effect of warfarin on PT and international normalised ratio (INR); INR may thus be used to monitor the effect of oral anticoagulants during co-administration of both fondaparinux and warfarin.

Since fondaparinux is nearly completely bound to AT, it is not immediately available for placental transfer [44]. In an *in vitro* placental model, fondaparinux did not cross the barrier at significant concentrations. Therefore fondaparinux is a theoretical alternative to current antithrombotic therapy in pregnant women. However, no clinical data are yet available on the effects of fondaparinux during pregnancy, therefore safe use in pregnancy is only theoretical and requires appropriate studies.

THROMBOCYTOPAENIA

The occurrence of moderate thrombocytopaenia (platelet count 50.000–100.000/mm^3) has been reported at a rate of 2.9% in clinical trials with a dose of 2.5 mg of fondaparinux. Severe thrombocytopaenia (<50.000/mm^3) is rare (0.2%) [38]. The small molecules of fondaparinux do not interact with platelet proteins, such as platelet factor 4, rendering unlikely the production of anti-heparin-platelet factor 4 antibodies [8]. Fondaparinux does not cross-react with serum of patients with heparin-induced thrombocytopaenia (HIT) [45, 46]. The absence of high sulphation content and the low molecular weight seems to be related to the lack of reactivity with the antibodies of HIT patients [47]. Although direct thrombin inhibitors would likely be preferred in patients with established HIT, use of fondaparinux may result in a lower incidence of HIT, and its associated thrombotic complications, than observed with the current widespread use of unfractionated and low-molecular-weight heparins [48].

EFFECTS ON BONE METABOLISM

Osteoporosis is a potential side-effect with long-term use of all heparins [49]. Usually heparins are administered for short periods and are followed by oral VKA when chronic anticoagulation therapy is required. However there are a number of settings where long-term heparin therapy is currently indicated. During pregnancy, UFH or LMWH may be used for treatment of thrombosis, for prophylaxis of systemic embolism in women with mechanical heart valves, and to prevent fetal loss in women with antiphospholipid syndrome. Fondaparinux *in vitro* did not show inhibitory effect on human osteoblasts [50]. Therefore fondaparinux could potentially avoid both osteoporosis in long-term treatment and negative influence on bone healing after orthopaedic surgery. Definitive conclusions on this issue will require data from appropriate clinical outcome studies.

NEUTRALISATION

Despite the ongoing development of antagonists, there is no currently available antidote for fondaparinux [38]. Even at high concentrations protamine is unable to reverse the anticoagulant effects of fondaparinux [8]. Similarly, protamine does not reverse anti-Xa activity after LMWH administration [51]. This is probably due to its inability to bind the very low molecular weight components of heparins that are responsible for their anti-fXa effect.

A candidate for reversal of the anticoagulant effect of fondaparinux is recombinant factor VIIa (rFVIIa – NovoSeven®). The efficacy of a single 90 μg/kg IV dose of rFVIIa to reverse the anticoagulant effects of a single 10 mg SC dose of fondaparinux was evaluated in a randomised, placebo-controlled clinical trial [26]. Injection of rFVIIa after fondaparinux normalised the mildly prolonged aPTT and PT and normalised the decrease in prothrombin activation fragments 1 + 2. rFVIIa rapidly restored the thrombin generation time and the endogenous thrombin potential. The duration of the effect of a single of rFVIIa ranged from 2 to 6 h.

The reversal effects of rFVIIa are not specific for fondaparinux, and have been observed also for other anticoagulants [52, 53]. It is unclear if the effects of rFVIIa on coagulation assays can be translated into a reduction of clinically relevant bleeding [54–57]. Moreover the potential prothrombotic effects of rFVIIa, particularly in patients at high risk for venous and/or arterial thrombosis, need to be evaluated.

CLINICAL STUDIES

The efficacy and safety of fondaparinux has been studied in phase II and phase III trials in the prevention (Table 8.2) and treatment (Table 8.3) of venous thromboembolism (VTE). In acute coronary syndromes (ACS), two dose-finding phase II trials have been published and two large phase III trials are ongoing in patients with non-ST-elevation acute coronary syndromes and ST elevation myocardial infarction (STEMI).

PROPHYLAXIS OF VTE

Despite the recommended use of antithrombotic drugs for VTE prophylaxis, the incidence of VTE after major orthopaedic surgery remains high [58]. Fondaparinux has been extensively studied in a series of trials that were designed to compare the efficacy and safety of fondaparinux with the current standard therapy for VTE prophylaxis, LMWH enoxaparin.

The dose of fondaparinux subsequently studied in phase III clinical trials was determined in a double-blind dose ranging study of 593 patients undergoing elective total hip replacement [59]. Patients were randomised to receive either 0.75 mg, 1.5 mg, 3.0 mg, 6.0 mg or 8.0 mg of fondaparinux subcutaneously six hours postoperatively, followed by daily injection for 5–10 days. The control group received enoxaparin subcutaneously, 30 mg twice a day, started 12 to 24 h after the end of surgery and continued for 5–10 days. The primary efficacy endpoint was the incidence of deep venous thrombosis (DVT) assessed by mandatory bilateral venography at day 10, or symptomatic VTE. The highest dosing regimens, 6.0 mg and 8.0 mg, were stopped prematurely due to high rates of major bleeding (respectively, 16.7 and 17.3%). The primary endpoints in the 0.75 mg, 1.5 mg and 3.0 mg groups were 11.8%, 6.7% and 1.7%, respectively, suggesting a dose–effect relationship. The rate of VTE with 3.0 mg of fondaparinux was significantly lower than with enoxaparin in the intention-to-treat population (1.7 vs. 9.4%, $P = 0.01$). Also, the risk of major bleeding was dose-related (0%, 0.5%, 4.5% in 0.75 mg, 1.5 mg and 3.0 mg groups, respectively; $P < 0.001$). The significant dose–response effects on both efficacy and safety endpoints were also associated with a clear dose–plasma level relationship. The results of this phase II study suggested a dose between 1.5 and 3.0 mg as the regimen with a reasonable benefit-to-risk ratio for prevention of VTE. Interpolation of these data lead to the choice of 2.5 mg as the dose to test in phase III trials in VTE prophylaxis after major orthopaedic surgery (Figure 8.3).

Four phase III trials comparing efficacy and safety of fondaparinux with enoxaparin in VTE prophylaxis after major orthopaedic surgery have been published: EPHESUS, PENTATHLON 2000, PENTHIFRA and PENTAMARKS (Table 8.2). These trials used the same comparative drug (subcutaneous enoxaparin 40 mg once daily starting 12 h prior to surgery or 30 mg twice daily starting 12 to 24 h after surgery), duration of therapy, and endpoints.

Table 8.2 Phase III randomised clinical trials evaluating fondaparinux in DVT prevention

Study	N	Population	Regimen	Control	End points	Efficacy outcome	Major bleeding
EPHESUS [60]	2309	Total hip replacement	2.5 mg qd Post-op	Enoxaparin 40 mg qd Pre-op	DVT at venography, or symptomatic VTE to day 11	Fondaparinux: 4.1% Enoxaparin: 9.2% ($P < 0.0001$)	Fondaparinux: 4.1% Enoxaparin: 2.8% ($P = 0.11$)
PENTATHLON 2000 [61]	2275	Total hip replacement	2.5 mg qd Post-op	Enoxaparin 30 mg bid Post-op		Fondaparinux: 6.1% Enoxaparin: 8.3% ($P = 0.099$)	Fondaparinux: 1.7% Enoxaparin: 0.9% ($P = 0.11$)
PENTAMARKS [63]	1049	Major knee surgery	2.5 mg qd Post-op	Enoxaparin 30 mg bid Post-op		Fondaparinux:12.5% Enoxaparin: 27.8% ($P < 0.001$)	Fondaparinux: 1.9% Enoxaparin: 0.2% ($P = 0.006$)
PENTHIFRA [62]	1711	Hip fracture surgery	2.5 mg qd Post-op	Enoxaparin 40 mg qd Pre-op		Fondaparinux: 8.3% Enoxaparin: 19.1% ($P < 0.001$)	Fondaparinux: 2.3% Enoxaparin: 2.3% ($P = 1.00$)
PENTHIFRA Plus [67]	646	Hip fracture surgery	2.5 mg qd x 3 weeks after initial 7 days of fondaparinux	After 7 days of fondaparinux placebo for 3 wks	DVT at venography or symptomatic VTE to 3 wks	Fondaparinux: 1.4% Placebo: 35% ($P < 0.001$)	Fondaparinux: 2.4% Placebo: 0.6% ($P = 0.06$)
PEGASUS [68]	2927	High-risk abdominal surgery	2.5 mg qd for 5–9 days Post-op	Dalteparin 5000 UI qd (2500 UI pre-op) for 5–9 days	DVT at venography or symptomatic VTE to day 10	Fondaparinux: 4.6% Dalteparin: 6.1% ($P = 0.14$)	Fondaparinux: 3.4% Dalteparin: 2.4% ($P = 0.12$)
ARTEMIS [69]	849	Acute medical	2.5 mg qd for 6–14 days	Placebo for 6–14 days	DVT at venography or symptomatic VTE to day 15	Fondaparinux: 5.6% Placebo: 10.5% ($P = 0.03$)	Fondaparinux: 0.2% Dalteparin 0.2% ($P = 1.00$)

Table 8.3 Phase III randomised clinical trials of fondaparinux in treatment of VTE

Study	N	Population	Regimen of fondaparinux†	Control	Outcome	Efficacy outcome*	Major bleeding
MATISSE-PE [71]	2213	Acute Symptomatic PE	7.5 mg qd for ≥5dd, then warfarin for 3 months	UFH (aPTT 1.5–2.5) for ≥5 dd, then warfarin for 3 months	Symptomatic recurrent PE, or new/recurrent DVT up to 3 months	Fondaparinux: 3.8% UFH: 5.0% (AD –1.2; 95% CI –0.7 to 1.1)	Fondaparinux: 1.3% UFH: 1.1% (AD –0.2%; 95% CI –0.7 to 1.1)
MATISSE-DVT [72]	2205	Acute DVT	7.5 mg qd for ≥5 dd, then warfarin for 3 months	Enoxaparin 1 mg/Kg bid for ≥5dd, then warfarin for 3 months	Symptomatic recurrent PE, or new/recurrent DVT up to 3 months	Fondaparinux: 3.9% Enoxaparin: 4.1% (AD –0.15, 95% CI –1.8 to 1.5)	Fondaparinux: 1.1% Enoxaparin: 1.2% (AD –0.1%; 95% CI –1.0 to 0.8%).

AD = absolute difference. *Non-inferiority margin set at 3.5% AD.
†Weight-adjusted doses (5.0 mg if <50 kg and 10.0 mg if weight >100 kg).

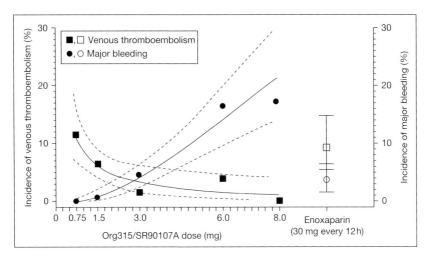

Figure 8.3 Dose–response curve for fondaparinux. The curves indicate an evident dose–response effect on both rate of VTE and rate of major bleeding. The lower VTE rate in 3.0 mg group compared to 0.75 mg, 1.5 mg and enoxaparin groups, and the lower rate of major bleeding in 0.75 mg and 1.5 mg groups indicate that a dose between 1.5 mg to 3.0 mg has the potential to have to best risk/benefit ratio. With permission from Turpie AG *et al*. *N Engl J Med* 2001; 344:619 [59].

The primary efficacy endpoint was defined as the presence of DVT, pulmonary embolism (PE) or both by day 11. DVT was assessed with mandatory bilateral venography of the legs between day 5 and day 11. The primary safety outcome was major bleeding defined as fatal bleeding, bleeding that was retroperitoneal, intracranial, intraspinal, or involving other critical organs, bleeding leading to re-operation and overt bleeding with a bleeding index ≥ 2. The dose of fondaparinux was 2.5 mg subcutaneous, started 4 to 8 h postoperatively, and followed by the same dose once daily for 5–9 days after the surgery. The similar design of these four trials was planned in order to perform a meta-analysis of their data.

The EPHESUS and PENTATHLON 2000 trials compared fondaparinux with enoxaparin in similar populations of patients undergoing elective hip-replacement surgery [60, 61]. In EPHESUS, 2309 European patients undergoing elective hip-replacement were randomised to receive either fondaparinux 2.5 mg or enoxaparin 40 mg started 12 h before surgery. The incidence of the primary endpoint was 4 and 9% respectively in the fondaparinux and enoxaparin groups ($P < 0.0001$). The rate of major bleeding did not differ between the fondaparinux and enoxaparin groups (4 vs. 3%; $P = 0.11$).

The PENTATHLON 2000 trial randomised 2275 North American patients to receive either fondaparinux 2.5 mg or enoxaparin 30 mg twice daily, with the first dose given 4–8 h after surgery. A non-significant trend in favour of fondaparinux in the primary efficacy endpoint was found (6 vs. 8%; $P = 0.099$). Major bleeding did not differ significantly between the groups (2 vs. 1%; $P = 0.11$).

In the PENTHIFRA study, 1711 patients undergoing surgery following hip fracture were randomised to either fondaparinux 2.5 mg or enoxaparin 40 mg once daily started post-operatively [62]. The incidence of VTE by day 11 was 8.3% in the fondaparinux group and 19.1% in the enoxaparin group ($P < 0.001$). The rate of major bleeding was nearly the same in the two groups (2.2 fondaparinux vs. 2.3% enoxaparin; $P = 1.00$). Interestingly, only 25.6% of patients received the pre-operative enoxaparin recommended in the protocol, illustrating the practical challenges in administration of LMWH pre-operatively under emergency situations.

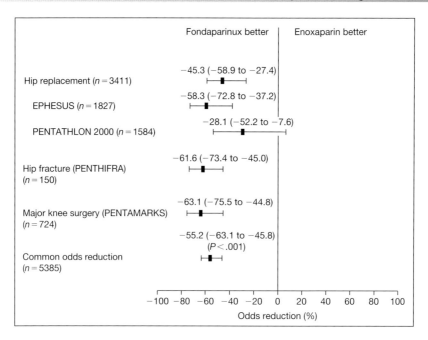

Figure 8.4 Incidence of VTE by day 11 in the 4 trials evaluating fondaparinux after major orthopaedic surgery, and the overall data from the meta-analysis. With permission from Turpie AG *et al. Arch Int Med* 2002; 162:1833 [64].

Finally, the PENTAMARKS trial evaluated the efficacy and safety of fondaparinux 2.5 mg once daily compared to enoxaparin 30 mg twice daily started immediately after surgery in 1049 patients undergoing major knee surgery [63]. The incidence of VTE by day 11 was 12.5 and 27.8% in the fondaparinux and enoxaparin groups respectively ($P < 0.001$). The prophylaxis with fondaparinux was associated with a significant increase in the rate of major bleeding (1.9 vs. 0.2%; $P = 0.006$).

A meta-analysis of these four trials included 7344 patients [64]. The overall incidence of VTE was 6.8% in the fondaparinux group and 13.7% in the enoxaparin group ($P < 0.001$) (Figure 8.4). The superiority of fondaparinux on the primary efficacy endpoint was consistent across multiple subgroups including, age, sex, obesity, type of anaesthesia, use of cement, and duration of surgery. Patients treated with fondaparinux, however, also had significantly more bleeding (2.7 vs. 1.7%; $P = 0.008$). In particular there was an increase of bleeding with a bleeding index ≥ 2 (2.3 vs. 1.5%) while the rate of re-intervention due to bleeding was similarly low in the two groups (0.3 vs. 0.2%). The rate of blood transfusions (not included in the major safety endpoint) was significantly higher in patients treated with fondaparinux compared to those treated with enoxaparin (53.9 vs. 51.5%; $P = 0.04$). Minor bleeding occurred in 3.0% of patients in the fondaparinux group and in 2.7% in the enoxaparin group. The death rate by day 49 was 1.3 and 1.4% in the fondaparinux and enoxaparin group, respectively.

One of the major criticisms of the results of these trials was that the primary endpoint used was a combination of a surrogate frequently but less clinically relevant endpoint (all DVT detected by routine venography) and a clinically relevant but less common endpoint (symptomatic DVT or PE) [65]. The superiority of fondaparinux over enoxaparin was shown using this composite endpoint, while no differences were found regarding the incidence of symptomatic VTE (0.6 fondaparinux vs. 0.4% enoxaparin; $P = 0.25$).

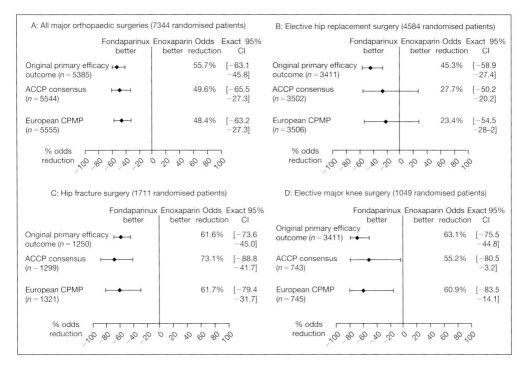

Figure 8.5 Common odds reduction using different efficacy end point definitions in DVT prophylaxis. With permission from Turpie AG *et al. Chest* 2004; 126:501 [66].

Recently, Turpie and colleagues re-evaluated in a *post hoc* analysis the results of the four DVT prevention trials using the efficacy endpoints established by the ACCP Consensus Conference on Antithrombotic Therapy (any proximal DVT, symptomatic proven DVT or PE, or fatal PE) and that established by the European CPMP (any proximal DVT, symptomatic proven PE, or death from any cause) [66]. Using these clinically more significant endpoints, fondaparinux retained superiority over enoxaparin in the meta-analysis of the four trials (Figure 8.5). The superior effect of fondaparinux was principally driven by the reduction of any proximal DVT (1.3 vs. 2.9%). No differences were observed regarding symptomatic VTE, fatal PE, or death. Moreover, using these endpoints fondaparinux was no longer significantly superior to enoxaparin among patients undergoing total hip replacement.

One proposed explanation for the higher incidence of major bleeding in fondaparinux-treated patients is the timing of the administration. In fact, in most of these trials, fondaparinux was administered 6 h after surgery, while enoxaparin was administered 12 to 24 h after surgery, with or without a dose 12 h prior the surgery. A *post hoc* analysis showed a statistically significant relationship between the incidence of major bleeding and timing of first fondaparinux injection (between 3 and 9 h after surgery) (Figure 8.6) [64]. On the other hand, the different timing of administration between fondaparinux and enoxaparin may also account for the superior efficacy seen with fondaparinux. The appropriate timing of fondaparinux following major orthopaedic surgery still remains unclear.

The PENTHIFRA Plus trial evaluated the efficacy and safety of extended use of fondaparinux after hip fracture surgery [67]. In this phase III, double-blind-multicentre trial, 656 patients undergoing hip fracture surgery were randomised to receive either fondaparinux 2.5 mg once daily or placebo for 19 to 23 days. Before randomisation all patients

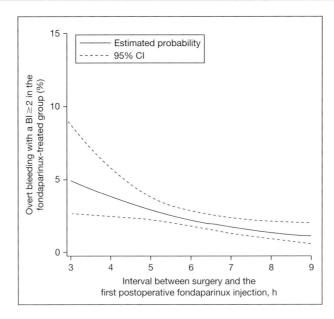

Figure 8.6 Incidence of bleeding and time of first postoperative injection of fondaparinux. (Logistic regression model; $P = 0.008$). With permission from Turpie AG et al. *Lancet* 2002; 359:1715 [61].

received post-operative fondaparinux for 6–8 days. All patients were evaluated by bilateral venography of legs between days 25 and 32. The primary efficacy endpoint was the same as that used in the four DVT prophylaxis trials previously described. Prolonged fondaparinux substantially reduced the incidence of VTE compared with placebo (1.4 vs. 35.0%; $P < 0.001$). More importantly, the extended use of fondaparinux also significantly reduced the incidence of symptomatic VTE (0.3 vs. 2.7%; $P = 0.02$). There was also a trend toward more bleeding in patient receiving extended fondaparinux (2.4 vs. 0.6%; $P = 0.06$). The majority (75%) of the bleeding was at the surgical site. No differences were seen in bleeding leading to re-operation (0.6%, in both groups). The rate of transfusions and minor bleeding were also higher with fondaparinux than with placebo (8.9 vs. 6.2% and 1.5 vs. 0.6%, respectively). These results demonstrate that patients remain at high risk for VTE for at least several weeks after major orthopaedic surgery and that prolonged prophylaxis with fondaparinux may substantially reduce this risk.

Two studies assessing fondaparinux in general medical and surgical patients have been conducted but not yet published. In the PEGASUS study, 2927 patients undergoing high-risk abdominal surgery were randomised to either fondaparinux 2.5 mg once daily started 6 h after surgery or dalteparin 2500 IU two hours before surgery, 2500 IU 12 h after the pre-operative dose, followed by 5000 IU once daily [68]. Both agents were given for 5 to 9 days. The primary efficacy outcome of the study was the composite of DVT detected by mandatory bilateral venography, or symptomatic VTE up to day 10. The primary endpoint occurred in 4.6% of patients in the fondaparinux group and 6.1% in the dalteparin group ($P = 0.14$). No differences were found regarding symptomatic VTE episodes (0.4 vs. 0.3%, in the fondaparinux and enoxaparin groups, respectively). Of interest and deserving further prospective evaluation is the finding regarding cancer patients (68.8% of the total population) in whom the incidence of VTE was significantly reduced in the fondaparinux group compared with the dalteparin group (4.7 vs. 7.7%; $P = 0.02$). The rate of major bleeding was 3.4 and 2.4% with fondaparinux and enoxaparin, respectively ($P = 0.12$).

The ARTEMIS study was designed to demonstrate efficacy and safety of fondaparinux in patients ≥60 years old hospitalised for acute cardiac, respiratory, infectious or inflammatory diseases, and expected to remain in bed for at least 4 days [69]. A total of 849 patients were randomly assigned to receive fondaparinux 2.5 mg subcutaneously once daily or placebo, starting within 48 h after admission, and continuing for 6–14 days. The primary efficacy outcome was the occurrence of any VTE (any DVT detected by mandatory venography or symptomatic VTE) up to day 15. The primary safety endpoint was the occurrence of major bleeding (fatal, involving critical organ, requiring surgery, associated with haemoglobin fall ≥2 g/dl and/or transfusion of ≥2 units). Fondaparinux significantly decreased the risk of VTE from 10.5 to 5.6% ($P = 0.029$); The rate of major bleeding was equally low in both the fondaparinux and control groups (0.2%); rates of minor bleeding are not yet publicly available. The use of a placebo control group in this population, which is at moderate risk of VTE, is somewhat controversial [58]. The authors justified use of a placebo arm based on the relatively low and inconsistent use of VTE prophylaxis in this population.

Finally, the APOLLO trial, which has just completed enrolment of 1070 patients at 80 US hospitals, aims to assess the benefit of adding fondaparinux to intermittent pneumatic compression in patients undergoing major abdominal surgery.

Based on the results of the four DVT prophylaxis clinical trials, the FDA approved use of fondaparinux for DVT prophylaxis after hip fracture, hip replacement, and knee replacement surgery, with the first doses to be given 6–8 h after the surgery [38]. In patients with creatinine clearance <30 ml/min and in patients with body weight <50 kg, prophylactic therapy with fondaparinux is contraindicated.

The recent Seventh ACCP Conference on Antithrombotic and Thrombolytic Therapy recommended the use of fondaparinux in the prophylaxis of DVT after orthopaedic surgery [58]. However, the ACCP did not specifically recommend the use of fondaparinux over LMWH or VKA, placing a relatively low value on the prevention of venographic thrombosis compared to a relatively high value on minimising bleeding complications.

TREATMENT OF VTE

Two randomised, phase III trials sought to demonstrate the non-inferiority of fondaparinux compared with UFH in patients with established PE and with enoxaparin in symptomatic DVT (Table 8.3). Initially, the REMBRANDT dose-finding study tested the efficacy and safety of three different doses (5 mg, 7.5 mg or 10 mg) of fondaparinux relative to dalteparin (100 IU/kg bid) in 456 patients with symptomatic VTE [70]. The primary efficacy outcome was the change in thrombus mass assessed by ultrasonography and perfusion lung scintigraphy, both performed at baseline and at day 6–8. No differences were observed among the three groups or compared to dalteparin. The rates of major bleeding were also similar among the groups. Based on the numerically lowest rate of worsening thrombosis on ultrasounds and lung perfusion observed in the 7.5 mg dose group, this dosing regimen was proposed to be evaluated in phase III trials.

The open-label MATISSE-PE trial randomised 2213 patients with symptomatic PE to receive either subcutaneous weight-adjusted fondaparinux once daily (5.0 mg for < 50 kg, 7.5 mg for 50–100 kg, 10 mg for >100 kg) or heparin (5000 UI bolus, followed by 1250 U/h infusion and adjusted for aPTT between 1.5 and 2.5 the control value) for at least 5 days [71]. Both groups received an oral VKA started within 72 h and continued for a minimum of 3 months. The primary efficacy outcome was the rate of symptomatic recurrent VTE at 3 months. The main safety outcome was major bleeding (clinically overt bleeding associated with ≥2 g/dl haemoglobin reduction or with transfusion of ≥2 units, retroperitoneal or intracranial bleeding, occurring in a critical organ, or contributing to death) during the initial treatment period and death during the 3 months.

The study was designed to assess non-inferiority of fondaparinux compared to UFH, with the non-inferiority limit set at 3.5% absolute difference in the primary efficacy outcome. The incidence of symptomatic recurrent VTE was 3.8% in the fondaparinux and 5.0% in the UFH group (absolute difference 1.2%; 95% CI −3.0 to 0.5), meeting the criterion for non-inferiority. The rate of major bleeding was 1.3% with fondaparinux and 1.1% with heparin (absolute difference 0.2%; 95% CI −0.7 to 1.1). The major or clinically relevant non-major bleeding rate was 4.5% with fondaparinux and 6.3% with UFH (absolute difference 1.8%; 95% CI −3.7 to 0.1).

In the MATISSE-DVT trial, 2205 patients with acute symptomatic DVT were randomised to either fondaparinux (weight-adjusted as in the MATISSE-PE) or enoxaparin (1 mg/kg twice daily) for 5 days followed by a minimum 3 months of oral VKA treatment. Both efficacy and safety primary endpoints were similar to the MATISSE-PE trial [72]. The non-inferiority margin was again set at 3.5%. The recurrence of symptomatic VTE at 3 months was 3.9 with fondaparinux and 4.1% with enoxaparin (absolute difference −0.15; 95% CI −1.8 to 1.5). The rate of major bleeding during the initial treatment period was 1.1% with fondaparinux and 1.2% with enoxaparin (absolute difference −0.1%; 95% CI −1.0 to 0.8). Major or clinically relevant non-major bleeding during initial treatment was 3.7% with fondaparinux and 4.2% with enoxaparin. Following these two studies the FDA approved fondaparinux for the treatment of acute DVT and PE when administered in hospital in conjunction with warfarin.

ACUTE CORONARY SYNDROMES AND PERCUTANEOUS CORONARY INTERVENTIONS

Fondaparinux has been evaluated in two phase II trials in patients with ACS. The PENTALYSE study was a randomised, open-label, dose-finding trial in 333 patients with acute STEMI comparing UFH, as adjunctive therapy to alteplase, with 3 weight-adjusted dose regimens of fondaparinux: 4 mg (6 mg if >90 kg); 8 mg (6 mg if <60 kg or 10 mg if >90 mg); 12 mg (10 mg if <60 kg) compared to UFH, as adjuncts to alteplase [73]. Fondaparinux was given intravenously on the first day, then subcutaneously for 5–7 days. UFH was administered by continuous infusion for 48 to 72 h. The primary efficacy endpoint was thrombosis in myocardial infarction (TIMI) flow in the culprit-vessel, evaluated by coronary angiography at 90 min and again on days 5–7. The primary safety endpoint was the combined incidence of intracranial haemorrhage (ICH) and bleeding requiring blood transfusion. The incidence of TIMI 3 flow at 90 min was 65%, 69%, 60% and 68% in the three fondaparinux and heparin groups, respectively (P = 0.6). On days 5–9 the rate of TIMI 3 flow was higher than at 90 min in all groups, without significant differences among the groups (81%, 88%, 89% and 75%; P = 0.1). The rate of ICH or blood transfusion was 4.9%, 9.1%, 7.2% and 7.1% in the 3 doses of fondaparinux and UFH groups respectively without statistically significant differences.

The dose-finding study PENTUA [74] randomised 1134 patients with unstable angina (UA) or non-ST elevation myocardial infarction (NSTEMI) to receive one of four doses of fondaparinux: 2.5 mg, 4 mg, 8 mg, or 12 mg (doses were adjusted for patients <50 kg or >100 kg) or enoxaparin (1 mg/kg twice daily). The primary efficacy endpoint was the composite of mortality, myocardial infarction (MI), recurrent symptomatic or asymptomatic ischaemia up to day 9. The primary safety endpoint was major bleeding (resulting in death, life-threatening, leading to an operation, retroperitoneal, intracranial, involving a critical organ, associated with ≥2 g/dl haemoglobin fall or requiring ≥2 unit transfusion). In a significant number of patients (211) the assigned treatment was prematurely discontinued mostly before a planned revascularisation. The primary endpoint occurred at a similar frequency among the four regimens of fondaparinux and enoxaparin (27.9%, 35.9%, 34.7%, 30.3% and 35.7% in the fondaparinux and enoxaparin groups respectively; P = 0.7). In the pre-protocol analysis, the rate of the primary endpoint was lower among patients receiving 2.5 mg of fondaparinux (30.0%) than among those receiving 4.0 mg (43.5%), 8.0 mg (41.0) and enoxaparin (40.2%). These data, based on multiple *post hoc* comparisons and not observed in the intention-to-treat analysis, should be interpreted cautiously. The incidence of major bleeding in PENTUA was 0%, 1.4%, 1.8%, 0.4% and 0% in the fondaparinux and enoxaparin groups, respectively. The rate of clinically relevant non-major bleeding was also similar among the groups (3.9%, 3.6%, 4.0%, 4.3% and 4.8%, respectively).

The lack of a dose–response effect in these two ACS trials both on efficacy and safety makes the choice of a dose to test in phase III trials difficult. Nevertheless, the 2.5 mg dose was chosen to be tested in phase III trials. Unlike enoxaparin for which the dose approved for ACS is 3–5 fold higher than that used for VTE prophylaxis, the dose of fondaparinux that is under investigation in the ongoing phase III trials in ACS is the same as that used in VTE prophylaxis.

Fondaparinux has also been assessed in a small pilot study in conventional balloon coronary angioplasty [75]. In this study, fondaparinux was administered as 12 mg IV bolus prior to angioplasty. Two of the 61 patients experienced acute vessel closure, the primary endpoint (3.3%; 95% CI 0.4 to 11.4%). No major bleeding occurred in this small sample. More recently, fondaparinux has also been evaluated as an alternative to heparin in patients undergoing percutaneous coronary intervention (PCI). The recently completed ASPIRE pilot study compared fondaparinux (either 2.5 mg or 5 mg IV) with UFH in 350 patients scheduled for PCI, including patients with NSTEMI and STEMI (primary PCI). The incidence of major and minor bleeding was 7.7% in the UFH group and 6.4% in the combined fondaparinux groups ($P = 0.61$). The bleeding rate was lower in the 2.5 mg fondaparinux group compared with the 5 mg fondaparinux group (3.4 vs. 9.6%; $P = 0.06$). The composite efficacy outcome of all-cause mortality, MI, urgent revascularisation, or need for a bailout glycoprotein IIb/IIIa antagonist was 6.0% in the UFH group and 6.0% in the fondaparinux group [76].

Two large phase III trials evaluating fondaparinux in ACS are currently ongoing. The OASIS-5 trial is an international, randomised, double-blind, double-dummy study evaluating the efficacy and safety of fondaparinux 2.5 mg once daily vs. enoxaparin 1.0 mg/kg bid in the treatment of non-ST-elevation acute coronary syndromes. The primary efficacy outcome endpoint is the occurrence of death, MI or refractory ischaemia up to day 9. The trial has recently completed the enrolment and the results were presented at the European Society of Cardiology Congress, 2005.

The OASIS-6 trial is an international randomised, double-blind, double-dummy trial designed to evaluate fondaparinux in a broad range of patients with STEMI, reperfused with either PCI or fibrinolytic therapy, or not eligible for reperfusion. Those eligible for reperfusion are randomised to either fondaparinux 2.5 mg or UFH. Those not eligible for reperfusion are randomised to either fondaparinux 2.5 mg or placebo. The primary efficacy endpoint is the first occurrence of death or recurrent MI up to day 9. Overall more than 20 000 patients will be enrolled in the OASIS-5 and -6 programs. The evaluation of fondaparinux in ACS and in PCI patients is still underway, therefore its use cannot be recommended in these settings at this time. Given the relatively long half-life of fondaparinux, management of arterial access for patients undergoing angiography, and appropriate timing of coronary artery bypass surgery for those patients who need it, will need to be addressed. Finally, given the effect of fondaparinux on thrombin generation, the role of potent antiplatelet therapy with clopidogrel or glycoprotein IIb/IIIa antagonists in conjunction with fondaparinux will need to be examined. Despite these potential issues, fondaparinux remains a promising alternative to current anticoagulants in ACS.

IDRAPARINUX

Idraparinux sodium (SANORG 34006, Sanofi-Aventis, Paris, France) is a synthetic, long-acting, highly sulfated analogue of fondaparinux. Like fondaparinux, it is a selective indirect fXa inhibitor [77].

The idraparinux affinity for AT is more than 10-fold higher than that of fondaparinux. The high affinity for AT probably explains its long plasma half-life. The plasma half-life is estimated at 80 h, close to the half-life of AT, based on data from animal models. Because of the long half-life, idraparinux can be given subcutaneously once a week [77].

The anti-fXa activity and inhibition of thrombin generation is dose dependent. Like fondaparinux, idraparinux has a limited effect on aPTT. In a clinical study on healthy subjects, aPTT was prolonged from 37.4 ± 3.8 sec to 46.5 ± 6.4 sec 2 h after the administration of idraparinux. The PT increased from 13.8 ± 0.9 sec at baseline to 15.4 ± 0.6 sec at 2 h [78].

Idraparinux showed a dose-dependent antithrombotic effect in animal thrombosis models and a lack of fibrinolytic properties, although it was able to enhance recombinant tissue-type plasminogen activator (rt-PA)-induced thrombolysis in a rabbit model [77].

rFVIIa, given both 3 h and one week after idraparinux, significantly reversed the effects of idraparinux on blood coagulation markers (increased thrombin generation time, prolongation of aPTT and PT, and reduction of prothrombin fragments 1 + 2 levels) [78].

Given the pharmacologic properties of idraparinux, this drug is being developed in long-term anticoagulation. In the phase-II PERSIST trial, 659 patients with established proximal DVT, after 5 to 7 days of enoxaparin treatment, were randomised to receive 2.5, 5.0, 7.5 or 10 mg of subcutaneous idraparinux once weekly, or warfarin (INR 2.0 to 3.0) for 12 weeks [79]. The primary efficacy outcome was the composite of change in thrombotic burden, as assessed by ultrasonography and perfusion lung scanning at baseline and at week 12 + 1, or symptomatic VTE. The primary outcome measure rates were similar in all idraparinux groups and did not differ from the warfarin group. However, there was a clear dose–response relationship for major bleeding among patients treated with idraparinux ($P = 0.003$). The 2.5 mg idraparinux group had a lower rate of combined minor and major bleeding than the warfarin group (2.3 vs. 8.3%, $P = 0.029$). Based on these results the 2.5 mg dose was chosen for phase III studies.

Currently, there are two phase III trials that will evaluate idraparinux in two different settings. The Van Gogh program comprises three phase III trials named Van Gogh PE, Van Gogh DVT, and Van Gogh Extension (EXT), which will compare idraparinux and oral VKA in long-term anticoagulation of patients with confirmed PE or DVT. The trials are designed to demonstrate that idraparinux is at least as effective as VKA. In both the Van Gogh PE and DVT, patients are randomised to receive either idraparinux or a VKA for 3–6 months. In the Van Gogh-EXT study, patients with previous PE or DVT, who completed 6 months of treatment with daily oral VKAs or once-weekly injections of idraparinux, receive either idraparinux or placebo for an additional 6 months.

AMADEUS (AF Trial of Monitored, Adjusted Dose VKA, Comparing Efficacy and Safety with Unadjusted SanOrg34006/idraparinux) is an ongoing trial enrolling patients with atrial fibrillation at high risk of stroke, with an indication for VKA. Patients are randomised to receive idraparinux 2.5 mg once weekly or VKA (INR 2.0–3.0) for 6–24 months.

Idraparinux is a potentially new advance in long-term anticoagulation, as an alternative to oral VKA, which is difficult to manage and can limit the quality of life of patients. The ongoing trials will give information about efficacy and safety of idraparinux. However, two issues can potentially affect the use of idraparinux. First, the repeated subcutaneous injections, in the long-term (from a few months to several years), may potentially cause local complications. Second, the very long duration of effect may be a major problem in case of bleeding complications or of urgent surgical intervention. Therefore, the clinical utility of idraparinux (even if its efficacy will be confirmed) could be potentially limited unless an effective and safe reversal agent becomes available.

DIRECT FACTOR Xa INHIBITORS

Direct fXa inhibitors act by direct binding and inhibition of fXa, without any cofactor, and blocking interaction between fXa and its substrates. A number of oral and parenteral direct fXa inhibitors are in various stages of development.

DX-9065A

DX-9065a (Daiichi Pharmaceutical, Tokyo, Japan) was the first of this family of drugs. DX-9065a is a small, non-peptidic molecule that specifically binds and neutralises fXa and exerts only a small effect on thrombin and other proteases [80, 81]. Unlike fondaparinux, DX-9065a also inhibits fXa bound into prothrombinase complex [82].

The antithrombotic effect of DX-9065a has been shown in animal models [82]. DX-9065a is largely eliminated by renal clearance without any evidence of a metabolic transformation [82, 83]. Although DX-9065a is orally bioavailable, its oral bioavailability is only 10–15%. Plasma half-life after an intravenous bolus is about 90 min [82].

Intravenous DX-9065a was tested in the XaNADU phase-Ib trial in 73 patients with stable coronary artery disease. Patients were randomly assigned to receive a fixed-dose of intravenous bolus, followed by a weight-adjusted infusion targeted to achieve four different plasma concentrations [84]. DX-9065a produced a dose-dependent increase in anti-Xa activity and PT. There was a strong correlation between DX-9065a concentration and anti-Xa level (Pearson correlation coefficient 0.97) and a weaker but still significant correlation between DX-9065a concentration and protime (0.77) and aPTT (0.56). Neither major bleeding nor significant changes of median haemoglobin, platelet count, and renal and hepatic function were observed.

Similar results were found in the XaNADU-PCI Pilot, where patients undergoing elective, native-vessel PCI were randomised in one of four sequential stages (4:1) to receive either a weight-adjusted double bolus and infusion dosing regimen of DX-9065a or UFH [85]. A fourth stage reinvestigated the DX-9065a regimen from the third stage, but in patients recently treated with UFH. Each stage enrolled a total of 56 patients. Plasma drug levels were predictable by dose and rapidly obtained. The significant correlation between DX-9065a and whole blood INR potentially makes this coagulation test useful to monitor therapies with DX-9065a. Ischaemic and bleeding events were rare and without a clear relationship with the dose.

XaNADU-ACS Trial is a phase II randomised trial that randomised 402 patients with non-ST-elevation ACS to either UFH (70 U/kg bolus, 15 U/kg/h infusion, target aPTT 50–85s), low dose of DX-9065a (0.025 mg/kg bolus, 0.04 mg/kg/h 3-h loading infusion, 0.012 mg/kg/h maintenance infusion) or high dose of DX-9065a (0.5 mg/kg bolus, 0.08 mg/kg/h 3-h loading infusion, 0.024 mg/kg/h maintenance infusion), in a double-blind, double-dummy fashion [86]. The primary efficacy endpoint was the composite of 30-day death, MI, urgent revascularisation, or ischaemia on continuous ST-segment monitoring. The main safety endpoint was TIMI major or minor bleeding. The primary efficacy endpoint occurred with equal frequency among patients in the DX-9065a high-dose group (31.3%), in the low-dose DX-9065a group (34.3%), and in the UFH-group (33.6%; $P = 0.91$; heparin vs. combined DX-9065a), however, there was a non-significant trend toward a lower rate of the composite of death, MI, or urgent revascularisation in the high dose of DX-9065a (11.9%) compared to low dose of DX-9065a (19.3%) and heparin (19.5%; $P = 0.125$ heparin vs. high-dose DX-9065a). The rate of TIMI major/minor bleeding was similar among the groups, but tended to be lower in patients treated with low dose of DX-9065a (4.2%, 7.0%, 7.7%, low and high dose of DX-9065a and UFH respectively; $P = 1.0$). The data of both XaNADU, PCI and ACS lay the foundations for adequately powered phase III trials, where higher doses seem to result in better efficacy but also more bleeding.

RAZAXABAN

Razaxaban (DPC-906, Bristol-Myers Squibb) is a synthetic, potent, direct selective inhibitor of fXa that is orally bioavailable. Razaxaban at the maximally effective antithrombotic dose moderately increased aPTT and PT (2.2 $\pm$ 0.1 and 2.3 $\pm$ 0.1 times control, respectively) [87]. It is orally well absorbed, reaching maximal concentration 1–6 h after administration and the steady state after 3–4 days. The maximal fXa inhibition was obtained with an oral dose of 200 mg followed by 100 mg twice daily [88].

Razaxaban has been compared with enoxaparin 30 mg twice daily, in a double-blind, phase II, dose-ranging trial enrolling 656 patients undergoing elective primary total knee replacement [89]. Patients were randomised to receive one of four doses of razaxaban: 25 mg, 50 mg, 75 mg, or 100 mg twice a day started 8 h after the end of surgery, or enoxaparin 30 mg twice a day started 12–24 h after the end of the surgery. The treatments were continued for 8–12 days and a mandatory bilateral venography was performed at the end of treatment. The primary efficacy outcome measure was a composite of asymptomatic DVT, symptomatic DVT, and PE during the treatment period. The three highest doses of razaxaban were stopped because of increased rate of major bleeding, mainly at the surgical site (0.7%, 4.1%, 3.5%, 5.8% and 0% for 25 mg, 50 mg, 75 mg, 100 mg and enoxaparin, respectively). A clear dose–response effect was seen on the efficacy endpoint. The rate of the primary efficacy endpoint was 8.6% in the razaxaban 25 mg group and 15.9% in the enoxaparin group.

SUMMARY

The inhibition of fXa is a promising alternative approach to targeting thrombin in the development of novel antithrombotics. Fondaparinux is the most extensively studied fXa inhibitor. It has been widely evaluated in the VTE prophylaxis of patients undergoing high-risk orthopaedic surgery. In this setting fondaparinux has received FDA approval and the recent ACCP guidelines have recommended its use as an alternative to LMWH and oral VKA in this setting. The current evidence from phase III trials suggested the superiority of fondaparinux on the surrogate endpoint of venographically detected DVT compared to enoxaparin, but with a significant increase of bleeding. This limitation is noteworthy in post-surgical patients, in particular since it is not counterbalanced by an improvement in clinically relevant outcomes.

In the two MATISSE trials, fondaparinux was also effective and safe in the treatment of symptomatic VTE and remains a reasonable alternative to UFH and LMWH.

The use of fondaparinux in arterial thrombosis is still under investigation. Initial results are promising but the results of the two large phase III randomised clinical trials, OASIS-5 and OASIS-6, will determine the role of this agent in patients presenting with coronary thrombosis.

A number of oral and parenteral, direct, selective fXa inhibitors, including DX-9065a and Razaxaban, are under investigation and may represent attractive alternatives to current antithrombotics.

REFERENCES

1. Koller F. History of factor X. *Thromb Diath Haemorrh* 1960; 4(suppl):58–65.
2. Telfer TP, Denson KW, Wright DR. A new coagulation defect. *Br J Haematol* 1956; 2:308–316.
3. Hougie C, Barrow EM, Graham JB. Stuart clotting defect. I. Segregation of an hereditary hemorrhagic state from the heterogeneous group heretofore called stable factor (SPCA, proconvertin, factor VII) deficiency. *J Clin Invest* 1957; 36:485–496.
4. Cooper DN *et al*. Inherited factor X deficiency: molecular genetics and pathophysiology. *Thromb Haemost* 1997; 78:161–172.
5. Mann KG, Butenas S, Brummel K. The dynamics of thrombin formation. *Arterioscler Thromb Vasc Biol* 2003. 23:17–25.
6. Hirsh J. Low-Molecular-Weight Heparin: A Review of the Results of Recent Studies of the Treatment of Venous Thromboembolism and Unstable Angina. *Circulation* 1998; 98:1575–1582.
7. Wong GC, Giugliano RP, Antman EM. Use of low-molecular-weight heparins in the management of acute coronary artery syndromes and percutaneous coronary intervention. *JAMA* 2003; 289:331–342.
8. Walenga JM *et al*. Biochemical and pharmacologic rationale for the development of synthetic heparin pentasaccharide. *Thrombosis Research* 1997; 86:1–36.
9. Thunberg L, Backstrom G, Lindahl U. Further characterisation of the antithrombin-binding sequence in heparin. *Carbohydr Res* 1982; 100:393–410.
10. Choay J *et al*. Structure-activity relationship in heparin: a synthetic pentasaccharide with high affinity for antithrombin III and eliciting high anti-factor Xa activity. *Biochem Biophys Res Commun* 1983; 116:492–499.
11. Petitou M *et al*. Binding of heparin to antithrombin III: a chemical proof of the critical role played by a 3-sulfated 2-amino-2-deoxy-D-glucose residue. *Carbohydr Res* 1988; 179:163–172.
12. Lindahl U, Backstrom G, Thunberg L. The antithrombin-binding sequence in heparin. Identification of an essential 6-O-sulfate group. *J Biol Chem* 1983; 258:9826–9830.
13. Petitou M *et al*. Synthesis of heparin fragments. A chemical synthesis of the pentasaccharide O-(2-deoxy-2-sulfamido-6-O-sulfo-alpha-D-glucopyranosyl)-(1–4)-O-(beta-D-glucopyranosyluronic acid)-(1–4)-O-(2-deoxy-2-sulfamido-3 6-di-O-sulfo-alpha-D-glu copyranosyl)-(1–4)-O-(2-O-sulfo-alpha-L-idopyranosyluronic acid)-(1–4)-2-deoxy-2-sulfamido-6-O-sulfo-D-glucopyranose decasodium salt, a heparin fragment having high affinity for antithrombin III. *Carbohydr Res* 1986; 147:221–236.
14. Paolucci F *et al*. Fondaparinux sodium mechanism of action: identification of specific binding to purified and human plasma-derived proteins. *Clin Pharmacokinet* 2002; 41(suppl 2):11–18.
15. Holmer E, Kurachi K, Soderstrom G. The molecular-weight dependence of the rate-enhancing effect of heparin on the inhibition of thrombin, factor Xa, factor IXa, factor XIa, factor XIIa and kallikrein by antithrombin. *Biochem J* 1981; 193:395–400.
16. Zitoun D *et al*. Plasma TFPI activity after intravenous injection of pentasaccharide (PS) and unfractionated heparin in rabbits. *Thromb Res* 1994; 75:577–580.
17. Olson ST *et al*. Role of the antithrombin-binding pentasaccharide in heparin acceleration of antithrombin-proteinase reactions. Resolution of the antithrombin conformational change contribution to heparin rate enhancement. *J Biol Chem* 1992; 267:12528–12538.
18. Gettins P, Choay J. Examination, by 1H-n.m.r. spectroscopy, of the binding of a synthetic, high-affinity heparin pentasaccharide to human antithrombin III. *Carbohydr Res* 1989; 185:69–76.
19. Bauer KA. New pentasaccharides for prophylaxis of deep vein thrombosis: pharmacology. *Chest* 2003; 124(suppl 6):364S–370S.
20. Boneu B *et al*. Pharmacokinetics and tolerance of the natural pentasaccharide (SR90107/Org31540) with high affinity to antithrombin III in man. *Thromb Haemost* 1995; 74:1468–1473.
21. Walenga JM *et al*. Functionality of pentasaccharide depends on endogenous antithrombin levels. *Blood* 2000; 96:817a (abstract).
22. Walenga JM *et al*. The inhibition of the generation of thrombin and the antithrombotic effect of a pentasaccharide with sole anti-factor Xa activity. *Thromb Res* 1988; 51:23–33.
23. Lormeau JC, Herault JP. Comparative inhibition of extrinsic and intrinsic thrombin generation by standard heparin, a low molecular weight heparin and the synthetic ATIII-binding pentasaccharide. *Thromb Haemost* 1993; 69:152–176.
24. Lormeau JC, Herault JP. The effect of the synthetic pentasaccharide SR 90107/ORG 31540 on thrombin generation *ex vivo* is uniquely due to ATIII-mediated neutralisation of factor Xa. *Thromb Haemost* 1995; 74:1474–1477.

25. Beguin S, Choay J, Hemker HC. The action of a synthetic pentasaccharide on thrombin generation in whole plasma. *Thromb Haemost* 1989; 61:397–401.
26. Bijsterveld NR *et al.* Ability of recombinant factor VIIa to reverse the anticoagulant effect of the pentasaccharide fondaparinux in healthy volunteers. *Circulation* 2002; 106:2550–2554.
27. Herault JP *et al.* Comparative effects of two direct and indirect factor Xa inhibitors on free and clot-bound prothrombinase. *J Pharmacol Exp Ther* 1997; 283:16–22.
28. Walenga JM, Fareed J. Preliminary biochemical and pharmacologic studies on a chemically synthesized pentasaccharide. *Semin Thromb Hemost* 1985; 11:89–99.
29. Walenga JM *et al.* Intravenous antithrombotic activity of a synthetic heparin pentasaccharide in a human serum induced stasis thrombosis model. *Thromb Res* 1986; 43:243–248.
30. Walenga JM *et al.* Antithrombotic activity of a synthetic heparin pentasaccharide in a rabbit stasis thrombosis model using different thrombogenic challenges. *Thromb Res* 1987; 46:187–198.
31. Amar J *et al.* Antithrombotic potencies of heparins in relation to their antifactor Xa and antithrombin activities: an experimental study in two models of thrombosis in the rabbit. *Br J Haematol* 1990; 76:94–100.
32. Hobbelen PM *et al.* Pharmacological profile of the chemically synthesized antithrombin III binding fragment of heparin (pentasaccharide) in rats. *Thromb Haemost* 1990; 63:265–270.
33. Carrie D *et al.* Pharmacokinetic and antithrombotic properties of two pentasaccharides with high affinity to antithrombin III in the rabbit: comparison with CY216. *Blood* 1994; 84:2571–2577.
34. Vogel GM *et al.* Pentasaccharide and Orgaran arrest, whereas heparin delays thrombus formation in a rat arteriovenous shunt. *Thromb Haemost* 1993; 69:29–34.
35. Vogel GM *et al.* Two new closely related rat models with relevance to arterial thrombosis – efficacies of different antithrombotic drugs. *Thromb Haemost* 1997; 77:183–189.
36. Bernat A *et al.* The synthetic pentasaccharide SR 90107A/Org 31540 enhances tissue-type plasminogen activator-induced thrombolysis in rabbits. *Fibrinolysis* 1996; 10:191–197.
37. Donat F *et al.* The pharmacokinetics of fondaparinux sodium in healthy volunteers. *Clin Pharmacokinet* 2002; 41(suppl 2):1–9.
38. http://www.fda.gov/cder/foi/nda/2001/21–345_Arixtra_prntlbl.pdf.
39. http://www.fda.gov/cder/foi/nda/2001/21–345_Arixtra_biopharmr.pdf.
40. Ollier C *et al.* Absence of interaction of fondaparinux sodium with aspirin and piroxicam in healthy male volunteers. *Clin Pharmacokinet* 2002; 41(suppl 2):31–37.
41. Mant T *et al.* Absence of interaction of fondaparinux sodium with digoxin in healthy volunteers. *Clin Pharmacokinet* 2002; 41(suppl 2):39–45.
42. Faaij RA *et al.* Absence of an interaction between the synthetic pentasaccharide fondaparinux and oral warfarin. *Br J Clin Pharmacol* 2002; 54:304–308.
43. Faaij RA *et al.* The synthetic pentasaccharide fondaparinux sodium does not interact with oral warfarin. *Clin Pharmacokinet* 2002; 41(suppl 2):27–29.
44. Lagrange F *et al.* Fondaparinux sodium does not cross the placental barrier: study using the *in vitro* human dually perfused cotyledon model. *Clin Pharmacokinet* 2002; 41(suppl 2):47–49.
45. Ahmad S *et al.* Synthetic pentasaccharides do not cause platelet activation by antiheparin-platelet factor 4 antibodies. *Clin Appl Thromb Hemost* 1999; 5:259–266.
46. Elalamy I *et al.* Absence of *in vitro* cross-reaction of pentasaccharide with the plasma heparin-dependent factor of twenty-five patients with heparin-associated thrombocytopenia. *Thromb Haemost* 1995; 74:1384–1385.
47. Jeske WP *et al.* Heparin-induced thrombocytopenic potential of GAG and non-GAG-based antithrombotic agents. *Clin Appl Thromb Hemost* 1999; 5(suppl 1):S56–S62.
48. Granger CB. CATCH Registry: Oral Communication. American Heart Association Scientific Session 2004.
49. Hirsh J *et al.* Heparin and low-molecular-weight heparin: mechanisms of action, pharmacokinetics, dosing, monitoring, efficacy, and safety. *Chest* 2001; 119(suppl 1):64S–94S.
50. Matziolis G *et al.* Effects of fondaparinux compared with dalteparin, enoxaparin and unfractionated heparin on human osteoblasts. *Calcif Tissue Int* 2003; 73:370–379.
51. Massonnet-Castel S *et al.* Partial reversal of low molecular weight heparin (PK 10169) anti-Xa activity by protamine sulfate: *in vitro* and *in vivo* study during cardiac surgery with extracorporeal circulation. *Haemostasis* 1986; 16:139–146.
52. Erhardtsen E *et al.* The effect of recombinant factor VIIa (NovoSeven) in healthy volunteers receiving acenocoumarol to an International Normalised Ratio above 2.0. *Blood Coagul Fibrinolysis* 1998; 9:741–748.

53. Friederich PW *et al*. Ability of recombinant factor VIIa to generate thrombin during inhibition of tissue factor in human subjects. *Circulation* 2001; 103:2555–2559.

54. Holm M, Andreasen R, Ingerslev J. Management of bleeding using recombinant factor VIIa in a patient suffering from bleeding tendency due to a lupus anticoagulant-hypoprothrombinemia syndrome. *Thromb Haemost* 1999; 82:1776–1778.

55. Meijer K *et al*. Successful treatment of massive hemoptysis in acute leukemia with recombinant factor VIIa. *Arch Intern Med* 2000; 160:2216–2217.

56. Arkin S *et al*. Human coagulation factor FVIIa (recombinant) in the management of limb-threatening bleeds unresponsive to alternative therapies: results from the NovoSeven emergency-use programme in patients with severe haemophilia or with acquired inhibitors. *Blood Coagul Fibrinolysis* 2000; 11:255–259.

57. Tarantino MD, Aberle R. Recombinant factor VIIa (NovoSeven) for post-prostatectomy hemorrhage in a patient with type I von Willebrand disease. *Am J Hematol* 2001; 68:62–63.

58. Geerts WH *et al*. Prevention of venous thromboembolism: the Seventh ACCP Conference on Antithrombotic and Thrombolytic Therapy. *Chest* 2004; 126(suppl 3):338S–400S.

59. Turpie AG, Gallus AS, Hoek JA. A synthetic pentasaccharide for the prevention of deep-vein thrombosis after total hip replacement. *N Engl J Med* 2001; 344:619–625.

60. Lassen MR *et al*. Postoperative fondaparinux versus preoperative enoxaparin for prevention of venous thromboembolism in elective hip-replacement surgery: a randomised double-blind comparison. *Lancet* 2002; 359:1715–1720.

61. Turpie AG *et al*. Postoperative fondaparinux versus postoperative enoxaparin for prevention of venous thromboembolism after elective hip-replacement surgery: a randomised double-blind trial. *Lancet* 2002; 359:1721–1726.

62. Eriksson BI *et al*. Fondaparinux compared with enoxaparin for the prevention of venous thromboembolism after hip-fracture surgery. *N Engl J Med* 2001; 345:1298–1304.

63. Bauer KA *et al*. Fondaparinux compared with enoxaparin for the prevention of venous thromboembolism after elective major knee surgery. *N Engl J Med* 2001; 345:1305–1310.

64. Turpie AG *et al*. Fondaparinux vs enoxaparin for the prevention of venous thromboembolism in major orthopedic surgery: a meta-analysis of 4 randomised double-blind studies. *Arch Intern Med* 2002; 162:1833–1840.

65. Lowe GD, Sandercock PA, Rosendaal FR. Prevention of venous thromboembolism after major orthopaedic surgery: is fondaparinux an advance? *Lancet* 2003; 362:504–505.

66. Turpie AG *et al*. Superiority of fondaparinux over enoxaparin in preventing venous thromboembolism in major orthopedic surgery using different efficacy endpoints. *Chest* 2004; 126:501–508.

67. Eriksson BI, Lassen MR. Duration of prophylaxis against venous thromboembolism with fondaparinux after hip fracture surgery: a multicenter, randomised, placebo-controlled, double-blind study. *Arch Intern Med* 2003 163:1337–1342.

68. Agnelli G *et al*. A randomised double-blind study to compare the efficacy and safety of fondaparinux with dalteparin in the prevention of venous thromboembolism after high-risk abdominal surgery: the Pegasus study. *J Thromb Haemost* 2003; 1(suppl 1):OC396.

69. Cohen AT *et al*. Fondaparinux vs. placebo for the prevention of venous thromboembolism in acutely ill medical patients (artemis). *J Thromb Haemost* 2003; 1(suppl 1):P2046.

70. Treatment of Proximal Deep Vein Thrombosis With a Novel Synthetic Compound (SR90107A/ORG31540) With Pure Anti-Factor Xa Activity: A Phase II Evaluation. *Circulation* 2000; 102:2726–2731.

71. Buller HR *et al*. Subcutaneous fondaparinux versus intravenous unfractionated heparin in the initial treatment of pulmonary embolism. *N Engl J Med* 2003; 349:1695–1702.

72. Buller HR *et al*. Fondaparinux or Enoxaparin for the Initial Treatment of Symptomatic Deep Venous Thrombosis: A Randomised Trial. *Ann Intern Med* 2004; 140:867–873.

73. Coussement PK *et al*. A synthetic factor-Xa inhibitor (ORG31540/SR9017A) as an adjunct to fibrinolysis in acute myocardial infarction. The PENTALYSE study. *Eur Heart J* 2001; 22:1716–1724.

74. Simoons ML *et al*. A dose-finding study of fondaparinux in patients with non-ST-segment elevation acute coronary syndromes: the Pentasaccharide in Unstable Angina (PENTUA) Study. *J Am Coll Cardiol* 2004; 43:2183–2190.

75. Vuillemenot A *et al*. Efficacy of a synthetic pentasaccharide, a pure factor Xa inhibitor, as an antithrombotic agent – a pilot study in the setting of coronary angioplasty. *Thromb Haemost* 1999; 81:214–220.

76. Mehta SR *et al*. Randomised, Blinded Trial Comparing Fondaparinux With Unfractionated Heparin in Patients Undergoing Contemporary Percutaneous Coronary Intervention: Arixtra Study in

Percutaneous Coronary Intervention: A Randomised Evaluation (ASPIRE) Pilot Trial. *Circulation* 2005; 111:1390–1397.

77. Herbert JM *et al.* Biochemical and pharmacological properties of SANORG 34006, a potent and long-acting synthetic pentasaccharide. *Blood* 1998; 91:4197–4205.

78. Bijsterveld NR *et al.* Recombinant factor VIIa reverses the anticoagulant effect of the long-acting pentasaccharide idraparinux in healthy volunteers. *Br J Haematol* 2004; 124:653–658.

79. A novel long-acting synthetic factor Xa inhibitor (SanOrg34006) to replace warfarin for secondary prevention in deep vein thrombosis. A Phase II evaluation. *J Thromb Haemost* 2004; 2:47–53.

80. Yamazaki M *et al.* Effects of DX-9065a, an orally active, newly synthesized and specific inhibitor of factor Xa, against experimental disseminated intravascular coagulation in rats. *Thromb Haemost* 1994; 72:392–396.

81. Herbert JM *et al.* DX 9065A a novel, synthetic, selective and orally active inhibitor of factor Xa: *in vitro* and *in vivo* studies. *J Pharmacol Exp Ther* 1996; 276:1030–1038.

82. Samama MM. Synthetic direct and indirect factor Xa inhibitors. *Thromb Res* 2002; 106:V267–V273.

83. Murayama N *et al.* Pharmacokinetics of the anticoagulant 14C-DX-9065a in the healthy male volunteer after a single intravenous dose. *Xenobiotica* 2000; 30:515–521.

84. Dyke CK *et al.* First experience with direct factor Xa inhibition in patients with stable coronary disease: a pharmacokinetic and pharmacodynamic evaluation. *Circulation* 2002; 105:2385–2391.

85. Alexander JH *et al.* Initial experience with factor-Xa inhibition in percutaneous coronary intervention: the XaNADU-PCI Pilot. *J Thromb Haemost* 2004; 2:234–241.

86. Alexander JH *et al.* First experience with direct, selective factor Xa inhibition in patients with non-ST-elevation acute coronary syndromes: results of the XaNADU-ACS Trial. *J Thromb Haemost* 2005; 3:439–447.

87. Wong PC *et al.* Antithrombotic Effects of Razaxaban, an Orally-Active Factor Xa Inhibitor, in Rabbit Models of Thrombosis. *Blood* 2003; 102:(abstract 3011).

88. Swaminathan A *et al.* Pharmacokinetic and pharmacodynamic characteristics in healthy volunteers of razaxaban, an orally-active, potent, selective inhibitor of Factor Xa. *Clin Pharmacol Ther* 2004; 75:P1–142,2004; 75:(abstract PI–12).

89. Lassen MR *et al.* A Phase II Randomised, Double-Blind, Five-Arm, Parallel-Group, Dose-Response Study of a New Oral Directly-Acting Factor Xa Inhibitor, Razaxaban, for the Prevention of Deep Vein Thrombosis in Knee Replacement Surgery – on Behalf of the Razaxaban Investigators. *Blood* 2003; 102:(abstract 41).

9

Direct thrombin inhibition – thromboprophylaxis, deep venous thrombosis, atrial fibrillation and coronary artery disease

S. Husted, L. C. Wallentin

INTRODUCTION

Until recently, anticoagulant treatment has been based on three classes of agents: unfractionated heparin (UFH), low-molecular-weight heparins (LMWH) and vitamin K antagonists (VKA). The heparins and VKA are effective drugs, but they have limitations. They are not selective, they are acting on a broad range of substances in the coagulation cascade, and heparins are a heterogenous mixture of different molecules purified from animal tissues with a variable antithrombotic activity.

The controversies concerning the use of UFH and LMWH, which are produced by chemical or enzymatic degradation of UFH, stem from the complex mechanism of action and structural heterogeneity. VKA has a well-defined mechanism of action, but the clinical use of these drugs is difficult because of inter- and intraindividual variation in response and numerous potential interactions with other drugs and food.

New molecules have been designed in order to be more selective in their target and more homogenous in their structure, thereby improving efficacy and safety of anticoagulant treatment.

A better understanding of the molecular mechanism underlying blood coagulation, advances in biotechnology and the isolation and characterisation of anticoagulant proteins from blood sucking organisms (such as leeches and ticks), as well as improvements in structure-based drug design have contributed to the development of new anticoagulant agents. These new agents have different targets in the coagulation cascade inhibiting the first stage in coagulation (tissue factor (TF), factor VIIa, Factor IXa), thrombin generation (Xa) and fibrin formation (thrombin) (Figure 9.1). The agents may be indirect coagulation inhibitors (heparins and synthetic pentasaccharides) acting by enhancing the inhibitory activity of antithrombin (AT) or direct inhibitors (recombinant hirudin, bivalirudin, argatroban, melagatran, dabigatran), which act directly on the target serine protease.

THROMBIN INTERACTION WITH DIRECT THROMBIN INHIBITORS

Thrombin is a trypsin-like serine protease and has many biological roles. It is procoagulant by hydrolyzing fibrinogen factors V, VIII, XI, XIII and the platelet protease activated

Steen Husted, Head of Department, University Department of Medicine-Cardiology, Aarhus Hospital, Aarhus, Denmark.

Lars C. Wallentin, Professor of Cardiology, University Hospital, Uppsala, Sweden.

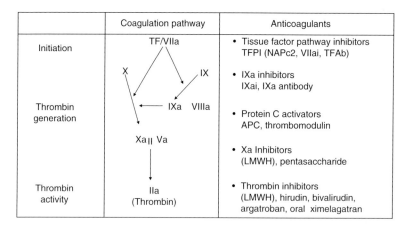

	Coagulation pathway	Anticoagulants

Initiation	TF/VIIa
	
	X IX
		• Tissue factor pathway inhibitors
		  TFPI (NAPc2, VIIai, TFAb)
		
		• IXa inhibitors
		  IXai, IXa antibody

Thrombin
generation
	IXa VIIIa
	
	Xa॥ Va
		• Protein C activators
		  APC, thrombomodulin
		
		• Xa Inhibitors
		  (LMWH), pentasaccharide

Thrombin
activity
	IIa
	(Thrombin)
		• Thrombin inhibitors
		  (LMWH), hirudin, bivalirudin,
		  argatroban, oral ximelagatran

Figure 9.1 New anticoagulants already established in the clinic or under development.

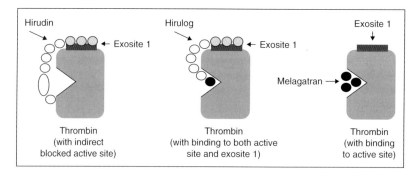

Figure 9.2 Site of action of the direct thrombin inhibitors. Adapted with permission from Lafkovits. *Circulation* 1994; **90**: 1522–1536.

receptors (PAR). Thrombin is the link between coagulation and fibrinolysis. Thrombin regulates after binding to thrombomodulin (TM) fibrinolysis via the zymogene activation of thrombin activatable fibrinolysis inhibitor (TAFI) [1]. The thrombin-TM complex has a dual role as it can also activate protein C, which in the presence of protein S, inhibits factors Va and VIIIa.

Thrombin's exquisite substrate specificity derives from surface binding sites (e.g., exosite 1) that are specific for its substrates (Figure 9.2). UFH and LMWH indirectly inhibit thrombin by catalyzing AT, which covalently binds to the active site of thrombin.

In contrast, the direct thrombin inhibitors (DTI) inhibit thrombin directly binding to exosite 1 and/or the active site of thrombin. The DTIs have potential advantages over heparin. Unlike heparin they produce a predictable anticoagulant response, because they exhibit minimal binding to plasma proteins. Furthermore, they do not bind platelet factor 4 and, thus, do not crossreact with autoantibodies that cause heparin-induced thrombocytopaenia (HIT). DTIs inhibit fibrin-bound thrombin as well as fluid-phase thrombin. There is no food interaction and the potential for drug–drug interaction is very low.

Table 9.1 Pharmacology of direct thrombin inhibitors (DTI)

DTI	Valence	Mol. weight (Daltons)	Half-life	Excretion
Lepirudin	Bivalent#	698	60–80 min (IV)	Renal
Desirudin			120 min (SC)	
Bivalirudin	Bivalent#	218	25 min	Non renal non hepatic
Argatroban	Univalent*	527	45 min	Biliary secretion
Melagatran	Univalent*	430	2–3 h	Renal
Ximelagatran	Univalent*	474	3–5 h	Renal
Dabigatran	Univalent*	–	14–17 h	Renal

Active site and exocite 1; *active site, non-covalent; IV = intravenous; SC = subcutaneous

Finally, the therapeutic window of the oral DTI's (e.g., ximelagatran and dabigatran etexilate) is so broad that routine laboratory monitoring and dose adjustment are not necessary.

DTIs have also potential disadvantages as there is no specific antidote for rapid reversal of their anticoagulant effect. In animal models, activated prothrombin complex concentrates (e.g., Feiba®, Autoplex®) are effective in reducing blood loss associated with high plasma DTI concentrations, as does recombinant activated factor VII (Novoseven®).

PHARMACOLOGY OF DIRECT THROMBIN INHIBITORS (TABLE 9.1)

RECOMBINANT HIRUDIN

A 65-amino acid polypeptide originally isolated from the medical leech, Hirudin inhibits thrombin in a bivalent fashion interacting both with the active site and exosite 1 (Figure 9.2). The hirudin/thrombin 1:1 stoichiometric complex is essentially irreversible.

Hirudins (e.g., lepirudin and desirudin) must be administered parenterally and have a half-life of 60 min after intravenous (IV) injection and 120 min after subcutaneous injection (SC). Elimination is renal. Lepirudin is used for anticoagulation in patients with HIT. The therapeutic window is narrow and the anticoagulant effect must be monitored and dose adjusted to maintain the activated partial thromboplastin time (aPTT) within the therapeutic range (aPTT ratio of 1.5–2.0). There is not a linear relation between plasma hirudin concentration and aPTT, and at higher hirudin doses the ecarin clotting time (ECT) is used.

BIVALIRUDIN

Bivalirudin (hirulog) is a synthetic analogue of hirudin with 20 amino acids. It has an NH_2-terminal D-Phe-Pro-Arg-Pro sequence, which binds to the active site of thrombin and four Gly residues link this sequence to a carboxy-terminal dodecapeptide that interacts with exosite 1 [2]. However, once bound, thrombin cleaves the Pro-Arg bond within the NH_2-terminal of bivalirudin, thereby allowing the recovery of thrombin activity. Bivalirudin must be administered parenterally and has a half-life of 25 min. Elimination is via degradation by endogenous peptidases and only a small fraction is excreted via the kidneys. It is administered intravenously in a weight-adjusted bolus dose followed by a continuous weigh-adjusted infusion. It is used as an alternative to UFH in patients undergoing percutaneous coronary intervention (PCI) and the anticoagulant effect is monitored using the activated clotting time (ACT) with a target of about 350 s. Bivalirudin seems to be safer than hirudin because of the reversible thrombin binding and shorter half-life.

ARGATROBAN

Argatroban is a synthetic, competitive inhibitor that binds noncovalently to the active site of thrombin. Its plasma half-life is 45 min and it is metabolised in the liver. It is used intravenously in patients with HIT and therapy is monitored by aPTT with a target aPTT ratio of 1.5–3.0.

XIMELAGATRAN (MELAGATRAN)

Ximelagatran is a prodrug of the active site thrombin inhibitor melagatran (Figure 9.2) [3]. Ximelagatran is absorbed from the small intestine with an absorption fraction of 20% and is rapidly transformed to melagatran, which has a half-life of about 4 h. Melagatran has a poor oral availability and must be administred subcutaneously. About 80% of melagatran is excreted via the kidneys.

Ximelagatran is administered orally twice daily and no food or drug interactions have been documented. Based on the predictable anticoagulant response routine monitoring is not necessary. Of patients treated with ximelagatran about 7.6% develop an increase in alanine aminotransferase (ALAT) that is usually asymptomatic and reversible, whether or not treatment is continued. Ximelagatran has been tested in numerous phase trials in orthopaedic surgery, venous thromboembolism, and atrial fibrillation.

DABIGATRAN ETEXILATE (DABIGATRAN)

Dabigatran etexilate is an orally administered prodrug that is converted to the thrombin inhibitor, dabigatran. The half-life of dabigatran is 14–17 h, which might allow for a once daily dosing. Elimination is primarily renal. Phase 3 trials in orthopedic surgery, venous thromboembolism and atrial fibrillation are ongoing.

CLINICAL TRIALS

VENOUS THROMBOEMBOLISM PROPHYLAXIS

Desirudin, bivalirudin, melagatran/ximelagatran and ximelagatran alone have been tested in fixed doses without laboratory monitoring in venous thromboembolism (VTE) prophylaxis in elective total hip replacement (THR) and/or total knee replacement (TKR). Endpoints in all studies were symptomatic VTE and DVT detected by routine venography. In a phase III trial, desirudin SC was evaluated against routine SC treatment with enoxaparin in THR, and the desirudin group had the lowest incidence of VTE with no increase in bleeding complications [4].

Ximelagatran
The efficacy and safety of ximelagatran/melagatran in preventing VTE after major orthopaedic surgery of the lower limbs has been studied in a large phase II and phase III clinical program including at least 14 000 patients (Table 9.2).

Despite this extensive clinical program, the optimal dosage regimen of ximelagatran/melagatran in preventing VTE after TKR or THR remains uncertain. Two different approaches have been used in Europe and North America. The European studies used both the SC form melagatran and the oral form ximelagatran, whereas in the North American studies only the oral form was used, initiated in the morning after surgery. SC melagatran was initiated either at the 'time of surgery', defined as 'knife-to-skin' (Melagatran for Thrombin Inhibition in Orthopaedic Surgery II [METHRO II] and Expanded Prophylaxis Evaluation Surgery Study Conclusion [EXPRESS]) or between 4 and 12 h after surgery (METHRO III), at the dose of 3 mg (METHRO II and III) or 2 mg (EXPRESS) and followed

Table 9.2A Ximelagatran *versus* low-molecular-weight heparin (LMWH) or warfarin in the prevention of venous thromboembolism (VTE)

Surgery	Variable	Ximelagatran BID				LMWH or Warfarin
TKR	Dose (mg)	8	12	18	24	Enoxaparin 30 mg BID
(n=600)	Overall VTE (%)	27.0	19.8	28.7	15.8	22.7
	Proximal DVT (%)	6.6	2.0	5.8	3.2	3.1
	Major bleeding (%)	0	0	2.4	0	0.8
THR	Dose (mg)	24				Enoxaparin 30 mg BID
(n=1838)	Overall VTE (%)	7.9				4.6
	Proximal DVT (%)	3.6				1.2
	Major bleeding (%)	0.8				0.9
TKR	Dose (mg)	24				Warfarin INR 2.5, range 1.8-3.0
(n=680)	Overall VTE (%)	19.2				25.7
	Proximal DVT (%)	3.3				5.2
	Major bleeding (%)	1.7				0.9
TKR	Dose (mg)	24				Warfarin INR 2.5, range 1.8-3.0
(n=2301)	Overall VTE (%)	24.9				27.6
EXULT	Proximal DVT (%)	2.5				4.1
	Major bleeding (%)	4.8				4.5

TKR = Total knee replacement; THR = total hip replacement

Table 9.2B Melagatran/ximelagatran *versus* low-molecular-weight heparin (LMWH) in the prevention of venous thromboembolism (VTE)

Surgery	Variable	Melagatran SC/ximelagatran PO BID				LMWH
TKR or THR	Dose (mg/mg)	1/8	1.5/12	2.25/18	3/24	Dalteparin 5000 IU QD
(n=1900)	Overall VTE (%)	37.8	24.1	23.7	15.1	28.2
METHRO II	Proximal DVT (%)	8.5	6.2	3.3	2.1	5.5
	Major bleeding (%)	0.8	1.2	3.5	5.5	2.3
TKR or THR	Dose (mg/mg)	3/24				Enoxaparin 40 mg QD
(n=2788)	Overall VTE (%)	31.0				27.3
METHRO III	Proximal DVT (%)	5.7				6.2
	Major bleeding (%)	1.4				1.7
TKR or THR	Dose (mg/mg)	2/3(M)/24(X)				Enoxaparin 40 mg QD
(n=2764)	Overall VTE (%)	20.3				26.7
EXPRESS	Proximal DVT (%)	2.3				6.3
	Major bleeding (%)	3.3				1.2

TKR = Total knee replacement; THR = total hip replacement

by ximelagatran [5–7]. Ximelagatran was administered in all studies twice daily at the dose of 24 mg, starting within the second postoperative day. In the METHRO III study [6], in which melagatran was initiated subcutaneously between 4 and 12 h after surgery, ximelagatran/melegatran tended to be less effective than enoxaparin 40 mg QD ($P = 0.052$) in preventing total VTE with no difference in major bleeding. In the EXPRESS study [7] in which 2 mg melagatran was initiated 'knife-to-skin', followed by 3 mg 4–12 h postoperatively, ximelagatran/melagatran was significantly more effective than enoxaparin ($P < 0.001$) but with a significant increase in bleeding (Table 9.2; $P < 0.05$).

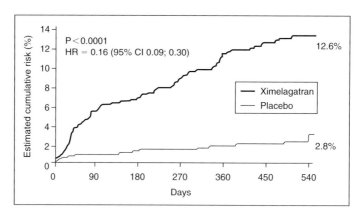

Figure 9.3 The THRIVE III study. Effect of ximelagatran against placebo on recurrent venous thromboembolic (VTE) events (intention to treat analysis = ITT).

In a North American TKR dose-finding study [8], ximelagatran 24 mg BID was as effective and safe as enoxaparin 30 mg BID SC, while a similar study in THR showed less effectivity of ximelagatran [9]. In TKR (PLATINUM Knee and Exanta Used to Lessen Thrombosis A [EXULT A] studies) ximelagatran 24 mg BID was at least as effective as warfarin [10, 11], and with ximelagatran 36 mg BID in the EXULT A [11], and EXULT B [12] studies, ximelagatran was more effective ($P < 0.001$) than warfarin in preventing VTE and/or death. There was a trend to an increased bleeding risk in the ximelagatran treated patients [10, 12].

TREATMENT OF ACUTE VENOUS THROMBOEMBOLISM

Only one phase II trial has evaluated recombinant hirudin for the initial treatment of VTE [13]. Hirudin was administered at different weight-based dosage levels SC BID and was tested against adjusted dose IV UFH; no difference in the rates of VTE progression/regression after 5 days of treatment was seen.

Ximelagatran

Two major phase III VTE treatment trials with a fixed oral dose of ximelagatran without laboratory monitoring or dose adjustment have been performed [14, 15]. The Thrombin Inhibitor in Venous Thromboembolism (THRIVE) study is a blinded, placebo-controlled trial randomising 2489 patients with VTE to ximelagatran 36 mg BID for 6 months or enoxaparin 1 mg/kg SC BID followed by warfarin (international normalised ratio [INR] 2–3) for 6 months [14]. After 6 months the cumulative incidence of recurrent objectively verified VTE was 2% in the warfarin group and 2.1% in the ximelagatran group. Major bleeding was 2.2% and 1.3%, respectively ($P =$ NS), and all-cause mortality 3.4% and 2.3% ($P =$ NS).

In THRIVE III, 1233 VTE patients, who had previously been treated for 6 months with warfarin, were randomised to receive ximelagatran 24 mg BID or placebo for an additional 18 months [15]. Recurrent VTE occurred in twelve patients in the ximelagatran group and 71 in the placebo group (hazard ratio 0.16; 95% CI: 0.09–0.30; $P < 0.001$) (Figure 9.3). All-case mortality, major and minor bleeding rates did not differ significantly between the groups. A rise in ALAT was seen in 6.4% and 1.2%, respectively. For Dabigatran etexilate, major phase III trials with similar design and once daily dosing are planned. No trial has tested efficacy and safety of oral DTI against warfarin in long-term secondary prophylaxis beyond 6 months of treatment in VTE patients.

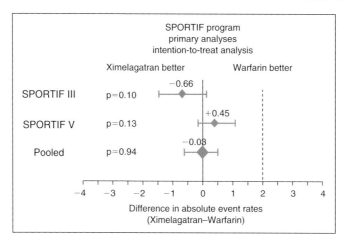

Figure 9.4 The SPORTIF III and V studies. Effect of ximelagatran against warfarin (INR 2.0–3.0) on cerebral and systemic embolic events.

ATRIAL FIBRILLATION

VKA is the routine treatment for stroke prevention in patient with atrial fibrillation (AF) and has been shown to reduce the risk by two-thirds in a number of major clinical trials. However, the management of VKA therapy is cumbersome and the treatment has a high risk of bleeding complications in daily practice. Therefore, it is used in only half the AF patients who are candidates for anticoagulation.

Dabigatran etexilate has been tested in a phase II dose-finding trial, and a phase III trial with Dabigatran etexilate against warfarin is now planned.

Ximelagatran

Two phase III trials have evaluated ximelagatran against warfarin for stroke prevention in patients with nonvalvular AF and at least one additional risk factor [16, 17]. The Stroke Prevention using an Oral Direct Thrombin Inhibitor in Atrial Fibrillation (SPORTIF) III trial, which used an open-label design, was conducted in Europe [16], whereas the blinded SPORTIF V trial was conducted in North America [17].

The SPORTIF III trial randomised 3410 AF patients to receive ximelagatran 36 mg BID or warfarin (INR 2–3) for 12 to 36 (mean 17.4) months. Stroke and systemic arterial embolism rates were 2.3% and 1.6% per year for ximelagatran and warfarin, respectively ($P = 0.10$). An on-treatment analysis showed fewer events in the ximelagatran group ($P = 0.018$). While rates for disabling or fatal stroke, mortality and major bleeding were similar, combined major and minor bleeding rates were significantly lower in the ximelagatran group (25.8% *vs.* 29.8% per year; $P = 0.007$).

SPORTIF V enrolled 3922 patients in a randomised, double-blind study. In the ximelagatran group receiving 36 mg BID event rate was 1.6% per year, and in the warfarin group (INR 2–3) event rate was 1.2% per year with a mean follow-up period of 20 months ($P = 0.13$). Overall mortality was the same. Rates of major bleeding were 3.1% per year and 2.4% per year with warfarin and ximelagatran, respectively ($P = $ NS), while total bleeding (major and minor) were 47% and 37%, respectively ($P < 0.001$). Increase in serum levels of ALAT occurred with ximelagatran in 6% of patients (0.8% with warfarin), typically within the first 6 months, and returned to baseline spontaneously or after stopping the drug.

The quality of warfarin therapy was very good in both trials with 81% and 83% of the measured INR within the range 1.8–3.2.

When the results of SPORTIF III and SPORTIF V are combined, ximelagatran was associated with a 0.3% absolute risk reduction in the rate of stroke and systemic embolism relative to warfarin ($P = 0.94$) (Figure 9.4) and a 0.6% reduction in the rate of major haemorrhage ($P = 0.05$).

The results of the SPORTIF trials indicate that the efficacies of ximelagatran and warfarin in preventing arterial emboli in patients with nonvalvular AF are comparable, and total bleeding events were somewhat lower with ximelagatran.

ACUTE CORONARY SYNDROMES

Acute coronary syndromes (ACS) contain a spectrum of cardiac disorders of increasing severity, from unstable angina pectoris (UAP) through non-ST-elevation myocardial infarction (NSTEMI) and ST-elevation myocardial infarction (STEMI). These disorders are pathophysiologically linked to intracoronary thrombus formation that causes complete or partial occlusion of the artery, imparing the supply of blood to the heart. Given the key roles of thrombin generation and platelet activation in the pathophysiology of ACS, antithrombotic treatment strategies commonly target one or both of these elements using anticoagulants and/or antiplatelet agents. Recurrent events after myocardial infarction (MI) are common owing to persistent activation of platelets and the coagulation cascade for several weeks to months after a coronary event [18]. Antithrombotic treatment, therefore, needs to be appropriate for use in the long-term management of ACS.

Recombinant hirudin and bivalirudin
Recombinant hirudin for 72 h has been compared against UFH in patients with UAP and NSTEMI in the major Organisation to Assess Strategies for Ischaemic Syndromes (OASIS)-2 trial randomising 10 141 patients [19]. Hirudin significantly reduced the incidence of death and MI at 7 days but the significance was not observed at 35 days. Risk of major bleedings was increased during hirudin treatment as compared to UFH. A major trial, Acute Catheterization and Urgent Intervention Triage Strategy (ACUITY) comparing bivalirudin with heparin is now ongoing in these patients.

Recombinant hirudin was tested against UFH adjunct to thrombolytic therapy in two major trials, the GUSTO-IIB trial [20] and the TIMI 9B trial [21]. Taken together, these trials suggest that hirudin therapy is at least as effective as UFH when used as an adjunct to thrombolytic therapy. The bleeding risk during hirudin and UFH therapy was similar in both trials. Given the lack of a clear benefit hirudin has not been licensed for this indication. The Hirulog and Early Reperfusion or Occlusion (HERO)-2 randomised trial [22] compared the benefits of UFH and bivalirudin in STEMI patients treated with streptokinase. The two treatments exhibited similar efficacy for the primary endpoint 30-day mortality. However, there were significantly fewer reinfarctions within 96 h in the bivalirudin group compared to the UFH group, with no significant increase in severe or intracerebral bleeding.

Ximelagatran
In the phase II Efficacy and Safety of the Oral Direct Thrombin Inhibitor Ximelagatran in Patients with Recent Myocardial Damage (ESTEEM) trial, 1883 patients with documented STEMI or NSTEMI within the past 14 days were randomised to ximelagatran 24, 36, 48 or 60 mg BID or placebo for 6 months as secondary prevention [23]. Routine therapy included aspirin 160 mg daily.

Ximelagatran significantly reduced the cumulative risk for cardiovascular death, MI, ischaemic stroke and severe recurrent ischaemia from 16.3% to 12.7% compared to placebo ($P = 0.036$; Figure 9.5). There was no dose-response relationship for the reduction of

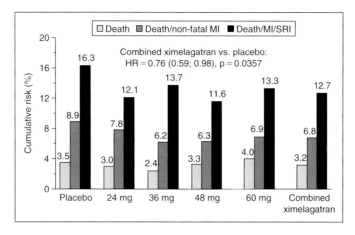

Figure 9.5 The ESTEEM study. Dose-related effect of ximelagatran against placebo on the combined endpoint of death, non-fatal myocardial infarction (MI) and severe refractory ischaemia (SRI).

coronary events. Major bleeding was not significantly increased in the individual or combined ximelagatran groups relative to placebo.

In agreement with previous studies, transient elevated ALAT levels were detected after 2 to 6 months, peaked after 60 to 120 days, and then returned to normal, irrespective of whether the patient continued or stopped treatment. Elevation of ALAT in this study was dose-dependent.

PERCUTANEOUS CORONARY INTERVENTION

Bivalirudin has been tested in a major phase III study (Randomized Evaluation in PCI Linking Angiomax to Reduced Clinical Events [REPLACE]-2) against UFH in 6010 low-to moderate-risk patients undergoing elective PCI [24]. All patients in the heparin group received a glycoprotein IIb/IIIa inhibitor (eptifibatide or abciximab), while it was provisional in the bivalirudin group. There was no difference in the composite endpoint of death, MI or urgent revascularization, but the rate of major bleeding was significantly lower in patients treated with bivalirudin than in those treated with heparin (2.4% and 4.1%, respectively; $P < 0.001$).

CONCLUSIONS

Routine thromboprophylaxis in high-risk orthopaedic patients is LMWH during hospitalisation. Though several clinical trials have indicated a need for a more extended prophylaxis in these patients, this strategy is not generally accepted partly because of the need of parenteral drug administration. An oral anticoagulant that does not need monitoring would be optimal for this purpose and ongoing studies will demonstrate whether ximelagatran will be useful for this indication.

In patients with unprovoked VTE or in high-risk patients with cancer and important thrombophilia, such as antiphospholipid antibodies, long-term anticoagulation is of benefit. However, the benefit of warfarin treatment may be offset in part by bleeding risk and a careful management of therapy with close monitoring of INR is needed to ensure an acceptable quality of treatment.

Promising results have been obtained by ximelagatran in long-term secondary prophylaxis of VTE patients with no need of monitoring, but studies comparing efficacy and safety against warfarin therapy are still needed. In VTE treatment ximelagatran has been shown to be as effective and safe as enoxaparin/warfarin, and may be an alternative to the routine anticoagulant therapy for this indication. When used in this setting there will be a need of measuring liver enzymes for at least 6 months during ongoing therapy.

Further major studies in VTE patients with another oral DTI, Dabigatran etexilate, are planned.

The risk of cerebral and systemic embolism in patients with AF is high and increases with age, and when one or more risk factors like hypertension, diabetes mellitus, previous stroke, congestive heart failure etc. are present. VKA effectively reduces this risk, but the use of VKA is problematic, especially in the elderly with the highest prevalence of AF. It is estimated that only half of the eligible AF patients receive anticoagulant therapy.

Ximelagatran therapy is as effective as warfarin in these patients and the risk of major and minor bleeding is lower. With no need for coagulation monitoring, ximelagatran is more convenient than warfarin and this feature may increase the use of anticoagulant therapy in high-risk AF patients. During long-term therapy with ximelagatran, there will be a need of measuring liver enzymes for at least 6 months.

Major studies in AF patients with the oral DTI Dabigatran etexilate are planned.

In patients with ACS an intense antithrombotic therapy with antiplatelet drugs and anticoagulants is indicated, and many patients are treated with acute/early revascularization. Long-term thrombosis prophylaxis to reduce the risk of death, recurrent ischaemic coronary events and stroke is indicated, and often aspirin in combination with clopidogrel is used. In addition, long-term warfarin therapy has been shown to be effective, but the risks and benefits from a combined therapy with warfarin and the two antiplatelet drugs are unknown.

Ximelagatran combined with aspirin following MI has shown to be more effective than aspirin alone in preventing recurrent ischaemic events without an increase in bleeding risk. Further studies are needed to evaluate the role of oral DTI following MI in the modern era of antiplatelet and revascularization therapy.

Revascularization, especially PCI, are increasingly used in modern cardiology, both electively in stable patients and acute/early in ACS patients. The optimal antithrombotic treatment regimen during PCI is still controversial, but recent studies with bivalirudin in low-to moderate-risk patients indicate that this DTI may be used as an alternative to routine therapy with UFH and a glycoprotein IIb/IIIa inhibitor. However, the efficacy and safety of DTIs in high-risk patients remains to be settled.

REFERENCES

1. Bajzar L, Manuel R, Nesheim ME. Purification an characterization of TAFI, a thrombin activatable fibrinolysis inhibitor. *J Biol Chem* 1995; 270:144777–144784.
2. Maraganore JM, Bourdon P, Jablonski J *et al*. Design and characterization of hirologs: a novel class of bivalent peptide inhibitors of thrombin. *J Clin Invest* 1990; 29:7095–7101.
3. Gustafsson D, Nyström JE, Carlsson S *et al*. The direct thrombin inhibitor melagatran and its oral prodrug H376795: intestinal absorption properties, biochemical and pharmacodynamic effects. *Thromb Res* 2001; 101:171–181.
4. Eriksson BI, Wille-Jørgensen P, Kälebo P *et al*. A comparison of recombinant hirudin with a low-molecular-weight heparin to prevent thromboembolic complications after total hip replacement. *N Engl J Med* 1997; 337:1329–1335.
5. Eriksson BI, Bergqvist D, Kärlebo P, *et al*. Ximelagatran and melagatran compared with dalteparin for prevention of venous thromboembolism after total hip or knee replacement: the METHRO II randomised trial. *Lancet* 2002; 360:1441–1447.
6. Eriksson BI, Agnelli GA, Cohen AT *et al*. Direct thrombin inhibitor melagatran followed by oral ximelagatran in comparison with enoxaparin for prevention of venous thromboembolism after total hip or knee replacement. The METHRO III Study Group. *Thromb Haemost* 2003; 89:288–296.

7. Eriksson BI, Agnelli GA, Cohen AT *et al*. The direct thrombin inhibitor melagatran followed by oral ximelagatran compared with enoxaparin for the prevention of venous thromboembolism after total hip or knee replacement: The EXPRESS Study Group. *J Thromb Haemost* 2003; 1:2490–2496.

8. Heit JA, Colwell CW Jr, Francis CW *et al*. Comparison of the oral direct thrombin inhibitor ximelagatran with enoxaparin as prophylaxis against venous thromboembolism after total knee replacement: a phase 2 dose-finding study. *Arch Int Med* 2001; 161:2215–2221.

9. Collwell CW, Berkowitz SD, Davidson BL *et al*. Comparison of ximelagatran, an oral direct thrombin inhibitor, with enoxaparin for the prevention of venous thromboemb olism following total hip replacement. A randomized, double-blind study. *J Thromb Haemost* 2003; 1:2119–2130.

10. Francis CW, Davidson BL, Berkowitz SD *et al*. Ximelagatran *versus* warfarin for the prevention of venous thromboembolism after total knee arthroplasty. A randomized double-bind trial. *Ann Intern Med* 2002; 137:648–655.

11. Francis CW, Berkowitz SD, Comp PC *et al*. Comparison of ximelagatran and warfarin for the prevention of venous thromboembolism after total knee replacement. *N Engl J Med* 2003; 349:1703–1712.

12. Colwell CW, Berkowitz SD, Comp PC *et al*. Randomized double-blind comparison of ximelagatran, an oral direct thrombin inhibitor, and warfarin to prevent venous thromboembolism after total knee replacement: *EXULT B. Blood* 2003; 102:Abstract 39.

13. Schiele F, Lindgaerde F, Eriksson H *et al*. Subcutaneous recombinant hirudin (HBW 023) *versus* intravenous sodim heparin in treatment of established acute deep vein thrombosis of the legs: a multicentre prospective dose-ranging randomized trial. *Thromb Haemost* 1997; 77:834–838.

14. Fiessinger J-N, Huisman MV, Davidson BL *et al*. for the THRIVE Treatment Study Investigators. Ximelagatran vs low-molecular-weight heparin and warfarin for the treatment of deep vein thrombsis: a randomized trial. *JAMA* 2005; 293:681–689.

15. Schulman S, Wåhlander K, Lundström T *et al*. Secondary prevention of venous thromboembolism with the oral direct thrombin inhibitor ximelagatra. *N Engl J Med* 2003; 349:1713–1721.

16. Olsson SB; Executive steering Committee on behalf of the SPORTIF III Investigators. Stroke prevention with the oral direct thrombin inhibitor ximelagatran compared with warfarin in patients with non-valvular atrial fibrillation (SPORTIF III); randomized controlled trial. *Lancet* 2003; 362:1691–1698.

17. Sportif Executive Steering Committee for the SPORTIF V Investigators. Ximelagatran vs warfarin for stroke prevention in patients with nonvalvular atrial fibrillation: a randomized trial. *JAMA* 2005; 293:298.

18. Merlini PA, Bauer KA, Oltrona L *et al*. Persistent activation of coagulation mechanism in unstable angina and myocardial infarction. *Circulation* 1994; 90:61–68.

19. Organisation to Assess Strategies for Ischemic Syndromes (OASIS-2) Investigators. Effects of recombinant hirudin (lepirudin) compared with heparin on death, myocardial infarction, refractory angina, and revascularization procedures in patients with acute myocardial ischaemia without ST-elevation: a randomised trial. *Lancet* 1999; 353:429–438.

20. The Global Use of Strategies to Open Occluded Coronary Arteries (GUSTO) IIb Investigators. A comparison of recombinant hirudin with heparin for the treatment of acute coronary syndromes. *N Engl J Med* 1996; 335:775–782.

21. Antman EM, for the TIMI 9B Investigators. Hirudin in acute myocardial infarction. Thrombolysis and thrombin inhibition in myocardial infarction (TIMI) 9B trial. *Circulation* 1996; 94:911–921.

22. White H. Thrombin-specific anticoagulation with bivalirudin versus heparin in patients receiving fibrinolytic therapy for acute myocardial infarction: the HERO-2 randomised trial. *Lancet* 2001; 358:1855–1863.

23. Wallentin L, Wilcox RG, Weaver WD *et al*. Oral ximelagatran for secondary prophylaxis after myocardial infarction; the ESTEEM randomised controlled trial. *Lancet* 2003; 362:789–797.

24. Lincoff AM, Bittl JA, Harrington RA *et al*. Bivalirudin and provisional GPIIb/IIIa blockade compared with heparin and planned GPIIb/IIIa blockade during percutaneous coronary intervention: REPLACE-2 randomised trial. *JAMA* 2003; 289:853–863.

10

Warfarin after acute myocardial infarction

F. W. A. Verheugt, M. A. Brouwer

INTRODUCTION

Early angiographic observations in the seventies have shown that most cases of acute trans-mural myocardial infarction (MI) are caused by an occlusion of a major epicardial coronary artery [1]. Since the introduction of intracoronary fibrinolytic therapy for acute MI it became clear that the nature of this occlusion is thrombotic [2]. It also became clear that after lytic therapy many coronary stenoses that had produced acute occlusion probably may not have been very severe to start with [3]. From these observations the hypothesis emanated that coronary thrombosis is an acute phenomenon and may occur on not very tight coronary stenoses (Figure 10.1). From histopathology it became clear that rupture of a lipid-laden coronary plaque may initiate acute coronary thrombosis [4]. Three types of coronary throm-bosis in acute coronary syndromes (ACS) have been distinguished: occlusive, non-occlusive and dispersive coronary thrombosis. Occlusive coronary thrombosis usually causes ST-elevation myocardial infarction (STEMI) with Q-wave formation. Non-occlusive throm-bosis is most seen in non-ST-segment elevation ACS without Q-wave formation, and may or may not lead to myocardial necrosis: the former being a non-Q-wave MI and the latter unstable angina pectoris. Dispersive thrombosis has been observed downstream of a rup-tured atherosclerotic plaque in patients with sudden cardiac death, apparently resulting in malignant electric instability.

The cause of plaque rupture remains unclear. Interestingly, a circadian variation is observed in the occurrence of acute MI [5]. The incidence of arterial thrombosis peaks in the early morning hours leading to an increased incidence of acute MI, malignant ventricular arrhythmia, sudden cardiac death and stroke. The mechanisms involved in the circadian variation may be two-fold: in the early part of the day, beta-adrenergic stimulation is more pronounced than in the other parts of the day, and there is also hypercoagulability of the blood and hyperreactivity of the platelets in the morning hours [6]. Possibly, the combina-tion of increased vascular tone, blood pressure and hypercoagulability may precipitate arte-rial thrombosis.

Fibrinolytic therapy has become standard therapy in most cases of acute ST-segment ele-vation coronary syndromes. Fibrinolytic therapy is easy to administer in most institutions, where patients with acute ST-elevation coronary syndromes are presented. The costs are moderate and the benefit is marked, especially in very early, and preferably, pre-hospital

Freek W. A. Verheugt, Professor of Cardiology, Heartcenter, Department of Cardiology, Nijmegen, The Netherlands.

M. A. Brouwer, Heartcenter, Department of Cardiology, Nijmegen, The Netherlands.

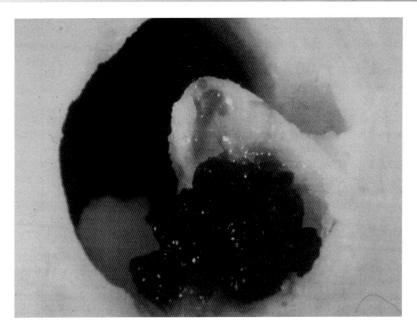

Figure 10.1 Coronary thrombosis on a ruptured atherosclerotic plaque.

treatment. Fibrinolysis can be improved by adjuvant antiplatelet therapy like aspirin and, very likely, also by anticoagulant treatment. The alternative to fibrinolysis is primary balloon angioplasty (with or without stenting) of the infarct artery. This therapy has been shown to be superior to fibrinolysis [7], but has logistic drawbacks, such as transport to a tertiary center.

Current anticoagulant therapy in MI can be divided in parenteral and oral treatment. Parenteral therapy is mainly aimed at thrombin inhibition, and oral treatment at inhibition of the formation of coagulation factors involved in the generation and propagation of coronary thrombosis.

ANTITHROMBIN THERAPY IN ACUTE MYOCARDIAL INFARCTION

Since fibrinolytic therapy is accompanied by intensive thrombin generation and activation, immediate and continuous adjunctive therapy with intravenous unfractionated heparin (UFH) is recommended [8]. Heparin is thought to block the thrombin activity observed in acute coronary thrombosis and counteract thrombin generated by the fibrinolytic treatment. The paradoxical pro-coagulant state induced by fibrinolytic therapy is considered responsible for the occurrence of coronary re-occlusion [9], although neither angiographic nor clinical benefit of heparin against re-occlusion has ever been firmly established [8, 9]. Heparin therapy needs close monitoring using repeated measurements of the activated partial thromboplastin time (aPTT) to provide efficacy and safety. In any case, heparin increases bleeding, in particular cerebral bleeding, after lytic therapy [8]. Lowering the dose of heparin results in reduction of intracranial haemorrhage without loss of clinical efficacy [10]. The recommended dose in the current guidelines is a bolus of 60 U/kg to a maximum of 4000 U followed by a continuous infusion 12 U/kg/h for at least 48 h with a target aPTT of 50–70 seconds, measured 3, 6, 12 and 24 h after first dose [11]. The maximum infusion dose is 1000 U/hour.

For these and other reasons direct thrombin inhibition has been studied extensively in patients undergoing fibrinolytic therapy for acute infarction. In two large clinical trials with over 20 000 patients hirudin showed only marginal improvement of mortality over heparin at the expense of increased bleeding [12, 13]. The same has been observed recently in a 12 000-patient trial with the less expensive, specific thrombin inhibitor hirulog [14].

Low-molecular-weight heparins (LMWH) have a better bioavailability, induce less platelet activation and can be given longer than UFH as the result of their subcutaneous administration. They have been tested in acute MI treated with fibrinolytic therapy against UFH in two relatively small angiographic trials [15, 16] and against placebo in one somewhat larger angiographic study [17]. Coronary patency is equivalent to UFH and re-occlusion seems less [16]. The specific Xa inhibitor pentasaccharide has also been tested in this setting (Table 2) [18]. In the PENTALYSE trial, re-occlusion was favourable with the agent (8% with the pentasaccharide vs. 18% with UFH; $P = 0.06$).

The angiographic trials on novel anticoagulant strategies in fibrinolysis were much too small for clinical conclusions on safety. In the large ASSENT-3 trial bolus enoxaparin (followed by subcutaneous injections twice daily until discharge) has been compared to UFH (bolus followed by infusion for at least 48 h) as adjunct to the bolus lytic agent TNK-tPA (tenecteplase) in over 4000 patients [19]. Enoxaparin turned out to be superior to UFH with regard to mortality, re-infarction and re-ischaemia with a 40% increase in severe, but not cerebral bleeding. However, in the recently presented ASSENT-3 PLUS study, in which patients were randomised pre-hospitally to bolus UFH (bolus followed by in-hospital infusion for at least 48 h) or bolus enoxaparin (followed by in-hospital subcutaneous injections twice daily) as adjunctive to TNK, cerebral bleeding was unacceptably increased by bolus enoxaparin [20].

Thus, current antithrombin therapy after fibrinolytic therapy seems to be optimal with UFH, which is given as a bolus together with the lytic (preferably TNK) and continued for at least 48 h. An alternative after the bolus UFH could be enoxaparin subcutaneously until hospital discharge. These recommendations originate from several randomised angiographic observations and two large clinical trials. Definite guidelines should be funded on more clinical data, especially those on safety. These issues will be studied in the giant EXTRACT-TIMI 25 clinical trial, where enoxaparin bolus and subcutaneous injections will be compared to UFH bolus plus infusion after lytic therapy either with alteplase, TNK, reteplase or streptokinase.

Also non-ST-elevation myocardial infarction (NSTEMI) should be treated with LMWH [11], although the evidence is not impressive.

The major drawback of both unfractionated and low-molecular-weight heparin is rebound activation of thrombosis [21]. This is the rationale for continuation of anticoagulation with oral anticoagulants after cessation of parenteral anticoagulants.

ORAL ANTICOAGULATION AFTER MYOCARDIAL INFARCTION

After MI oral anticoagulation has been tested extensively in the past three decades [22]. However, the combination of oral anticoagulation with the standard antiplatelet regimen after MI (aspirin) has only recently been evaluated [23]. Combining anticoagulants with aspirin has become more appealing, since the introduction of lower doses of aspirin (maximum 325 mg daily), and the newer insights with respect to the safety window of oral anticoagulation after the introduction of the international normalised ratio (INR). The benefit and risk of oral anticoagulants on top of aspirin vs. aspirin alone after MI are given in Tables 10.1 and 10.2.

Table 10.1 Randomised aspirin-controlled studies of warfarin plus aspirin after myocardial infarction

Study	Year	n	INR target	INR reached	Aspirin dose (mg)	Death/re-infarction Warfarin + aspirin	Aspirin	RR	P	F/U (months)
ATACS[24]	1994	214	2.0–3.0	2.3	163	4/105 (3.8%)	9/109 (8.3%)	0.46 (0.14–1.49)	0.22	3
CARS[25]	1997	8803	1 mg qd	1.1	80	173/2028 (8.6%)*	332/3393 (9.8%)	0.87 (0.73–1.04)	0.18	14
			3 mg qd	1.5	160	328/3382 (9.7%)		0.99 (0.90–1.09)	0.94	14
OASIS-2[26]	2001	3712	2.0–2.5	na	80	129/1848 (7.0%)***	137/1864 (7.4%)***	0.95 (0.75–1.20)	0.75	5
CHAMP[27]	2002	5059	1.5–2.5	1.9	na	778/2522 (30.9%)	771/2537 (30.4%)	1.02 (0.94–1.10)	0.82	33
APRICOT-2 [28]	2002	300	2.8–4.5	2.6	160/80**	4/153 (2.6%)	10/147 (6.8%)	0.41 (0.11–1.57)	0.17	3
ASPECT-2[29]	2002	668	2.8–4.8	2.4	80	19/332 (5.7%)	27/336 (8.0%)	0.71 (0.40–1.26)	0.34	12
WARIS-2[30]	2002	2414	2.8–4.2	2.2	160/75**	181/1208 (15.0%)	241/1206 (20.0%)	0.71 (0.58–0.86)	0.0005	48
LOWASA[32]	2004	3300	1.25 mg qd	na	75	466/1659 (28.1%)***	473/1641 (28.8%)***	0.98 (0.88–1.09)	0.67	60
Total		24 470				2082/13 237 (15.7%)	2000/11 233 (17.8%)	0.88 (0.84–0.93)		0.00001

*Estimate for 14 months follow-up; **the aspirin alone/combination groups; ***including stroke.
INR = international normalised ratio; RR = relative risk; F/U = follow-up; na = not available; P = P-value.

Table 10.2 Major bleeding in the randomised aspirin-controlled studies of warfarin plus aspirin after myocardial infarction

Study	Year	n	INR target	INR reached	Aspirin dose*	Major bleeding		RR	P	F/U (months)
						Warfarin + aspirin	Aspirin			
ATACS[24]	1994	214	2.0–3.0	2.3	163	3/105 (2.9%)	0/109 (0.0%)		0.24	3
CARS[25]	1997	8803	1 mg qd	1.1	80	31/2028 (1.5%)**	57/3393 (1.7%)	0.88 (0.57–1.36)	0.65	14
			3 mg qd	1.5	160	75/3382 (2.2%)		1.32 (0.93–1.84)	0.14	14
OASIS-2[26]	2001	3712	2.0–2.5	na	80	49/1848 (2.7%)	25/1864 (1.3%)	1.98 (1.24–3.17)	0.01	5
CHAMP[27]	2002	5059	1.5–2.5	1.9	na	86/2522 (3.4%)	48/2537 (1.9%)	1.80 (1.27–2.56)	0.001	33
APRICOT-2[28]	2002	300	2.8–4.5	2.6	160/80***	1/153 (0.6%)	0/147 (0.0%)	0.98	0.98	3
ASPECT-2[29]	2002	668	2.8–4.8	2.4	80	7/332 (2.1%)	3/336 (0.9%)	2.41 (0.63–9.24)	0.34	12
WARIS-2[30]	2002	2414	2.8–4.8	2.2	160/75***	28/1208 (2.3%)	8/1206 (0.7%)	3.49 (1.60–7.64)	0.001	48
LOWASA[32]	2004	3300	1.25 mg qd	na	na	36/1659 (2.2%)	16/1641 (1.0%)	2.23 (1.23–4.00)	0.006	60
Total		24 470				316/13 237 (2.4%)	157/11 233 (1.4%)	1.71 (1.41–2.07)	0.00001	

*Daily dose in milligrams; **estimate for 14 months follow-up; ***the aspirin alone/combination groups.
INR = international normalised ratio; RR = relative risk; na = not available; F/U = follow-up; P = P-value.

Oral anticoagulation on top of aspirin was found to be superior in the small ATACS study [24], in which 214 patients with unstable angina pectoris or NSTEMI were randomised to aspirin alone or to aspirin plus heparin followed by warfarin with a mean INR of 2.3. In the CARS trial [25] over 9000 patients early after MI were randomised to aspirin alone (daily dose 160 mg), or to aspirin (80 mg daily) combined with warfarin 1 or 3 mg daily (reached INR 1.1 and 1.5, respectively). After 1.2 years no differences were observed in death and recurrent MI.

In a large multinational trial (OASIS-2) with 3712 patients with unstable angina pectoris or NSTEMI, no specific benefit of oral anticoagulation on top of aspirin was found [26]. However, in the countries with good compliance (nearly 50% of patients had INR >2.0), death, infarction and stroke were reduced by more than 30%.

More or less the same results were seen after 2.5 years in the CHAMP study of >5000 patients [27], where the INR reached was 1.8. In that trial patients were randomised to aspirin alone (160 mg daily) or to aspirin (80 mg daily) plus warfarin, which was laboratory-monitored to an INR of 1.5–2.5.

Recently, two trials from the Netherlands on this topic have been published. The APRICOT-2 study [28] investigated the role of combined anticoagulant (median INR 2.6)/ antiplatelet therapy vs. aspirin alone (80 mg daily) after angiographically successful fibrinolytic therapy in over 300 patients with acute MI. So far, this is the only study with oral anticoagulation and aspirin vs. aspirin alone specifically in patients treated with fibrinolysis. The combined treatment reduced angiographic re-occlusion at 3 months from 28% with aspirin to 15% ($P < 0.02$). Also this trial was too small for the evaluation of clinical events: recurrent infarction and the need for revascularisation were about 50% less with the coumadin/aspirin combination and safety was excellent (only minor bleedings were doubled by coumadin plus aspirin). The ASPECT-2 trial [29] studied full intensity (mean INR 3.2) coumadin without aspirin, the combination coumadin (mean INR 2.4) and aspirin (80 mg daily), and aspirin (80 mg daily) alone in 993 patients randomised within 2 weeks after MI. About 50% of the patients had received fibrinolytic therapy in the acute phase. Death and re-infarction at 1 year were reduced from 8% in the aspirin alone group to 5.7% in the combination and coumadin alone groups ($P = 0.05$). Also in this trial bleeding was astonishingly low (1.8% major bleeding for the combination, for aspirin alone 0.9%). On the other hand both trials are far too small to be conclusive on safety issues.

The WARIS-2 trial carried out in Norway had 3600 patients who had survived MI, and compared aspirin (160 mg daily) alone with either full-intensity oral anticoagulation (target INR 2.8–4.2) alone or the combination of low-dose aspirin (75 mg daily) with medium-intensity oral anticoagulation (target INR 2.0–2.5). The results showed a 30% reduction of death, re-infarction and stroke with medium-intensity warfarin (mean INR 2.2) plus aspirin compared to aspirin alone [30].

None of the above trials specifically established the role of coumadin preceded by heparin in patients treated with fibrinolysis for acute MI except for the APRICOT-2 trial [26], which was especially designed to evaluate coronary re-occlusion. The only other, but small angiographic trial on the combination of warfarin plus aspirin vs. aspirin alone was done in a mixed patient population recovering from ACS, and found the same results [31]. The protective effect of coumadin against vessel re-occlusion corroborates well with the clinical benefit seen with LMWH in the angiographic studies [15–17] and clinical ASSENT-3 trial [19].

Recently, a post-MI study evaluated combined, fixed low dose of oral anticoagulation (1.25 mg warfarin daily) and antiplatelet therapy (aspirin 75 mg daily) in comparison to aspirin (75 mg daily) alone in 3300 patients in Sweden over 4 years. This regimen did not show clinical benefit of the combined treatment, but increased severe bleeding [32].

Thus, adding oral anticoagulants to antiplatelet therapy does not seem to show a benefit when the INR reached is below 2.0 (Table 10.3, Figure 10.2). Adequate anticoagulation

Table 10.3 Randomised aspirin-controlled studies of warfarin plus aspirin after myocardial infarction with reached INR <2.0

Study	Year	n	INR target	INR reached	Aspirin dose*	Death/re-infarction		RR	P	F/U (months)
						Warfarin + aspirin	Aspirin			
CARS[25]	1997	8803	1 mg qd	1.1	80	173/2028 (8.6%)**	332/3393 (9.8%)	0.87 (0.73–1.04)	0.18	14
			3 mg qd	1.5	160	328/3382 (9.7%)		0.99 (0.90–1.09)	0.94	14
OASIS-2[26]	2001	1891	2.0–2.5	<2.0	80	85/940 (9.0%)	74/1864 (7.8%)	1.17 (0.86–1.60)	0.33	5
CHAMP[27]	2002	5059	1.5–2.5	1.9	160/80***	778/2522 (30.9%)	771/2537 (30.4%)	1.02 (0.94–1.10)	0.82	33
LOWASA[32]	2004	3300	1.25 mg qd	na	75	446/1659 (28.1%)*	473/1641 (1.0%)*	0.98 (0.88–1.09)	0.67	60
Total		19 053				1810/10 531 (17.3%)	1650/9435 (19.4%)	0.90 (0.85–0.95)	0.0001	

*Including stroke; **estimate for 14 months follow-up; ***the aspirin alone/combination groups.
INR = international normalised ratio; RR = relative risk; F/U = follow-up; na = not available; P = P-value.

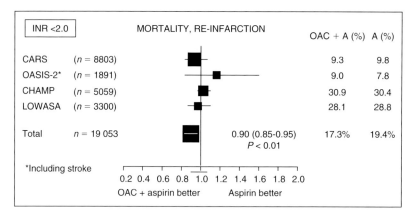

Figure 10.2 Meta-analysis of trials of oral anticoagulants plus aspirin vs. aspirin alone with a mean INR under 2.0 (see also Table 10.3).

with INRs over 2.0 improves angiographic and clinical outcome consistently (Table 10.4, Figure 10.3). Bleeding is significantly increased not only with INRs over 2.0 (Table 10.5), but also under 2.0 (Table 10.6). Cerebral haemorrhage, often considered the most dangerous complication of oral anticoagulants in combination with aspirin, is not significantly increased (Table 10.7), whereas ischaemic stroke is dramatically reduced by the combination of warfarin and aspirin.

Little is known about the cost-effectiveness of warfarin after MI. Does the benefit of warfarin outweigh its laboriousness and associated bleeding risk when compared to the simple and inexpensive aspirin alone therapy? In Italy the cost of warfarin monotherapy including monitoring and bleeding are similar to aspirin alone, suggesting a favourable cost-effectiveness for warfarin given the net clinical benefit of warfarin over aspirin [33].

ORAL ANTICOAGULANTS IN SPECIFIC SUB-GROUPS OF PATIENTS AFTER MYOCARDIAL INFARCTION

Warfarin is thought to be especially efficacious in post-MI patients with left ventricular dilatation and/or clinical heart failure [34], in those with left ventricular aneurysm, and those with atrial fibrillation complicating MI. None of the above trials have specifically evaluated the benefit in the above subgroups. Therefore, there is no evidence to support anticoagulants in these patients in the guidelines on MI.

There is no consensus on warfarin in heart failure in general. One of the unsolved issues is the suggested interaction of aspirin with angiotensin-converting enzyme (ACE) inhibitors, which is standard therapy in heart failure. Earlier observations have cast doubt on this relationship [35], but there has never been a large randomised trial with aspirin in heart failure patients on ACE inhibitors. The WATCH trial was recently presented and addressed the issues of the optimal antithrombotic strategy to prevent thromboembolism in patients with heart failure in sinus rhythm, as well as clinical interaction between aspirin and ACE inhibitors [36]. A total of 1587 patients with New York Heart Association class II–IV heart failure and a left ventricular ejection fraction of less than 35%, who were in sinus rhythm, were randomised between aspirin (162 mg daily), or clopidogrel (75 mg daily), or warfarin with a target INR between 2.5 and 3.0. The only significant outcome was that admission for heart failure was seen in 16.1% in patients on warfarin, 18.3% on clopidogrel

Table 10.4 Randomised aspirin-controlled studies of warfarin plus aspirin after myocardial infarction with reached INR >2.0

Study	Year	n	INR target	INR reached	Aspirin dose*	Death/re-infarction Warfarin + aspirin	Death/re-infarction Aspirin	RR	P	F/U (months)
ATACS[24]	1994	214	2.0–3.0	2.3	163	4/105 (3.8%)	9/109 (8.3%)	0.46 (0.14–1.49)	0.22	3
OASIS-2[26]	2001	1821	2.0–2.5	>2.0	na	55/908 (6.1%)*	81/913 (7.8%)*	0.68 (0.48–0.95)	0.01	5
APRICOT-2[28]	2002	300	2.8–4.5	2.6	80	4/153 (2.6%)	10/147 (6.8%)	0.41 (0.11–1.57)	0.17	3
ASPECT-2[29]	2002	668	2.8–4.8	2.4	80	19/332 (5.7%)	27/336 (8.0%)	0.71 (0.40–1.26)	0.34	12
WARIS-2[30]	2002	2414	2.8–4.2	2.2	160/75**	181/1208 (15.0%)	241/1206 (20.0%)	0.71 (0.58–0.86)	0.0005	48
Total		5417				263/2706 (9.7%)	368/2711 (13.6%)	0.72 (0.62–0.82)	0.0001	

*Including stroke; **aspirin alone/combination group.
INR = international normalised ratio; RR = relative risk; F/U = follow-up; na = not available; P = P-value.

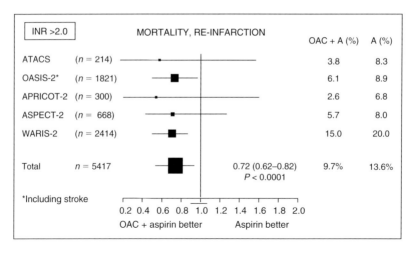

Figure 10.3 Meta-analysis of trials of oral anticoagulants plus aspirin versus aspirin alone with a mean INR over 2.0 (see also Table 10.4).

and in 22.2% in patients on aspirin (aspirin vs. warfarin $P < 0.01$). This strongly suggests that aspirin interacts with the beneficial effects of ACE inhibitors. The same was observed in the small randomised WASH trial [37], but could not be confirmed in a small substudy of the WARIS-2 trial [38]. In this respect, warfarin can be advised to heart failure patients on ACE inhibitors in general. It is likely that postinfarction patients with heart failure benefit from warfarin similarly.

Another substudy of warfarin after MI was carried out in patients with diabetes in the double-blind placebo-controlled WARIS-1 study on warfarin after MI [39]. It turned out that diabetics do not benefit from oral anticoagulation after MI, but it should be noted that this was a non-prespecified *post hoc* analysis. Thus, little is known of any interaction between diabetes and oral anticoagulation.

Finally, in postinfarction patients with a strong indication for oral anticoagulants like those with artificial heart valves and/or atrial fibrillation, warfarin should never be withheld [22].

FUTURE PERSPECTIVES

Although beneficial, oral anticoagulation is a laborious and potentially unsafe treatment. Self-management of oral anticoagulation is a major leap forward and may even improve overall quality of the therapy [40]. This approach, however, requires thorough patient instruction and will never be applicable in disabled or less cooperative patients.

Recently, an oral direct thrombin inhibitor ximelagatran, which lacks the need of monitoring, has been tested in post-MI patients and turned out to be effective with an acceptable bleeding profile [41]. However, up to 6% of patients experienced (transient) liver enzyme elevations, to the same extent as in two megatrials with the same agent in patients with atrial fibrillation [42]. Whether this will be the Achilles' heel of the agent, or just a cosmetic problem in analogy with the statins, remains to be established.

Finally, oral direct factor Xa inhibitors are on the horizon. These are currently tested in phase II trials in atrial fibrillation, but their appearance in the MI arena is likely in the future.

Table 10.5 Major bleeding in the randomised aspirin-controlled studies of warfarin plus aspirin after myocardial infarction with reached INR >2.0

| | | | | | Major bleeding | | | | |
Study	Year	n	INR target	INR reached	Aspirin dose*	Warfarin + aspirin	Aspirin	RR	P	F/U (months)
ATACS[24]	1994	214	2.0–3.0	2.3	163	3/105 (2.9%)	0/109 (0.0%)		0.24	3
OASIS-2[26]	2001	1821	2.0–2.5	>2.0	na	24/908 (2.6%)	9/913 (1.0%)	2.71 (1.26–5.83)	0.008	5
APRICOT-2[28]	2002	300	2.8–4.5	2.6	80	1/153 (0.6%)	0/147 (0.0%)		0.98	3
ASPECT-2[29]	2002	668	2.8–4.8	2.4	80	7/332 (2.1%)	3/336 (0.9%)	2.41 (0.63–9.24)	0.34	12
WARIS-2[30]	2002	2414	2.8–4.8	2.2	160/75**	28/1208 (2.3%)	8/1206 (0.7%)	3.49 (1.60–7.64)	0.001	48
Total		5417				63/2706 (2.3%)	20/2711 (0.7%)	3.15 (1.91–5.20)	0.0001	

*Daily dose in milligrams; **the aspirin alone/combination groups.
INR = international normalised ratio; RR = relative risk; F/U = follow-up; na = not available; P = P-value.

Table 10.6 Major bleeding in the randomised aspirin-controlled studies of warfarin plus aspirin after myocardial infarction with reached INR <2.0

Study	Year	n	INR target	INR reached	Aspirin dose*	Major bleeding — Warfarin + aspirin	Aspirin	RR	P	F/U (months)
CARS[25]	1997	8803	1 mg qd	1.1	80	31/2028 (1.5%)** 160	57/3393 (1.7%)	0.88 (0.57–1.36)	0.65	14
OASIS-2 [26]	2001	1891	3 mg qd	1.5	80	75/3382 (2.2%)	16/951 (1.6%)	1.32 (0.93–1.84)	0.14	14
			2.0–2.5	<2.0	na	25/940 (2.7%)		1.58 (0.84–3.00)	0.11	5
CHAMP[27]	2002	5059	1.5–2.5	1.9	160/80***	86/2522 (3.4%)	48/2537 (1.9%)	1.80 (1.27–2.56)	0.001	33
LOWASA [32]	2004	3300	1.25 mg qd	na	75	36/1659 (2.2%)	16/1641 (1.0%)	2.23 (1.23–4.00)	0.006	60
Total		19 053				253/10 531 (2.4%)	137/8522 (1.6%)	1.49 (1.22–1.84)	0.0001	

*Daily dose in milligrams; **estimate for 14 months follow-up; ***the aspirin alone/combination groups.
INR = international normalised ratio; RR = relative risk; F/U = follow-up; na = not available; P = P-value.

Table 10.7 Stroke and stroke types in six randomised aspirin-controlled studies of warfarin plus aspirin after myocardial infarction*

Stroke type	Warfarin + aspirin	Aspirin	RR	P
Ischaemic	131/7712 (1.7%)	199/7731 (2.6%)	0.65 (0.53–0.82)	0.0001
Haemorrhagic	35/7712 (0.5%)	25/7731 (0.3%)	1.40 (0.84–2.34)	0.24
Total	166/7712 (2.2%)	224/7731 (3.3%)	0.75 (0.61–0.90)	0.004

*From the six trials in this chapter (OASIS-2 [26], CHAMP [27], APRICOT-2 [28], ASPECT-2 [29], WARIS-2 [30] and LOWASA [32]), of which specific data on the nature of strokes which occurred are available. RR = relative risk.

SUMMARY

Anticoagulants are important to the acute treatment and probably also to the chronic phase of MI. Acutely, UFH is used widely for this purpose and does not seem to be inferior to specific thrombin inhibitors like hirudin and hirulog. So far, the best clinical results are obtained with LMWH, but its safety in association with fibrinolytic therapy is still a matter of debate. Furthermore, (low-molecular-weight) heparin shows a rebound phenomenon. The logical follow-up treatment after cessation of LMWH is oral anticoagulation. Warfarin in addition to aspirin is more effective after acute MI, when compared to aspirin alone. Important issues are timing and adequacy of the intensity of therapy. INRs below 2.0 do not lead to better outcomes following MI. The rate of bleeding is acceptable with combination therapy when lower doses of aspirin are used. Whether novel anticoagulant therapy is superior to warfarin after MI remains to be established.

REFERENCES

1. DeWood MA, Spores J, Notske R *et al*. Prevalence of total coronary occlusion during the early hours of transmural myocardial infarction. *N Engl J Med* 1980; 303:897–902.
2. Rentrop KP, Blanke H, Karsch KR *et al*. Acute myocardial infarction: intracoronary application of nitroglycerin and streptokinase. *Clin Cardiol* 1979; 2:354–363.
3. Serruys PW, Arnold AE, Brower RW *et al*. Effect of continued rt-PA admission on the residual stenosis after initially successful recanalization in acute myocardial infarction. A quantitative coronary angiography study of a randomized trial. *Eur Heart J* 1987; 8:1172–1181.
4. Davies MJ, Thomas AC. Thrombosis and acute coronary artery lesions in sudden cardiac ischemic death. *N Engl J Med* 1984; 310:1137–1140.
5. Willich SN, Linderer T, Wegschneider K, Leizorovicz A, Alamercery I, Schröder R. Increased morning incidence of myocardial infarction in the ISAM study: absence with prior β-adrenergic blockade. *Circulation* 1989; 80:853–858.
6. Andreotti F, Kluft C, Davies GJ, Huisman LG, De Bart AC, Maseri A. Effect of propranolol (long-acting) on the circadian fluctuation of tissue-plasminogen activator and plasminogen activator inhibitor-1. *Am J Cardiol* 1991; 68:1295–1299.
7. Keeley EC, Boura JA, Grines CL. Primary coronary angioplasty versus intravenous fibrinolytic therapy for acute myocardial infarction: a quantitative review of 23 randomised trials. *Lancet* 2003; 361:13–20.
8. Collins R, Peto R, Baigent C, Sleight P. Aspirin, heparin, and fibrinolytic therapy in acute myocardial infarction. *N Engl J Med* 1997; 336:847–860.

9.   Verheugt FWA, Meijer A, Lagrand WK, Van Eenige MJ. Reocclusion, the flipside of coronary
     thrombolysis. *J Am Coll Cardiol* 1996; 27:766–773.
10. Gugliano RP, McCabe CH, Antman EM *et al*. Lower-dose heparin with fibrinolysis is associated with
     lower rates of intracranial haemorrhage. *Am Heart J* 2001; 141:742–750.
11. Van de Werf F, Ardissino D, Betriu A *et al*. Management of acute myocardial infarction in patients
     presenting with ST-elevation. *Eur Heart J* 2003; 24:28–66.
12. GUSTO-IIb Investigators. A comparison of recombinant hirudin with heparin for the treatment of
     acute coronary syndromes. *N Engl J Med* 1996; 335:775–782.
13. OASIS-2 Investigators. Effects of recombinant hirudin (lepirudin) compared with heparin on death,
     myocardial infarction, refractory angina and revascularisation procedures in patients with acute
     myocardial ischemia without ST-elevation: randomised trial. *Lancet* 1999; 353:429–438.
14. HERO-2 Investigators. Thrombin-specific anticoagulation with bivalirudin versus heparin in patients
     receiving fibrinolytic therapy for acute myocardial infarction: the HERO-2 trial. *Lancet*
     2001; 358:1855–1863.
15. Wallentin L, Dellborg DM, Lindahl B, Nilsson T, Pehrsson K, Swahn E. The low-molecular-weight
     heparin dalteparin as adjuvant therapy in acute myocardial infarction: the ASSENT PLUS study. *Clin
     Cardiol* 2001; 24(suppl 1):12–14.
16. Ross AM, Molhoek P, Lundergan C *et al*. Randomised comparison of enoxaparin, a low molecular weight
     heparin, with unfractionated heparin adjunctive to tissue plasminogen activator thrombolysis and aspirin:
     second trial of Heparin and Aspirin Reperfusion Therapy (HART II). *Circulation* 2001; 104:648–652.
17. Simoons ML, Alonso A, Krzeminska-Pakula M *et al*. Early ST segment elevation resolution: predictor
     of outcome and angiographic patency in patients with acute myocardial infarction. Results of the
     AMI-SK study. *Eur Heart J* 2002; 23:1282–1290.
18. Coussement PK, Bassand JP, Convens C *et al*. A synthetic factor-Xa inhibitor (ORG13540/SR9017A) as
     an adjunct to fibrinolysis in acute myocardial infarction. The PENTALYSE-study. *Eur Heart J*
     2001; 22:1716–1724.
19. ASSENT-3 Investigators. Efficacy and safety of tenecteplase with enoxaparin, abciximab or unfractionated
     heparin: the ASSENT-3 randomised trial in acute myocardial infarction. *Lancet* 2001; 358:605–613.
20. Wallentin L, Goldstein P, Armstrong PW *et al*. Efficacy and safety of tenecteplase in combination
     with the low-molecular weight heparin enoxaparin, or unfractionated heparin in the pre-hospital
     setting: the ASSENT-3 PLUS randomized trial in acute myocardial infarction. *Circulation*
     2003; 108:135–142.
21. Bahit MC, Topol EJ, Califf RM *et al*. Reactivation of ischemic events in acute coronary syndromes:
     results from GUSTO-IIb. *J Am Coll Cardiol* 2001; 37:1001–1007.
22. Brouwer MA, Verheugt FWA. Oral anticoagulants in acute coronary syndromes. *Circulation*
     2002; 105:1270–1274.
23. Anand SS, Yusuf S. Oral anticoagulants in patients with coronary artery disease. *J Am Coll Cardiol*
     2003; 41(suppl S):62S–69S.
24. Cohen M, Adams PC, Parry G *et al*. Combination antithrombotic therapy in unstable rest angina and
     non-Q-wave infarction in nonprior aspirin users. Primary end-points analysis from the ATACS trial.
     Circulation 1994; 89:81–88.
25. Coumadin Aspirin Reinfarction Study (CARS) Investigators. Randomised double-blind trial of fixed
     low-dose warfarin with aspirin after myocardial infarction. *Lancet* 1997; 350:389–396.
26. The Organization to Assess Strategies for Ischemic Syndromes (OASIS-2) Investigators. Effects of long-
     term, moderate-intensity oral anticoagulation in addition to aspirin in unstable angina. *J Am Coll
     Cardiol* 2001; 37:475–484.
27. Fiore LD, Ezekowitz MD, Brophy MT *et al*. for the Combination Hemotherapy and Mortality
     Prevention (CHAMP) Study Group. Department of veteran affairs cooperative studies program
     clinical trial comparing combined warfarin and aspirin with aspirin alone in survivors of acute
     myocardial infarction. Primary results of the CHAMP study. *Circulation* 2002; 105:557–563.
28. Brouwer MA, Van den Bergh PJPC, Vromans RPJW *et al*. Aspirin plus medium intensity coumadin
     versus aspirin alone in the prevention of reocclusion after successful thrombolysis for suspected acute
     myocardial infarction: results of the APRICOT-2 study. *Circulation* 2002; 106:659–665.
29. Van Es RF, Jonker JJC, Verheugt FWA, Deckers JW, Grobbee DE. Aspirin, coumadin or both after acute
     coronary syndromes: results of the ASPECT-2 trial. *Lancet* 2002; 360:109–113.
30. Hurlen M, Abdelnoor M, Smith P, Erikssen J, Arnesen H. Warfarin, aspirin, or both after myocardial
     infarction. *N Engl J Med* 2002; 347:969–974.

31. Williams MJA, Morison IM, Parker JH, Stewart RH. Progression of the culprit leasion in unstable coronary artery disease with warfarin and aspirin versus aspirin alone: preliminary study. *J Am Coll Cardiol* 1997; 30:364–369.

32. Herlitz J, Holm J, Peterson M, Karlson B, Evander M, Erhardt L. Effect of low dose warfarin added to aspirin long term after acute myocardial infarction on cardiovascular death, reinfarction and stroke. *Eur Heart J* 2004; 25:232–239.

33. Gianetti G, Gensini G, De Caterina R. A cost-effectiveness analysis of aspirin versus oral anticoagulants after acute myocardial infarction in Italy: equivalence of costs as a possible case for oral anticoagulants. *Thromb Haemost* 1998; 80:887–893.

34. Loh E, St John Sutton M, Wun CC *et al*. Ventricular dysfunction and the risk of stroke after myocardial infarction. *N Engl J Med* 1997; 336:251–257.

35. Teo KK, Yusuf S, Pfeffer M *et al*. Effects of long-term treatment with angiotensin-converting enzyme inhibitors in the presence or absence of aspirin: a systematic review. *Lancet* 2002; 360:1037–1043.

36. Massie B. The WATCH trial. Presented American College of Cardiology, New Orleans, March 2004.

37. Cleland JGF. The WASH trial. Presented European Society of Cardiology, Amsterdam, September 2000.

38. Hurlen M, Hole T, Seljeflot I, Arnesen H. Aspirin does not influence the effect of angiotensin-converting enzyme inhibition on left ventricular ejection fraction 3 months after acute myocardial infarction. *Eur J Heart Fail* 2001; 3:203–207.

39. Smith P, Arnesen H, Abdelnoor M. Effects of of long-term anticoagulant therapy in subgroups after myocardial infarction. *Arch Intern Med* 1992; 152:993–997.

40. Cromheecke ME, Levi M, Colly LP *et al*. Oral anticoagulation self-management and management by a specialist anticoagulation clinic: a randomised cross-over comparison. *Lancet* 2000; 356:97–102.

41. Wallentin L, Wilcox RG, Weaver WD *et al*. Oral ximelagatran for secondary prophylaxis after myocardial infarction: the ESTEEM randomised controlled trial. *Lancet* 2003; 362:789–797.

42. Verheugt FWA. Can we pull the plug for warfarin in atrial fibrillation? *Lancet* 2003; 362:1686–1687.

11

Thrombolytic therapy and concomitant antithrombotic therapy

P. R. Sinnaeve, F. J. Van de Werf

INTRODUCTION

Acute myocardial infarction (MI), the leading cause of death in industrialised countries, is generally caused by rupture of an atherosclerotic plaque, triggering the formation of an occlusive coronary thrombus. When the occlusion persists, typical ST-segment elevations appear on the ECG. Coronary artery occlusion sets off a wave front of myocardial necrosis spreading from endocardium to epicardium, with an inverse relation between the time to perfusion and the ultimate extent of the infarct. To rescue myocardial muscle at risk from undergoing necrosis, rapid restoration of coronary blood flow is critical. Various studies during the past decades have established the paradigm of achieving early, complete and sustained infarct-related artery patency, resulting in a reduction in an average 30-day mortality of 18% in the pre-thrombolytic era to less than 6% in the context of contemporary clinical thrombolytic trials [1].

In ST-elevation myocardial infarction (STEMI), infarct-related coronary artery patency can be achieved by administration of fibrinolytic agents or by primary percutaneous coronary intervention (PCI). While primary PCI achieves higher patency rates and carries a lower risk of intracranial bleeding complications, pharmacological reperfusion can not only be given earlier, but is also less costly, widely available and less dependent on operator experience. Recent guidelines recommend primary PCI if the procedure can be performed by an experienced team within 90 min after initial medical contact [2, 3]. Because of limited access to catheterisation laboratory facilities, however, fibrinolytic therapy is still used for acute MI in the majority of centres worldwide. Results from the Global Registry of Acute Coronary Events (GRACE) indicate that, while only 7 out of 10 patients eligible for reperfusion therapy actually receive treatment, 43% of these patients receive lytic therapy as opposed to 17% who undergo mechanical intervention [4].

FIBRINOLYTIC THERAPY – RATIONALE AND INDICATION

Clot lysis can be achieved by activating the endogenous fibrinolytic system using intravenous plasminogen-activating agents. Plasminogen activators convert plasminogen to plasmin, which then degrades fibrin, a major constituent of clots (Figure 11.1). Fibrin-selective fibrinolytic drugs, such as alteplase or its derivatives and staphylokinase, digest the clot in

Peter R. Sinnaeve, Professor, Department of Cardiology, University Hospital Gasthuisberg, Leuven, Belgium.

Frans J. Van de Werf, Chairman, Department of Cardiology, University Hospital Gasthuisberg, Leuven, Belgium.

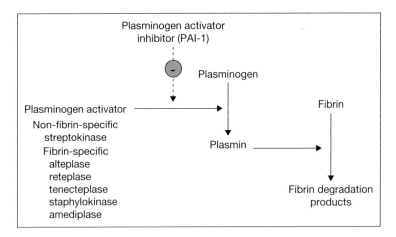

Figure 11.1 Mechanism of fibrinolytic agents.

the absence of systemic plasminogen activation, in contrast to non-fibrin-selective agents, such as streptokinase, which activates both systemic and clot-bound plasminogen. Fibrin-selective drugs are more efficient in dissolving thrombi and they do not deplete systemic coagulation factors, in contrast with non-fibrin-selective agents. This potential asset can increase the risk of re-occlusion, however [5]. As a consequence, concomitant antithrombotic treatment with heparin is needed in patients receiving fibrin-specific fibrinolytics.

Administration of fibrinolytic drugs should be considered in patients with typical chest pain and/or other infarct-related symptoms, and presenting with typical electro-cardiographic changes. Treatment has to be initiated as soon as possible, preferably within 6 h of symptom onset. Although administering fibrinolytic agents up to 12 h after the onset of symptoms may still be beneficial in terms of outcome [6], every minute that reperfusion is postponed will inevitably lead to more extensive necrosis. Early in the course of STEMI, the thrombus may be smaller and easier to lyse. In a meta-analysis, the proportional mortality reduction following fibrinolytic therapy was 44% in patients treated within 2 h vs. 20% in those treated later [7]. Also, treatment delay is associated with less successful ST-segment recovery and subsequent higher long-term mortality rates [8]. Fibrinolytic therapy is *not* recommended for non-ST elevation myocardial infarction (NSTEMI) or unstable angina. Although a substantial reduction of thrombus formation with alteplase compared to placebo was observed in the TIMI IIIa acute coronary syndrome trial [9], the Fibrinolytic Therapy Trialists' overview showed an increased mortality in patients with ST-segment depression treated with fibrinolytics [6].

Standard fibrinolytic regimens suffer from several limitations. Fibrinolytics need up to 45 min to recanalise the infarct-related artery, and complete patency (TIMI grade 3 flow) is only achieved in 60 to 80% of patients. Re-occlusion due to prothrombotic side-effects is also common, occurring in 5 to 15% of successfully recanalised arteries [10]. To prevent re-occlusion, antithrombotic agents are usually given concomitantly with fibrinolytic agents. Furthermore, even when blood flow to the infarct-related artery is restored, micro-circulatory reperfusion might be insufficient ('no-reflow' phenomenon). Finally, bleeding complications, especially intracranial haemorrhages continue to be a concern in high-risk patients.

FIBRINOLYTIC AGENTS

STREPTOKINASE

Streptokinase is a non-fibrinogen-specific fibrinolytic that indirectly activates plasminogen. Because it is produced by haemolytic streptococci, patients who receive streptokinase invariably develop antistreptococcal antibodies, precluding re-administration. In addition, pre-existing anti-streptokinase antibodies may reduce fibrinolytic activity and consequently impede reperfusion in patients with acute MI. Although newer fibrin-specific fibrinolytics have theoretical advantages, streptokinase remains widely used in part because of its low cost. The first trial to show a significant reduction in mortality with a fibrinolytic agent was the landmark Gruppo Italiano per lo Studio della Streptochinasi nell'Infarto Miocardio (GISSI-1) trial [11]. In this study, patients with a STEMI presenting within 12 h of symptom onset were randomised to either streptokinase or standard non-fibrinolytic therapy. In-hospital mortality was 10.7% in patients treated with intravenous streptokinase vs. 13.1 in control patients, representing 23 lives saved per 1000 patients treated. This difference remained significant after 10 years of follow-up [12].

Anisoylated plasminogen streptokinase activator complex (anistreplase or APSAC) is a complex of streptokinase and lys-plasminogen with its active site protected by an acyl group, increasing its half-life. Anistreplase did not improve outcome compared to streptokinase in the ISIS-3 study, and was associated with more bleeding complications [13].

ALTEPLASE

Recombinant tissue-type plasminogen activator (alteplase, rt-PA) is a single-chain tissue-type plasminogen activator molecule, manufactured by recombinant DNA technology. Due to its short half-life, alteplase requires a continuous infusion. It has considerable greater fibrin-specificity than streptokinase, but still induces systemic fibrinogen depletion to some extent. Because the re-occlusion rate with alteplase given alone is almost twice as high as that with non-fibrin specific drugs [5], concomitant antithrombin treatment is required in patients receiving alteplase.

The question whether alteplase is superior to streptokinase in terms of mortality reduction was answered in the first Global Utilisation of Streptokinase and Tissue Plasminogen Activator for Occluded Coronary Arteries (GUSTO-1) trial [14]. In this trial that included over 40 000 patients, a 'front-loaded' 90 min dosing regimen of alteplase was used, which had been shown to achieve higher patency rates than the 3 h scheme [15]. 30-day mortality was 6.3% in patients receiving alteplase compared to 7.4% in patients treated with streptokinase (P=0.001) [14]. This 1% lower 30-day mortality with alteplase over streptokinase could be explained by a significantly higher TIMI flow grade 3 at 90 min: 54% vs. 32% with streptokinase [16].

RETEPLASE

Reteplase, a second-generation fibrinolytic agent, was a first attempt to improve on the shortcomings of alteplase. It is a mutant of alteplase in which the finger, the kringle-1 domain and epidermal growth factor domains were removed, resulting in decreased plasma clearance. In contrast with alteplase, which requires a continuous 90 min infusion, reteplase can be given as a double bolus. Unfortunately, the removal of the finger domain reduces fibrin specificity [17], although inactivation by plasminogen activator inhibitor (PAI-1) remains similar as with alteplase. In an open-label randomised pilot trial, TIMI 3 flow rates were higher with reteplase than with front-loaded alteplase [18].

Double-bolus reteplase was shown to be at least equivalent to streptokinase in the double-blind International Joint Efficacy Comparison of Thrombolytics (INJECT) trial [19]. In the GUSTO-III trial [20], which was designed as a superiority trial, 15 059 patients were randomised to double-bolus reteplase (10 MU) given 30 min apart, or front-loaded alteplase. Mortality at 30 days was again similar for both treatment arms (7.47 vs. 7.24%, respectively), as was the incidence of haemorrhagic stroke or other major bleeding complications. Similar mortality rates were maintained for both treatment groups at one-year follow-up [21]. Thus, higher TIMI-3 rates at 90 min with reteplase, as seen in pilot studies, were not associated with lower short-term mortality rates. This might be explained in part by increased platelet activation and surface receptor expression with reteplase compared to alteplase [22].

TENECTEPLASE

Tenecteplase (TNK-tPA) is also derived from alteplase. Mutations at three places (T103, N117, KHRR296–299) increase the plasma half-life, increase fibrin binding and specificity, and increase resistance to PAI-1. Its slower clearance allows convenient single-bolus administration [23]. The efficiency of tenecteplase to activate plasminogen is reduced in the presence of fibrinogen and fibrin degradation products, while efficiency in the presence of fibrin remains equivalent, explaining its improved fibrin specificity [24]. TNK also has higher thrombolytic potency than its parent molecule [25] or rPA [26]. As a consequence, TNK leads to faster recanalisation compared to alteplase [27, 28]. TIMI 3 flow rates were found to be identical after single-bolus administration of 40 mg TNK compared with standard alteplase in the TIMI-10B trial [29].

In the double-blind Assessment of the Safety and Efficacy of a New Thrombolytic Regimen (ASSENT-2) trial [30], 16 949 patients were randomised to single-bolus TNK or weight-adjusted front-loaded alteplase. Specifically designed as an equivalency trial, this study showed that TNK and alteplase had equivalent 30-day mortality (6.18 vs. 6.15%; 90% CI 0.917–1.104). Mortality rates remained similar at one year follow-up [31]. The two treatments did not differ significantly in any subgroup analysis, except for a lower 30-day mortality with TNK in patients treated after 4 h of symptom onset. Although the rates of intracranial haemorrhage were similar for TNK (0.93%) and alteplase (0.94%), female patients, elderly >75 years and patients weighing less than 67 kg tended to have lower rates of intracranial haemorrhage after treatment with TNK [32]. Non-cerebral bleeding complications occurred less frequently in the TNK group and, as a consequence, there was less need for blood transfusion after TNK. Differences were even more apparent in high-risk women. Thus, increased fibrin specificity of TNK may induce both a better outcome in late-treated patients and fewer bleeding complications especially in high-risk patients.

STAPHYLOKINASE

Staphylokinase (STAR), a bacterial profibrinolytic agent, is a 136 amino acid single-chain polypeptide with a unique structure and mechanism of action and of fibrin specificity [33]. In contrast with streptokinase, staphylokinase is highly fibrin-selective [34]. Staphylokinase variants with reduced immunogenicity and preserved lytic potency have been derivatised with maleimide-polyethylene glycol (PEG) to reduce the plasma clearance by 2.5-fold [35]. PEGylated variants detected only one-third of the antibodies generated by wild-type Sak in patients with STEMI. In a pilot trial, PEG-staphylokinase was shown to be associated with promising patency rates. In an angiography-controlled dose-finding trial (Collaborative Angiographic Patency Trial of Recombinant Staphylokinase [CAPTORS II]), patency rates for the highest doses of PEG-staphylokinase were lower than those in the pilot trial, but remained comparable to those achieved with tPA [36]. Further clinical studies are currently being conducted.

AMEDIPLASE

Amediplase is a chimeric fusion protein consisting of the kringle 2 domain of tPA and the catalytic domain of urokinase-PA. It is fibrin-specific, non-immunogenic and can be given as a single bolus. In two angiographic studies (2k2 and 3k2) [37, 38], TIMI flow grade 3 was obtained in more than 50% of the patients in a dose of ± 1 mg/kg with a good safety profile. Currently, a phase III trial investigating the safety and efficacy of this fibrinolytic agent is being prepared.

ANTITHROMBOTIC CO-THERAPY IN FIBRINOLYSIS

ASPIRIN

The landmark ISIS-2 (Second International Study of Infarct Survival) study clearly showed a benefit of adding aspirin to streptokinase. In ISIS-2 17 187 patients received 1.5 MU streptokinase, 160 mg aspirin daily for one month, both treatments, or neither [39]. Treatment with aspirin or streptokinase alone resulted in a significant reduction in mortality (23% and 24%, respectively), an effect that was additive, as shown by a 43% reduction in the combination group. Re-infarction rate was higher when streptokinase was used alone, an effect that was abolished when aspirin was added.

The benefit of aspirin in the setting of acute MI appears to be time-dependent. In a small trial, patients who received aspirin before fibrinolysis ($n = 346$) had a lower 7-day mortality than patients who received the first dose of aspirin after administration of the fibrinolytic agent ($n = 836$) (2.5 vs. 6.0%; $P = 0.01$) [40]. Similarly, patients with an acute MI had a better survival rate at 30 days when they received aspirin before hospital admission compared to in-hospital initiation [41].

THIENOPYRIDINES

The thienopyridine clopidogrel inhibits platelet aggregation *via* adenosine diphosphate (ADP)-dependent activation of the GPIIb/IIIa complex. Clopidogrel has similar antiplatelet activity but a better safety profile than ticlopidine. According to recent guidelines, clopidogrel can be considered in patients receiving fibrinolytic treatment who are unable to take aspirin due to hypersensitivity or gastrointestinal intolerance [2]. Currently, clopidogrel is being investigated as an antithrombotic adjuvant to fibrinolysis in the Clopidogrel as Adjunctive to Reperfusion Therapy (CLARITY) trial.

UNFRACTIONATED HEPARIN

Initially, clinical trials investigating subcutaneous heparin failed to show a clear benefit in patients with STEMI treated with fibrinolytics [42, 43]. Intravenous unfractionated heparin (UFH), however, has been the standard adjunctive antithrombotic therapy with fibrin-specific fibrinolytics since GUSTO-I, although an effect on outcome has not been observed [44]. Even though intravenous UHF does not improve early patency rates [45], patency after alteplase is enhanced by UHF at later time-points because it reduces the likelihood of re-occlusion [46, 47].

The optimal dosing regimen of UFH in combination with fibrinolytic therapy remains unclear. A retrospective analysis of UFH in fibrinolytic therapy suggested that a reduced and fully weight-adjusted dose of heparin, together with earlier monitoring of the activated partial thromboplastin time (aPTT), may further reduce the risk of intracranial haemorrhage [48]. The reduced, weight-adjusted dosing scheme in ASSENT-3 was associated with less major bleeding when compared to the previously recommended dose in ASSENT-2, without significantly affecting outcome [49].

Still, the use of UFH suffers from several drawbacks. The effectiveness of UFH is highly variable in patients, due to low bioavailability and variable clearance. UFH is also relatively ineffective in inhibiting clot-associated thrombin and factor X, and does not reduce thrombin generation associated with fibrinolysis. This can result in rebound activation of the coagulation cascade after cessation of an infusion, increasing the risk of re-occlusion [50]. When combined with fibrinolysis, short-term use of UFH is also associated with a two-fold increase in major bleeding. Because of the large variability in bioavailability of UFH, the anticoagulant effect has to be monitored *via* aPTT measurements.

LOW-MOLECULAR-WEIGHT HEPARIN

Low-molecular-weight heparin (LMWH) offers several advantages over conventional UFH, including greater bioavailability, better resistance to inhibition by activated platelets, lower incidence of heparin-induced thrombocytopaenia (HIT) and increased anti-factor Xa activity. LMWHs are also easier to administrate, and have a more stable and predictable anticoagulant response that eliminates the need for aPTT monitoring. Also, a better anti-Xa:IIa ratio than that of UFH more efficiently promotes the inhibition of thrombin generation. Furthermore, subcutaneous administration and a longer half-life greatly facilitate administration when compared to UFH. Studies have shown a reduction in re-infarction rates and enhanced late patency with the use of LMWH in acute coronary syndromes (ACS) [51]. Compared to UFH, TIMI 3 flow rates after alteplase administration tended to be higher with dalteparin or enoxaparin in the ASSENT PLUS trial and Heparin Aspirin Reperfusion Trial (HART II) [52, 53]. In the ENTIRE-TIMI (ENoxaparin and Tenecteplase with or without glycoprotein IIb/IIIa Inhibitor as Reperfusion strategy in ST-elevation MI – Thrombolysis in Myocardial Infarction) 23 trial, enoxaparin plus full-dose TNK achieved similar TIMI 3 flow rates compared to UFH plus TNK at 60 min. Although this study was relatively small, a significant reduction in the composite endpoint of death and re-infarction at 30 days was seen with enoxaparin compared to UFH, largely due to a substantial reduction in re-infarction rates. Major haemorrhages were less frequent in the enoxaparin group. Enoxaparin has also been tested in combination with streptokinase in the AMI-SK (Acute Myocardial Infarction – Streptokinase) trial [54]. Compared to placebo, enoxaparin was associated with higher patency rates and faster and more complete ST-segment resolution.

In the ASSENT-3 study, enoxaparin, UFH and abciximab were compared in combination with TNK [55]. A total of 6095 patients with STEMI received either full-dose weight-adjusted single-bolus TNK with weight-adjusted enoxaparin (30 mg intravenous bolus followed by 1 mg/kg immediately and every 12 h subcutaneous for 7 days) or UFH, or half-dose TNK with abciximab and weight-adjusted low-dose UFH. Primary endpoints were the composites of 30-day mortality, in-hospital re-infarction or refractory ischaemia at 30 days (primary efficacy endpoint), and the above plus in-hospital intracranial haemorrhage or major bleeding (primary efficacy points plus safety endpoint). Enoxaparin and full-dose TNK significantly reduced the risk for ischaemic complications (re-infarction and refractory ischaemia) (Figure 11.2). A significant improvement in the primary efficacy and safety endpoint was seen with TNK and enoxaparin when compared to standard TNK and UFH, but 30-day and one-year mortality rates were similar in the three groups [56]. Enoxaparin in combination with TNK was also evaluated in the pre-hospital setting in the ASSENT-3 PLUS trial [57]. A non-significant reduction in ischaemic complications with enoxaparin was observed, at the expense of an increase in intracranial haemorrhage in elderly patients (>75 years).

A recent meta-analysis of six trials comparing enoxaparin with UFH as adjunct therapy to fibrinolysis confirmed that enoxaparin is associated with improved outcome [58]. Unfortunately, a significantly higher incidence of minor bleeding complications with enoxaparin was also noted. As a consequence, although enoxaparin reduces ischaemic

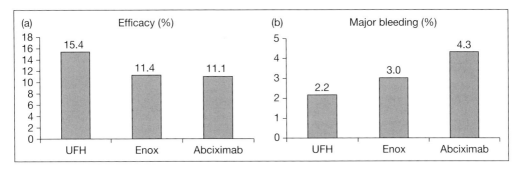

Figure 11.2 Results from ASSENT-3 [55] (a) Efficacy (30-day mortality, in-hospital reinfarction and in-hospital recurrent angina) (b) Major bleeding complications. (UFH = Unfractionated Heparin, Enox = Enoxaparin).

complications in randomised clinical trials, current guidelines await further studies investigating the benefit and risk of LMWH in all patients (including the elderly) before fully endorsing the use of these agents in combination with fibrinolysis [2, 3]. According to the most recent AHA/ACC guidelines, however, LMWH can be considered as an alternative to UFH in low-risk patients less than 75 years of age receiving fibrinolytic therapy (class IIb indication) [2]. Currently, enoxaparin is further evaluated in patients with STEMI receiving fibrinolytic therapy in the 21 000-patient ExTRACT-TIMI 25 study. In this trial, given the results of ASSENT-3 PLUS, patients over 75 years of age will receive a reduced dose of enoxaparin (0.75 mg SC twice a day and no bolus).

FACTOR Xa INHIBITOR

Fondaparinux, a synthetic pentasaccharide, is a selective antithrombin-dependent factor Xa inhibitor [59]. Compared to UFH and LMWH, fondaparinux is associated with less biological variability, immunogenic reactivity and risk of contamination. Also, in contrast with UFH or LMWH, fondaparinux does not bind to platelet factor 4 and thus reduces the risk of platelet activation. In the PENTALYSE trial, fondaparinux was compared to UFH in 333 patients with STEMI [60]. Epicardial patency rates at 90 min and 5 days were similar for both groups, but there was a trend towards less re-occlusion of the infarct-related artery and fewer revascularisations during the 30-day follow-up in patients receiving fondaparinux. The bleeding rate was similar for both groups. The efficacy and safety of fondaparinux in STEMI is currently further evaluated in the MICHELANGELO (OASIS) 6 trial.

GLYCOPROTEIN IIb/IIIa INHIBITORS

The addition of glycoprotein (GP)IIb/IIIa inhibitors to fibrinolytic regimens might also overcome some of the drawbacks of fibrinolysis. The combination of half-dose lytic and a GPIIb/IIIa inhibitor was shown to induce less systemic plasminogen activation [61] and to reverse the platelet activating effect of fibrinolytic drugs [62, 63]. This results in a reduction in angiographically evident thrombus, which is thought to improve epicardial and tissue perfusion [64]. Initially, GPIIb/IIIa inhibitors were tested in combination with full-dose fibrinolytics, but this was associated with an increased risk in major bleeding complications, especially in patients requiring early PCI [65]. In the Integrilin and low-dose Thrombolysis in acute myocardial infarction (INTRO-AMI), the highest 60-min reperfusion rates were seen in patients treated with double-bolus eptifibatide (10 min apart) followed by a 48-h

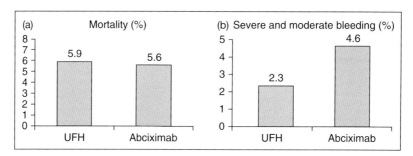

Figure 11.3 Results from GUSTO-V [104] (a) Primary endpoint (mortality) (b) Severe and moderate bleeding complications.

infusion and half-dose tPA (60-min TIMI 3 flow rate of 65 vs. 40% for full-dose alteplase alone [66]. In the TIMI (Thrombolysis in Myocardial Infarction) 14 study, reperfusion rates were evaluated after half-dose alteplase with standard dose abciximab vs. standard dose alteplase alone in 888 patients [67]. Abciximab with half-dose alteplase significantly enhanced reperfusion at 90 min in the TIMI-14 trial, with TIMI 3 flow in 74%, compared to 57% with alteplase alone. The effect of low-dose reteplase with abciximab on early reperfusion was tested in 528 patients in the SPEED (Strategies for Patency Enhancement in the Emergency Department) trial [68]. TIMI 3 flow rate was significantly higher with reduced-dose reteplase in combination with abciximab and heparin (61%) compared to abciximab in monotherapy (27%) or to full-dose reteplase alone (47%). Unfortunately, this benefit was at the expense of a substantial increase in major bleedings [69].

The efficacy and safety of abciximab in combination with reduced-dose fibrinolysis was evaluated in GUSTO-V and ASSENT-3. In the GUSTO-V trial, an open-label non-inferiority trial, 16 588 patients were randomised to either reteplase or half-dose reteplase with weight-adjusted abciximab (Figure 11.3) [70]. The primary endpoint was mortality at 30 days, while secondary endpoints were recurrent ischaemia and re-infarction at 7 days and safety at 30 days. Thirty-day mortality rates were 5.9% for reteplase and 5.6% for the combined reteplase–abciximab group, thus fulfilling the criteria for non-inferiority. One-year follow-up mortality rates were 8.4% in both cases [71]. The overall risk of bleeding, however, was significantly higher with reteplase and abciximab than with reteplase alone. Intracranial haemorrhage (ICH) rates were equally low in the overall study population for both treatment arms, although in patients above 75 years of age the rate of ICH was almost twice as high in the combination treatment arm. In the ASSENT-3 study, a significant decrease in ischaemic complications with abciximab was also offset by an increase in bleeding complications (Figure 11.2) [55]. Although ICH rates were very similar in the three treatment arms, major and minor bleeding complications, thrombocytopaenia and transfusion rates were more frequent in the half-dose TNK plus abciximab arm. Like in the GUSTO-V trial, patients older than 75 years experienced significantly more bleeding complications. Taken together, combination therapy with fibrinolysis and abciximab results in a significant reduction in ischaemic complications after acute MI, but this benefit is offset by an increased risk of bleeding complications, particularly in elderly patients.

DIRECT THROMBIN INHIBITORS

In contrast with UFH, which only inhibits fluid-phase thrombin, direct thrombin inhibitors inhibit both fibrin-bound and fluid-phase thrombin [72]. Because inadequately inactivated thrombin at the site of the thrombus is in part responsible for the procoagulant side-effect of fibrinolysis, direct inhibition of thrombin might reduce the occurrence of ischaemic complications after reperfusion.

Hirudin was shown to improve early patency rates with streptokinase [73]. In fact, results from GUSTO-IIb suggest that hirudin only interacts favorably with streptokinase, not with alteplase [74]. In the TIMI-9B study, the primary composite endpoint of death, re-infarction, heart failure or shock at 30 days was similar for hirudin and UFH in patients receiving streptokinase or alteplase [75]. Hirudin was also associated with a higher rate of complete ST-segment recovery at 90 min compared to UFH in the HIT-4 study [76]. In the first HERO (Hirulog and Early Reperfusion or Occlusion) study, reperfusion rates were assessed in 412 patients receiving streptokinase with UFH or bivalirudin, a semi-synthetic variant of hirudin [77]. Patency rates were higher in the bivalirudin group (48%) than in the UFH group (35%), while no increase in bleeding complications in patients receiving bivalirudin was observed.

In the HERO-2 (Hirulog and Early Reperfusion or Occlusion) trial, 17 073 patients with STEMI were randomised to streptokinase and UFH or streptokinase and bivalirudin [78]. Mortality at 30 days was no different for bivalirudin (10.5%) or for UFH (10.9%). On the other hand, re-infarction rate within 96 h was significantly lower in the bivalirudin group (1.6% vs. 2.3% for UFH), suggesting that early and more efficient inhibition of thrombin can inhibit re-occlusion. Mild to moderate bleeding complications were higher in the bivalirudin group, but ICH occurred infrequently in both groups. The current ACC/AHA guidelines recommend bivalirudin as an alternative to UFH in patients with HIT treated with streptokinase [2].

Ximelagatran, the first oral direct thrombin inhibitor, has recently been evaluated in 1900 patients with a recent NSTEMI or STEMI in the ESTEEM (Efficacy and safety of the oral direct thrombin inhibitor ximelagatran in patients with recent myocardial damage) trial [79]. Patients were randomised to aspirin plus placebo or aspirin plus ximelagatran. Ximelagatran was associated with a significant reduction in the composite primary endpoint of death, MI and recurrent ischaemia. In a *post hoc* analysis, the 'thrombotic' endpoint of death, MI and stroke was reduced by 34% (hazard ratio [HR] 0.66; 95% CI 0.48–0.90) in the overall ximelagatran group.

PRE-HOSPITAL FIBRINOLYSIS

Time lost between symptom onset and treatment initiation remains a crucial contributor to treatment delay in STEMI. Since mortality rates in randomised fibrinolytic trials are consistently lower when patients are treated within two hours of symptom onset, pre-hospital treatment might be an attractive approach to improve outcome in STEMI. Bolus fibrinolytic agents undoubtedly facilitate pre-hospital reperfusion protocols. The combination of single-bolus TNK plus enoxaparin, which emerged as a convenient and attractive therapy in the ASSENT-3 study, has been investigated in the pre-hospital setting in the ASSENT-3 PLUS trial. In ASSENT-3 PLUS 1639 patients with acute MI received pre-hospital TNK and were randomised to either enoxaparin or UFH [57]. A time gain of 47 min was observed, increasing the fraction of patients treated within two hours of symptom onset from 29% in ASSENT-3 to 52% in ASSENT-3 Plus. Early treatment (<2 h) was associated with a lower 30-day mortality (4.4 vs. 6.2 [2–4 h] and 10.4% [4–6 h]), but no significant difference in outcome was observed between enoxaparin and heparin. Pre-hospital initiation of reteplase, which needs to be administered in double-bolus injections, has also been shown to be associated with faster treatment initiation [80, 81]. A meta-analysis of six trials including 6434 patients showed that the time gained with pre-hospital treatment resulted in a significant 17% mortality reduction compared to in-hospital fibrinolysis [82].

The question of whether pre-hospital fibrinolysis compares favourably with transport to a centre with interventional facilities for primary PCI was addressed in the Comparison of

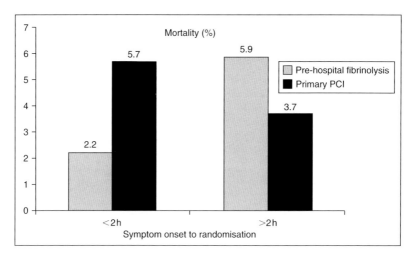

Figure 11.4 Mortality in CAPTIM in patients randomised before and after 2 h after symptom onset.

Angioplasty and Prehospital Thrombolysis in Acute Myocardial Infarction (CAPTIM) trial [83]. Primary PCI was not found to be superior to pre-hospital fibrinolysis in terms of outcome. It is important to note that 26% of the patients randomised to pre-hospital fibrinolysis subsequently underwent rescue PCI in the tertiary care hospital, which might have contributed to the favourable outcomes in the pre-hospital group. Also, pre-hospital fibrinolysis was associated with a mortality reduction in patients randomised within two hours of symptom onset [84] (Figure 11.4). These findings emphasise the importance of initiation of reperfusion therapy as soon as possible after symptom onset.

PHARMACO-INVASIVE STRATEGIES

A recent meta-analysis indicated that primary PCI is superior to fibrinolysis in randomised trials with regard to short-term and long-term outcome [85]. Primary PCI allows immediate treatment of the culprit lesion, and is associated with lower mortality rates in qualified high-volume centres. Although the efficacy of primary PCI appears to be less dependent on the time elapsed between symptom onset and treatment initiation than fibrinolysis, symptom-onset-to balloon-time also appears to be related to outcome in primary PCI [86]. Recent guidelines therefore recommend primary PCI if the procedure can be performed by an experienced team within 90 min after initial medical contact [2, 3]. Unfortunately, much time is often lost between diagnosis and PCI in daily practice due to transport to another centre or while waiting for a catheterisation lab or team to become available.

In primary PCI studies, 10 to 20% of patients with STEMI appear to have spontaneous epicardial reperfusion before the intervention [87–89], which is an independent predictor of outcome [90]. Patients with reperfusion before the procedure also have better preserved left ventricular function, and less progression to heart failure and cardiogenic shock [87, 89]. Similarly, adequate tissue perfusion before a primary PCI is associated with improved outcome, irrespective of epicardial reperfusion [91].

Therefore, the next logical step in treatment for acute MI is to combine the advantages of both primary PCI and fibrinolysis. The rationale behind this approach is that reperfusion can be obtained sooner than with PCI alone, while PCI allows immediate recanalisation when fibrinolysis fails. Surprisingly, earlier trials comparing routine angioplasty immediately following fibrinolysis with more conservative treatment showed that the invasive

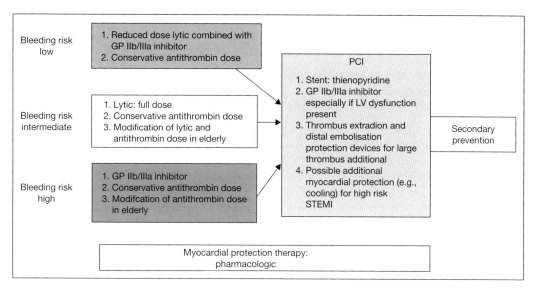

Figure 11.5 Proposal for a unifying pharmacoinvasive approach to patients with STEMI: Potential roles for pharmacological and myocardial protection [105] (E Antman and F Van de Werf, *Circulation* 2004 ;109:2480–2486, reproduced with permission).

approach was associated with a higher complication rate, including abrupt artery closure, re-infarction and death [92–97]. One explanation for these findings is that traditional fibrinolytic strategies activate platelets and the coagulation system, promoting thrombotic complications in the setting of angioplasty. It is likely that the availability of more potent antithrombotic agents like GPIIb/IIIa inhibitors, the increased experience of interventional cardiologists, the use of stents and better catheters and guide wires have significantly reduced the risk of early interventions. More recent studies such as Southwest German Interventional Study in Acute Myocardial Infarction (SIAM)-III and GRACIA-2 indeed indicate that early contemporary invasive treatment immediately following fibrinolysis appears to be safe [98, 99]. In the GRACIA-1 study, immediate planned PCI after fibrinolysis not only appeared to be safe, but was also associated with improved one-year outcome [100]. In the SPEED trial, the combined endpoint of death, re-infarction and urgent revascularisation was significantly lower in patients treated with reteplase and abciximab who had an intervention within 60 to 90 min than in patients who did not undergo early PCI [101]. The Plasminogen-activator Angioplasty Compatibility Trial (PACT) has also shown that, even in the absence of a GPIIb/IIIa antagonist, coronary interventions can be safely performed immediately following a single bolus of 50 mg rt-PA The ongoing ASSENT-4 PCI and Facilitated Intervention with Enhanced Reperfusion Speed to Stop Events (FINESSE) trials will give more insight into the benefits and risks of early pharmacological reperfusion followed by planned mechanical intervention [102]. Awaiting the results of these trials, a unifying pharmacoinvasive approach tailoring fibrinolytic and concomitant antithrombotic therapy to the estimated risk of bleeding has been proposed (Figure 11.5).

SUMMARY

Fibrinolytic therapy significantly improves outcome after STEMI. Over the last years, new fibrinolytics with several theoretical advantages over standard agents have been developed. Although they do not seem to have an impact on mortality, they are easier to administer and induce fewer side-effects. Further improvement can be expected from novel antithrombotic drugs, reduction of reperfusion injury, and reduced time-to-reperfusion through facilitated percutaneous intervention and pre-hospital treatment.

REFERENCES

1. de Vreede JJ, Gorgels AP, Verstraaten GM , Vermeer F, Dassen WR, Wellens HJ. Did prognosis after acute myocardial infarction change during the past 30 years? A meta-analysis. *J Am Coll Cardiol* 1991; 18:698–706.
2. Antman EM, Anbe DT, Armstrong PW *et al.* ACC/AHA guidelines for the management of patients with ST-elevation myocardial infarction – executive summary: a report of the American College of Cardiology/American Heart Association Task Force on Practice Guidelines (Writing Committee to Revise the 1999 Guidelines for the Management of Patients With Acute Myocardial Infarction). *Circulation* 2004; 110:588–636.
3. Van de Werf FJ, Ardissino D, Betriu A *et al.* Management of acute myocardial infarction in patients presenting with ST-segment elevation. The Task Force on the Management of Acute Myocardial Infarction of the European Society of Cardiology. *Eur Heart J* 2003; 24:28–66.
4. Eagle KA, Goodman SG, Avezum A, Budaj A, Sullivan CM, Lopez-Sendon J. Practice variation and missed opportunities for reperfusion in ST-segment-elevation myocardial infarction: findings from the Global Registry of Acute Coronary Events (GRACE). *Lancet* 2002; 359:373–377.
5. Granger CB, Califf RM, Topol EJ. Thrombolytic therapy for acute myocardial infarction. A review. *Drugs* 1992; 44:293–325.
6. Indications for fibrinolytic therapy in suspected acute myocardial infarction: collaborative overview of early mortality and major morbidity results from all randomised trials of more than 1000 patients. Fibrinolytic Therapy Trialists' (FTT) Collaborative Group. *Lancet* 1994; 343:311–322.
7. Boersma E, Maas AC, Deckers JW, Simoons ML. Early thrombolytic treatment in acute myocardial infarction: reappraisal of the golden hour. *Lancet* 1996; 348:771–775.
8. Fu Y, Goodman S, Chang WC, Van de Werf FJ, Granger CB, Armstrong PW. Time to treatment influences the impact of ST-segment resolution on one-year prognosis: insights from the assessment of the safety and efficacy of a new thrombolytic (ASSENT-2) trial. *Circulation* 2001; 104:2653–2659.
9. Early effects of tissue-type plasminogen activator added to conventional therapy on the culprit coronary lesion in patients presenting with ischaemic cardiac pain at rest. Results of the Thrombolysis in Myocardial Ischemia (TIMI IIIA) Trial. *Circulation* 1993; 87:38–52.
10. Topol EJ. Acute myocardial infarction: thrombolysis. *Heart* 2000; 83:122–126.
11. Effectiveness of intravenous thrombolytic treatment in acute myocardial infarction. Gruppo Italiano per lo Studio della Streptochinasi nell'Infarto Miocardico (GISSI). *Lancet* 1986; 1:397–402.
12. Franzosi MG, Santoro E, De Vita C *et al.* Ten-year follow-up of the first megatrial testing thrombolytic therapy in patients with acute myocardial infarction: results of the Gruppo Italiano per lo Studio della Sopravvivenza nell'Infarto-1 study. The GISSI Investigators. *Circulation* 1998; 98:2659–2665.
13. ISIS-3: a randomised comparison of streptokinase vs. tissue plasminogen activator vs. anistreplase and of aspirin plus heparin vs. aspirin alone among 41,299 cases of suspected acute myocardial infarction. ISIS-3 (Third International Study of Infarct Survival) Collaborative Group. *Lancet* 1992; 339:753–770.
14. An international randomised trial comparing four thrombolytic strategies for acute myocardial infarction. The GUSTO investigators. *N Engl J Med* 1993; 329:673–682.
15. Neuhaus KL, Feuerer W, Jeep-Tebbe S, Niederer W, Vogt A, Tebbe U. Improved thrombolysis with a modified dose regimen of recombinant tissue-type plasminogen activator. *J Am Coll Cardiol* 1989; 14:1566–1569.
16. The effects of tissue plasminogen activator, streptokinase, or both on coronary-artery patency, ventricular function, and survival after acute myocardial infarction. The GUSTO Angiographic Investigators. *N Engl J Med* 1993; 329:1615–1622.

17. Hoffmeister HM, Kastner C, Szabo S *et al.* Fibrin specificity and procoagulant effect related to the kallikrein-contact phase system and to plasmin generation with double-bolus reteplase and front-loaded alteplase thrombolysis in acute myocardial infarction. *Am J Cardiol* 2000; 86:263–268.

18. Bode C, Smalling RW, Berg G *et al.* Randomised comparison of coronary thrombolysis achieved with double-bolus reteplase (recombinant plasminogen activator) and front-loaded, accelerated alteplase (recombinant tissue plasminogen activator) in patients with acute myocardial infarction. The RAPID II Investigators. *Circulation* 1996; 94:891–898.

19. Randomised, double-blind comparison of reteplase double-bolus administration with streptokinase in acute myocardial infarction (INJECT): trial to investigate equivalence. International Joint Efficacy Comparison of Thrombolytics. *Lancet* 1995; 346:329–336.

20. A comparison of reteplase with alteplase for acute myocardial infarction. The Global Use of Strategies to Open Occluded Coronary Arteries (GUSTO III) Investigators. *N Engl J Med* 1997; 337:1118–1123.

21. Topol EJ, Ohman EM, Armstrong PW *et al.* Survival outcomes 1 year after reperfusion therapy with either alteplase or reteplase for acute myocardial infarction: results from the Global Utilization of Streptokinase and t-PA for Occluded Coronary Arteries (GUSTO) III Trial. *Circulation* 2000; 102:1761–1765.

22. Gurbel PA, Serebruany VL, Shustov AR *et al.* Effects of reteplase and alteplase on platelet aggregation and major receptor expression during the first 24 hour of acute myocardial infarction treatment. GUSTO-III Investigators. Global Use of Strategies to Open Occluded Coronary Arteries. *J Am Coll Cardiol* 1998; 31:1466–1473.

23. Leah V, Clark C, Doyle K, Coats TJ. Does a single bolus thrombolytic reduce door to needle time in a district general hospital? *Emerg Med J* 2004; 21:162–164.

24. Stewart RJ, Fredenburgh JC, Leslie BA, Keyt BA, Rischke JA, Weitz JI. Identification of the mechanism responsible for the increased fibrin specificity of TNK-tissue plasminogen activator relative to tissue plasminogen activator. *J Biol Chem* 2000; 275:10112–10120.

25. Collen D, Stassen JM, Yasuda T *et al.* Comparative thrombolytic properties of tissue-type plasminogen activator and of a plasminogen activator inhibitor-1-resistant glycosylation variant, in a combined arterial and venous thrombosis model in the dog. *Thromb Haemost* 1994; 72:98–104.

26. Al Shwafi KA, de Meester A, Pirenne B, Col JJ. Comparative fibrinolytic activity of front-loaded alteplase and the single-bolus mutants tenecteplase and lanoteplase during treatment of acute myocardial infarction. *Am Heart J* 2003; 145:217–225.

27. Binbrek A, Rao N, Absher PM, Van de Werf FJ, Sobel BE. The relative rapidity of recanalization induced by recombinant tissue-type plasminogen activator (r-tPA) and TNK-tPA, assessed with enzymatic methods. *Coron Artery Dis* 2000; 11:429–435.

28. Binbrek AS, Rao NS, Neimane D, Hatou E, Abdulali S, Sobel BE. Comparison of rapidity of coronary recanalization in men with tenecteplase versus alteplase in acute myocardial infarction. *Am J Cardiol* 2004; 93:1465–1468.

29. Cannon CP, Gibson CM, McCabe CH *et al.* TNK-tissue plasminogen activator compared with front-loaded alteplase in acute myocardial infarction: results of the TIMI 10B trial. Thrombolysis in Myocardial Infarction (TIMI) 10B Investigators. *Circulation* 1998; 98:2805–2814.

30. Single-bolus tenecteplase compared with front-loaded alteplase in acute myocardial infarction: the ASSENT-2 double-blind randomised trial. Assessment of the Safety and Efficacy of a New Thrombolytic Investigators. *Lancet* 1999; 354:716–722.

31. Sinnaeve P, Alexander J, Belmans A *et al.* One-year follow-up of the ASSENT-2 trial: a double-blind, randomised comparison of single-bolus tenecteplase and front-loaded alteplase in 16,949 patients with ST-elevation acute myocardial infarction. *Am Heart J* 2003; 146:27–32.

32. Van de Werf FJ, Barron HV, Armstrong PW *et al.* Incidence and predictors of bleeding events after fibrinolytic therapy with fibrin-specific agents: a comparison of TNK-tPA and rt-PA. *Eur Heart J* 2001; 22:2253–2261.

33. Collen D, Vanderschueren S, Van de Werf FJ. Fibrin-selective thrombolytic therapy with recombinant staphylokinase. *Haemostasis* 1996; 26(suppl 4):294–300.

34. Collen D, Moreau H, Stockx L, Vanderschueren S. Recombinant staphylokinase variants with altered immunoreactivity. II: Thrombolytic properties and antibody induction. *Circulation* 1996; 94:207–216.

35. Vanwetswinkel S, Plaisance S, Zhi-Yong Z *et al.* Pharmacokinetic and thrombolytic properties of cysteine-linked polyethylene glycol derivatives of staphylokinase. *Blood* 2000; 95:936–942.

36. Armstrong PW, Burton J, Pakola S *et al.* Collaborative Angiographic Patency Trial Of Recombinant Staphylokinase (CAPTORS II). *Am Heart J* 2003; 146:484–488.

37. Charbonnier B, Pluta W, De Ferrari G, Ceddia F, Capriati A, Van de Werf FJ. Evaluation of Two
    Weight-Adjusted Single Bolus Doses of Amediplase to Patients with Acute Myocardial Infarction: the
    3k2 Trial (Abstract). *Circulation* 2001; 107:II-538.

38. Vermeer F, Oldrovd K, Pohl J, Gianelli S, Charbonnier B. Safety and angiography data of Amediplase,
    a new fibrin specific thrombolytic agent, given as a single bolus to patients with acute myocardial
    infarction: the 2K2 Dose Finding Trial (Abstract). *Circulation* 2001; 104:II-538.

39. Mechanisms for the early mortality reduction produced by beta-blockade started early in acute
    myocardial infarction: ISIS-1. ISIS-1 (First International Study of Infarct Survival) Collaborative Group.
    Lancet 1988; 1:921–923.

40. Freimark D, Matetzky S, Leor J *et al*. Timing of aspirin administration as a determinant of survival of
    patients with acute myocardial infarction treated with thrombolysis. *Am J Cardiol* 2002; 89:381–385.

41. Barbash IM, Freimark D, Gottlieb S *et al*. Outcome of myocardial infarction in patients treated with
    aspirin is enhanced by pre-hospital administration. *Cardiol* 2002; 98:141–147.

42. GISSI-2: a factorial randomised trial of alteplase versus streptokinase and heparin versus no heparin
    among 12,490 patients with acute myocardial infarction. Gruppo Italiano per lo Studio della
    Sopravvivenza nell'Infarto Miocardico. *Lancet* 1990; 336:65–71.

43. Randomised trial of intravenous streptokinase, oral aspirin, both, or neither among 17,187 cases of
    suspected acute myocardial infarction: ISIS-2. ISIS-2 (Second International Study of Infarct Survival)
    Collaborative Group. *Lancet* 1988; 2:349–360.

44. Mahaffey KW, Granger CB, Collins R *et al*. Overview of randomised trials of intravenous heparin in
    patients with acute myocardial infarction treated with thrombolytic therapy. *Am J Cardiol* 1996;
    77:551–556.

45. Topol EJ, George BS, Kereiakes DJ *et al*. A randomised controlled trial of intravenous tissue plasminogen
    activator and early intravenous heparin in acute myocardial infarction. *Circulation* 1989; 79:281–286.

46. Bleich SD, Nichols TC, Schumacher RR, Cooke DH, Tate DA, Teichman SL. Effect of heparin on
    coronary arterial patency after thrombolysis with tissue plasminogen activator in acute myocardial
    infarction. *Am J Cardiol* 1990; 66:1412–1417.

47. Hsia J, Hamilton WP, Kleiman N, Roberts R, Chaitman BR, Ross AM. A comparison between heparin and
    low-dose aspirin as adjunctive therapy with tissue plasminogen activator for acute myocardial infarction.
    Heparin-Aspirin Reperfusion Trial (HART) Investigators. *N Engl J Med* 1990; 323:1433–1437.

48. Giugliano RP, McCabe CH, Antman EM *et al*. Lower-dose heparin with fibrinolysis is associated with
    lower rates of intracranial haemorrhage. *Am Heart J* 2001; 141:742–750.

49. Curtis JP, Alexander JH, Huang Y *et al*. Efficacy and safety of two unfractionated heparin dosing
    strategies with tenecteplase in acute myocardial infarction (results from Assessment of the Safety and
    Efficacy of a New Thrombolytic Regimens 2 and 3). *Am J Cardiol* 2004; 94:279–283.

50. Antman EM, Braunwald E. A second look at bivalirudin. *Am Heart J* 2001; 142:929–931.

51. Turpie AG, Antman EM. Low-molecular-weight heparins in the treatment of acute coronary
    syndromes. *Arch Intern Med* 2001; 161:1484–1490.

52. Wallentin L, Dellborg DM, Lindahl B, Nilsson T, Pehrsson K, Swahn E. The low-molecular-weight
    heparin dalteparin as adjuvant therapy in acute myocardial infarction: the ASSENT PLUS study. *Clin
    Cardiol* 2001; 24:I12–I14.

53. Ross AM, Molhoek P, Lundergan C *et al*. Randomised comparison of enoxaparin, a low-molecular-weight
    heparin, with unfractionated heparin adjunctive to recombinant tissue plasminogen activator
    thrombolysis and aspirin: second trial of Heparin and Aspirin Reperfusion Therapy (HART II). *Circulation*
    2001; 104:648–652.

54. Simoons M, Krzeminska-Pakula M, Alonso A *et al*. Improved reperfusion and clinical outcome with
    enoxaparin as an adjunct to streptokinase thrombolysis in acute myocardial infarction. The AMI-SK
    study. *Eur Heart J* 2002; 23:1282.

55. Efficacy and safety of tenecteplase in combination with enoxaparin, abciximab, or unfractionated
    heparin: the ASSENT-3 randomised trial in acute myocardial infarction. *Lancet* 2001; 358:605–613.

56. Sinnaeve PR, Alexander JH, Bogaerts K *et al*. Efficacy of tenecteplase in combination with enoxaparin,
    abciximab, or unfractionated heparin: one-year follow-up results of the Assessment of the Safety of a
    New Thrombolytic-3 (ASSENT-3) randomised trial in acute myocardial infarction. *Am Heart J* 2004;
    147:993–998.

57. Wallentin L, Goldstein P, Armstrong PW *et al*. Efficacy and safety of tenecteplase in combination
    with the low-molecular-weight heparin enoxaparin or unfractionated heparin in the pre-hospital

setting: the Assessment of the Safety and Efficacy of a New Thrombolytic Regimen (ASSENT)-3 PLUS randomised trial in acute myocardial infarction. *Circulation* 2003; 108:135–142.

58. Theroux P, Welsh RC. Meta-analysis of randomised trials comparing enoxaparin versus unfractionated heparin as adjunctive therapy to fibrinolysis in ST-elevation acute myocardial infarction. *Am J Cardiol* 2003; 91:860–864.

59. Samama MM, Gerotziafas GT. Evaluation of the pharmacological properties and clinical results of the synthetic pentasaccharide (fondaparinux). *Thromb Res* 2003; 109:1–11.

60. Coussement PK, Bassand JP, Convens C *et al.* A synthetic factor-Xa inhibitor (ORG31540/SR9017A) as an adjunct to fibrinolysis in acute myocardial infarction. The PENTALYSE study. *Eur Heart J* 2001; 22:1716–1724.

61. Szabo S, Etzel D, Ehlers R *et al.* Increased fibrin specificity and reduced paradoxical thrombin activation of the combined thrombolytic regimen with reteplase and abciximab versus standard reteplase thrombolysis. *Drugs Exp Clin Res* 2004; 30:47–54.

62. Bertram U, Moser M, Peter K *et al.* Effects of Different Thrombolytic Treatment Regimen with Abciximab and Tirofiban on Platelet Aggregation and Platelet-Leukocyte Interactions: A Subgroup Analysis from the GUSTO V and FASTER Trials. *J Thromb Thrombolysis* 2002; 14:197–203.

63. Coulter SA, Cannon CP, Ault KA *et al.* High levels of platelet inhibition with abciximab despite heightened platelet activation and aggregation during thrombolysis for acute myocardial infarction: results from TIMI (thrombolysis in myocardial infarction) 14. *Circulation* 2000; 101:2690–2695.

64. Gibson CM, de Lemos JA, Murphy SA *et al.* Combination therapy with abciximab reduces angiographically evident thrombus in acute myocardial infarction: a TIMI 14 substudy. *Circulation* 2001; 103:2550–2554.

65. Jong P, Cohen EA, Batchelor W *et al.* Bleeding risks with abciximab after full-dose thrombolysis in rescue or urgent angioplasty for acute myocardial infarction. *Am Heart J* 2001; 141:218–225.

66. Brener SJ, Zeymer U, Adgey AA *et al.* Eptifibatide and low-dose tissue plasminogen activator in acute myocardial infarction: the integrilin and low-dose thrombolysis in acute myocardial infarction (INTRO AMI) trial. *J Am Coll Cardiol* 2002; 39:377–386.

67. Antman EM, Giugliano RP, Gibson CM *et al.* Abciximab facilitates the rate and extent of thrombolysis: results of the thrombolysis in myocardial infarction (TIMI) 14 trial. The TIMI 14 Investigators. *Circulation* 1999; 99:2720–2732.

68. Trial of abciximab with and without low-dose reteplase for acute myocardial infarction. Strategies for Patency Enhancement in the Emergency Department (SPEED) Group. *Circulation* 2000; 101:2788–2794.

69. Herrmann HC, Moliterno DJ, Ohman EM *et al.* Facilitation of early percutaneous coronary intervention after reteplase with or without abciximab in acute myocardial infarction: results from the SPEED (GUSTO-4 Pilot) Trial. *J Am Coll Cardiol* 2000; 36:1489–1496.

70. Topol EJ, Moliterno DJ, Herrmann HC *et al.* Comparison of two platelet glycoprotein IIb/IIIa inhibitors, tirofiban and abciximab, for the prevention of ischaemic events with percutaneous coronary revascularization. *N Engl J Med* 2001; 344:1888–1894.

71. Lincoff AM, Califf RM, Van de Werf FJ *et al.* Mortality at 1 year with combination platelet glycoprotein IIb/IIIa inhibition and reduced-dose fibrinolytic therapy vs. conventional fibrinolytic therapy for acute myocardial infarction: GUSTO V randomised trial. *JAMA* 2002; 288:2130–2135.

72. Weitz JI. Biological rationale for the therapeutic role of specific antithrombins. *Coron Artery Dis* 1996; 7:409–419.

73. Molhoek GP, Laarman GJ, Luz CM *et al.* Angiographic dose-finding study with r-hirudin (HBW 023) for the improvement of thrombolytic therapy with streptokinase (HIT-SK). Interim results. *Eur Heart J* 1995; 16(suppl D):33–37.

74. Metz BK, White HD, Granger CB *et al.* Randomised comparison of direct thrombin inhibition versus heparin in conjunction with fibrinolytic therapy for acute myocardial infarction: results from the GUSTO-IIb Trial. Global Use of Strategies to Open Occluded Coronary Arteries in Acute Coronary Syndromes (GUSTO-IIb) Investigators. *J Am Coll Cardiol* 1998; 31:1493–1498.

75. Antman EM. Hirudin in acute myocardial infarction. Thrombolysis and Thrombin Inhibition in Myocardial Infarction (TIMI) 9B trial. *Circulation* 1996; 94:911–921.

76. Neuhaus KL, Molhoek GP, Zeymer U *et al.* Recombinant hirudin (lepirudin) for the improvement of thrombolysis with streptokinase in patients with acute myocardial infarction: results of the HIT-4 trial. *J Am Coll Cardiol* 1999; 34:966–973.

77. White HD, Aylward PE, Frey MJ *et al*. Randomised, double-blind comparison of hirulog versus heparin in patients receiving streptokinase and aspirin for acute myocardial infarction (HERO). Hirulog Early Reperfusion/Occlusion (HERO) Trial Investigators. *Circulation* 1997; 96:2155–2161.

78. White H. Thrombin-specific anticoagulation with bivalirudin versus heparin in patients receiving fibrinolytic therapy for acute myocardial infarction: the HERO-2 randomised trial. *Lancet* 2001; 358:1855–1863.

79. Wallentin L, Wilcox R, Weaver WD *et al*. Oral ximegalatran for secondary prophylaxis after acute myocardial infarction: the ESTEEM randomised controlled trial. *Lancet* 2003; 362:789–797.

80. Lamfers EJ, Schut A, Hooghoudt TE *et al*. Prehospital thrombolysis with reteplase: the Nijmegen/Rotterdam study. *Am Heart J* 2003; 146:479–483.

81. Morrow DA, Antman EM, Sayah A *et al*. Evaluation of the time saved by pre-hospital initiation of reteplase for ST-elevation myocardial infarction: results of The Early Retavase-Thrombolysis in Myocardial Infarction (ER-TIMI) 19 trial. *J Am Coll Cardiol* 2002; 40:71–77.

82. Morrison LJ, Verbeek PR, McDonald AC, Sawadsky BV, Cook DJ. Mortality and pre-hospital thrombolysis for acute myocardial infarction: A meta-analysis. *JAMA* 2000; 283:2686–2692.

83. Bonnefoy E, Lapostolle F, Leizorovicz A *et al*. Primary angioplasty versus pre-hospital fibrinolysis in acute myocardial infarction: a randomised study. *Lancet* 2002; 360:825–829.

84. Steg G, Bonnefoy E, Chabaud S *et al*. Impact of time to treatment on mortality after pre-hospital fibrinolysis or primary angioplasty – Data from the CAPTIM randomised clinical trial. *Circulation* 2003; 108:2851–2856.

85. Keeley EC, Boura JA, Grines CL. Primary angioplasty versus intravenous thrombolytic therapy for acute myocardial infarction: a quantitative review of 23 randomised trials. *Lancet* 2003; 361:13–20.

86. De Luca G, Suryapranata H, Zijlstra F *et al*. Symptom-onset-to-balloon time and mortality in patients with acute myocardial infarction treated by primary angioplasty. *J Am Coll Cardiol* 2003; 42:991–997.

87. Brodie BR, Stuckey TD, Hansen C, Muncy D. Benefit of coronary reperfusion before intervention on outcomes after primary angioplasty for acute myocardial infarction. *Am J Cardiol* 2000; 85:13–18.

88. Stone GW, Brodie BR, Griffin JJ *et al*. Prospective, multicenter study of the safety and feasibility of primary stenting in acute myocardial infarction: in-hospital and 30-day results of the PAMI stent pilot trial. Primary Angioplasty in Myocardial Infarction Stent Pilot Trial Investigators. *J Am Coll Cardiol* 1998; 31:23–30.

89. Stone GW, Cox D, Garcia E *et al*. Normal flow (TIMI-3) before mechanical reperfusion therapy is an independent determinant of survival in acute myocardial infarction: analysis from the primary angioplasty in myocardial infarction trials. *Circulation* 2001; 104:636–641.

90. De Luca G, Ernst N, Zijlstra F *et al*. Preprocedural TIMI flow and mortality in patients with acute myocardial infarction treated by primary angioplasty. *J Am Coll Cardiol* 2004; 43:1363–1367.

91. Gibson CM, Cannon CP, Murphy SA, Marble SJ, Barron HV, Braunwald E. Relationship of the TIMI myocardial perfusion grades, flow grades, frame count, and percutaneous coronary intervention to long-term outcomes after thrombolytic administration in acute myocardial infarction. *Circulation* 2002; 105:1909–1913.

92. Immediate vs delayed catheterization and angioplasty following thrombolytic therapy for acute myocardial infarction. TIMI II A results. The TIMI Research Group. *JAMA* 1988; 260:2849–2858.

93. Comparison of invasive and conservative strategies after treatment with intravenous tissue plasminogen activator in acute myocardial infarction. Results of the thrombolysis in myocardial infarction (TIMI) phase II trial. The TIMI Study Group. *N Engl J Med* 1989; 320:618–627.

94. SWIFT trial of delayed elective intervention v conservative treatment after thrombolysis with anistreplase in acute myocardial infarction. SWIFT (Should We Intervene Following Thrombolysis?) Trial Study Group. *BMJ* 1991; 302:555–560.

95. Califf RM, Topol EJ, Stack RS *et al*. Evaluation of combination thrombolytic therapy and timing of cardiac catheterization in acute myocardial infarction. Results of thrombolysis and angioplasty in myocardial infarction–phase 5 randomised trial. TAMI Study Group. *Circulation* 1991; 83:1543–1556.

96. Simoons ML, Arnold AE, Betriu A *et al*. Thrombolysis with tissue plasminogen activator in acute myocardial infarction: no additional benefit from immediate percutaneous coronary angioplasty. *Lancet* 1988; 1:197–203.

97. Topol EJ, Califf RM, George BS *et al*. A randomised trial of immediate versus delayed elective angioplasty after intravenous tissue plasminogen activator in acute myocardial infarction. *N Engl J Med* 1987; 317:581–588.

98. Fernandez-Aviles F, Alonso J, Castro-Beiras A *et al*. Randomised trial comparing stenting within 24 h of thrombolysis versus conservative ischaemia-guided approach to thrombolysed ST-elevated acute myocardial infarction. Final results of the GRACIA trial (abstract). *Eur Heart J* 2003; 24(suppl):704.

99. Scheller B, Hennen B, Hammer B *et al*. Beneficial effects of immediate stenting after thrombolysis in acute myocardial infarction. *J Am Coll Cardiol* 2003; 42:634–641.

100. Fernandez-Aviles F, Alonso J, Castro-Beiras A *et al*. Routine invasive strategy within 24 h of thrombolysis versus ischaemia-guided conservative approach for acute myocardial infarction with ST-segment elevation. (GRACIA-1): a randomised controlled trial. *Lancet* 2004; 364:1045–1053.

101. Herrmann HC, Moliterno DJ, Ohman EM *et al*. Facilitation of early percutaneous coronary intervention after reteplase with or without abciximab in acute myocardial infarction: results from the SPEED (GUSTO-4 Pilot) Trial. *J Am Coll Cardiol* 2000; 36:1489–1496.

102. Ellis SG, Armstrong P, Betriu A *et al*. Facilitated percutaneous coronary intervention versus primary percutaneous coronary intervention: design and rationale of the Facilitated Intervention with Enhanced Reperfusion Speed to Stop Events (FINESSE) trial. *Am Heart J* 2004; 147:E16.

12

Pre-hospital reperfusion therapy

K. Huber, R. De Caterina, S. D. Kristensen

INTRODUCTION

Over the past years, 4–6 week mortality from acute ST-elevation myocardial infarction (STEMI) has decreased from more than 20% in the pre-thrombolytic area to 8% using fibrin-specific thrombolytic agents, and down to 4% with the use of primary percutaneous coronary intervention (PPCI) in controlled trials under optimal conditions. Data from registries have shown 4–6 week mortality rates of >20% non-reperfused patients, of 10% in thrombolysed patients (fibrin-specific agents), and of up to 8% in patients treated with PPCI. The increased mortality rate in registries might be due to the general higher risk of patients in registries as compared with patients in controlled trials, where patients in shock or the elderly are frequently excluded [1, 2]. With thrombolytic therapy, concerns remain related to suboptimal patency, early re-occlusion, and failure of myocardial reperfusion at the microcirculatory level [3]. Lack of operator experience and excessive treatment delays might decrease efficacy of PPCI [4]. The mean door-to-balloon time in registries often expands up to 120 min, depending on the availability of a cath lab and experienced interventionists [5].

At present, in most regions in the world thrombolytic therapy is still the fastest and most accessible reperfusion treatment for most patients presenting with acute STEMI, as indicated in the international guidelines [4, 6], while PPCI covers only up to 20% of patients except in areas where 24 h around-the-clock available catheter facilities have been well organised. As demonstrated recently, thrombolysis and PPCI are not mutually exclusive therapies, and attempts at combining them are ongoing.

For an optimal organisation of reperfusion therapy in acute STEMI the most important questions currently appear to be:

1) what kind of reperfusion therapy is immediately available, dependent on the local situation;
2) how can time from onset of symptoms to reperfusion be reduced; and
3) whether 'facilitated PCI', i.e., the combination of early pharmacologic reperfusion followed immediately by PCI, can further improve efficacy of therapy.

Besides these questions, however, the most burning goal today is to increase the number of STEMI patients who are treated with any type of reperfusion therapy, since data from

Kurt Huber, Professor of Cardiology and Internal Medicine, 3rd Medical Department (Cardiology and Emergency Medicine), Wilhelminenhospital, Vienna, Austria.

Raffaele De Caterina, Professor of Cardiology, Institute of Cardiology, "G. d'Annunzio" University – Chieti, Ospedale San Camillo de Lellis, Chieti, Italy.

Steen Dalby Kristensen, Head of Cardiology, University Department of Cardiology, Skejby Hospital, Aarhus University Hospital, Aarhus, Denmark.

registries have shown that about one-third of eligible patients is not given reperfusion therapy at all [7].

REPERFUSION STRATEGIES AND IMPORTANCE OF TIME-TO-TREATMENT

Thrombolytic therapy is most effective if initiated within the first 1–3 h from symptom onset (the 'golden hour' concept) [8–11]. Compared with the huge amount of data generated in more than 58 000 patients undergoing thrombolytic therapy, the importance of early reperfusion with PPCI is less well investigated and frequently denied by interventionists, who often prefer to intervene on patients despite longer organisation times based on the assumption that mechanical reperfusion is superior to pharmacological reperfusion in any case. Indeed, randomised trials comparing timely performed PPCI in experienced centres with thrombolytic therapy have demonstrated higher patency rates, fewer early re-occlusion rates, better residual left ventricular function, and better clinical outcome [12–30, 31]. In particular, several prospective, randomised trials have shown a significant benefit of PPCI vs. lysis in acute STEMI of up to 12 h duration [14, 28, 29, 31].

The PRAGUE trial randomised 300 patients with STEMI and symptoms of <6 h to treatment with streptokinase, treatment with streptokinase and transferral for 'facilitated' PCI, or transferral for PPCI [28]. Transfer was safe, and transferral for PPCI was associated with a significantly lower incidence of the composite endpoint of death/re-infarction/stroke at 30 days compared with the other treatment groups. This difference was mainly due to a very low incidence of re-infarction in the PPCI group.

In the AIRPAMI study, 138 high-risk acute STEMI patients with <12 h from symptom onset were randomised to either tPA (plus 48 h of unfractionated heparin [UFH] infusion) in the local hospital, or transferred for PPCI [31]. The primary endpoint was the combination of death, re-infarction and disabling stroke within 30 days. The trial was stopped prematurely because of difficulties in recruiting patients. The transfer group had a 38% reduction in the primary endpoint, but this difference was not statistically significant. The time-to-treatment was delayed in the PPCI group, mainly due to a delay in the inititation of transport.

PRAGUE-2 was a multicentre trial performed in the Czech Republic [29]. Here 850 patients with acute STEMI presenting within 12 h from symptom onset admitted to the nearest community hospital without PCI facilities were randomised to either thrombolysis (streptokinase) in the local hospital or immediate transport for PPCI. The primary endpoint (30-day mortality) occurred in 6.8% in the PPCI group compared with 10.0% in the streptokinase group ($P = 0.12$).

DANAMI-2 was a randomised multicentre Danish controlled trial that assigned 1572 patients to alteplase (plus 48 h of UFH) or PPCI [14, 32]. The primary endpoint was a combination of death, clinical re-infarction and disabling stroke at 30 days. A total of 1129 patients were enrolled at referral hospitals and 443 patients were randomised in centres with PCI facilities. Among patients who underwent randomisation at referral centres, the primary endpoint occurred in 8.5% of the patients transferred for PPCI and in 14.2% of the patients treated with alteplase ($P = 0.002$). In patients randomised in the hospitals with PCI facilities, 6.7% in the PPCI group reached the primary endpoint compared with 12.3% in the thrombolysis group ($P = 0.05$). Among all patients, the better outcome of PPCI was driven by a reduction in re-infarction (1.6% in the PPCI vs. 6.3% in the thrombolysis group; $P < 0.001$). No significant differences were observed in the rate of death (6.6 vs. 7.8%; $P = 0.35$) or the rate of stroke (1.1 vs. 2.0%; $P = 0.15$). The superiority of PPCI over thrombolysis was present in patient subgroups randomised <2 h, between 2 and 4 h, and >4 h from the onset of symptoms. Unfortunately, <2% of patients in the alteplase group underwent 'rescue' PCI.

Since DANAMI-2 showed that transferral for primary PCI (allowed up to 3 h, on the average happening within 2 h) was superior to thrombolytic therapy, it might be argued that the useful window for transfer to a PPCI centre indicated in guidelines might theoretically be extended to 120 min. However, based on the results of an analysis of the randomised controlled trials comparing fibrinolysis with a fibrin-specific agent vs. PPCI (showing that the mortality benefit of PPCI only exists when treatment is delayed by no more than 60 min [33]), and based on data showing that the mortality benefit associated with primary PCI in acute STEMI may be lost if door-to-balloon time is delayed by >1 h compared with the door-to-needle time in thrombolytic therapy with tissue-type plasminogen activator [34, 35], the recent American College of Cardiology/American Heart Association (ACC/AHA) Guidelines have also reduced the medical contact-to-balloon or door-to-balloon time goal to 90 min, in an attempt to maximise the benefits of reperfusion with PPCI [4]. The Writing Committee of the recent ACC/AHA Guidelines also openly stated that there is legitimate evidence-based concern that routine PPCI for patients with acute STEMI will result in unacceptable delays in achieving reperfusion in a substantial number of patients and also lead to suboptimal outcomes if performed by less-experienced interventionists [4]. Accordingly, in patients in whom PPCI is performed by non-specialised centres, outcome data for PPCI are not so impressive: TIMI 3 flow rates were below 90% [36]. In-hospital and 3-year mortality rates were comparable with those of thrombolytic therapy even in high-risk patients, and treatment costs were significantly higher [36].

Keely *et al.* [37] combined most of the published trials in an overview of fibrinolysis vs. PPCI ($n = 2909$) by additional inclusion of the SHOCK study, which compared medical stabilisation with immediate revascularisation for cardiogenic shock [38]. This analysis showed that PCI-treated patients experienced lower short-term mortality rates, fewer non-fatal myocardial infarctions (MIs), and fewer haemorrhagic strokes than those treated with fibrinolysis, at the cost of an increased risk of major bleeding [37]. Transfer for PPCI in this meta-analysis was also associated with a non-significant trend towards a decrease in death rate compared with thrombolytic therapy ($P = 0.057$), even when the SHOCK trial was excluded from calculations (PPCI 5.5 vs. lysis 6.7%; $P = 0.081$) [39].

In another meta-analysis, Dalby and co-workers [40] analysed the data from various trials comparing on-site thrombolyis with transferrals for PPCI ($n = 3750$). The combined endpoint of death, re-infarction and stroke was significantly reduced, by 42%, in the group transferred for PPCI compared with the group that received on-site thrombolysis. Looking at the endpoints separately, re-infarction was significantly reduced by 68%, and stroke by 56%. There was a trend towards a reduction of all-cause mortality by 19% at 30 days ($P = 0.08$) in the PPCI group, despite the time delay for transferral.

However, despite these beneficial effects shown in patients who had to be transferred for PPCI, the loss of time during the organisation of PPCI (door-to-needle time) was also associated with an increase in mortality. The Analyses of the National Registry of Myocardial Infarction-2 trial (NRMI-2) indeed demonstrated a 41–62% increase in mortality with increases in the door-to-balloon time [41]. Similar data were obtained from the GUSTO-IIb study [42]. In an analysis of the randomised controlled trials comparing a fibrin-specific agent with PPCI, Juliard *et al.* demonstrated that mortality increases significantly with each 15 min delay in the time between patient's arrival and restoration of TIMI 3 flow [33]. Furthermore, time from symptom onset to balloon inflation was significantly correlated with 1-year mortality in patients undergoing PPCI (8% increase of relative risk for each 30-min delay; $P = 0.04$) [43, 44].

In the discussion of these trials comparing PPCI with thrombolysis, it has frequently not been taken into account that thrombolytic therapy is only highly effective in infarctions with short symptom onset (up to 2–3 h), when salvage of myocardium is the goal of reperfusion, while PPCI has benefits also in infarctions of longer duration, most possibly based on the 'open artery' hypothesis [45, 46]. Accordingly, recent studies have clearly demonstrated that mortality is in general low and not different for both treatment strategies in the early phase of acute STEMI [15, 29, 47] (Figure 12.1).

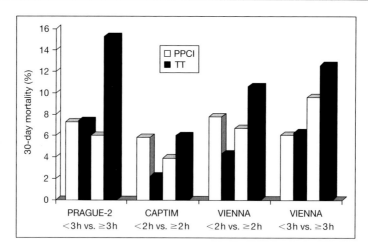

Figure 12.1. Thirty-day mortality in dependence of time between symptom onset and start of therapy. comparison between primary percutaneous coronary intervention (PPCI) and thrombolytic therapy (TT) in acute ST-elevation myocardial infarction up to 12 h from onset of symptoms.
Data represent results from the PRAGUE-2 trial [29], the CAPTIM trial [15], and the VIENNA Registry [47]

In the PRAGUE-2 trial, among 299 patients who were randomised after >3 h from symptom onset, the 30-day mortality for primary PCI was 6 vs. 15.3% in the thrombolysis group ($P < 0.02$) whereas for patients randomised within 3 h from symptom onset ($n = 551$) there was no difference in mortality between the two groups (PPCI 7.3%; thrombolysis 7.4%) [29].

Similarily, patients of the CAPTIM trial [15] treated with thrombolysis within 2 h of onset of symptoms had a better mortality outcome compared with patients treated with PPCI, while after two hours from symptom onset the efficacy benefit was better for PPCI.

Recently, in the Vienna Registry for Optimisation of Reperfusion Strategies in Acute STEMI [47], it could be shown that, with respect to in-hospital mortality, thrombolytic therapy is slightly, but not significantly, better than PPCI when treatment is started within 2 h from symptom onset, while both reperfusion strategies turned out to be equal when started within 3 h from symptom onset. After 3 h from symptom onset, PPCI was always better than thrombolytic therapy [47].

The pathophysiologic evidence of the increase in myocardial necrosis over time and of the related increase in mortality with both treatment options clearly underscores the impact of time delay, regardless of whether pharmacologic or mechanical reperfusion is used. The increase in mortality over time in relation with the start of reperfusion therapy with pharmacological vs. mechanical means is shown in Figure 12.2 [46], compiling data from a meta-analysis of thrombolysis trials [9] and the NRMI-2 results for mechanical reperfusion [41]. Also in these older studies mortality rates after thrombolysis and PPCI have been comparable if both procedures were started within the first 2–3 h from symptom onset. Afterwards, mortality increased dramatically after thrombolysis, whereas there is a slighter increase of mortality over time with PPCI. This might be explained by the fact that successful PPCI immediately leads to optimal recanalisation (TIMI 3 flow) in >90% of patients, while thrombolysis is less effective on 'older' clots, resulting in a TIMI 3 flow rate of only 50% or less. Furthermore, if successful, fibrinolysis requires at least an additional 30–45 min from initiation of treatment until vessel reperfusion [48]. This makes the 'golden hour' so important for thrombolytic therapy, and still important – albeit less – for PPCI.

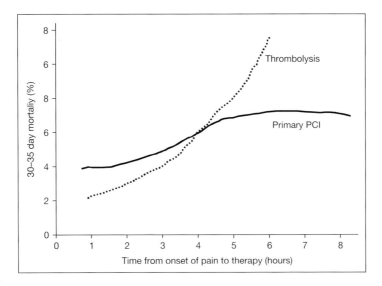

Figure 12.2. Impact of time on 30- to 35-day mortality: primary PCI vs. thrombolytic therapy. Mortality rates, as related to time of pain onset to initiation of therapy, are given from a meta-analysis of thrombolysis trials [9] and from the NRMI-2 Registry [41].

TIME DELAYS IN REPERFUSION THERAPY

The overall time delay between the onset of chest pain and initiation of reperfusion therapy on average is 2.5–3 h [49]. It is composed of the pre-hospital patient decision delay (1.5 to 3 h), the pre-hospital transportation delay (30 to 130 min), and the in-hospital organisation delay, respectively. The latter is either composed of the 'door-to-needle' time (up to 60–90 min in non-specialised hospitals) or the 'door-to-balloon' time (up to two hours and more in non-specialised hospitals with catheter facilities) [49]. Since in many cases patients with an acute MI are initially admitted to a community hospital without catheterisation facilities and then transferred to a tertiary medical centre for mechanical intervention, a further delay for transportation between hospitals has to be added.

The first of these three components, the pre-hospital patient decision delay, can be reduced to <1 h by community programs of improved patient information [50]. Unfortunately, the initial benefit seen in these programs is not sustained, and also its cost-effectivenes has been questioned [51, 52]. Other investigations based on media campaigns have resulted in increased use of medical services without significant reduction of the individual patient's delay [53].

The last component of treatment delay, in-hospital delay, has been shortened to about 20–30 min by establishing special in-hospital structures, e.g., by building-up emergency departments with special equipment and specifically trained personnel, as well as by allowing emergency physicians to administer thrombolytic therapy [54].

A further substantial shortening of time delays is, therefore, only possible by bringing reperfusion therapy to the patient before the patient reaches the hospital. This will now be analysed in greater detail.

RISK STRATIFICATION FOR STEMI

It has recently been demonstrated that the time-dependence of the outcome after PPCI is higher in 'not-low-risk' STEMI patients than in patients at low risk (Figure 12.4) [55].

'Not-low'-risk patients include those with at least one of the following three clinical parameters at presentation: age >70 years, heart rate >100 b.p.m., and the anterior wall as infarct localisation [55]. Other authors have also described the existence of similar high-risk subgroups of patients with STEMI who might especially benefit from timely reperfusion [19, 56]. The logical conclusion, therefore, is that STEMI patients with an early presentation (within 2–3 h from symptom onset) should be recanalised with the method that can be offered fastest – at present in most cases world-wide thrombolytic therapy. This can be followed by transportation to a tertiary centre for 'facilitated' PCI of an already recanalised vessel (still currently under investigation) or 'rescue' PCI for failed thrombolysis. Transportation for PPCI is the other option if transportation times are expected to result in a sufficiently short treatment delay.

Patients with signs of cardiogenic shock especially are at high-risk concerning outcome [38]. In shock patients an absolute 9% reduction in 30-day mortality with coronary revascularisation compared with immediate medical stabilisation was reported [38]. In general, PPCI should be the preferred method in patients with shock [4, 57].

PRE-HOSPITAL THROMBOLYSIS

Pre-hospital thrombolytic therapy in STEMI has led to an additional reduction of the delay time between 33 and 130 min, as demonstrated in three high-quality pre-hospital thrombolysis trials: the EMIP, MITI, and GREAT trials [10, 58, 59]. This overall reduction in delay time was associated with a significant 1.7% absolute (17% relative) risk reduction of 30-day mortality. No significant safety risk was demonstrated for pre-hospital vs. in-hospital thrombolysis [60].

Despite these interesting and favourable data, pre-hospital thrombolysis has only been organised on a widespread basis in a few countries [61]. The underuse of pre-hospital thrombolysis can be explained by different reasons, namely 1) by the inability of responsible persons or institutions to organise pre-hospital treatment in a quality-controlled fashion, and 2) by budgetary restriction and selective preference for in-hospital allocations of resources. Pre-hospital thrombolysis has been shown to be beneficial especially in rural areas with long transportation delays, while transportation times are considered to be short in urban areas. Therefore, minimisation of in-hospital delays appeared to many cardiologists and hospital administrators in urban areas to be more important and effective, involving fewer logistics and expenditures than implementing pre-hospital thrombolysis. In contrast, it has been shown that, at present also in urban areas, time from first medical contact to first balloon inflation with PPCI often exceeds the optimal pre-intervention period of <90 min [4, 57, 62] recommended in the recent guidelines [4, 57].

Efficacy and safety of pre-hospital thrombolysis depend on the likelihood of diagnosis, well-trained personnel, monitoring during transporation, as well as optimal information of the referring hospital: STEMI has to be diagnosed by a 12-lead-ECG, which helps to initate treatment appropriately, even in the hands of paramedics with or without computer assistance [63–67]. Ambulance personnel (physicians, nurses, paramedics) have to be well trained for symptom recognition and management of STEMI and its early complications. Intravenous access has to be established and IV therapy has to be administered according to a reperfusion therapy checklist. During transportation, rhythm monitoring and advanced cardiac life support are mandatory. Finally, early contact with the referring hospital (e.g., by electronic transmission of the 12-lead ECG), appears to be necessary, allowing early preparation of further care, which also contributes to improving the outcome [61].

The specific value of a mobile coronary care unit (MCCU) (i.e., an ambulance equipped with a defibrillator, which can also record the 12-lead ECG, and with facilities to transmit the ECG digitally to the referring hospital, all manned by a trained, even junior, doctor and a coronary care nurse) has recently been emphasised [68]. With such MCCUs, the response time to a call has been shown to be as low as 10 min [69]. As mentioned by the authors, the patients managed pre-hospitally showed a significantly shorter median delay time from call for help to receiving thrombolytic therapy (1.0 vs. 1.8 h; $P < 0.001$), resulting in a shorter pain-to-needle time (2.3 vs. 4.0 h; $P < 0.001$) and consequently a lower in-hospital mortality rate (7 vs. 13%; $P = 0.02$). Patients aged ≥75 years who received pre-hospital thrombolytic therapy had a significantly lower mortality than those first treated in hospital (21 vs. 43%; $P = 0.02$).

The administration of thrombolytics by infusion, as it was mostly available over the past years has been, until recently, another obstacle for the implementation of quicker pre-hospital reperfusion strategies. The administration of thrombolysis by infusion resulted in 13.5% medication errors in the streptokinase arm, and 11.5% in the tissue plasminogen activator (tPA) arm in GUSTO-1, and this was associated with a more than doubling of the 24-h mortality rate, and a significant increase in 30-day mortality [70]. A similar experience comes from the TIME-II trial, indicating that dosing errors with tPA infusion were mostly seen in patients with a low body weight, and suggesting that the need for weight adjustments in only a fraction of patients for tPA was the major source of incorrect dosing, resulting in a higher number of intracranial haemorrhages (ICH) [70]. These data provide support for the observation that appropriate dosing of the fibrinolytic agent is important to optimise outcomes in acute MI, and that the use of simpler weight-adjusted dosing regimens, such as those associated with the single-bolus fibrinolytic agent tenecteplase, might improve the accuracy of dosing and, in turn, the therapeutic outcome.

The availability of thrombolytic agents suitable for double- or single-bolus injection has, therefore, led to a new interest in the setting-up of clinical pre-hospital thrombolysis trials. Furthermore, new adjunct antithrombotic treatment options have been tested in order to increase efficacy of thrombolysis, including low-molecular-weight heparins (LMWH) and clopidogrel.

The Early Retavase-Thrombolysis in Myocardial Infarction 19 (ER-TIMI-19) trial planned inclusion of 1000 patients, comparing open-label pre-hospital thrombolytic therapy (r-PA, double bolus 10 + 10 mg) with a retrospective group [69]. The trial was stopped after only 315 patients had been recruited, because a 31 min reduction of the delay time compared with a historical control group was demonstrated [71].

The third Assessment of the Safety and Efficacy of New Thrombolytic Regimens Pre-hospital Substudy (ASSENT-3+) enrolled more than 1600 patients, randomised to pre-hospital tenecteplase (TNK-tPA) and either UFH or the LMWH enoxaparin as an adjunct antithrombotic agent [72]. The impact of pre-hospital thrombolysis was compared with the results of a similar population from the ASSENT-3 main trial [73] in a non-randomised comparison. Time-to-treatment was reduced in the pre-hospital treatment group by about 45 min. Treatment with enoxaparin resulted in a 3.2% absolute risk reduction ($P = 0.08$). However, intracerebral bleeding rate was significantly higher in enoxaparin-treated patients compared with UFH (2.2% vs. 0.97%; $P = 0.047$), which was primarily a function of age (enoxaparin group: >75 years 6.8% vs. ≤75 years 1.2%; $P = 0.01$) and gender (higher bleeding rates in women; $P = 0.02$). Accordingly, pre-hospital thrombolytic therapy with TNK-tPA and enoxaparin has been demonstrated to be beneficial and safe in patients ≤75 years of age compared with UFH. In older patients (>75 years) the optimal dosage of adjunct enoxaparin is still unknown. The recently published ACC/AHA Guidelines for the Management of Patients With ST-Elevation Myocardial Infarction have taken these results into account: accordingly, LMWH is considered an acceptable alternative to UFH as ancillary therapy for patients of <75 years of age, while it is not recommended for patients over the age of 75 [4]. The Thrombosis in Myocardial Infarction (TIMI) group has suggested that the dose of enoxaparin be reduced to 75% of the full dose (0.75 mg/kg SC twice a day) and the initial bolus avoided in the elderly. This regimen is currently being tested in the TIMI-25 ExTRACT trial, which also involves a pre-hospital treatment arm.

Conversely, favourable results concerning efficacy and safety with clopidogrel as an adjunct to thrombolytic therapy together with UFH or LMWH have been published recently. The CLARITY-TIMI-28 trial, which also offered the possibility of performing pre-hospital thrombolytic therapy [74], enrolled 3491 patients 75 years of age or younger who presented within 12 h after onset of STEMI and were randomly assigned to receive clopidogrel (300 mg loading dose, followed by 75 mg once daily) or placebo. Patients received a fibrinolytic agent (in 70% a fibrin-specific agent, in 30% streptokinase), aspirin, as well as heparin or LMWH, and were scheduled to undergo angiography 48–120 h after the initiation of study medication. The primary efficacy endpoint consisted of an occluded infarct-related artery (TIMI flow grade 0 or 1) on angiography or death, or recurrent MI before angiography (after 2–8 days). Clopidogrel-treated patients reached this endpoint in 15.0 vs. 21.7% in the placebo group (36% relative risk reduction; $P < 0.001$). By 30 days, clopidogrel reduced the odds of the composite endpoint of cardiovascular death, recurrent MI, or urgent revascularisation due to recurrent ischaemia by 20% (11.6 vs. 14.1%; $P = 0.03$). Bleeding complications (intracerebral or major) were comparable in the two groups.

'FACILITATED'-PCI IN STEMI

Studies have shown smaller infarct size, better left ventricular function and fewer complications when reperfusion occurs before PCI [75–77]. Therefore, early triage of candidates to PPCI and the pre-hospital initiation of pharmacologic reperfusion therapy with subsequent transfer to coronary angiography (and angioplasty) might improve the efficacy of treatment. 'Facilitated'-PCI, the fixed combination of early pharmacological reperfusion with subsequent mechanical optimisation of the initial result, is a very attractive therapeutic concept that deserves further investigation. Facilitation thereby can be achieved by the use of thrombolytic agents, glycoprotein IIb/IIIa antagonists, or a combination of the two. In addition, the early administration of high-dose clopidogrel is currently being tested.

Earlier trials combining full-dose thrombolytic therapy with subsequent PCI in order to improve reperfusion and/or reduce re-occlusion all showed an unfavourable trend to more complications and an increased mortality rate [78–80]. Due to improved interventional methods and devices, PCI following thrombolytic therapy has become more effective and relatively safe. A combination of different antithrombotic agents, however, which is often necessary in these situations, may lead to excessive bleeding complications [81], and careful dosing and patient selection is recommended. A meta-analysis of all published trials using combination therapy of thrombolytic agents and abciximab has shown that combination therapy leads to severe bleeding rates, which are increased by more than 50% in the combination arm compared with thrombolytic monotherapy, without improving efficacy outcomes [82]. Extremely high bleeding complications have been shown for streptokinase in combination with abciximab (TIMI-14 trial [83]), which should therefore no longer be used.

FACILITATION WITH THROMBOLYTIC AGENTS

In the PACT trial, patients with acute STEMI were treated with a bolus of 50 mg tPA and subsequently underwent coronary angiography. A higher percentage of TIMI 2 and 3 flow at diagnostic angiography, no excess need for mechanical intervention due to TIMI 3 flow and low residual stenosis after successful thrombolysis could be demonstrated. Furthermore, PCI was unproblematic from the technical point of view. Moreover, complication rates due to the combined treatment (thrombolysis plus PCI) were low and acceptable [84].

In the GRACIA-2 trial, PPCI (108 patients) was compared with fibrinolysis with TNK-tpA (and enoxaparin) and subsequent PCI (104 patients) [85]. Primary endpoints were infarct size, time until ST-segment resolution, and the development of left ventricular dysfunction. The secondary combined endpoints consisted of death, non-fatal MI, or acute revascularisation after 6 weeks and 6 months, respectively. Diagnostic angiography revealed an open infarct-related artery in 59% of patients pre-treated with TNK-tPA, but in only 14% of patients initially randomised to PPCI. Patients in the facilitated-PCI group showed at 6 h a significantly faster reduction of initial ST-segment elevation (61% vs. 43%; $P = 0.03$). No significant differences could be demonstrated as to infarct size and the secondary combined endpoints. There was a trend, however, towards lower mortality, re-infarctions and re-intervention rates in patients facilitated with thrombolysis (9 vs. 14%).

In the ASSENT-4 PCI trial (Assessment of the Safety and Efficacy of a New Treatment Strategy for Acute Myocardial Infarction trial; 4000 patients planned; PPCI vs. TNK-tPA/enoxaparin-facilitated PCI), which was initiated to investigate the effectiveness and safety of PPCI facilitated with full-dose TNK-tPA, inclusion of patients has been recently suspended due to a lower mortality rate in patients treated with PPCI only. The concept of facilitated-PCI with thrombolytc agents is, therefore, still a matter of discussion and open questions.

FACILITATION WITH GPIIb/IIIa-RECEPTOR BLOCKERS WITH/WITHOUT HALF-DOSE THROMBOLYTICS

In the BRAVE-1 trial, pre-treatment of patients with acute STEMI during transfer from the secondary hospital to the cath lab in a tertiary hospital was performed either with a combination therapy of half-dose reteplase plus full-dose abciximab or with abciximab alone [86]. Although TIMI 2 and 3 flow was higher at first diagnostic angiogram in the combination therapy group, immediate outcome of PCI and myocardial salvage was similar in both groups. However, bleeding complications were significantly increased in the combination therapy group [86].

Facilitated-PCI combining the glycoprotein (GP)IIb/IIIa-receptor blocker abciximab (full dose) and reteplase (half dose) is currently being tested in the FINESSE and CARESS trials, both of which show slow patient inclusion.

FACILITATION WITH GPIIb/IIIa-RECEPTOR BLOCKERS

Randomised trials with abciximab as adjunctive antiplatelet therapy during PCI of the infarct-related artery demonstrated the usefulness of this GPIIb/IIIa-blocker.

In the RAPPORT trial (482 patients), abciximab significantly improved the immediate clinical outcome (combination of death, MI, and urgent revascularisation) and reduced the need for 'bail-out' stenting [87]. However bleeding complications also increased significantly in the abciximab group, likely as a result of the relatively high doses of adjunct intravenous UFH.

In the ISAR-2 trial (401 patients), the use of abciximab in combination with a reduced dose of UFH resulted in a significant reduction of the combined endpoint (death, re-infarction, target lesion revascularisation after 30 days), but did not reduce angiographic restenosis [88].

In the double-blind ADMIRAL trial (300 patients), abciximab was given before sheath insertion in all patients, and one-fourth of the patients received the study drug early, either in the emergency room or in the ambulance on the way to the cath lab [89]. The drug improved angiographic and clinical outcomes in the global population, with a particular benefit in the subgroup of patients treated early. Recent data have shown that there is a long-term benefit at 3 years in patients treated early with abciximab [90].

In the CADILLAC trial (2082 patients), a beneficial effect of abciximab could only be demonstrated for patients with balloon dilatation, but not for patients receiving stents [91]. There was some benefit of abciximab vs. no abciximab on the combined endpoint of death, re-infarction and target vessel revascularisation at 30 days in this study, but the primary

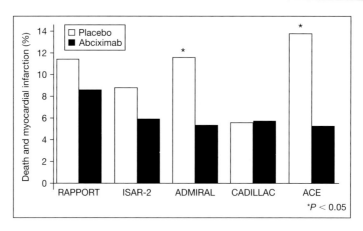

Figure 12.3. Abciximab in primary PCI: Death or myocardial infarction at 6 months. Data are presented from the five largest trials performed with the adjunctive use of this drug.

endpoint of death and re-infarction, both at 30 days and 6 months, was reduced non-significantly [92]. In this study, a high-risk subgroup that was not included into the main trial (long, complicated lesions, multivessel disease, small vessels, visible thrombus) showed some advantage of abciximab.

Recently, the ACE trial, performed in 400 patients with acute STEMI, reported on the use of abciximab in high-risk patients (cardiogenic shock, massive coronary thrombus load, main stem lesions, and significant stenoses of side branches related to the culprit lesion) that had been excluded in most other trials [93]. The combined primary endpoint (death, re-infarction, urgent target vessel revascularisation and stroke at 30 days) was significanlty reduced in the abciximab group (4.5% vs. 10.5%; $P = 0.023$). Early ST-segment resolution ($\geq 50\%$ after 30 min) occurred significantly more often (85% vs. 68%; $P = 0.001$) in abciximab-treated patients, in some of whom smaller infarct size was also shown at 30 days. After 6 months, the rate of the combined endpoint was still significantly lower in the abciximab arm of the trial (5.5% vs. 13.5%). Restenosis rate was comparable in the two groups.

One should remember that inclusion criteria differed markedly in these five trials: patients with shock were only incuded in the ISAR-2, ADMIRAL, and ACE trials, while patients in the CADILLAC trial had a relatively low-risk profile, as confirmed by the low event rate in the placebo group. Figure 12.3 summarises the combined endpoint of death and MI for the five above-mentioned trials. With the exception of CADILLAC, all trials showed some benefit for patients treated with abciximab, which was statistically significant in those trials (ADMIRAL, ACE) in which abciximab was initiated early before PPCI.

Three smaller trials have investigated surrogate parameters, which could help in understanding mechanisms underlying the benefit of early abciximab use:

Zorman *et al.* demonstrated a higher patency rate at diagnostic angiography in patients with acute MI pre-treated with abciximab as compared with patients without pre-treatment [94]. In the REOMOBILE trial, Arntz *et al.* studied 100 patients randomised to an early administration of abciximab in the mobile intensive care unit vs. administration at the time of intervention in the cath lab. Only a moderate trend in favour of early initiation of abciximab was shown for ST-segment resolution after 60–90 min, TIMI 2+3 flow and TIMI blush score at diagnostic angiography, as well as TIMI-3 flow after PCI [95].

In contrast, the ReoPro-BRIDGING trial [96] showed significantly improved surrogate parameters for early reperfusion when abciximab was administered in the emergency room

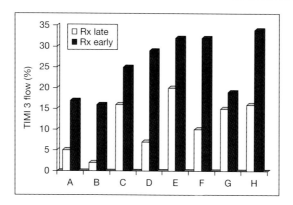

Figure 12.4. Early vs. late use of GPIIb/IIIa-antagonists in patients with ST-elevation myocardial infarction treated with primary PCI: TIMI 3 flow at diagnostic angiogram. Black bars represent early treatment groups (initiation of treatment in the emergency room or pre-hopsital), white bars represent late treatment groups (initiation of treatment immediatley before PCI). Abciximab was used in trials A–D (A: ADMIRAL [89]; B: Zorman *et al.* [94]; C: ReoMobile [95]; D: ReoPro-BRIDGING [96]), tirofiban in trials E-G (E: Cutlip *et al.* [99]; F: TIGER-PA [100]; G: OnTIME [101]), and eptifibatide in trial H (INTAMI [102]), respectively.

compared to immediately before PPCI: pre-PPCI ST-segment resolution: 55 ± 21.4% vs. 42.4 ± 18.2%; $P = 0.005$; TIMI 3 flow grade 29 vs. 7%; $P = 0.042$; corrected TIMI frame count 58.4 ± 32.7 vs. 78.9 ± 28.4 frames; $P = 0.018$); percent diameter stenosis (median 76.3 vs. 100; $P = 0.023$) [96].

Recently, a meta-analysis of the different trials comparing early adminstration of abciximab vs. administration in the cath lab confirmed the favourable outcome of early abciximab use on surrogate parameters and clinical endpoints (especially on re-infarction), but failed to demonstrate a significant reduction of mortality [97].

In a larger meta-analysis [98], a positive influence from early administration of abciximab, a significant reduction in mortality could also be demonstrated.

Overall, these data on the use of abciximab before PPCI are promising, but its routine administration before PPCI is still a matter of discussion.

Compared with abciximab, less data on tirofiban (Cutlip *et al.* [99]; TIGER-PA pilot trial [100]; OnTime Trial [101]) and eptifibatide (INTAMI trial [102]) in PPCI are currently available, but have demonstrated similar improvements in the TIMI-3 flow rate at first diagnostic angiogram when treatment with the GPIIb/IIIa-antagonist was initiated early (Figure 12.4).

FACILITATION WITH CLOPIDOGREL

Clopidogrel as an adjunctive antithrombotic agent has been shown to be effective in patients with non-ST-elevation acute coronary syndrome at low, medium and high risk for thromboembolic complications. In the CREDO trial a beneficial effect of clopidogrel 300 mg loading dose followed by 75 mg/day if administered >6 h before PCI with stent implantation, compared with later administration, was shown [103]. Data from experimental studies suggest a much faster (within 2 h) maximum action of clopidogrel if the drug is given with a high loading dosage, which has also been demonstrated to be safe [104]. Whether the early use of clopidogrel might reduce the need for GPIIb/IIIa-blockers, is still unknown.

Based on promising preliminary data [105, 106], high-dose clopidogrel (600 mg loading dose, followed by 150 mg/day) given before PCI has been investigated in chronic stable low-risk patients in the ISAR-REACT-1 trial [107], showing that it may render the use of abciximab before PCI in these patients unnecessary. Moreover, the ISAR-SWEET study, performed in clinically stable but otherwise high-risk diabetic patients, also demonstrated the decreasing importance of abciximab if high-dose clopidogrel was used before the intervention [108].

At present, early use of clopidogrel with or without the addition of abciximab is being tested in patients with NSTEMI (ISAR-REACT-2 study), as well as in patients with STEMI (BRAVE-3 study). The use of clopidogrel in the pre-hospital setting in patients with STEMI is of potential interest, but clearly needs further testing.

SUMMARY

Although the medical and technological revolution in the last three decades has improved clinical outcome in patients presenting with acute STEMI, residual morbidity and mortality are still high. The critical role of treatment delay and optimal sustained patency as pre-requisites of successful reperfusion have to be underlined. Clinical efficacy of successful reperfusion has been repeatedly demonstrated. Nevertheless, the ideal pharmacologic and mechanical reperfusion methods are still a matter of major debate.

Depending on the local situation, either immediate thrombolytic therapy or fast transfer to an experienced high-volume tertiary care centre for PPCI may be preferred. According to mortality data, pre-hospital and in-hospital thrombolysis have success rates comparable with PPCI when intitiated within the first 2 to 3 h after the onset of pain. Therefore, in these patients, thrombolytic therapy should not be withheld in favour of mechanical reperfusion if it cannot be offered within 90 min from first medical contact [4, 57]. The situation seems to be somewhat different in patients presenting later than 3 h after the onset of pain. These patients, have a mortality rate of about 6–8% when treated by mechanical reperfusion. In contrast, mortality rates increase exponentially with every hour delay when treated with thrombolysis. Therefore, for patients with a longer delay from symptom onset, a further time delay for transfer to a tertiary care hospital with catheter facilities seems to be acceptable and less deleterious.

Outcomes can be further improved by pre-hospital administration of thrombolytic therapy whether or not immediate PCI ('facilitated'-PCI) is performed following hospital arrival. Although the advantages of pre-hospital thrombolysis have been well-known for many years, this therapy has not become common practice for various reasons. This is a missed opportunity for many patients, especially those in rural areas requiring long transportation times to the referral hospitals, although thrombolysis, when left alone, is still a suboptimal therapy. Efforts should therefore be made to improve this situation wherever possible, by organising quick transportation to centres equipped for PCI and with an experienced staff. Investigations have clearly shown that a well-organised pre-hospital pharmacologic reperfusion strategy can save lives and positively influence other clinical outcomes.

Besides pre-hospital thrombolysis, and because of better overall results in first pilot studies, pre-hospital 'facilitation' of PCI is currently under investigation. Facilitation can be performed by using either thrombolytic drugs, a combined approach (thrombolytics half-dose + GPIIb/IIIa inhibition; now decreased in credit due to higher bleeding rates but similar in efficacy to monotherapy), or by pre-treatment with GPIIb/IIIa-blockers alone. The combined use of pharmacologic and mechanical reperfusion might be the optimal treatment principle, but open questions with regard to safety still remain (see the increase in bleeding complications and in mortality rates compared with PPCI alone in the ASSENT IV-PCI study). Changes in dose of the various antithrombotic agents need to be further tested before pre-PCI pharmacological treatment can become a general treatment option.

REFERENCES

1. Granger CB, Goldberg RJ, Dabbous O *et al.* for the Global Registry of Acute Coronary Events Investigators. Predictors of hospital mortality in the Global Registry of Acute Coronary Events. *Arch Int Med* 2003; 163:2345–2353.
2. Morrow DA, Antman EM, Charlesworth A *et al.* TIMI risk score for ST-elevation myocardial infarction: a convenient, bedside, clinical score for risk assessment at presentation: an intravenous nPA for treatment of infarcting myocardium early II trial substudy. *Circulation* 2000; 102:2031–2037.
3. Roe MT, Ohman EM, Maas AC *et al.* Shifting the open artery hypothesis downstream: the quest for optimal reperfusion. *J Am Card Cardiol* 2001; 37:9–18.
4. Antman EM, Anbe DT, Armstrong P *et al.* ACC/AHA Guidelines for the Management of Patients With ST-Elevation Myocardial Infarcion-Executive Summary. *Circulation* 2004; 110:588–636.
5. Tiefenbrunn AJ, Chandra NC, French WJ, Gore JM, Rogers WJ. Clinical experience with primary percutaneous transluminal angioplasty compared with alteplase (recombinant tissue-type plasminogen activator) in patients with acute myocardial infarction. A report from the Second National Registry of Myocardial Infarction (NRMI-2). *J Am Coll Cardiol* 1998; 31:1240–1245.
6. Van de Werf F, Ardissino D, Betriu A *et al.* Management of acute myocardial infarction in patients presenting with ST-segment elevation. The Task Force on the Management of Acute Myocardial Infarction of the European Society of Cardiology. *Eur Heart J* 2003; 24:28–66.
7. Barron HV, Bowlby LJ, Breen T *et al.* Use of reperfusion therapy for acute myocardial infarction in the United States: data from the National Registry of Myocardial Infarction 2. *Circulation* 1998; 97:1150–1156.
8. Boersma E, Maas ACP, Deckers JW, Simoons ML. Early thrombolytic treatment in acute myocardial infarction: reappraisal of the golden hour. *Lancet* 1996; 348:771–775.
9. Cannon CP, Antman EM, Walls R, Braunwald E. Time as an adjunctive agent to thrombolytic therapy. *J Thrombos Thrombolys* 1994; 1:27–34.
10. Weaver WD, Cerqueira M, Hallstrom AP *et al.* for the Myocardial Infarction Triage and Intervention Project Group. Prehospital-initiated vs hospital-initiated thrombolytic therapy. The Myocardial Infarction Triage and Intervention Trial. *JAMA* 1993; 270:1211–1216.
11. Fu Y, Goodman S, Chang WC *et al.* Time to treatment influences the impact of ST-segment resolution on one-year prognosis: insights from the assessment of the safety and efficacy of a new thrombolytic (ASSENT-2) trial. *Circulation* 2001; 104:2653–2659.
12. Akhras F, Ousa AA, Swann G *et al.* Primary coronary angioplasty or intravenous thrombolysis for patients with acute myocardial infarction? Acute and late follow-up results in a new cardiac unit. *J Am Card Cardiol* 1997; 29:A235–A236 (abstract).
13. Andersen HR, Nielsen TT, Rasmussen K *et al.* for the DANAMI-2 Investigators. Thrombolytic therapy versus primary percutaneous coronary intervention for myocardial infarction in patients presenting to hospitals without on-site cardiac surgery: a randomised controlled trial. *JAMA* 2003; 287:1943–1951.
14. Andersen HR, Nielsen TT, Rasmussen K *et al.* for the DANAMI-2 Investigators. A comparison of coronary angioplasty with fibrinolytic therapy in acute myocardial infarction. *N Engl J Med* 2003; 349:733–742.
15. Bonnefoy E, Lapostolle F, Leizorovicz A *et al.* for the Comparison of Angioplasty and Prehospital Thrombolysis in Acute Myocardial Infarction (CAPTIM) study group. Primary angioplasty versus prehospital fibrinolysis in acute myocardial infarction: a randomised study. *Lancet* 2002; 360:825–829.
16. de Boer MJ, Ottervanger JP, van t' Hof AW *et al.* for the Zwolle Myocardial Infarction Study Group. Reperfusion therapy in elderly patients with acute myocardial infarction: a randomised comparison of primary angioplasty and thrombolytic therapy. *J Am Card Cardiol* 2002; 39:1723–1728.
17. Garcia E, Elizaga J, Perez-Castellano N *et al.* Primary angioplasty versus systemic thrombolysis in anterior myocardial infarction. *J Am Coll Cardiol* 1999; 33:605–611.
18. Gibbons RJ, Holmes DR, Reeder GS, Bailey KR, Hopfenspirger MR, Gersh BJ. Immediate angioplasty compared with the administration of a thrombolytic agent followed by conservative treatment for myocardial infarction. *N Engl J Med* 1993; 328:685–691.
19. Grines CL, Browne KF, Marco J *et al.* A comparison of immediate angioplasty with thrombolytic therapy for acute myocardial infarction. *N Engl J Med* 1993; 328:673–679.
20. Grinfield L, Berrocal D, Bellardi J *et al.* Fibrinolytics versus primary angioplasty in acute myocardial infarction (FAP): a randomised trial in a community hospital in Argentina. *J Am Card Cardiol* 1996; 27:A222 (abstract).

21. The Global Use of Strategies to Open Occluded Coronary Arteries in Acute Coronary Syndromes (GUSTO IIb) Angioplasty Substudy Investigators. A clinical trial comparing primary coronary angioplasty with tissue plasminogen activator for acute myocardial infarction. *N Engl J Med* 1997; 336:1621–1628.

22. Kastrati A, Mehilli J, Dirschinger J *et al.* for the Stent versus Thrombolysis for Occluded Coronary Arteries in Patients with Acute Myocardial Infarction (STOPAMI-2) Study. Myocardial salvage after coronary stenting plus abciximab versus fibrinolysis plus abciximab in patients with acute myocardial infarction: a randomised trial. *Lancet* 2002; 359:920–925.

23. Le May MR, Labinaz M, Davies RF *et al.* Stenting versus thrombolysis in acute myocardial infarction (STAT). *J Am Coll Cardiol* 2001; 37:985–991.

24. Ribeiro EE, Silva LA, Carneiro R *et al.* Randomised trial of direct coronary angioplasty versus intravenous streptokinase in acute myocardial infarction. *J Am Coll Cardiol* 1993; 22:376–380.

25. Ribichini F, Steffenino G, Dellavalle A *et al.* Comparison of thrombolytic therapy and primary coronary angioplasty with liberal stenting for inferior myocardial infarction with precordial ST-segment depression: immediate and long-term results of a randomised study. *J Am Coll Cardiol* 1998; 32:1687–1694.

26. Schömig A, Kastrati A, Dirschinger J *et al.* for the Stent versus Thrombolysis for Occluded Coronary Arteries in Patients with Acute Myocardial Infarction Study Investigators. Coronary stenting plus platelet glycoprotein IIb/IIIa blockade compared with tissue plasminogen activator in acute myocardial infarction. *N Engl J Med* 2000; 343:385–391.

27. Vermeer F, Oude Ophuis AJ, van den Berg EJ *et al.* Prospective randomised comparison between thrombolysis, rescue PTCA, and primary PTCA in patients with extensive myocardial infarction admitted to a hospital without PTCA facilities: a safety and feasibility study. *Heart* 1999; 82:426–431.

28. Widimsky P, Groch L, Zelizko M *et al.* Multicentre randomised trial comparing transport to primary angioplasty vs immediate thrombolysis vs combined strategy for patients with acute myocardial infarction presenting to a community hospital without a catheterization laboratory. The PRAGUE Study. *Eur Heart J* 2000; 21:823–831.

29. Widimsky P, Budesinsky T, Vorac D *et al.* on behalf of the PRAGUE Study Group Investigators. Long distance transport for primary angioplasty vs immediate thrombolysis in acute myocardial infarction. Final results of the randomised national multicentre trial – PRAGUE-2. *Eur Heart J* 2003; 24:94–104.

30. Zijlstra F, de Boer MJ, Hoorntje JC, Reiffers S, Reiber JH, Suryapranata H. A comparison of immediate coronary angioplasty with intravenous streptokinase in acute myocardial infarction. *N Engl J Med* 1993; 328:680–684.

31. Grines CL, Westerhausen DRJ, Grines LL *et al.* A randomised trial of transfer for primary angioplasty versus on-site thrombolysis in patients with high-risk myocardial infarction: the Air Primary Angioplasty in Myocardial Infarction study. *J Am Coll Cardiol* 2002; 39:1713–1719.

32. Andersen HR, Nielsen TT, Vesterlund T *et al.* The Danish multicenter randomised study on fibrinolytic therapy versus acute coronary angioplasty in acute myocardial infarction: rationale and design of the DANAMI-2 trial. *Am Heart J* 2003; 146:234–241.

33. Juliard JM, Feldman LJ, HGolmard JL *et al.* Relation of mortality of primary angioplasty during acute myocardial infarction to door-to-Thrombolyis in Myocardial Infarction (TIMI) time. *Am J Cardiol* 2003; 91:1401–1405.

34. Nallamothu BK, Antman EM, Bates ER. Primary percutaneous coronary intervention versus fibrinolytic therapy in acute myocardial infarction: does the choice of fibrinolytic agent impact on the importance of time-to-treatment? *Am J Cardiol* 2004; 94:772–774.

35. Nallamothu BK, Bates ER. Percutaneous coronary intervention versus fibrinolytic therapy in acute myocardial infarction: is timing (almost) everything? *Am J Cardiol* 2003; 92:824–826.

36. Every NR, Parsons LS, Hlatky M, Martin JS, Weaver WD. A comparison of thrombolytic therapy with primary coronary angioplasty for acute myocardial infarction. *N Engl J Med* 1996; 335:1253–1261.

37. Keely EC, Boura JA, Grines CL. Primary angioplasty versus intravenous thrombolytic therapy for acute myocardial infarction: a quantitative review of 23 randomised trials. *Lancet* 2003; 361:13–20.

38. Hochman JS, Sleeper LA, Webb JG *et al.* for the SHOCK Investigators. Early revascularization in acute myocardial infarction complicated by cardiogenic shock. *N Engl J Med* 1999; 341:625–634.

39. Melandri G. The obsession with primary angioplasty. *Circulation* 2003; 108:e162.

40. Dalby M, Bouzamando A, Lechat P *et al.* Transfer for primary angioplasty versus immediate thrombolysis in acute myocardial infarction. *Circulation* 2003; 108:1809–1814.

41. Cannon CP, Gibson CM, Lambrew CT. Relationship of symptom-onset-to-balloon time and door-to-balloon time with mortality in patients undergoing angioplasty for acute myocardial infarction. *JAMA* 2000; 283:2941–2947.

42. Berger PB, Ellis SG, Holmes DR. Relationship between delay in performing direct coronary angioplasty and early clinical outcome in patients with acute myocardial infarction: results from the Global Use of Strategies To Open Occluded Arteries in Acute Coronary Syndromes (GUSTO-IIb) trial. *Circulation* 1999; 100:14–20.

43. De Luca G, Suryapranata H, Ottervanger JP, Antman EM. Time delay to treatment and mortality in primary angioplasty for acute myocardial infarction. Every minute of delay counts. *Circulation* 2004; 109:1223–1225.

44. Willimas DO. Treatment delayed is treatment denied. *Circulation* 2004; 109:1806–1808.

45. Gersh BJ, Stone GW, White HD, Holmes DR, Jr. Pharmacological facilitation of primary percutaneous coronary intervention for acute myocardial infarction: is the slope of the curve the shape of the future? *JAMA* 2005; 293:979–986.

46. Huber K, De Caterina R, Kristensen SD *et al.* Prehospital reperfusion therapy: a strategy to improve therapeutic outcome in patients with ST-elevation myocardial infarction. *Eur Heart J* 2005; 26:2063–2074.

47. Kalla K, Kozanli I, Unger G *et al.* Relation of time to treatment and in-hospital mortality in patients with ST-segment elevation myocardial infarction: Vienna pilot study on mechanical versus medication reperfusion strategies. *Circulation* 2004; 110:III-538 (abstract 2511).

48. Collen D. Thrombolytic therapy. *Thromb Haemost* 1997; 78:742–746.

49. Huber K, Maurer G. Thrombolytic therapy in acute myocardial infarction. *Semin Thromb Haemost* 1996; 22:12–23.

50. Herlitz J, Hartford M, Blohm M *et al.* Effect of a media campaign on delay times and ambulance use in suspected acute myocardial infarction. *Am J Cardiol* 1989; 64:90–93.

51. Blohm M, Herlitz J, Hartford M *et al.* Consequences of a media campaign focusing on the delay in acute myocardial infarction. *Am J Cardiol* 1992; 69:411–413.

52. Ho MT, Eisenberg MS, Litwin PE *et al.* Delay between onset of chest pain and seeking medical care: the effect of public education. *Ann Emerg Med* 1989; 18:727–731.

53. Luepker RV, Raczynski JM, Osganian S *et al.* for the REACT Study Group. Effect of a community intervention on patient delay and emergency medical service use in acute coronary heart disease: the Rapid Early Action for Coronary Treatment (REACT) trial. *JAMA* 2000; 284:60–67.

54. MacCallum AG, Stafford PJ, Jones C, Vincent R, Perez-Avila C, Chamberlain DA. Reduction in hospital time to thrombolytic therapy by audit of policy guidelines. *Eur Heart J* 1990; 11:48–52.

55. Antoniucci D, Valenti R, Migliorini A *et al.* Relation of time to treatment and mortality in patients with acute myocardial infarction undergoing primary coronary angioplasty. *Am J Cardiol* 2002; 89:1248–1252.

56. Stone GW, Grines CL, Browne KF *et al.* Predictors of in-hospital and 6-months outcome after acute myocardial infarction in the reperfusion era: the Primary Angioplasty in Myocardial Infarction (PAMI) Trial. *J Am Coll Cardiol* 1995; 25:370–377.

57. Silber S, Albertsson P, Aviles F *et al.* Guidelines for percutaneous coronary interventions. The Task Force for Percutaneous Coronary Interventions of the European Society of Cardiology. *Eur Heart J* 2005; 26:804–847.

58. European Myocardial Infarction Project Group. Prehospital thrombolytic therapy in patients with suspected acute myocardial infarction. *N Engl J Med* 1993; 329:383–389.

59. Rawles J on behalf of the GREAT Group. Halving of mortality at 1 year by domiciliary thrombolysis in the Grampian Region Early Anistreplase Trial (GREAT). *J Am Coll Cardiol* 1994; 23:1–5.

60. Morrison LJ, Verbeek PR, McDonald AC, Sawadsky BV, Cook DJ. Mortality and prehospital thrombolysis for acute myocardial infarction: a meta-analysis. *JAMA* 2000; 283:2686–2692.

61. Welsh RC, Ornato J, Armstrong PW. Prehospital management of acute ST-elevation myocardial infarction: A time for reappraisal in North America. *Am Heart J* 2003; 145:1–8.

62. Nallam othu BK, Bates ER, Herrin J, Wang Y, Bradley EH, Krumholz HM. Times to treatment in transfer patients undergoing primary percutaneous coronary intervention in the United States: National Registry of Myocardial Infarction (NRMI)-3/4 analysis. *Circulation* 2005; 111:761–767.

63. Canto JG, Rogers WJ, Bowlby U *et al.* The prehospital electrocardiogram in acute myocardial infarction: Is its full potential being realized? National Registry of Myocardial Infarction 2 Investigators. *J Am Card Cardiol* 1997; 29:498–505.

64. Karagounis L, Ipsen SK, Jessop MR *et al.* Impact of field-transmitted electrocardiography on time to in-hospital thrombolytic therapy in acute myocardial infarction. *Am J Cardiol* 1990; 66:786–791.

65. Kudenchuk PJ, Ho MT, Weaver WD et al. Accuracy of computer-interpreted electrocardiography in selecting patients for thrombolytic therapy: MITI project investigators. *J Am Card Cardiol* 1991; 17:486–491.

66. O'Rourke MF, Cook A, Carroll G et al. Accuracy of a portable interpretive ECG machine in diagnosis of acute evolving myocardial infarction. *Aust N Z J Med* 1992; 22:9–13.

67. Weaver WD, Eisenberg MS, Martin JS et al. Myocardial Infarction Triage and Intervention Project-phase I: patient characteristics and feasibility of pre-hospital initiation of thrombolytic therapy. *J Am Card Cardiol* 1990; 15:925–931.

68. Mathew TP, Menown IBA, McCarthy D, Gracey H, Hill L, Adgey AAJ. Impact of pre-hospital care in patients with acute myocardial infarction compared with those first managed in-hospital. *Eur Heart J* 2003; 24:161–171.

69. Adgey AAJ, Zaidi SA. Mobile coronary care teams. *Br Med J* 1969; 4:427.

70. Cannon CP. Exploring the issues of appropriate dosing in the treatment of acute myocardial infarction: Potential benefits of bolus fibrinolytic agents. *Am Heart J* 2000; 140:154–160.

71. Morrow DA, Antman EM, Sayah AJ et al. Evaluation of the time saved by pre-hospital initiation of reteplase for ST-elevation myocardial infarction: results of the early retavase-thrombolysis in myocardial infarction (ER-TIMI) 19 trial. *J Am Card Cardiol* 2002; 40:71–77.

72. Wallentin L, Goldstein P, Armstrong PW et al. Efficacy and safety of tenecteplase in combination with the low-molecular-weight heparin enoxaparin or unfractionated heparin in the prehospital setting. The Assessment of the Safety and Efficacy of a New Thrombolytic Regimen (ASSENT)-3 PLUS Randomised Trial in Acute Myocardial Infarction. *Circulation* 2003; 108:r1–r8.

73. The Assessment of the Safety and Efficacy of a New Thrombolytic Regimen (ASSENT)-3 Investigators. Efficacy and safety of tenecteplase in combination with enoxaparin, abciximab, or unfractionated heparin: the ASSENT-3 randomised trial in acute myocardial infarction. *Lancet* 2001; 358:605–613.

74. Sabatine MS, Cannon CP, Gibson M et al. for the CLARITY-TIMI 28 Investigators. Addition of clopidogrel to aspirin and fibrinolytic therapy for myocardial infarction with ST-segment elevation. *N Engl J Med* 2005; 352:1179–1189.

75. Brodie BR, Stuckey TD, Hansen C et al. Benefit of coronary reperfusion before intervention on outcomes after primary angioplasty for acute myocardial infarction. *Am J Cardiol* 2000; 85:13–18.

76. Clements IP, Christian TF, Higano ST et al. Residual flow to the infarct zone as a determinant of infarct size after direct angioplasty. *Circulation* 1993; 88:1527–1533.

77. Stone GW, Cox DA, Garcia EJ et al. Normal flow (TIMI-3) before mechanical reperfusion therapy is an independent determinant of survival in acute myocardial infarction: analysis from the primary angioplasty in myocardial infarction trials. *Circulation* 2000; 104:636–641.

78. Simoons ML, Arnold AE, Betriu A et al. Thrombolysis with tissue plasminogen activator in acute myocardial infarction: no additional benefit from immediate PTCA. *Lancet* 1988; 1:197–203.

79. The TIMI Research Group. Immediate vs delayed catheterization and angioplasty following thrombolytic therapy for acute myocardial infarction. *JAMA* 1988; 260:2849–2858.

80. Topol EJ, Califf RM, George BS et al. A randomised trial of immediate versus delayed elective angioplasty after intravenous tissue plasminogen activator in acute myocardial infarction. *N Engl J Med* 1987; 317:581–588.

81. Verheugt FWA. Acute coronary syndromes: drug treatments. *Lancet* 1999; 353:SII20–SII23.

82. Verheugt FWA, Brouwer MA. Half dose lytic plus abciximab compared to full dose lytic in acute myocardial infarction; a meta-analysis. *Eur Heart J* 2002; 23(supp):637.

83. Antman EM, Giugliano RP, Gibson M et al. for the TIMI 14 Investigators. Abciximab facilitates the rate and extent of thrombolysis: Results of the Thrombolysis In Myocardial Infarction (TIMI) 14 Trial. *Circulation* 1999; 99:2720–2732.

84. Ross AM, Coyne KS, Reiner JS for the PACT-Investigators. A randomised trial comparing primary angioplasty with a strategy of short-acting thrombolysis and immediate planned rescue angioplasty in acute myocardial infarction: the PACT Trial. *J Am Coll Cardiol* 1999; 34:1954–1962.

85. Fernandez-Avilés F, Alonso JJ, Castro-Beiras A et al. for the GRACIA-2 Investigators. Primary angioplasty versus facilitated intervention (tenecteplase plus stenting) in patients with ST elevation acute myocardial infarction: Final results of the GRACIA-2 trial. *J Am Coll Cardiol* 2004; 43: 289A–290A (abstract 1118–78).

86. Kastrati A, Mehilli J, Schlotterbeck K et al. Early administration of reteplase plus abciximab vs abciximab alone in patients with acute myocardial infarction referred for percutaneous coronary intervention: a randomised controlled trial. *JAMA* 2004; 291:947–954.

87. Brener SJ, Barr LA, Burchenal JE *et al.* on behalf of the ReoPro and Primary PTCA Organization and Randomised Trial (RAPPORT) Investigators. Randomised, placebo-controlled trial of platelet glycoprotein IIb/IIIa blockade with primary angioplasty for acute myocardial infarction. *Circulation* 1998; 98:734–741.

88. Neumann F-J, Kastrati A, Schmitt C. Effect of glycoprotein IIb/IIIa receptor blockade with abciximab on clinical and angiographic restenosis rate after the placement of coronary stents following acute myocardial infarction. *J Am Coll Cardiol* 2000; 35:915–921.

89. Montalescot G, Barragan P, Wittenberg O. Platelet glycoprotein IIb/IIIa inhibition with coronary stenting for acute myocardial infarction (ADMIRAL). *N Engl J Med* 2001; 344:1895–1903.

90. Montalescot G, Barragan P, Wittenberg O *et al.* Three years follow-up after primary stenting with or without abciximab in acute myocardial infarction (the ADMIRAL trial). *Circulation* 2003; 106:332–333 (abstract).

91. Stone GW, Grines CL, Cox DA *et al.* for the CADILLAC Investigators. Comparison of angioplasty with stenting, with or without abciximab, in acute myocardial infarction. *N Engl J Med* 2002; 346:957–966.

92. Tcheng JE, Kandzari DE, Grines CL *et al.* Benefits and risks of abciximab use in primary angioplasty for acute myocardial infarction: the Controlled Abciximab and Device Investigation to Lower Late Angioplasty Complications (CADILLAC) Trial. *Circulation* 2003; 108:1316–1323.

93. Antoniucci D, Rodriguez A, Hempel A *et al.* A randomised trial comparing primary infarct artery stenting with or without abciximab in acute myocardial infarction. *J Am Coll Cardiol* 2003; 42:1879–1885.

94. Zorman S, Zorman D, Noc M. Effects of abciximab pretreatment in patients with acute myocardial infarction undergoing primary angioplasty. *Am J Cardiol* 2002; 90:533–536.

95. Arntz H-R, Schröder J, Schwimmbeck P *et al.* Is early prehospital administration of abciximab superior to periprocedural therapy in patients with ST-segment elevation myocardial infarction and planned percutaneous coronary intervention? Early and late results from the randomised REOMOBILE pilot study. *J Am Coll Cardiol* 2004; 43:(abstract 1002–1079).

96. Gyöngyösi M, Domanovits H, Benzer W *et al.* Use of abciximab prior to primary angioplasty in STEMI results in early recanalization of the infarct-related artery and improved myocardial tissue reperfusion. Results of the Austrian multicenter randomised ReoPro-BRIDGING Study. *Eur Heart J* 2004; 25:2125–2133.

97. Montalescot G, Borentain M, Payot L, Collet JPH, Thomas D. Early versus late administration of glycoprotein IIb/IIIa inhibitors in primary percutaneous coronary intervention of acute ST-segment elevation myocardial infarction. *JAMA* 2004; 292:362–366.

98. Gödicke J, Flather M, Arntz H-R *et al.* Meta-Analysis of Early versus Peri-Procedural Administration of Abciximab for Primary Angioplasty. *Am Heart J* 2005; in press.

99. Cutlip DE, Ricciardi MJ, Frederick SL *et al.* Effect of tirofiban before primary angioplasty on initial coronary flow and early ST segment resolution in patients with acute myocardial infarction. *Am J Cardiol* 2003; 92:977–980.

100. Lee DP, Herity NA, Hiatt BL *et al.* for the Tirofiban Given in the Emergency Room before Primary Angioplasty Investigators. Adjunctive platelet glycoprotein IIb/IIIa receptor inhibition with tirofiban before primary angioplasty improves angiographic outcomes: results of the TIrofiban Given in the Emergency Room before Primary Angioplasty (TIGER-PA) pilot trial. *Circulation* 2003; 107:1497–1501.

101. van't Hof AW, Ernst N, de Boer MJ *et al.* for the On-TIME study group. Facilitation of primary angioplasty by early start of a glycoprotein 2b/3a inhibitor: results of the ongoing tirofiban in myocardial infarction evaluation (On-TIME) trial. *Eur Heart J* 2004; 25:837–846.

102. Zeymer U, Zahn R, Schiele R, Jansen W, Girth E, Gitt A. Early eptifibatide improves TIMI 3 patency before primary percutaneous coronary intervention for acute ST elevation myocardial infarction. Results of the randomised INTegrilin in Acute Myocardial Infarction (INTAMI) Pilot trial. *Eur Heart J* 2005; 111:in press.

103. Steinhubl SR, Berger PB, Mann III JT *et al.* for the CREDO Investigators. Early and sustained dual oral antiplatelet therapy following percutaneous coronary intervention. A randomised controlled trial. *JAMA* 2002; 288:2411–2420.

104. Müller I, Seyfarth M, Rudiger S *et al.* Effect of a high loading dose of clopidogrel on platelet function in patients undergoing coronary stent placement. *Heart* 2001; 85:92–93.

105. Müller I, Besta F, Schulz C *et al.* Prevalence of clopidogrel non-responders among patients with stable angina pectoris scheduled for elective coronary stent placement. *Thromb Haemost* 2003; 89:783–787.

106. Pache J, Kastrati A, Mehilli J *et al.* Clopidogrel therapy in patients undergoing coronary stenting: Value of a high-loading-dose regimen. *Catheter Cardiovasc Interv* 2002; 55:436–441.

107. Schömig A, Mehilli J, Dotzer F *et al*. Glycoprotein IIb/IIIa inhibition with abciximab in patients undergoing coronary stenting after pretreatment with a high loading dose of clopidogrel (ISAR-REACT). *N Engl J Med* 2004; 350:232–238.

108. Mehili J, Kastrati A, Schühlen H *et al*. Randomised clinical trial of abciximab in diabetic patients undergoing elective percutaneous coronary interventions after treatment with a high loading dose of clopidogrel. *Circulation* 2004; 110:3627–3635.

13

Antithrombotic strategies in patients undergoing primary percutaneous intervention

S. D. Kristensen, J. F. Lassen, H. R. Andersen

INTRODUCTION

In acute ST-elevation myocardial infarction (STEMI) the major initial therapeutic challenge is rapid and complete restoration of blood flow. The prognosis is dependent on the time to reperfusion, on the TIMI flow rate obtained in the infarct-related coronary artery and also on the flow in the microcirculation [1, 2]. Randomised trials have shown that primary or direct percutaneous coronary intervention (PCI) is superior to fibrinolytic therapy [2, 3, 4]. Recent trials such as the DANAMI-2 and the PRAGUE-2 studies demonstrated that transferral of patients with acute STEMI from a district hospital to a tertiary centre for primary PCI (PPCI) is safe and superior to thrombolysis [5, 6]. In the largest of the studies (DANAMI-2) it was demonstrated that transferral for PPCI caused a significant reduction in the composite endpoint of death, re-infarction and disabling stroke [6]. Meta-analysis of the transferral trials performed so far showed that this approach was associated with a significant reduction in mortality [4, 7]. Therefore, if a system for rapid and safe refer is available or can be established, acute transferral is an attractive option [8]. Current guidelines recommend the use of PPCI if this can be performed within 60–90 min.

One of the reasons for the success with PPCI is the technical improvement in device technology, especially implantation of stents in the culprit lesion. Although implantation of stents causes a higher degree of low/no flow in the infarct-related artery than plain old balloon angioplasty, several trials have shown that stent implantation over-all leads to a better outcome [8, 9]. Therefore, at the present time, implantation of stents in the culprit lesion is recommended when this approach is possible. So far, implantation of bare metal stents is the evidence-based therapy, but trials comparing bare metal with drug-eluting stents are ongoing and may change clinical practice.

ANTITHROMBOTIC THERAPY IN PRIMARY PCI

Another major reason for the good results now obtained with PPCI is the development and optimisation of adjunctive medical therapy, in particular in the field of potent antithrombotics drugs. Clearly, implantation of metal stents in a thrombus-containing disrupted atherosclerotic

Steen Dalby Kristensen, Head of Cardiology, University Department of Cardiology, Skejby Hospital, Aarhus University Hospital, Aarhus, Denmark.

Jens Flensted Lassen, Consultant Cardiologist, Associate Professor, Department of Cardiology, Skejby Hospital, Aarhus University Hospital, Aarhus, Denmark.

Henning Rud Andersen, Associate Professor of Cardiology, University Department of Cardiology, Skejby Hospital, Aarhus University Hospital, Aarhus, Denmark.

Table 13.1 Immediate antithrombotic therapy in patients undergoing primary PCI with stenting, 2005

Aspirin: 300–500 mg bolus followed by 75–325 mg daily lifelong.
Clopidogrel: 300–600 mg bolus followed by 75 mg daily for 9–12 months.
Heparin: Intravenous bolus dose 70–100 IU/kg.
Abciximab: Intravenous bolus followed by 12 h of infusion.

lesion in a patient with ongoing myocardial infarction (MI) is a challenge that needs optimal antithrombotic therapy as a back-up in the catheterisation laboratory. These patients also benefit from antithrombotic therapy after the PPCI [8, 9]. Finally, the time interval from diagnosis to first balloon inflation, now further widened by the concept of transferral, calls for improvement in prognosis by the introduction of potent antithrombotic therapy prior to angioplasty to facilitate this procedure. This issue is, however, covered in chapter 12 [10].

PRIMARY PCI: ANTITHROMBOTIC THERAPY IN THE CATHETERISATION LABORATORY

The options are inhibition of platelet aggregation with aspirin, clopidogrel or glycoprotein GPIIb/IIIa blockers, inhibition of the coagulation system with unfractionated heparin (UFH) or heparin-like drugs and dissolution/removal of the thrombus with fibrinolytics or mechanical devices (Table 13.1).

Platelet inhibition

Aspirin causes irreversible blockade of the cyclooxygenase-1 enzyme and thereby inhibition of the production of the pro-aggregatory and vasoconstrictive thromboxane A2. Aspirin has been shown to be of benefit in acute coronary syndromes and in chronic ischaemic heart disease, and is the cornerstone of antithrombotic therapy in these patients [11]. Randomised trials with aspirin in the setting of PPCI have not been and probably never will be performed. The recommendation of aspirin is therefore based on clinical experience and extrapolation from other trials including the trials performed with other drugs or devices in these patients, where aspirin always has been used as standard adjunctive therapy [11].

In patients with acute STEMI, aspirin should be administered as soon as the diagnosis is suspected, with an initial loading dose of 300–500 mg given as dissoluble or chewing tablets. In the catheterisation laboratory aspirin can be given as a bolus of 300–500 mg intravenously. After the intervention, aspirin 75–150 mg orally is recommended as life-long therapy [11].

Clopidogrel and ticlodipine inhibit the platelet adenosine diphosphate (ADP) $P2Y_{12}$ receptor and causes inhibition of platelet aggregation. Ticlopidine has many side-effects, and therefore clopidogrel is now the recommended drug for antiplatelet therapy in patients who cannot tolerate aspirin [12]. Also, the combination of aspirin and clopidogrel has been proven to be beneficial prior to and after coronary stenting and in patients suffering from unstable angina/non-STEMI [12].

Clopidogrel has not been tested in randomised trials in patients undergoing PPCI, and therefore there is no evidence-based recommendation. However, as a large majority of patients undergoing PPCI receive a stent, it is logical to treat these patients with clopidogrel in combination with aspirin. Steinhubl *et al.* have shown a beneficial effect of a loading dose of 300 mg of clopidogrel followed by 75 mg/day if administered >6 h before PCI with stent implantation, compared with later administration [13]. Data from experimental studies suggest a much faster (within 2 h) maximum action of clopidogrel if the drug is given with a high-dosage load, which has been demonstrated to be safe [14]. High-dose clopidogrel (600 mg loading dose, followed by 150 mg/day) given before PCI has been investigated in chronic stable low-risk patients in the ISAR-REACT trial [15] and in the ARMYDA-2 trial (600 mg loading dose of clopidogrel prior to PCI reduced incidence of periprocedural infarction compared to 300 mg) [16], and is at the moment being tested in patients with NSTEMI in the ongoing

ISAR-REACT-2 study, as well as in patients with STEMI (BRAVE-3 trial). Our approach is to recommend an oral bolus dose of 300 mg or 600 mg of clopidogrel to be given as soon as the patient is diagnosed and sent for PPCI. The potential drawback of this approach could be the increased bleeding risk if the angiogram reveals that the patient should go to acute by-pass surgery. However, in 2005 almost all STEMI patients with need for revascularisation therapy are handled with modern PCI technology (e.g., stenting of the left main).

For how long should patients undergoing PPCI with stent implantation be treated with clopidogrel? No trials are available and again we have to extrapolate from other studies. First of all there are no data to support life-long combination therapy. The PCI CURE and the CREDO trials showed that patients with stable angina and unstable angina/NSTEMI with implanted stents did benefit from a longer therapy than one month [12, 13]. In PCI CURE the duration of treatment was 3–12 (average 9) months and in CREDO patients were treated for 12 months [12, 13]. We recommend that patients in whom stents are implanted receive 12 months of clopidogrel therapy, but a more individualised approach for assessing the duration of clopidogrel therapy based on benefit/risk of bleeding could also be taken.

In patients treated with PPCI without stenting, the evidence for giving clopidogrel is non-existent. However, based on data from the CLARITY trial showing benefit of clopidogrel on top of aspirin in acute STEMI we recommend the use of clopidogrel for 1–12 months [17].

GLYCOPROTEIN IIb/IIIa RECEPTOR BLOCKERS

Of the three intravenous compounds on the market only the large molecule monoclonal antibody abciximab has been tested in major in-catheterisation laboratory trials in patients with STEMI. An intravenous bolus followed by infusion of abciximab for 12 h was used in the RAPPORT [18], ISAR-2 [19], ADMIRAL [20], CADILLAC [21] and ACE trials [22].

In the RAPPORT trial (482 patients) [18], abciximab improved the immediate clinical outcome (combination of death, myocardial infarction (MI), and urgent revascularisation) and significantly reduced the need for 'bail-out' stenting. However, bleeding complications also increased significantly in the abciximab group, likely as a result of the relatively high doses of adjunct intravenous unfractionated heparin (UFH).

In the ISAR-2 trial (401 patients) [19], the use of abciximab in combination with a reduced dose of UFH resulted in a significant reduction of the combined endpoint (death, re-infarction, target lesion revascularisation after 30 days) but did not reduce angiographic restenosis rate.

In the double-blind ADMIRAL trial (300 patients) [20], abciximab was given before sheath insertion in all patients. One-quarter of patients received the study drug early, either in the emergency room or in the ambulance on the way to the catheterisation laboratory. The drug improved angiographic and clinical outcomes with a particular benefit in the subgroup of patients treated early.

However, the largest study, the CADILLAC trial (2082 patients) [21], demonstrated a beneficial effect of abciximab only for patients with balloon dilatation, but not for patients receiving stents. There was some benefit of abciximab vs. no abciximab on the combined endpoint of death, re-infarction and target vessel revascularisation at 30 days in this study, but the primary endpoint of death and re-infarction, both at 30 days and 6 months, was not significantly reduced [21]. In this study, a high-risk subgroup that was not included in the main trial (long, complicated lesions, multivessel disease, small vessels, visible thrombus) had some advantage over abciximab.

Recently, the ACE trial, performed in 400 patients, reported on the use of abciximab in high-risk patients (cardiogenic shock, massive coronary thrombus load, main stem lesions, and significant stenoses of side branches related to the culprit lesion) with acute STEMI that had been excluded in most other trials [22]. The combined primary endpoint (death,

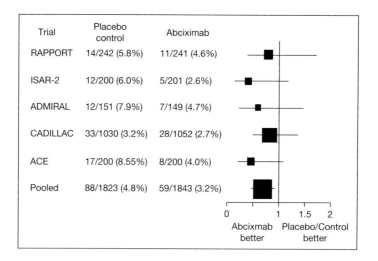

Figure 13.1 Meta-analysis of trials on abciximab in PPCI showing a decrease in the incidence of the combined endpoint of death/MI. With permission from [9].

re-infarction, urgent target vessel revascularisation, and stroke at 30 days) was significantly reduced in the abciximab group (4.5 vs. 10.5%). Early ST-segment resolution ($\geq$50% after 30 min) occurred significantly more often (85 vs. 68%) in abciximab-treated patients in whom a reduction in infarct size was also shown after 30 days. After 6 months, the rate of the combined endpoint was still significantly lower in the abciximab arm of the trial (5.5 vs. 13.5%). Restenosis rate was comparable in the two groups.

The inclusion criteria differed markedly in these five trials. Patients with cardiogenic shock were only included in the ISAR-2, ADMIRAL, and ACE trials, while patients in the CADILLAC trial had a relatively low-risk profile, as confirmed by the low event rate in the placebo group. The combined endpoint of death and MI for the five above-mentioned trials has been summarised. With the exception of CADILLAC, all trials showed a clear benefit for patients treated with abciximab. This was statistically significant in trials (ADMIRAL, ACE) in which abciximab was initiated early before PPCI.

The result of a meta-analysis of these trials is shown in Figure 13.1. The use of abciximab was associated with a significant reduction in the composite endpoint of death/MI/target vessel revascularisation and of death/MI at 30 days [9]. There was a trend towards a reduction in mortality at 30 days, but this did not reach statistical significance [9].

Compared with abciximab, the data on tirofiban [23, 24, 25] and eptifibatide (INTAMI trial), [26] in PPCI are limited. Eptifibatide and tirofiban have not been studied in larger randomised trials in STEMI patients undergoing PPCI, and can therefore not be recommended in these patients.

Currently, we recommend that patients with STEMI undergoing PPCI are treated with abciximab. Clearly, the benefit should be weighed against the risk of bleeding. It has been recommended to start the therapy as quickly as possible [27]. However, some experts prefer to use abciximab in the catheterisation laboratory-based on a benefit/risk assessment for the individual patient after the first angiogram is performed.

Inhibition of coagulation system

Standard therapy for inhibition of the coagulation system is an intravenous bolus dose of UFH. The dose originally recommended was 10 000 IU of heparin followed by additional bolus doses during the intervention given in sufficient doses to keep activated clotting time (ACT) between 250 and 350 seconds. In the HEAP study a mega dose of heparin (15 000 IU) was found to be of no benefit [28]. With the introduction of GPIIb/IIIa inhibitors, lower doses of heparin are recommended [29]. We recommend that a bolus dose of heparin 70–100 IU/kg is given as soon as the decision to do PPCI is made and and that an ACT is kept between 200 and 250 seconds during the procedure if a GPIIb/IIIa blocker is used.

The evidence for the use of low-molecular-weight heparins in PPCI is limited. A task force has suggested that a subcutaneous dose of enoxaparin can be given at the time the diagnosis is made [30], but this concept has not been tested in published clinical trials. Intravenous administration of the direct thrombin inhibitor bivalirudin in patients undergoing PPCI is currently being tested in the HORIZONS trial.

Fibrinolytics in the catheterisation lab
In the past, fibrinolytics such as streptokinase, urokinase or alteplase were used in the catheterisation laboratory in cases where thrombi were thought to be present. Fibrinolytics have not been shown to be efficient in randomised trials and should not be used on a routine basis in the catheterisation laboratory during PPCI.

Mechanical devices
Based on the concept that fragmentation of the thrombus and distal embolisation is an important risk factor for bad outcome during PPCI mechanical devices for thrombectomi and distal protection of the peripheral coronary circulation have been designed [31]. These devices are currently being tested in this setting. The first major randomised trial showed that distal protection with the Guard wire was not better than no distal protection [32]. A smaller recent trial showed some benefit of thrombectomy with manual aspiration [33]. However, at the present time the evidence to recommend use of these devices on a routine basis during PPCI is limited. Ongoing trials may tell us whether thrombectomy, distal protection, or the combination of both may be of benefit in some patients.

Primary PCI in patients with increased risk for bleeding
In patients with ongoing bleeding or recent major surgery, abxicimab should be avoided. Heparin use should be carefully controlled and clopidogrel should be used with great caution. Often a shorter duration of clopidogrel therapy should be considered. Aspirin should be used if possible, if stents are implanted.

In patients already on warfarin therapy, it is recommended that aspirin and clopidogrel be added if coronary stents are implanted. Anticoagulation should be carefully controlled and in some patients clopidogrel therapy should be shortened. In patients with a very high risk of bleeding, the use of balloon angioplasty without stenting is recommended in order to reduce the need for antithrombotic therapy.

FACILITATED-PCI

FACILITATED-PCI: ANTITHROMBOTIC THERAPY PRIOR TO THE INTERVENTION

Facilitation of the outcome after PPCI with potent antithrombotic drugs is a tempting challenge. Drugs with the potential of quick opening of the artery could save myocardium and therefore lead to a better prognosis. Trials with thrombolytics and GPIIb/IIIa blockers given at the time of diagnosis is made have been published recently and larger trials are ongoing. This interesting concept is discussed elsewhere in this book [10].

RESCUE PCI: FAILED THROMBOLYTIC THERAPY

Thrombolytic therapy is still widely used as the primary therapy in patients with acute STEMI with symptom onset within 12 h [34]. Thrombolytic therapy is less effective than PPCI in opening the infarct-related artery. TIMI flow 3 will only be present in 60–70% of patients even with the use of modern thrombolytic agents.

The obvious question is how to diagnose and treat the group of patients in which thrombolysis fails? Diagnosis is made on persisting clinical problems including chest pain, heart failure, arrhythmias and haemodymanic instability and the lack of regression of ST-segment elevation in the ECG usually recorded 60–90 min after start of thrombolytic therapy.

In patients with failed thrombolysis a new bolus dose (half or full) has been advocated, but the evidence is very limited. Immediate transport to a cath lab for acute coronary arteriography and rescue PCI is currently recommended. This is mainly based on the REACT trial reported by Gerschlik and coworkers at the 2004 AHA [35]. In this British multicentre trial patients with failure after thrombolytic therapy (judged mainly on ST-segment regression 90 min after start of thrombolysis) were randomised to conventional medical therapy, a second dose of thrombolytic or invasive therapy with rescue PCI. The patients randomised to rescue PCI with stent implantation had a better outcome than patients randomised to conventional medical therapy or a second dose of thrombolytics.

The choice of antithrombotic therapy in patients undergoing rescue PCI is based on clinical assessment and experience and extrapolation from studies with PPCI. In patients who have received alteplase, reteplase or TNK-tPA, heparin therapy should be continued and controlled carefully with ACT values around 250 seconds. Usually heparin therapy is stopped immediately after successful rescue PCI. Aspirin therapy should be continued and clopidogrel bolus and continuing therapy should usually be started. We tend to make a clinical judgement in the catheterisation laboratory as to whether aciximab should be given. The decision will mainly rely on the presence of major thrombus material and the overall risk of bleeding. In cases with thrombus, the use of thrombectomy and distal protection devices may also be considered.

Bleeding risk is particular high in patients treated with streptokinase and, in our opinion, abciximab should not be used in a setting where thrombolytic failure is treated with rescue PCI. In cases where streptokinase has been given, we would be reluctant to give heparin and abciximab. Aspirin should be given and clopidogrel used in case stents are implanted.

REFERENCES

1. Boersma E, Mercado N, Poldermans D et al. Acute myocardial infarction. *Lancet* 2003; 361:847–858.
2. Van de Werf F, Ardissino D, Betriu A et al. Management of acute myocardial infarction in patients presenting with ST-segment elevation. *Eur Heart J* 2003; 24:28–66. The current ESC Guidelines accepted for publication 7th August 2002.
3. Antman EM, Anbe DT, Armstrong P et al. ACC/AHA Guidelines for the Management of Patients With ST-Elevation Myocardial Infarcion-Executive Summary. *Circulation* 2004; 110:588–636.
4. Keeley EC, Boura JA, Grines CL. Primary angioplasty versus intravenous thrombolytic therapy for acute myocardial infarction: a quantitative review of 23 randomised trials. *Lancet* 2003; 361:13–20.
5. Widimsky P, Budesinsky T, Vorac D et al. Long distance transport for primary angioplasty vs. immediate thrombolysis in acute myocardial infarction. *Eur Heart J* 2003; 24:94–104.
6. Andersen HR, Nielsen TT, Rasmussen K et al. A comparison of coronary angioplasty with fibrinolytic therapy in acute myocardial infarction. *New Engl J Med* 2003; 349: 733–742.
7. Dalby M, Bouzamando A, Lechat P et al. Transfer for primary angioplasty versus immediate thrombolysis in acute myocardial infarction. *Circulation* 2003; 108:1809–1814.
8. Kristensen SD, Andersen HR, Thuesen L et al. Should patients with acute ST elevation myocardial infarction be transferred for primary PCI? *Heart* 2004; 90:1358–1363.

9.   Topol EJ, Neumann FJ, Montalescot G. A preferred reperfusion strategy for acute myocardial infarction. *J Am Coll Cardiol* 2003; 42:1886–1889.

10. Huber K, De Caterina R, Kristensen SD. Chapter 12 (this book).

11. Patrono C. Chapter 2 (this book).

12. Fathi RB, Bhatt DL, Topol EJ. Chapter 3 (this book).

13. Steinhubl SR, Berger PB, Mann III JT *et al.* for the CREDO Investigators. Early and sustained dual oral antiplatelet therapy following percutaneous coronary intervention. A randomized controlled trial. *JAMA* 2002; 288:2411–2420.

14. Muller I, Seyfarth M, Rudiger *et al.* Effect of high loading dose of clopidogrel on platelet function in patients undergoing coronary stent placement. *Heart* 2001; 85:92–93.

15. Kastrati A, Mehilli J, Schuhlen H *et al.* A clinical trial of abciximab in elective percutaneous coronary intervention after pre-treatment with clopidogrel. *N Engl J Med* 2004; 350:232–238.

16. Patti G, Colonna G, Pasceri V *et al.* Randomized trial of high loading dose of clopidogrel for reduction of periprocedural myocardial infarction in patients undergoing coronary intervention (ARMYDA-2). *Circulation* 2005; 111:2099–2106.

17. Sabatine MS, Cannon CP, Gibson CM *et al.* Addition of clopidogrel to aspirin and fibrinolytic therapy for myocardial infarction with with ST-segment elevation. *N Engl J Med* 2005; 352: 1179–1189.

18. Brener SJ, Barr LA, Burchenal JE *et al.* on behalf of the ReoPro and Primary PTCA Organization and Randomized Trial (RAPPORT) Investigators. Randomized, placebo-controlled trial of platelet glycoprotein IIb/IIIa blockade with primary angioplasty for acute myocardial infarction. *Circulation* 1998; 98:734–741.

19. Neumann F-J, Kastrati A, Schmitt C *et al.* Effect of glycoprotein IIb/IIIa receptor blockade with abciximab on clinical and angiographic restenosis rate after the placement of coronary stents following acute myocardial infarction. *J Am Coll Cardiol* 2000; 35:915–921.

20. Montalescot G, Barragan P, Wittenberg O. Platelet glycoprotein IIb/IIIa inhibition with coronary stenting for acute myocardial infarction (ADMIRAL). *N Engl J Med* 2001; 344:1895–1903.

21. Tcheng JE, Kandzari DE, Grines CL *et al.* Benefits and risks of abciximab use in primary angioplasty for acute myocardial infarction: the Controlled Abciximab and Device Investigation to Lower Late Angioplasty Complications (CADILLAC) Trial. *Circulation* 2003; 108:1316–1323.

22. Antoniucci D, Rodriguez A, Hempel A *et al.* A randomized trial comparing primary infarct artery stenting with or without abciximab in acute myocardial infarction. *J Am Coll Cardiol* 2003; 42:1879–1885.

23. Cutlip DE, Ricciardi MJ, Frederick SL *et al.* Effect of tirofiban before primary angioplasty on initial coronary flow and early ST segment resolution in patients with acute myocardial infarction. *Am J Cardiol* 2003; 92:977–980.

24. Lee DP, Herity NA, Hiatt BL *et al.* for the TIrofiban Given in the Emergency Room before Primary Angioplasty Investigators. Adjunctive platelet glycoprotein IIb/IIIa receptor inhibition with tirofiban before primary angioplasty improves angiographic outcomes: results of the TIrofiban Given in the Emergency Room before Primary Angioplasty (TIGER-PA) pilot trial. *Circulation* 2003; 107:1497–1501.

25. van't Hof AW, Ernst N, de Boer MJ *et al.* for the On-TIME study group. Facilitation of primary angioplasty by early start of a glycoprotein 2b/3a inhibitor: results of the ongoing tirofiban in myocardial infarction evaluation (On-TIME) trial. *Eur Heart J* 2004; 25:837–846.

26. Zeymer U, Zahn R, Schiele R *et al.* Early eptifibatide improves TIMI 3 patency before primary percutaneous coronary intervention for acute ST elevation myocardial infarction. Results of the randomised INTegrilin in Acute Myocardial Infarction (INTAMI) Pilot trial. *Eur Heart J* 2005; 111; in press.

27. Montalescot G, Borentain M, Payot L, Collet JPH, Thomas D. Early versus late administration of glycoprotein IIb/IIIa inhibitors in primary percutaneous coronary intervention of acute ST-segment elevation myocardial infarction. *JAMA* 2004; 292:362–366.

28. Liem A, Zijlstra F, Ottervanger JP *et al.* High dose heparin as pre-treatment for primary angioplasty in acute myocardial infarction: the Heparin in Early Patency trial (HEAP) randomized trial. *J Am Coll Cardiol* 2000; 35:600–604.

29. Brown B, Moliterno DJ. Chapter 4 (this book).

30. Kereiakis DJ, Montalescot G, Antman EM *et al.* Low-molecular-weight heparin for non-ST-elevation myocardial infarction and during percutaneous coronary intervention: an expert consensus. *Am Heart J* 2002; 144:615–624.

31. Topol EJ, Yadav JS. Recognition of the importance of embolization in atherosclerotic vascular disease. *Circulation* 2000; 101:570–580.

32. Stone GW, Webb J, Cox DA *et al*. Distal microcirculatory protection during percutaneous coronary intervention in acute ST-segment elevation myocardial infarction. A randomized controlled trial. *JAMA* 2005; 293:1063–1072.

33. Burzotta F, Trani C, Romagnoli E *et al*. Manual thrombus-aspiration improves myocardial reperfusion. *J Am Coll Cardiol* 2005; 46:371–376.

34. Sinnaeve PR, Van de Werf FJ. Chapter 11 (this book).

35. Gerschlik *et al*. REACT trial AHA 2004.

14

Antithrombotic management in patients with prosthetic valves

E. G. Butchart, C. Gohlke-Baerwolf, R. De Caterina

INTRODUCTION

Antithrombotic management in patients with prosthetic valves should be individualised for each patient, depending on the type of prosthesis and the patient's own risk factors, bearing in mind that thrombosis and embolism may have other sources in addition to a replaced valve, and that some patients may be more prone to thrombosis or more prone to bleeding. This concept of patient-specific and prosthesis-specific antithrombotic management requires an understanding of the basic mechanisms of thrombosis and embolism in valve surgery patients, the limitations of anticoagulation and antiplatelet therapy and the subtle differences between one prosthesis and another, even within a broad design category. It thus involves much more detailed patient assessment and prosthesis evaluation than contained in previously published North American guidelines [1, 2]. An inappropriately high intensity of anticoagulation or the unnecessary addition of aspirin to anticoagulation in patients with low thrombogenicity mechanical valves and no risk factors for thromboembolism (TE) will increase the incidence of major bleeding without conferring any additional antithrombotic protection.

PATHOGENESIS OF THROMBOSIS AND EMBOLISM

Following prosthetic valve replacement, the pathogenetic mechanisms involved in thrombosis and embolism are complex and often interactive. Even optimum anticoagulation control does not prevent all 'thromboembolism', for three principal reasons. Firstly, many events are part of the background incidence of stroke and transient ischaemic attack (TIA) in the general population which varies considerably with age [3], geography (highest in Eastern Europe) [4] and even within different regions of the same country [5]. Secondly, many risk factors such as hypertension and diabetes exert their effects through mechanisms uninfluenced or little influenced by anticoagulation [6]. Thirdly, total prevention of thrombosis on very thrombogenic surfaces requires anticoagulation at such a high international normalised ratio (INR) [7] that its efficacy is outweighed by the risk of serious bleeding.

Eric Gordon Butchart, Senior Consultant Cardiothoracic Surgeon, University Hospital of Wales, Cardiff, Wales, UK.

Christa Gohlke-Baerwolf, Cardiologist and Senior Staff Physician, Herz-Zentrum Bad Krozingen, Bad Krozingen, Germany.

Raffaele De Caterina, Professor of Cardiology, Institute of Cardiology, "G. d'Annunzio" University – Chieti, Ospedale San Camillo de Lellis, Chieti, Italy.

Coronary artery disease increases the risk of stroke two- to three-fold depending on age [8], while carotid disease and aortic atheroma increase the risk still further [9]. Hypertension, diabetes, increased left ventricular mass and cigarette smoking each act as major independent stroke risk factors [10–14].

After aortic valve replacement (AVR) in a middle-aged and elderly population, the incidence of cerebrovascular events has been shown to be predominantly associated with established stroke risk factors, particularly hypertension and continued cigarette smoking [6], and to be relatively little influenced by differences in anticoagulation intensity [15]. In a series based on the Medtronic Hall tilting disc valve, patients who were normotensive, in sinus rhythm, non-diabetic and non-smokers with no evidence of arterial disease, suffered no cerebrovascular events during a 13-year follow-up period [6]. Whilst it may not be possible to extrapolate these data to other types of prosthesis, this series serves to underline the importance of taking stroke risk factors into account when planning antithrombotic management. The mechanism of cerebrovascular events in this series of patients after AVR remains speculative. The overall incidence is in keeping with epidemiological data on stroke in the age- and sex-matched general population without prosthetic valves, although the possibility of some interaction between the prosthesis and stroke risk factors remains.

Following valve replacement, abnormal flow conditions imposed by the prosthesis coexist with disturbed flow conditions due to abnormal cardiac function and/or with irregular roughened arterial surfaces due to atheromatous plaques. The latter and the prothrombotic endothelial dysfunction which accompanies them [16, 17] are in turn associated with established risk factors for arterial disease: hypertension, cigarette smoking, diabetes and hyperlipidaemia [18].

Prosthetic valves are associated with two types of abnormal flow conditions: relative stagnation and high velocity disturbed flow causing high shear stress [19]. Relative stagnation exists in areas of very low flow or even reversed flow adjacent to certain parts of the prosthesis according to its particular design (e.g., the hinge pockets of a bileaflet valve and the concave outflow surfaces of a bioprosthesis) [20]. High shear stress occurs during forward flow and in mechanical valves during regurgitant flow when high velocity jets of blood are forced through narrow gaps in the mechanism with the prosthesis in a closed position. The degree of shear stress also varies according to valve design [19]. Relative stagnation in any part of the circulation increases the risk of thrombosis [21] but is particularly dangerous in proximity to an artificial surface [22]. High shear stress is also deleterious in that it induces platelet activation [23–25]. Activated platelets may subsequently adhere to a prosthetic surface [26] or to an abnormal surface downstream from the prosthesis, e.g., an aortic atheromatous plaque, with subsequent microembolism [27].

Prostheses in different positions within the heart impose and are associated with different flow conditions which have implications for the mechanisms of thrombosis and embolism and for antithrombotic therapy. Aortic prostheses are associated with relatively little stagnation unless they are of inferior design or incorrectly implanted; the dominant feature rather is high shear stress [19]. In addition many aortic valves are implanted within aortas scarred by atherosclerosis. Mitral prostheses in contrast are associated with much more stagnation [20], not only because the velocity of forward flow is much lower, especially in atrial fibrillation, but also because they are situated facing into the left atrium which is itself an area of relative stagnation in many cases of mitral valve disease, due to chamber enlargement and atrial fibrillation [21]. Mitral valve disease, particularly rheumatic disease, is also usually associated with less arterial disease than aortic valve disease [6, 28].

These fundamental differences result in a higher incidence of both valve thrombosis and embolism after mitral valve replacement (MVR) than after AVR [29]. Because these complications are related to blood stagnation both in the left atrium and adjacent to the prosthesis, and because anticoagulation is particularly useful for reducing thrombosis under these conditions, a dose–response effect can be demonstrated with increasing intensity of

Table 14.1   Risk factor modification to reduce thromboembolic risk.

Modifiable Risk factors	Action required
Systemic hypertension	Good blood pressure control
Diabetes	Good diabetic control
Chronic chlamydial infection	Antibiotic treatment
Factor VII 'resistance' to warfarin	Monitor factor VII level in addition to INR to optimise warfarin dose Reduce fat intake/statin therapy
Increased mean platelet volume	Investigate causes of increased platelet consumption (see text) Consider antiplatelet drug
Raised eosinophil count	Investigate and treat cause e.g., allergic conditions, parasites, suspected malignant disease
Raised fibrinogen	Investigate and treat cause, e.g., chronic infection, chronic inflammation, dental disease
Raised reticulocyte count	Investigate cause of increased haemolysis and treat cause
Atrial fibrillation	Conversion to sinus rhythm pharmacologically or electrically
Cigarette smoking	Stop smoking
Poor left ventricular function/ NYHA class IV / heart failure	Optimise drug treatment including ACE inhibitors
Hypercholesterolaemia*	Statin therapy – anti-inflammatory and antithrombotic effects also beneficial
Obesity*	Reduce weight. Increase exercise
Pulmonary infection*‡ (as an acute trigger factor) [63, 64]	Treat pulmonary infections promptly and vigorously

*Identified as risk factors for stroke in general, through pro-thrombotic and/or athero-genic mechanisms.
‡Indirect evidence in prosthetic heart valve patients also [22].

anticoagulation [15]. In contrast, embolism after AVR appears to be less influenced by the intensity of anticoagulation [15], suggesting a dominant effect of either platelet activation or coexisting stroke risk factors [6]. Several randomised trials have failed to detect any significant difference in embolic incidence with different intensities of anticoagulation in populations in which AVR and sinus rhythm predominated [30–34].

Thus, in patients with prosthetic valves, anticoagulation is of most value in preventing thrombosis on the prosthesis itself and within the left atrium, and the embolism which arises from these sites, but of much less value in preventing 'embolism' arising as the result of high shear stresses or arterial disease or any interaction between the two.

Antithrombotic management should thus encompass other strategies in addition to anti-coagulation to reduce the risk of thromboembolism. A recent prospective observational study of patients undergoing valve replacement, based on factors at the time of surgery identified several risk factors predictive of future thromboembolism during follow-up on multivariate analysis [35]. These risk factors were additive in their effect, enabling a scoring system to be developed: the greater the number of risk factors, the higher the risk.

The measures that can be undertaken to reduce the effect of risk factors which can be modified, are shown in Table 14.1. Risk factors identified in other studies have also been included. It should be stressed, however, that no studies have yet been conducted to assess the effect of risk factor modification in patients with prosthetic heart valves.

Many of the modifiable risk factors in Table 14.1 are also acknowledged independent risk factors for stroke in the general population and their control is equally as important in patients with heart valve disease [11, 14, 37–39]. Diabetes enhances the effect of other risk factors [40], and the effect of atrial fibrillation is magnified by other factors which contribute to low intracardiac flow conditions, such as left atrial enlargement and impaired left ventricular function [41]. Obesity is associated with a prothrombotic state [42] and is an independent risk factor for stroke in both men [43, 44] and women [45].

Increased mean platelet volume has been identified as an independent risk factor for stroke in patients with known cerebrovascular disease [46]. It is also associated with diabetes [47]. In the absence of rare congenital platelet abnormalities associated with large size, increased platelet size is usually associated with greater than normal platelet turnover consequent upon excessive platelet consumption [48]. Thus increased platelet size as a marker of thromboembolic risk after MVR [35] may indicate a prothrombotic milieu within the left atrium and the necessity for further investigation with transoesophageal echocardiography (TEE). If no modifiable abnormalities are found on TEE (e.g., left atrial or prosthetic thrombus or spontaneous echocardiographic contrast (SEC) secondary to a high transprosthetic gradient), consideration should be given to prescribing antiplatelet therapy in addition to anticoagulation, particularly if the patient has already experienced a thromboembolic event, because larger than normal platelets are more reactive and therefore more 'sticky' [49]. (See Antiplatelet therapy, p. 232).

Raised levels of fibrinogen elevate thrombotic risk by increasing platelet activation and by raising plasma viscosity [36]. High plasma viscosity and areas of sluggish flow adjacent to a prosthesis are additive in their prothrombotic effect. Causes of hyperfibrinogenaemia should be sought and treated if possible [50]. Dehydration, which also raises plasma viscosity, should be particularly avoided in the presence of hyperfibrinogenaemia.

In the risk factor study referred to above, chronic infection with *Chlamydia pneumoniae* was the strongest overall predictor of stroke, the effect occurring after both AVR and MVR [35]. This new finding is in keeping with similar data for stroke in the general population [51, 52]. Whether antibiotic treatment for *C. pneumoniae* will be effective in reducing risk after valve replacement remains to be tested in prospective trials. Prolonged treatment may be necessary as infection in circulating monocytes is refractory to antibiotic treatment, although the organism can be more readily eliminated from endothelial cells [53].

In patients with concomitant vascular disease, treatment with angiotensin converting enzyme (ACE) inhibitors should be considered as these drugs have been shown to significantly reduce the incidence of stroke in patients with coronary disease, cerebrovascular disease or peripheral vascular disease. In the HOPE study, there was a 32% reduction in relative risk of stroke and a 61% reduction in relative risk of fatal stroke with ramipril [54]. Hypercholesterolaemia should be treated with statins which also have additional benefits in reducing the risk of stroke through antithrombotic, anti-inflammatory and anti-oxidant mechanisms [55]. Carotid endarterectomy should be considered in patients with carotid stenosis >70%, even if they are asymptomatic, as this has been shown to reduce stroke risk [56].

An insufficiently reduced level of factor VII despite oral anticoagulation is a newly described risk factor for thromboembolism and deserves special mention. In the study mentioned above, this was the second strongest independent risk factor for thromboembolism after MVR on multivariate analysis [35] and confirms the view of other investigators that the degree of reduction in factor VII by oral anticoagulants may be equally as important as the degree of reduction in prothrombin (factor II) [57, 58]. At lower levels of INR, there is relatively less reduction of factor VII levels than prothrombin levels [59]. Acenocoumarol, because of its short half-life, allows greater fluctuation of factor VII levels than phenprocoumon [57], and this may be an important consideration in choosing an oral anticoagulant drug, particularly for mitral patients (see below).

There is diurnal fluctuation in factor VII levels. Factor VII has a short half-life and levels are increased by a fatty meal [60]. Levels also tend to rise with age and in obesity, pregnancy, hypercholesterolaemia, hypertriglyceridaemia, and diabetes [60]. Raised levels of factor VII have been associated with increased coronary risk [61], although this has not been confirmed in all studies and mechanisms have yet to be clarified, particularly with respect to the effect of polymorphisms in the factor VII gene [62]. Nevertheless, it is acknowledged that elevated factor VII coagulant activity is prothrombotic and this is consistent with the finding that relative 'resistance' of factor VII to oral anticoagulation, with lack of the anticipated reduction in levels, appears to act as a risk factor for thromboembolism in patients with prosthetic mitral valves. Such patients might benefit from factor VII monitoring to optimise their INR and should be advised to reduce their dietary fat intake. Statin therapy should also be considered, in view of the close relationship between lipid levels and factor VII.

ANTITHROMBOTIC THERAPY ACCORDING TO VALVE TYPE

MECHANICAL VALVES

It is generally agreed that all patients with mechanical prosthetic heart valves require anticoagulation for life, and there is no doubt that this is the safest approach under most circumstances [1, 2, 65]. Trials without anticoagulation and trials with antiplatelet therapy only have resulted in high rates of thromboembolism and/or valve thrombosis [36]. The details of how the intensity of anticoagulation should be adjusted according to the thrombogenicity of each type of mechanical valve is discussed in the section on choosing the optimum intensity of anticoagulation (p. 226).

BIOPROSTHESES

Bioprostheses in general are considered to be less thrombogenic than mechanical prostheses. However, they are still subject to thrombus deposition, both on the sewing ring and the leaflets, especially in the early postoperative months, and gross obstructive prosthesis thrombosis can occur, even in stentless bioprostheses. One randomised trial between mechanical valves on anticoagulation and porcine valves predominantly without anticoagulation showed no significant difference in the incidence of valve thrombosis at 15 years [66], and valve thrombosis rates reported in the literature for mechanical valves and porcine valves in the mitral position are also very similar [29]. Bioprosthetic valve thrombosis, especially in the early postoperative period, is often related to low cardiac output [67]. Degenerating bioprostheses and homografts may also be subject to thrombus deposition which, through organisation and secondary calcification, may contribute to further stiffening of the leaflets [67]. Although warfarin has no effect on primary tissue calcification, one study has shown less secondary calcification in degenerating bioprostheses in patients treated with warfarin [68]. A retrospective study based on echocardiographic data suggests that statins may also delay the degenerative process [69], perhaps through antithrombotic and anti-inflammatory mechanisms [56, 70] and immunomodulation [71] in addition to reducing lipid infiltration. Prospective randomised trials are clearly required.

Whether patients with stented bioprostheses with no other indications for anticoagulation (e.g., atrial fibrillation) should receive anticoagulants during the first three months remains controversial, due to the absence of randomised trials. It is widely assumed that the thrombogenicity of a bioprosthesis will be less after three months, as by this time the sewing ring will be fully endothelialised. However, bioprosthetic sewing rings are sometimes incompletely covered by endothelium even years after implantation and it is doubtful whether the endothelium which is present actually functions normally in such an abnormal and hostile environment [67]. Thus the three-month period is somewhat arbitrary, although it has been shown that the risk of thromboembolism declines after this time-period [72, 73], as it does with mechanical valves.

Some retrospective studies have found no difference in thromboembolism in the first three months between anticoagulated and non-anticoagulated patients [72, 74] whilst others have found fewer thromboembolic events in anticoagulated patients [73, 75]. One randomised trial of two different intensities of anticoagulation (INR 2.0–2.25 vs. 2.5–4.0) found no difference in thromboembolism but a significantly higher incidence of bleeding with higher INRs [30]. Two retrospective comparisons of warfarin, aspirin and no treatment following hospital discharge from the pre-INR era in the USA [72, 76] are therefore difficult to evaluate without knowledge of achieved INRs; both studies found that any possible benefit of warfarin was outweighed by a high incidence of bleeding, but anticoagulation intensity may have been too high, as in many American studies of that era [77]. A recent European non-randomised study found no difference in either thromboembolism or bleeding events in the first 3 months between warfarin (INR 2.0–3.0) and aspirin (dose not stated) in patients following bioprosthetic aortic valve replacement who had no other risk factors for thromboembolism [78].

A recent internet survey by CTSNet of 726 cardiac surgeons worldwide (45% from the USA, 33% from Europe) revealed that approximately 60% of respondents believed that antiplatelet therapy is an acceptable alternative to warfarin for the first three months after bioprosthetic AVR in patients without comorbidities. Almost 70% believed that warfarin for three months should no longer be the standard of care. This survey underlines the current uncertainty about optimum antithrombotic management and the inescapable conclusion that randomised trials in this situation are long overdue [79].

In the absence of firm guidance from randomised trials, recommendations can only be derived from basic principles and some observational studies:

1. If there are no contraindications to anticoagulation, the use of low-intensity anticoagulation (target INR 2.5) is recommended for all patients for the first three months.
2. In patients with chronic atrial fibrillation and otherwise normal cardiac function a target INR of 2.5 should be maintained indefinitely.
3. In patients with low cardiac output and heart failure due to impaired ventricular function, irrespective of whether they are in sinus rhythm or atrial fibrillation, a higher target INR should be used (3.0).
4. In patients with a high risk of bleeding on anticoagulation (Table 14.2), it is safer to avoid anticoagulation altogether even in the first 3 months if the patient is in sinus rhythm. In the presence of atrial fibrillation low-intensity anticoagulation (INR 2.0) should be considered. Age *per se* is not a contraindication to anticoagulation.

Controversy also surrounds the long-term antithrombotic management for bioprosthetic valve patients after the first 3 months. Current American guidelines recommend aspirin alone if the patient is in sinus rhythm [1, 2] but the evidence is weak, being derived from relatively small observational studies [80–82]. In one series of bioprosthetic AVR, the TE rate after 3 months was 1.3%/year on aspirin and 5.2%/year with no treatment ($P < 0.02$), although concerns were raised in discussion about data collection methods and event definitions [81]. Other series have found no differences between aspirin therapy and no treatment [72, 83]. In the absence of strong evidence, long-term antithrombotic management should be patient-specific, using aspirin for patients with established arterial disease and other stroke risk factors (diabetes, coronary disease, persistent smoking, etc.) and no contraindication to aspirin therapy (see section on Antiplatelet therapy, p. 232).

The evidence for aspirin following bioprosthetic MVR is even weaker. Nunez *et al.* found an overall TE rate of 0.5%/year on high-dose aspirin (500 mg or 1 g) among 768 mitral valve

Table 14.2   Risk factors for anticogulation-related bleeding [145–149]

> ■ INR >4.0
>> ■ Poor anticoagulation control
>> ■ Drugs which potentiate the effect of oral anticoagulants
> ■ Underlying pathological conditions prone to bleeding
>> ■ peptic ulcer
>> ■ angiodysplasia
>> ■ diverticulitis
>> ■ bladder papilloma
>> ■ menorrhagia
>> ■ cerebrovascular disease (history of stroke)
>> ■ untreated hypertension
>> ■ microvascular disease (diabetes)
> ■ Abnormal haemostasis
>> ■ coagulation disorders
>> ■ anaemia
>> ■ renal failure
>> ■ concomitant antiplatelet therapy
> ■ Past history of major bleeding
> ■ Occupational or sports-related risk of trauma
>
> Note: Many risk factors are additive, e.g., history of stroke, history of GI
> bleeding, anaemia and renal failure [149].

replacement (MVR) and double valve replacement (DVR) patients in Spain, 76% of whom were in atrial fibrillation (AF) [80]. This surprisingly low TE rate may possibly be explained by the young age of the patients (mean age 44), as the Atrial Fibrillation, Aspirin Anticoagulation Study (AFASAK) and Stroke Prevention in Atrial Fibrillation (SPAF) study in patients with non-valvular AF found TE rates of 5.0%/year and 3.6%/year respectively in older patients on aspirin [84, 85]. In the SPAF study, aspirin was also found to be much less effective in preventing cardioembolic stroke than non-cardioembolic stroke [86]. Thus, the study of Nunez *et al.* cannot be used to support the recommendation of aspirin alone, particularly for patients in their 70s and 80s undergoing bioprosthetic MVR, if they are in AF. If the patient is in sinus rhythm, the recommendation for the use of aspirin is the same as for AVR (see above).

Regular follow-up of patients with bioprostheses is required not only to detect early signs of degeneration but also to detect the development of AF. The Edinburgh valve trial has shown that 33% of bioprosthetic AVR patients and 57% of MVR patients require anticoagulation by 15 years, mainly because of AF [87]. Risk factors for AF include older age, mitral valve disease, hypertension, diabetes, ischaemic heart disease and congestive heart failure [88]. Patients with these conditions will require extra vigilance. Patients with mitral bioprostheses who are not anticoagulated require particularly close follow-up as routine echocardiography reveals that a small percentage will develop thrombosis on the ventricular side of the bioprosthetic cusps, which may not always be symptomatic initially [89]. Patients who have had chordal preservation may be at higher risk [90, 91].

HOMOGRAFTS AND AUTOGRAFTS

Homografts and autografts in the aortic position have no sewing ring and do not require anticoagulation if they are functioning normally, unless there are other indications [92].

However, degenerating homografts are subject to thrombus deposition [67, 93, 94] and antithrombotic treatment should be considered in this situation. Stentless aortic bioprostheses fall midway between homografts and stented bioprostheses in terms of potential thrombogenicity. They have no bulky sewing rings but do have artificial fabric exposed to the blood stream at annular level and the cusps are susceptible, albeit rarely, to thrombosis [95] usually associated with low cardiac output or technical factors leading to deformation of one or more cusps as the result of distortion at implantation or haematoma formation between the prosthesis and the aortic wall [96, 97]. In the absence of trials, the same principles should be applied to stentless bioprostheses as apply to their stented counterparts.

VALVE REPAIR INVOLVING PROSTHETIC MATERIALS

Mitral valve repair for regurgitation nearly always involves the use of a prosthetic ring, closely resembling the sewing ring of a prosthetic valve, to support the repair and/or reduce the size of the annulus. As with prosthetic valves, this represents a thrombogenic surface until it becomes endothelialised and on general principles a strong case can be made for anticoagulation for the first three postoperative months.

Other factors increasing thrombotic risk also need to be taken into account. The intensity of spontaneous echo contrast in the left atrium on echocardiography will provide a guide to the degree of stasis [98] and haematological evidence of coagulation activation may give further guidance for anticoagulation [99]. If AF or congestive heart failure remain after mitral valve repair, long-term anticoagulation with a minimum INR of 2.0 will be necessary as antiplatelet therapy alone [100, 101] or combined with ultra-low anticoagulation (INR <2.0) [102] provides insufficient protection against thromboembolism in AF. The recent Euro Heart Survey of current practice in 25 European countries revealed that approximately half of all patients following mitral valve repair are on chronic anticoagulation, mainly because of AF [103, 104]. Increasing interest in the concomitant use of various ablation procedures [105, 106] to restore sinus rhythm as an adjunct to mitral valve repair [107] may reduce the proportion of patients requiring anticoagulation in the future, although at present it remains uncertain whether restoration of electrical sinus rhythm corrects left atrial endothelial and contractile dysfunction and reduces thromboembolic risk [108, 109], or indeed whether correction of AF will remain stable in the long term [110].

EARLY POSTOPERATIVE ANTICOAGULATION

Following all cardiac operations performed on cardiopulmonary bypass, the immediate concern is prevention of excessive bleeding. Haemodilution, blood loss and platelet consumption caused by adherence to the bypass circuit result in moderate anaemia and a reduced platelet count. Platelet function is abnormal, fibrinogen levels are usually lower than normal, and coagulation may be deranged in other ways also [111, 112]. Consequently the risk of bleeding from surgical sites is usually greater than the risk of thromboembolic complications at this time. Nevertheless, foreign surfaces exposed to the blood stream will attract thrombus at a very early stage. Within seconds of exposure to blood, artificial surfaces are covered with a thin layer of plasma proteins and platelet deposition follows rapidly [113]. In areas subject to conditions of low flow, macroscopic thrombus may develop. It is not unusual to see thrombus on the sewing ring of a prosthetic valve on TEE soon after implantation for example [114]. Similarly, thrombus may form in the left atrial appendage very soon after surgery in patients in AF, especially if the cardiac output is low, underlining the need for TEE monitoring in the early postoperative period if possible [115].

Anticoagulation in the early postoperative period is thus a matter of balancing the risks of bleeding and thromboembolism. After the first 24 h, the risk of bleeding is usually very small, whilst the risk of thromboembolism progressively increases, as levels of fibrinogen and other coagulation proteins are restored, often exceeding pre-operative levels as part of the physiological response to trauma [116], and monocyte tissue factor expression increases [117]. Similarly, both platelet count and platelet aggregability may rise considerably above pre-operative levels, an effect persisting up to three weeks [116].

As currently available oral anticoagulants work indirectly by suppressing the carboxylation of vitamin-K dependent coagulation proteins (prothrombin, factor VII, factor IX and factor X) by the liver, effective anticoagulation usually takes several days to establish [59]. In fact, in patients not taking oral anticoagulants pre-operatively a steady-state in the level of prothrombin (factor II) in plasma may not be reached for 10–15 days, due to its long half-life (60–100 h) [57]. Relative resistance to oral anticoagulants, with the necessity for very large doses, can be due to interaction with other drugs, impaired absorption, gross obesity, hypothyroidism, excessive vitamin K intake (unusual in a hospital setting) or genetic factors [59]. The latter is very rare. Asian patients on average require lower doses of oral anticoagulant drugs than patients of other ethnic origins [59].

Three protocols of anticoagulation initiation postoperatively are in widespread use, and no randomised comparison has yet been performed:

1. Intravenous heparin commenced as soon as postoperative bleeding from drainage tubes moderates, maintained until simultaneously or later commenced oral anticoagulation achieves a therapeutic level of INR [65]. This strategy has the potential to increase the risk of bleeding and tamponade.
2. Oral anticoagulation commenced on the first postoperative day, supplemented by intravenous heparin only if an effective INR is not achieved by the third postoperative day. If the patient is unable to take oral medication, or if there is doubt about absorption from the gastrointestinal tract (e.g., paralytic ileus, vomiting and diarrhoea), an intravenous preparation of warfarin can be substituted, although this is not available in all countries. This strategy has the potential to increase the risk of thromboembolism although in practice the risk is very small for the first two postoperative days. A study from Sweden in 534 patients using intravenous warfarin commenced the morning after surgery, and only supplemented by heparin if the INR was not therapeutic on the second postoperative day, reported no thromboembolic events in patients who followed the protocol [118]. However, this approach may not have wide applicability due to lack of availability of intravenous warfarin and in any case would need to be tested in other large series of patients, preferably randomised to other methods of initiating anticoagulation before it could be recommended.
3. In recent years, subcutaneous low-molecular-weight heparin (LMWH) has been used increasingly as a bridge to therapeutic oral anticoagulation. This strategy is recommended as an alternative to intravenous unfractionated heparin (UFH) by the American College of Chest Physicians (ACCP) Guidelines [2]. Part of the motivation for using LMWH is to decrease length of stay in hospital and to reduce costs [119]. However, it must be emphasised that patient safety should be paramount and at present there are no randomised studies to support the use of LMWH in this setting. If LMWH is used, factor Xa monitoring should ideally be employed to ensure optimum anticoagulation [120], particularly in patients with renal failure or obesity, in whom dosage may be difficult to determine [121], and particularly immediately after surgery when the risk of bleeding will be higher at anti-Xa levels higher than 0.8 U/ml [121].

Until randomised studies are available with echocardiographic control and adequate follow-up beyond the period of hospitalisation to detect thromboembolism after discharge, no particular method can be recommended. Whichever strategy is employed, it must be emphasised that inadequate anticoagulation beyond the second or third postoperative day in the presence of increasing prothrombotic conditions is potentially dangerous. The hazard function curve for thromboembolism shows the incidence to be highest during the first 30 days, only falling to a steady long-term level after six months [116].

Initiation of oral anticoagulation after valve surgery requires care, particularly in elderly patients whose dosage requirement is usually less than younger patients due to decreased metabolic clearance of the unbound drug [122]. No loading dose should be given [123]. Patients who have taken oral anticoagulants pre-operatively can usually resume their previous dose, although drug interactions and reduced dietary intake may necessitate a slightly lower dose initially [124]. More frequent INR measurements are necessary in the first few weeks until a steady state is reached.

THE OPTIMUM INTENSITY OF ANTICOAGULATION

GENERAL PRINCIPLES AND CHOICE OF DRUG

The new oral direct antithrombin drug ximelagatran has been shown to be equally as effective as vitamin K antagonists in the prevention of postoperative venous thromboembolism, stroke in AF, and further events in acute coronary syndromes (ACS), with a slightly lower incidence of bleeding [125], but has not yet been approved by the Food and Drug Administration (FDA) due to concern about liver damage in long-term use in about 6% of patients. Until this issue is resolved and until trials are performed in patients with prosthetic valves, all patients will require anticoagulation using oral vitamin K antagonists. These drugs act indirectly by blocking the carboxylation of four coagulation proteins, factors II (prothrombin), VII, IX and X, which confers their procoagulant activity. The carboxylation of these factors is not blocked to an equal extent and there is also considerable interindividual variation in their plasma level at a given INR [57–59]. This biological variation, coupled with imprecision in measurement of the INR for technical reasons results in some uncertainty as to the precise extent of anticoagulation achieved [59, 126, 127]. Further variation can occur between INR measurements due to fluctuation in dietary vitamin K, poor compliance, impaired absorption during gastrointestinal disturbance or drug interactions [59]. It is therefore important to appreciate that selection of a particular target INR level or a range of INR values is not an exact science, and that it is unrealistic to expect that a target INR will be maintained by all patients. INR variability is unfortunately very common, often due to poor compliance [128], and is a major determinant of thromboembolic events [129] and reduced survival after valve replacement [130]. Furthermore, because of the many different pathogenetic mechanisms involved in thromboembolism after valve surgery [6, 35], it is also unrealistic to believe that anticoagulation at a particular INR will prevent all events. In general, it is preferable to aim for a specific INR rather than a range when monitoring anticoagulation.

Although warfarin is the most commonly used vitamin K antagonist worldwide, two other drugs should be mentioned, one shorter-acting and one longer-acting. The half-life of warfarin is 15–50 h, that of acenocoumarol (widely used in France, Italy and Spain) about 10 h and that of phenprocoumon (widely used in Germany and the Netherlands) 4–9 days [59]. Smoother control of the INR may be achieved with phenprocoumon in a steady state but the disadvantages of this drug are the slower response to a dosage change, the necessity to stop the drug well in advance of any planned interruption in anticoagulation and its manufacture in tablets of only one dose. Two non-randomised studies have shown a higher incidence of bleeding complications with phenprocoumon in comparison to acenocoumarol [131, 132], possibly because a high INR will take longer to return to the target range [132]. (See section on Management of the high INR, p. 230).

Given the increasing risk of bleeding with increasing anticoagulation intensity, the ideal INR for patients after valve surgery is the lowest which achieves effective reduction in the incidence of thromboembolic events, bearing in mind that the incidence cannot be lowered to zero in any large series of patients for the reasons discussed above. Evidence from several laboratory and clinical studies both in patients with non-valvular AF [102, 133, 134] and in patients with prosthetic valves [135, 136] indicates that an INR in the range 2.0–2.5 is the **minimum** requirement for adequate prophylaxis against thrombosis occurring under conditions of relative stasis, but many patients will require a higher INR than this if adverse intracardiac conditions or a more thrombogenic prosthesis impose a greater risk of thrombosis (see below).

In a study of 1608 patients with a variety of different mechanical valves (3% caged ball/disc, 77% tilting disc, 20% bileaflet) followed for a mean of 4 years per patient in four anticoagulation clinics in the Netherlands, Cannegieter and colleagues found the lowest incidence of all events (thromboembolic and bleeding) occurred in the INR range 2.5–4.9 [137]. However, this is a very broad range and almost certainly reflects not only the heterogeneity of the patient population in terms of age, risk factors, valve position (aortic or mitral) and valve type, but also the inherent limitations of the study: the assumption that the change in INR from one measurement to the next (up to 8 weeks apart) would be linear, as this was the basis for calculating event rates for particular INR ranges.

A recent meta-analysis of heterogeneous observational series from the literature, comparing mean target INRs above and below 3.0, came to the conclusion that all patients, irrespective of individual risk factors, valve position and valve type, should have an INR between 3.0 and 4.5 [138]. However, the methodology of the meta-analysis did not take into account differences among the series analysed in terms of data collection methods, selection bias, follow-up accuracy, patient risk factors or anticoagulation variability, all of which have been shown to influence thromboembolic rates [139]. In reaching their conclusion, the authors ignored evidence for a contrary view, including randomised controlled trials (RCTs), current guidelines, the much higher mortality rate for anticoagulant-related intracerebral haemorrhage in comparison to ischaemic stroke and the finding that the risk of intracerebral haemorrhage rises steeply above an INR of 4.0 (see sections on Management of the high INR, p. 230 and Antiplatelet therapy, p. 232). Nor did they take into account that many thromboembolic and bleeding events occur when the INR is outside the target range. Whilst having a unified approach to anticoagulation management may have advantages for anticoagulation clinics, this approach will not benefit individual patients who may be exposed to the risks of unnecessarily high anticoagulation intensity. In contrast, the trend in recent years has been towards lower intensity anticoagulation, prosthesis- and patient-specific anticoagulation [116] and greater concentration on the management of patient risk factors as discussed above [6, 35].

PATIENT-SPECIFIC AND PROSTHESIS-SPECIFIC ANTICOAGULATION

Unfortunately, currently available randomised trials of different INR ranges fail to provide widely applicable guidelines or to address the requirements of individual patients. All the randomised trials comparing different intensities of anticoagulation in patients with prosthetic heart valves suffer from limitations imposed by their selection criteria, their patient population or their methodology [30–34, 140]. Almost all involve relatively small numbers of patients with short follow-up and, because of their fundamental differences and lack of uniformity of INR ranges compared, they are not suitable for meta-analysis. The AREVA (Anticoagulation et Remplacement Valvulaire) trial for example, although providing useful recommendations for selected low-risk patients with the St. Jude Medical valve in the aortic position, specifically excluded all patients with risk factors for thromboembolism, including AF, left atrial enlargement or thrombosis, and a previous history of thromboembolism [33].

The most recently published randomised trial (German Experience with Low Intensity Anticoagulation – GELIA), a larger multicentre study based on patients with the St. Jude Medical prosthesis [34, 140], attempted to compare three overlapping INR ranges, 2.0–3.5, 2.5–4.0 and 3.0–4.5, for patients undergoing AVR, MVR or DVR, beginning three months after surgery. The relatively low event rates reported reflect the exclusion of the first three months, the period of highest risk. Unfortunately, the impact of the trial was also severely blunted by the finding that many patients (57% in one subgroup) failed to maintain INR within their allocated range. Each subgroup also contained a mixture of conventional anti-coagulation management and patient self-managed anticoagulation. Not surprisingly per-haps, the trial failed to find any differences in either thromboembolic or bleeding rates among the three INR ranges. This trial amply illustrates the problem inherent in all trials of different target ranges of INR; that most events occur whilst the INR is outside the target range, emphasising the importance of good quality INR control (see below).

Despite the lack of uniformity in INR ranges, patient characteristics and prostheses type in the various randomised trials, all trials share the same conclusions (in patients who were predominantly in sinus rhythm and who mostly had an aortic prosthesis): that the lower range of INR tested did not increase the risk of embolism but did reduce the risk of bleed-ing. In the case of mechanical valve trials, the selected lower INR range equated with a mean INR of about 2.5 and this value has been accepted in recently published guidelines as suitable for most patients with an aortic prosthesis in sinus rhythm [1, 2, 65].

The randomised trials offer much less useful guidance on the ideal INR for patients with a mitral prosthesis. The AREVA trial [33] largely excluded mitral patients, the trial from Saudi Arabia [42] was mainly in very young patients in sinus rhythm and the GELIA trial excluded from analysis the high-risk period of the first three months and had a high pro-portion of patients with INRs outside the target ranges [34, 140].

Following MVR, there are often additional prothrombotic conditions in the left atrium due to AF, left atrial enlargement, poor contractile performance of the appendage (even in sinus rhythm) or residual mitral valve gradient [115]. Hence anticoagulation intensity must be sufficient to combat conditions of relative stasis in the left atrium in addition to prevent-ing thrombus deposition on the prosthesis. Evidence from experimental laboratory studies [7] and retrospective comparison of different mean INR levels following isolated MVR [141] suggest that the lowest target INR for most MVR patients is 3.0, and this has also been rec-ommended by recently published guidelines [1, 2, 65]. This additional anticoagulation intensity is probably sufficient to combat adverse left atrial conditions as it has been shown to permit spontaneous regression of left atrial thrombus with return of elevated fibrinopep-tide A levels to normal in previously un-anticoagulated patients [142]. Patients with tricus-pid or pulmonary prostheses will also be at higher risk and require a minimum INR of 3.0 (Table 14.3). In the case of some prostheses of higher thrombogenicity, an INR of 3.0 may not be high enough to prevent valve thrombosis, particularly in the presence of low flow con-ditions or trigger factors for thrombosis such as dehydration or pulmonary infection. In some patients with prostheses of higher thrombogenicity or in newly introduced prostheses of uncertain thrombogenicity, it is probably safer to maintain a mean INR of 3.5 or 4.0. Thus in selecting an appropriate INR for patients after valve replacement it is necessary to take into account both patient-related and prosthesis-related factors (Table 14.3).

It is not possible to define low, medium and high thrombogenicity prostheses in exact scientific terms. Nor is it possible to assign the degree of thrombogenicity only on the basis of the broad design category or age of the prosthesis. One recently introduced bileaflet valve, for example, had to be withdrawn from the market before trials had been completed because of a high incidence of valve thrombosis. Unstratified thromboembolic rates pro-vide little guidance as they can be influenced by so many non-prosthetic factors. Prosthesis thrombosis rates on the other hand are less influenced by extraneous factors apart from the number of patients in the series who have had a period of anticoagulation interruption. Relating the prosthesis thrombosis rate to mean INR gives a better indication of specific prosthesis thrombogenicity, if sufficient large series exist in the literature for that prosthe-sis to provide the necessary data. For many prostheses on the market these data do not exist. In practical terms, from available data [29, 33, 34, 36, 140, 141, 143] the Medtronic

Table 14.3 Anticoagulation for valve replacement

		With risk factors	Without risk factors
Adjust target INR to: intracardiac conditions prosthesis thrombogenecity		SR LA 0 MVgr 0 LV normal SEC 0 AVR	AF LA > 50 mm MVgr+ EF < 35% SEC+ MVR TVR PVR
Prosthesis thrombogenecity	Low	2.5	3.0
	Medium	3.0	3.5
	High	3.5	4.0

Low = Medtronic Hall, St. Jude Medical (without Silzone), Carbomedics AVR; Medium = Bileaflet valves with insufficient data, Bjork-Shiley valves; High = Lillehei Kaster, Omniscience, Starr Edwards; SR = sinus rhythm; AF = atrial fibrillation; LA = left atrium; MVgr = mitral valve gradient; EF = ejection; fraction; SEC = spontaneous echo contrast.

Hall tilting disc valve, the St. Jude Medical bileaflet valve (without Silzone coating), the Carbomedics aortic prosthesis and all bioprostheses can be regarded as low thrombogenicity prostheses.

However, in comparing the St. Jude Medical and Carbomedics valves there is a paradox and a caution. Average prosthesis thrombosis rates in the mitral position are higher with the Carbomedics valve, but in the aortic position the opposite is the case [143]. A possible explanation is that the raised pivot guard of the St. Jude valve projects into the left ventricle in the aortic position, where it can come into contact with peri-annular tissue, particularly if implanted in a supra-annular position. This makes the pivot guard more susceptible to tissue ingrowth, which was the explanation for a relatively high incidence of incomplete leaflet excursion among asymptomatic patients identified on cinefluoroscopy in one Japanese series [144].

The Omniscience tilting disc valve has been shown to have a high susceptibility to valve thrombosis when exposed to low intensity anticoagulation [67] and should be regarded as a high thrombogenicity prosthesis in Table 14.3. It is no longer manufactured. Other tilting disc valves and other bileaflet valves not mentioned above probably occupy intermediate positions in terms of thrombogenicity and further data on valve thrombosis rates in relation to achieved INR are awaited in order to characterise them more accurately. In general terms, the thrombogenicity of bileaflet valves is primarily determined by their hinge design, as this is the point at which thrombosis usually begins. Hinge design varies considerably from one bileaflet valve to another. In tilting disc valves, thrombogenicity is primarily determined by the degree of flow through the minor orifice as thrombosis usually begins in an area of relatively stagnant flow. Modern tilting disc valves, such as the Medtronic Hall valve, exhibit good flow through the minor orifice, in contrast to early tilting disc designs [67], and this is almost certainly the explanation for their low thrombogenicity.

The ideal INR for patients following mitral valve repair using prosthetic ring annu-loplasty depends primarily on left atrial conditions. On general principles, if the patient is in sinus rhythm, has no significant left atrial enlargement and good left ventricular function, an INR of 2.5 is probably sufficient, although there are no clinical data from trials to support this recommendation. On the other hand, if the patient is in AF, has moderate to severe left atrial enlargement or poor left ventricular function, a target INR of 3.0 is safer.

MANAGEMENT OF THE HIGH INR

The risk of major bleeding begins to rise when the INR exceeds 4.5 and rises steeply and exponentially above an INR of 6.0 [145]. Patients with risk factors for bleeding (Table 14.2) [145–149] are at higher risk. Among 23 patients experiencing fatal intracerebral haemorrhage in a recent large 20-year prosthetic valve series [150], all had an INR >4.0, 74% had an INR >6.0, 39% were hypertensive and 39% were taking antiplatelet therapy in addition to warfarin. Other authors have also shown that the risk of intracerebral haemorrhage rises steeply above an INR of 4.0 [151]. Intracerebral haemorrhage is associated with the highest mortality among bleeding complications, with mortality directly related to haematoma volume [152]. Pre-existing cerebrovascular disease is a risk factor [146, 149, 151].

One of the most common causes of an INR >6.0 is drug interaction with the oral anticoagulant [59, 153]. Great care should be exercised when prescribing drugs known to enhance the anticoagulant effect. The dose of the anticoagulant drug will almost certainly need to be reduced and more frequent INR measurements will need to be made until a steady state is achieved. Some drugs should be avoided altogether because of the danger of a very high INR. These include azapropazone, ketorolac and intravenous diclofenac. Cranberry juice should also be avoided for the same reason. Paracetamol (acetominophen) should be used with caution. In prolonged use it was the most common cause of an INR >6.0 in one study [153]. Medical conditions that can enhance the effect of oral anticoagulants include advanced malignant disease and recent diarrhoeal illness [153].

An INR >6.0 is regarded as the threshold for reversal of anticoagulation, even in the absence of bleeding, either by discontinuation alone or by giving vitamin K in addition. However the recommendation to give vitamin K is based upon analyses of this treatment in groups of patients with very varied indications for anticoagulation [123, 154, 155]. In some literature series, follow-up is limited to a few days only. No publications have addressed the issue specifically in patients with prosthetic heart valves, other than making risk calculations based on average valve thrombosis rates in non-anticoagulated patients [155]. No echocardiographic studies have been performed to identify early valve thrombosis in patients treated with vitamin K. The most common cause of valve thrombosis is anticoagulation interruption (see section on Valve thrombosis, p. 237). Valve thrombosis is associated with a high mortality and prosthetic valve patients are therefore at higher risk than the average anticoagulated patient. Although, on average, the INR falls gradually to the therapeutic range with vitamin K [154], the response in individual patients is unpredictable [156] and herein lies the danger.

It is therefore recommended that a high INR (>6.0) without bleeding in prosthetic valve patients on warfarin or acenocoumarol should not be treated with intravenous vitamin K. In patients on phenprocoumon, it is permissible to use oral vitamin K, given in increments of 1 mg, as the long half-life of phenprocoumon allows the INR to fall more gradually following the administration of vitamin K. Because of the long half-life however, additional doses may be necessary as the INR often begins to rise again after the second day [156]. The response among individual patients is variable [156].

All patients with an INR >6.0 should be admitted to hospital for observation and their anticoagulation temporarily discontinued until the INR is <5.0. If the INR is >10.0, and the patient has risk factors for bleeding (Table 14.4) consideration should be given to the use of fresh frozen plasma at a dose of 15 ml/kg body weight, bearing in mind the very small risk of transmission of viruses [155] and variant Creutzfeldt–Jacob Disease [157]. A pathogen inactivation process is now available for treating fresh frozen plasma without reducing its effectiveness [158, 159]

In patients who are bleeding with a high INR, a risk assessment must be made according to the severity, site and controllability of bleeding. If the risk to life from continued bleeding, inaccessible to local control, is greater than that of valve thrombosis (e.g., intracranial bleeding), cessation of anticoagulation should be accompanied by prothrombin complex concentrate. Intravenous vitamin K may also be necessary if bleeding continues, as the half-life of factor VII is only 6 h. However, it should be recognised that both factor concentrates and vitamin K increase the risk of valve thrombosis [155]. Intracranial and, in particular intracerebral, haemorrhage always necessitates reversal of anticoagulation [160]. The exact timing of the resumption of anticoagulation remains controversial but most agree that it should be resumed after one week [161, 162] as the long-term risk of further intracranial bleeding is lower than that of valve thrombosis and thromboembolism.

Bleeding with a therapeutic INR is often related to an underlying pathological cause and it is important to identify and treat it. Anticoagulation often unmasks occult pathology which is why 'anticoagulant-related' bleeding is more common in the first few months [146]. Patients with intermittent major bleeding from the gastrointestinal tract sometimes represent a difficult problem. Peptic ulceration can usually be successfully treated but if intermittent bleeding is due to angiodysplasia not amenable to endoscopic ablation or surgery [163], effective treatment is much more difficult. Bleeding in angiodysplasia has been linked to von Willebrand syndrome type 2A [164]. If local measures or hormone therapy with oestrogens [163] or ocreotide [165] fail to control bleeding, lower intensity anticoagulation or, in extreme cases with ongoing severe bleeding from widespread diffuse angiodysplasia, discontinuation of anticoagulation may be necessary. Fortunately this is a very rare occurrence.

ANTICOAGULATION SELF-MANAGEMENT

The service provision for anticoagulation management varies considerably in different countries, ranging from specialised anticoagulation clinics to general physicians managing anticoagulation in their individual patients. The introduction of the INR in 1983 represented a marked improvement in measurement of intensity of oral anticoagulation and in comparability of test results, but anticoagulation-related bleeding and thromboembolism remain the most common complications after heart valve replacement. Better anticoagulation control has been shown to improve survival after valve replacement with anticoagulation variability being the strongest independent predictor of reduced survival [130].

Anticoagulation control therefore is of prognostic importance and poor control has significant healthcare costs. It has been calculated that life-time management of cerebrovascular events caused by inadequate anticoagulation adds up to $85 000 in the USA [166, 167].

There is great variation in both the delivery [103] and the quality [168, 169] of anticoagulation control. This was the impetus for the introduction of patient self-management, first in Germany [170, 171]. and then in the United States [172, 173]. Patients can be trained to test a capillary sample for the INR using a portable monitor. Advice on dose can then be given by a physician or alternatively the patient can be trained to adjust the anticoagulant dose also. Nevertheless, despite the availability and accuracy [169, 174–177] of this system the recent Euro Heart Survey on Valvular Heart Disease revealed that self-assessment was used by less than 1% of patients [103].

Hence, much still needs to be done to educate physicians, patients and healthcare providers about the benefits of anticoagulation self-management. Only patients on long-term anticoagulation, who are able to follow a teaching course of 6–12 h should be considered for self-management. They should have some manual skills to be able to puncture the finger, have no visual impairment and sufficient understanding to recognise values outside the therapeutic range. The consent of their physician should be obtained [169, 178, 179]. Teaching should include theoretical aspects, as well as practical skills in the use of the coagulation monitor.

EFFECTIVENESS OF SELF-MANAGEMENT

In seven randomised studies comparing conventional testing with self-testing, patients employing self-management were more frequently within the therapeutic range than with conventional testing, with 70–80% of INR values considered to be in range [173, 180–185] It has been shown that more frequent testing of the INR results in a higher percentage of INRs in the therapeutic range [186], although for practical purposes a test interval of 8 days is considered sufficient.

Quality control of anticoagulation is an important determinant of prognosis [130], and event-free survival in patients after valve replacement performing self-assessment has been shown to be significantly higher than in patients with conventional control [185]. Patients capable of performing self-assessment of anticoagulation are usually well educated and motivated and can be trained to be experts in anticoagulation. The frequency of testing (usually once per week in comparison to 4–13 weeks in physician-directed management) adds to improvement in control and also allows the flexibility to adjust testing intervals according to intercurrent events or diseases and changes in medication.

Nearly all studies have shown that most patients prefer self-management. Those who have been successfully trained consider their quality of life markedly improved. In one study, only 8.3% of those trained after valve surgery were unable to continue with self-management [185].

Although the cost of the monitors, the test strips and the training course for the patient must be taken into account, these costs must be weighed against the high costs of treating the complications of conventionally managed anticoagulation, such as valve thrombosis, thromboembolism, stroke and bleeding complications [177].

ANTIPLATELET THERAPY

The use of antiplatelet therapy either alone or in combination with anticoagulation remains controversial, particularly for patients with mechanical valves. There has been much less enthusiasm for combined therapy in Europe than in North America. One recent multicentre randomised trial, comparing two types of prosthesis, reported significant differences in antithrombotic management between the European and North American trial centres. Use of concomitant aspirin was zero in Europe, but 54.6% in the early postoperative period and 23.5% on discharge from hospital in North America [187]. Similarly, the recent Euro Heart Survey on Valvular Heart Disease in 25 European countries [103] found that only 9.2% of mechanical valve patients attending outpatient clinics were taking antiplatelet drugs in combination with anticoagulation.

In determining whether an antiplatelet agent should be added to anticoagulation in patients with prosthetic valves, it is important to distinguish between the possible benefits in cardiovascular disease in general and those specific to prosthetic valves, when computing the benefit-risk ratio. Trials showing a benefit from antiplatelet drugs in vascular disease and trials showing apparent benefit in groups of patients with prosthetic valves and vascular disease should not be taken as evidence that patients with prosthetic valves and no vascular disease will also benefit.

It is also important to distinguish between the mechanisms of action of different antiplatelet drugs rather than amalgamating them for the purposes of meta-analysis or extrapolating from the results of one drug when making recommendations about another. Aspirin for example does not significantly inhibit shear-induced platelet aggregation [188] and experimental work in animals has shown that it does not prevent platelet adhesion to prosthetic surfaces, whereas dipyridamole does [189].

BASIC MECHANISMS

Antiplatelet agents are widely believed to be effective in preventing thrombotic events in the arterial, but much less in the venous circulation. However, this is not completely true, since deep vein thrombosis and pulmonary embolism were reduced by 36% by aspirin in the PEP trial in which almost half the patients also received heparin [190]. In AF, a condition in which left atrial thrombi mostly occur because of blood stasis, aspirin alone has been shown to be effective in reducing the thromboembolic risk by 22% (95% confidence interval [CI] 0–38%; $P = 0.05$) in a combined analysis of six trials comparing aspirin with placebo. However, many of these patients also had arterial disease. In comparison, warfarin reduced the risk of thromboemboli in AF by 61% (95% CI 47–71%; $P < 0.001$) [191]. Since the pathogenesis of thrombosis in patients with prosthetic valves also involves shear-induced platelet activation [192], especially in the case of aortic valve replacement, the use of an appropriate antiplatelet agent in addition to oral anticoagulants seems to have a sound theoretical basis. This must however be balanced against the additional risk of bleeding associated with the addition of antiplatelet agents to oral anticoagulant therapy.

Used alone, antiplatelet agents are known to provoke lower rates of intracranial haemorrhage than agents interfering with coagulation (anticoagulants and fibrinolytics) [193]. While the combination of the two is expected to result in more bleeding, some trials have addressed the hypothesis that a safe decrease in the intensity of anticoagulation might be possible whilst preserving optimal antithrombotic effect. In a direct comparison of high-INR warfarin (2.8–4.2) vs. intermediate-INR warfarin (2.0–2.5) + aspirin 75 mg/day in patients after myocardial infarction (MI) (the Warfarin-Aspirin Reinfarction Study-II, WARIS II) [194], the combined therapy group had a slight trend to a better outcome (15.0% rate of death, MI and cerebrovascular accidents) than the warfarin arm (16.7%) in a 4-year follow-up, combined with a trend towards less major bleeding (0.52% vs. 0.68%) [194], although differences were small and non-significant.

A pooled analysis of all aspirin trials in cardiovascular disease concluded that the benefit from low-dose aspirin (75–150 mg/day) was not inferior to that with higher doses (160–325 mg/day) with no difference in the rate of bleeding [195], but this analysis did not address the issue of combined therapy with warfarin. Although gastrointestinal bleeding with aspirin has been shown to be dose-dependent [196], this is not the case with intracerebral haemorrhage [195–197]. Meta-analysis of RCTs shows an 84% increase in the risk of intracerebral haemorrhage with aspirin (RR 1.84; 95% CI 1.24–2.74; $P < 0.001$) [198].

Apart from aspirin, dipyridamole is the only other agent which has been studied in clinical trials in combination with anticoagulation. The mechanism of action of dipyridamole is controversial [199], but probably involves the inhibition of adenosine reuptake and potentiation of the effect of nitric oxide [200]. The inhibition of platelet adhesion to artificial surfaces by dipyridamole is of potential usefulness in patients with prosthetic heart valves [189]. Several studies have shown some therapeutic benefit with this drug in patients with prosthetic heart valves [201]. However most of these studies were carried out many years ago, mostly in patients with the Starr–Edwards caged ball valve (which is unique in featuring high shear rates, causing ADP release, and areas of low shear at the apex of the cage), and with a formulation of dipyridamole now thought not to be very effective [199]. Renewed interest in dipyridamole after the publication of a large stroke prevention trial with a newer higher-dose and longer-acting formulation [202, 203] should prompt new trials of this drug in the management of artificial heart valves. In a trial of 6602 patients, dipyridamole was equally as effective as aspirin but with half the risk of bleeding (no difference from placebo) [202, 203]. This absence of excess bleeding is in keeping with a meta-analysis of dipyridamole + warfarin trials [204] and the Mayo Clinic trial comparing warfarin alone, warfarin + dipyridamole and warfarin + aspirin after heart valve replacement [205]. A recent meta-analysis has also confirmed dipyridamole to be effective in reducing stroke recurrence in patients with previous cerebrovascular disease [206].

Clopidogrel is a new thienopyridine, blocking the platelet $P2Y_{12}$ ADP receptor, with proven antithrombotic efficacy in a number of settings involving atherothrombosis. This drug has efficacy at least comparable to aspirin in patients with a previous MI or a previous stroke/TIA, or with peripheral arterial disease [207]. The drug also has effects additive to those of aspirin in unstable coronary syndromes and after coronary stenting, reducing the combination of death, MI and stroke. Clopidogrel is now being investigated in combination with aspirin in comparison to warfarin in patients with AF at high risk of thromboembolic events (the ACTIVE trial, De Caterina R, personal communication).

CRITIQUE OF PREVIOUS RECOMMENDATIONS

Recommendations for the use of antiplatelet therapy in patients with bioprostheses have already been discussed above. Recent American guidelines have broadened the indications for antithrombotic therapy with aspirin in the treatment of patients with prosthetic heart valves in general and mechanical heart valves in particular [1, 2]. However, the evidence for many of the recommendations is relatively weak, particularly as there was no stratification according to vascular disease in any of the trials cited.

In older trials, combining anticoagulation with aspirin tended to decrease the incidence and severity of embolic episodes, but caused increased, mainly gastrointestinal, bleeding [205, 208, 209]. This was particularly true when aspirin at doses greater than 500 mg/day was combined with high-intensity oral anticoagulation, as there is evidence that gastro-intestinal symptoms and bleeding associated with aspirin are dose-dependent, and that low doses of aspirin provide equal cardiovascular benefits [195].

Turpie et al. in 1993 reported on a comparison of aspirin 100 mg in association with oral anticoagulation (at INR 3.0–4.5) vs. anticoagulation alone at the same INR range, with a 4-year follow-up [210]. In this small study with only ~300 follow-up years in each group, a high proportion of concomitant coronary artery surgery, and only 40% INRs in the target range, the authors showed that, in patients with mechanical heart valves and high-risk patients with prosthetic tissue valves, the addition of aspirin to warfarin therapy reduced mortality, particularly mortality from vascular causes, together with major systemic embolism, compared to oral anticoagulants alone (1.9/year vs. 8.5%/year; $P < 0.001$). However, in patients without coronary disease, this benefit could not be demonstrated. Although the increase in the rate of major bleeding with aspirin was not statistically signi-ficant (8.5/year vs. 6.6%/year), the rate of bleeding in both groups was considerably higher than that reported in most recent prosthetic valve series in the literature (average 1.5–2.0%/year) [29]. Of more concern, the rate of intracranial bleeding was doubled in the warfarin + aspirin group [148, 211].

After this study, a meta-analysis pooling data from six trials (including Turpie's trial) with either aspirin or dipyridamole as antiplatelet agents [205, 208–210, 212, 213], supported the contention that the rate of thromboembolism is further reduced with antiplatelet agents added to oral anticoagulants, by about two-thirds, in patients with mechanical prosthetic heart valves [211]. Major bleeding was however also increased. There was a 2.5-fold increase in major gastrointestinal haemorrhage from combination therapy. An analysis of the bene-fit–risk ratio at that time concluded that for about every 1.6 patients in whom stroke was prevented by combination therapy, there was an excess of one major gastrointestinal bleed-ing. There was also a suggestion that aspirin plus oral anticoagulants resulted in some increase in intracranial bleeding, which might not have occurred in studies using dipyri-damole plus oral anticoagulants. These conclusions, while not supported by statistically sig-nificant differences [211], are nevertheless in keeping with the meta-analysis of aspirin trials referred to above [198].

In this context, it is important to emphasise that ischaemic stroke and intracerebral haem-orrhage should not be considered events of equivalent severity and prognosis. The 1-year survival after ischaemic stroke is about 80%, in comparison to about 20% after intracerebral haemorrhage [214]. Immediate (30-day) mortality from intracerebral haemorrhage ranges from 40% in the general population, through 60% in anticoagulated patients and 64% in patients with vascular disease on no treatment, to 76% in patients on antiplatelet drugs for vascular disease [148, 195]. In contrast, immediate mortality from ischaemic stroke is in the range 15–25% [148, 195].

The meta-analysis by Cappelleri *et al.* in 1995 [211] and the subsequent meta-analysis of Massel *et al.* published in 2001 [215] illustrate the problems of attempting to apply meta-analysis to disparate trial settings. Meta-analysis was originally devised as a technique for amalgamating data from several RCTs which had used the same methodology. The trials utilised in both meta-analyses had numerous important differences between them, including differences in event definition, patient selection, antiplatelet drug used, drug dose, target anticoagulation intensity, and prosthetic type studied, with a predominance of older design caged ball valves. Differences in patient risk factors, particularly the prevalence of vascular disease, probably also existed as the majority of trials did not provide this information.

There was bias in the selection of the trials as well; most were small and of short duration. The meta-analysis of Cappelleri *et al.* [211] utilised five trials performed between 1971 and 1993, including that of Chesebro *et al.* reporting one of the largest trials from the Mayo Clinic, comparing warfarin alone, warfarin plus aspirin and warfarin plus dipyridamole [205]. Massel *et al.* [215] added only one more trial after 1993 (that of Meschengieser *et al.* see below), and five more from the 1970s and 1980s (including abstracts with limited information), but specifically excluded the Chesebro study which warned of the increased risk of major bleeding associated with the warfarin/aspirin (500 mg) combination in comparison to warfarin alone (6.1/year vs. 1.8%/year; $P < 0.001$), and showed no difference in bleeding risk between warfarin and warfarin plus dipyridamole [205].

A separate meta-analysis of the dipyridamole trials only, supplemented by additional data submitted to the FDA by the trial centres [204], confirmed the benefit of dipyridamole suggested by the Massel meta-analysis (equivalent to aspirin) [215] but reached the different conclusion that there was no increased bleeding risk with dipyridamole, in keeping with the results of other trials [202, 203, 205].

The most recent trial to address the issue of combined therapy (included in Massel's meta-analysis) requires particular mention as it is widely quoted to support the safety of combined therapy with aspirin. Meschengieser *et al.* compared the combination of 100 mg of aspirin in association with lower-intensity anticoagulation (INR 2.5–3.5) to higher-intensity anticoagulation alone (INR 3.5–4.5) [216]. This study was performed in 503 patients receiving mostly aortic valve replacement, and mostly with tilting disc valves, and reported that the association of lower-intensity anticoagulation and low-dose aspirin therapy (100 mg/day) offered similar antithrombotic protection compared to higher-intensity anticoagulation alone, in terms of a composite rate of thromboembolism and valve thrombosis (1.3/year vs. 1.5%/year), without any increase in major bleeding (1.1/year vs. 2.3%/year). However, these results must be interpreted with caution because patients were randomised at various different time intervals between operation and the start of the study, switching from a different therapy to one of the two arms of the study (thereby excluding the early peak in the hazard function curve for both anticoagulant-related bleeding and thromboembolism), and patients with previous gastrointestinal bleeding (presumably whilst on a different therapy) or a 'suspected haemorrhagic tendency' (undefined) and patients with previous thromboembolism were excluded. Thus, the study was not only blunted by the exclusion criteria but also biased in favour of the aspirin arm of the trial.

Combination therapy during pregnancy has been recommended by the ACC/AHA Guidelines on Management of Patients with Valvular Heart Disease [1], but this is not based on any trials and ignores the increased risk of fetal and neonatal intracranial haemorrhage with aspirin [217, 218]. Furthermore, aspirin may cause premature closure of the ductus arteriosus [219]. Dipyridamole is not approved for use in pregnancy due to lack of data.

In view of the lack of any data showing benefit and the potential risks to both mother and foetus, antiplatelet therapy should not be prescribed during pregnancy.

American guidelines (ACC/AHA and ACCP) base their recommendations for the wider use of aspirin in combination with oral anticoagulants for patients with mechanical valves largely on the trials of Turpie et al. and Meschengieser et al. and the meta-analyses referred to above, the flaws of which have already been discussed. There is thus insufficient evidence to recommend aspirin in combination with oral anticoagulants for all patients with mechanical valves. Until further evidence from RCTs in various subsets of patients becomes available (e.g., patients with no concomitant vascular disease, patients with AF, patients with concomitant coronary artery bypass graft (CABG), etc.) it is recommended that antiplatelet therapy in addition to anticoagulation should be reserved for specific indications only and that for each patient a balance should be struck between probable benefit and the increased risk of bleeding, particularly intracerebral haemorrhage, as the latter is such a lethal complication. All indications are thus relative rather than absolute. They represent situations in which antiplatelet therapy should be considered, rather than simply prescribed in all patients. In general, antiplatelet therapy should only be combined with a target INR of 3.0 or less, and aspirin should only be used in low dose formulations (≤100 mg). There are some arguments for preferring dipyridamole to aspirin, as discussed above.

Relative indications for antiplatelet therapy include:

1. Concomitant arterial disease, particularly coronary disease, aortic atheromatous plaques and carotid disease.
2. Following intracoronary stenting (although the safety of combining warfarin with two antiplatelet drugs has yet to be established).
3. Recurrent embolism, but only after full investigation and treatment of risk factors, and optimisation of anticoagulation control with self-management (if appropriate) has failed to abolish the problem (see section on Management of thromboembolism, p. 239).
4. Increase in mean platelet volume, particularly if an embolic event has already occurred and there is no remediable cause for increased platelet consumption (see text).
5. In patients with caged ball valves in particular, dipyridamole should be considered rather than aspirin in view of its apparent efficacy in prostheses of this unique design in trials from the 1970s, with less risk of bleeding than aspirin.

Contraindications (particularly to the use of aspirin) include:

1. Previous history of gastrointestinal bleeding, particularly from ulcer disease or angiodysplasia.
2. Poorly controlled hypertension, due to the increased risk of intracerebral haemorrhage [148] and the lack of efficacy of aspirin in preventing stroke in hypertension [220–222].
3. Elderly patients, particularly women aged >75 years [221].
4. Patients on multiple medications, patients who require frequent courses of antibiotics or patients whose anticoagulation control, despite all efforts, is extremely erratic. Frequent episodes of high INR due to drug interactions or poor compliance expose the patient to an increased risk if they are also taking aspirin.

Finally, it is important to remember that many drugs (other than conventional antiplatelet drugs) can have an adverse effect on platelet function and may prolong the bleeding time [48]. These include some antibiotics (penicillins, cephalosporins, tetracycline, gentamycin and nitrofurantoin) and non-steroidal anti-inflammatory drugs. Caution should be advised in prescribing these drugs in anticoagulated patients, particularly if they are also taking an antiplatelet agent. Patients should also be advised of food items and supplements which may affect platelet function if consumed in large quantities. These include n-3 fatty acids, garlic, onion, ginger, cloves, cumin, turmeric and vitamins C and E [48].

MANAGEMENT OF VALVE THROMBOSIS

Obstructive thrombosis is defined as a thrombotic occlusion of the prosthetic valve leading to severe haemodynamic compromise. It may begin as non-obstructive thrombosis which is defined as a thrombus located usually at the sewing ring of the prosthesis without significantly increased gradient across the prosthetic valve or interference with occluder movement. Peripheral or cerebral emboli are usually the only symptoms of this type of valve thrombosis, but many instances of non-obstructive thrombosis are silent, chronic and only discovered on routine TEE. Valve thrombosis is often associated with subtherapeutic or interrupted anticoagulation [223, 224], although other patient- and prosthesis-related factors may play a role also. The most frequent reasons for deliberate anticoagulation interruption leading to valve thrombosis are elective surgery or severe bleeding events [223].

The risk of valve thrombosis is determined by the inherent thrombogenicity and haemodynamic performance of the prosthesis, patient-related risk factors and trigger factors, such as infection, as well as by the quality of anticoagulation management [22, 28, 35, 130]. Among anticoagulated patients with mechanical valves the incidence varies from zero to 0.5%/year in the aortic position and from zero to 3%/year in the mitral position [29]. Thrombosis of a bileaflet prosthetic valve often leads more rapidly to severe haemodynamic impairment than thrombosis of a tilting disc valve, because even quite small amounts of thrombus at the hinge points can immobilise both leaflets [67]. Bioprostheses and homografts are less thrombogenic than mechanical prostheses, but bioprosthetic valve thrombosis may occur in the absence of anticoagulation [67, 225]. Predisposing factors include low cardiac output, chordal preservation in mitral valve replacement [90, 91] and structural valve deterioration [67]. Porcine valves appear to be more thrombogenic than pericardial valves [29] with thrombosis rates without anticoagulation similar to mechanical valves with anticoagulation [29, 66].

Acute obstructive valve thrombosis should be considered as the most likely diagnosis in all patients after valve replacement who present-in pulmonary oedema or shock, particularly if there is loss of mechanical valve clicks on auscultation or new stenosis or regurgitant murmurs. The diagnosis is confirmed by transthoracic and/or transoesophageal Doppler echocardiography [226, 227] or cinefluoroscopy [228, 229]. Transthoracic Doppler–echocardiography allows assessment of gradients across the valve, detection of regurgitation and occasionally demonstration of thrombus, while TEE is important for delineation of size, structure and location of thrombi. Cinefluoroscopy permits rapid assessment of leaflet motion of valves with radio-opaque occluders. In bileaflet valves it is possible to determine if one or both leaflets are involved and to what degree. Non-obstructive valve thrombosis is usually discovered only on TEE, often during investigation of an embolic event (see below).

Following diagnosis of valve thrombosis the patient should be transferred as soon as possible to a tertiary heart centre after intravenous injection of a bolus of heparin (5000 U) followed by continuous heparin infusion. Two therapeutic options are available: valve surgery or medical therapy with heparin or thrombolysis. Treatment strategy depends on several factors: presence or absence of obstruction, location of the prosthesis, acuteness of the thrombosis, severity of clinical symptoms, patient's age, and comorbidities. The degree of organisation of the thrombus and the presence of pannus also influence treatment. It is generally agreed that valve thrombosis in the right heart is best treated with fibrinolysis in the first instance because of the high success rate and low incidence of embolism [1, 230]. The following recommendations therefore apply primarily to aortic and mitral valve thrombosis.

OBSTRUCTIVE VALVE THROMBOSIS

Three treatment strategies need to be considered depending on the factors mentioned above:

1. Urgent or emergency valve replacement should be considered in critically ill patients without serious comorbidities if surgical treatment is readily available. Patients with a mechanical prosthesis should receive another mechanical prosthesis, preferably of lower thrombogenicity, providing that the long-term quality of anticoagulation can be assured. Bioprosthetic valve replacement should be considered in patients with high variability of anticoagulation level or in those with contraindications to anticoagulation due to recent intracranial haemorrhage, for example.
2. Fibrinolysis should be considered in critically ill patients with serious comorbidities (e.g., cancer or renal failure) or if surgery is not immediately available and the patient is *in extremis* and cannot be transferred. Contraindications to fibrinolysis include recent major surgery or recent intracranial bleeding. The overall success rate of fibrinolysis is 70–80% [231, 233], but is less likely to be successful in chronic thrombosis or in the presence of pannus. It is associated with a risk of systemic embolism and recurrent thrombosis (both about 20%). There is also a 5% risk of major bleeding. Success is less likely in mitral prostheses in comparison to aortic prostheses [231].
3. In haemodynamically stable patients with mild obstruction, in whom acute discontinuation of oral anticoagulation or recent inadequate anticoagulation is considered the most likely cause for valve thrombosis, a short treatment course of intravenous UFH, as a bolus, followed by infusion should be applied first, closely monitored by echocardiography and or cinefluoroscopy [228]. In patients with a good initial response, treatment should be continued until full resolution of the obstruction. If heparin (with activated partial thromboplastin time [aPTT] twice control) is not successful within 12–24 h, thrombolysis should be started. When fibrinogen level is above 0.5 g/l, UFH infusion should be recommended to obtain an aPTT 1.5 to 2.0 times the control value. In patients with no comorbidities, unsuccessful treatment with heparin should be followed by valve surgery rather than fibrinolysis.

Oral anticoagulation should be resumed as soon as clinical status is stable and heparin continued until the INR is within the therapeutic range for the mechanical valve and position (mitral valve 3.0 to 3.5, aortic valve 2.5. to 3.0).

NON-OBSTRUCTIVE VALVE THROMBOSIS

Initial treatment comprises optimisation of oral anticoagulation, if this was previously poorly controlled or subtherapeutic. Intravenous heparin should be used in the interim. Thereafter treatment should be directed to any underlying contributory factors, for example, prothrombotic intracardiac conditions caused by AF, dehydration, pulmonary infection, etc. Factors related to the prosthesis itself may also be important contributors and may necessitate re-operation. In the case of a large non-obstructive thrombus (>1 cm) which fails to regress with heparin and optimum oral anticoagulation, consideration should be given to re-operation or thrombolysis in patients with comorbidities at high risk for surgery.

If thrombus regresses with conservative treatment and correction of contributory factors, future management must be carefully considered. If the anticoagulation was previously adequate, it should be continued with a higher target INR. However, an INR of more than 4.0 has not been shown to be of benefit, and considerably increases the risk of bleeding. Although aspirin is often prescribed in this setting, there is no evidence to support its use for non-obstructive valve thrombosis and the risk of bleeding is further increased.

MANAGEMENT OF THROMBOEMBOLISM

Although always reported as a prosthesis-related (or in the case of valve repair, valve-related) event, as recommended by the reporting guidelines [234] and although often assumed to originate from the prosthesis, thromboembolism in fact is multifactoral both in its aetiology and its origin, as discussed at the beginning of this chapter. This underlines the importance of thorough investigation of each episode of thromboembolism, rather than simply increasing the target INR or adding an antiplatelet drug.

Clinical evaluation should be directed toward a search for evidence of subtherapeutic anticoagulation, endocarditis or new risk factors (e.g., hypertension, diabetes, AF), together with any change in auscultatory findings. Blood tests for prothrombotic factors should be part of a thrombophilia screen [35].

Transthoracic and transoesophageal echocardiography should be performed as soon as possible after an embolic event to evaluate the size of the left atrium, assess stasis and left ventricular function, and search for intracardiac or prosthetic thrombus. Cinefluoroscopy is a useful adjunct to echocardiography when early occlusive thrombosis is suspected in patients with prosthetic valves with radio-opaque occluders. A search should also be made for non-prosthetic causes of embolism, such as aortic or carotid atheroma or patent foramen ovale with aneurysm of the inter-atrial septum, particularly in patients with venous thrombosis.

Specific organ–orientated examinations will be necessary according to the location of the embolic complication. Cerebral imaging using computed tomography (CT) or magnetic resonance imaging (MRI) should be performed in the case of a cerebrovascular event in order to exclude intracerebral haemorrhage and to evaluate the size of the cerebral infarction. Doppler examination of the carotid arteries should also be performed. Coronary angiography is necessary in MI and Doppler evaluation or peripheral angiography in suspected limb embolism.

TREATMENT STRATEGIES

Remediable contributors to thromboembolism such as AF, hypercholesterolaemia, diabetes, smoking and prothrombotic blood test abnormalities should be sought and treated accordingly.

Antithrombotic therapy in patients with recent stroke still remains controversial and should take into account the balance between the risk of recurrence of embolism, on the one hand, and the risk of haemorrhagic transformation on the other. Overall the risk of early recurrence is lower than the risk of haemorrhage during the first two weeks. In patients with mechanical valve prostheses, anticoagulation should be restarted as soon as the initial CT scan, which is performed within 24 to 48 h of stroke, does not indicate haemorrhage and shows that the ischaemic stroke is of small to moderate size (less than 35% of the hemisphere). On the other hand, anticoagulation is contraindicated in cases of haemorrhage, large cerebral infarction, or uncontrolled systemic hypertension. In these cases, oral anticoagulation is usually postponed for at least five days or until hypertension is under control. This delay allows time to perform another CT scan to exclude haemorrhagic transformation. During this period, heparin therapy is usually recommended at a therapeutic range of 1.5 to 2 times the control value.

Patients who have suffered a thromboembolic event are at higher risk of further events. Regular follow-up echocardiographic examinations are recommended twice a year. Optimisation of anticoagulation control, if possible with patient self-management, should be a major component of the prevention strategy (see section on Anticoagulation self-management, p. 231). In the first instance, better control is preferable to simply increasing the target INR. Similarly, the prescription of antiplatelet drugs should not be a 'reflex response' to an embolic episode, but rather targeted to specific situations in which there is likely to be a benefit , e.g., in arterial disease. If aspirin is used, it should be prescribed in a low dose formulation (≤100 mg) and combined with low- or moderate-intensity anticoagulation depending on the site of the prosthesis and its thrombogenicity (INR 2.0–3.5). Alternatively, if the prosthesis is suspected to be the source, dipyridamole may be preferable to aspirin (see section on Antiplatelet therapy).

Surgery is only indicated in cases of recurrent thromboembolic episodes despite adequate anticoagulation and control of risk factors, in which the prosthesis appears to be not only the source but also the cause (e.g., a mechanical prosthesis of higher than average thrombogenicity or a degenerating bioprosthesis). The indication for surgery should be discussed on an individual patient basis after careful consideration of the risk to benefit ratio.

ANTICOAGULATION IN PREGNANCY

Antithrombotic management during pregnancy is discussed in general terms in Chapter 19. For the patient with a prosthetic heart valve, however, the optimal management of anticoagulation during pregnancy remains particularly controversial and problematic. The mother's safety must be weighed against that of the foetus. If the anticoagulation regime employed is less effective than their usual anticoagulation, pregnant patients with prosthetic heart valves have a much higher risk of valve thrombosis, arterial embolism and mortality.

Oral anticoagulants continued throughout pregnancy provide the greatest protection against prosthetic valve thrombosis and thromboembolism which are the most frequent causes of maternal mortality. If the daily dose of warfarin required to achieve a therapeutic INR of 2.5–3.0 is not more than 5 mg, this regime should be used up to the 36th week of pregnancy. If the patient who needs higher doses of warfarin opts for heparin to avoid embryopathy after having been informed in detail about her own increased risk, heparin should be given only for the first 12 weeks under strict aPTT control, prolonged to twice normal. Thereafter oral anticoagulants should be resumed. From the 36th week of pregnancy treatment should be changed to heparin under hospital conditions, because premature birth occurs often among these patients. Heparin should be discontinued at the onset of labour. Four to six h after delivery heparin therapy can be restarted. After 24 h oral anticoagulation may be resumed.

If premature labour occurs while the patient is still on oral anticoagulants, a Caesarean section should be performed after reducing the INR to 2.0 or less. A vaginal delivery should be avoided under oral anticoagulation because of the danger of fetal intracranial bleeding.

REFERENCES

1.   ACC/AHA Task Force on Practice Guidelines. ACC/AHA guidelines for the management of patients with valvular heart disease. *JACC* 1998; 32:1486–1588.
2.   Salem DN, Stein PD, Al-Ahmad A *et al*. Antithrombotic therapy in valvular heart disease – native and prosthetic. *Chest* 2004; 126(suppl):457S–482S.
3.   Oxford Community Stroke Project. Incidence of stroke in Oxfordshire: first year's experience of community stroke register. *BMJ* 1983; 287:713–717.
4.   Murray CJL, Lopez AD. Cerebrovascular disease. *Global Health Statistics*. World Health Organisation, 1996; 655–657.
5.   Gibbs RGJ, Newson R, Lawrenson R, Greenhalgh RM, Davies AH. Diagnosis and initial management of stroke and transient ischaemic attack across UK health regions from 1992 to 1996. *Stroke* 2001; 32:1085–1090.
6.   Butchart EG, Moreno de la Santa P, Rooney SJ, Lewis PA. Arterial risk factors and cerebrovascular events following aortic valve replacement. *J Heart Valve Dis* 1995; 4:1–8.
7.   Inauen W, Bombeli T, Baumgartner HR, Haeberli A, Straub PW. Effects of the oral anticoagulant phenprocoumon on blood coagulation and thrombogenesis induced by rabbit aorta subendothelium exposed to flowing human blood: role of dose and shear rate. *J Lab Clin Med* 1991; 118:280–288.

8. Wolf PA, Abbott RD, Kannel WB. Atrial fibrillation as an independent risk factor for stroke: the Framingham Study. *Stroke* 1991; 22:983–988.

9. Jones EF, Kalman JM, Calafiore P, Tonkin AM, Donnan GA. Proximal aortic atheroma – an independent risk factor for cerebral ischaemia. *Stroke* 1995; 26:218–224.

10. Wolf PA, Kannel WB, Cupples LA, D'Agostino RB. Risk factor interaction in cardiovascular and cerebrovascular disease. In: Furlan AJ (ed.). *The Heart and Stroke*. Springer–Verlag, London, 1987, pp 331–355.

11. MacMahon S, Peto R, Cutler J *et al.* Blood pressure, stroke and coronary heart disease; part 1, prolonged differences in blood pressure: prospective observational studies corrected for the regression dilution bias. *Lancet* 1990; 335:765–774.

12. Bowler JV, Hachinski V. Epidemiology of cerebral infarction. In: Gorelick PB (ed.). *Atlas of Cerebrovascular Disease*. Philadelphia, *Current Medicine* 1996; 1.2–1.22.

13. Manolio TA, Kronmal RA, Burke GL, O'Leary DH, Price TR. Short-term predictors of incident stroke in older adults. *Stroke* 1996; 27:1479–1486.

14. Shinton R, Beevers G. Meta-analysis of relation between cigarette smoking and stroke. *Br Med J* 1989; 298:789–794.

15. Butchart EG, Lewis PA, Bethel JA, Breckenridge IM. Adjusting anticoagulation to prosthesis thrombogenicity and patient risk factors: recommendations for the Medtronic Hall valve. *Circulation* 1991; 84(suppl III):III-61–III-69.

16. Harrison DG, Minor RL, Guerra R, Wuillen JE, Sellke FW. Endothelial dysfunction in atherosclerosis. In: Rubanyi GM (ed.). *Cardiovascular Significance of Endothelium-Derived Vasoactive Factors*. Futura, Mount Kisco, 1991, pp 263–280.

17. Burrig KF. The endothelium of advanced arteriosclerotic plaques in humans. *Arteriosclerosis Thromb* 1991; 11:1678–1689.

18. Packham MA, Kinlough-Rathbone RL. Mechanisms of atherogenesis and thrombosis. In: Bloom AL, Forbes CD, Thomas DP, Tuddenham EGD (eds). *Haemostasis and Thrombosis*, 3rd edition. Churchill Livingstone, Edinburgh, 1994; 1107–1138.

19. Yoganathan AP, Wick TM, Reul H. The influence of flow characteristics of prosthetic valves on thrombus formation. In: Butchart EG, Bodnar E. *Current Issues in Heart Valve Disease: Thrombosis, Embolism and Bleeding*. ICR Publishers, London, 1992, pp 123–148.

20. Jones M, Eidbo EE. Doppler color flow evaluation of prosthetic mitral valves: experimental epicardial studies. *J Am Coll Cardiol* 1989; 13:234–240.

21. Yasaka M, Beppu S. Hypercoagulability in the left atrium, Part II: Coagulation factors. *J Heart Valve Dis* 1993; 2:25–34.

22. Butchart EG. Fibrinogen and leukocyte activation – the keys to understanding prosthetic valve thrombosis? *J Heart Valve Dis* 1997; 6:9–16.

23. Ruggeri ZM. Mechanisms of shear-induced platelet adhesion and aggregation. *Thromb Haemost* 1993; 70:119–123.

24. Alkhamis TM, Beissinger RL, Chediak J. Artificial surface effect on red blood cells and platelets in laminar shear flow. *Blood* 1990; 75:1568–1575.

25. Kroll MH, Hellums JD, McIntyre LV, Schaefer AI, Moake JL. Platelets and shear stress. *Blood* 1996; 88:1525–1541.

26. Okazaki Y, Wika KE, Matsuyoshi T *et al.* Platelets are deposited early postoperatively on the leaflet of a mechanical valve in sheep without postoperative anticoagulants or antiplatelet agents. *ASAIO Journal* 1996; 42:M750–M754.

27. Janicek MJ, van den Abbeele AD, DeSisto WC *et al.* Embolization of platelets after endothelial injury to the aorta in rabbits. Assessment with [111] Indium-labelled platelets and angiography. *Invest Radiol* 1991; 26:655–659.

28. Butchart EG, Moreno de la Santa P, Rooney SJ, Lewis PA. The role of risk factors and trigger factors in cerebrovascular events after mitral valve replacement: implications for antithrombotic management. *J Card Surg* 1994; 9(suppl):228–236.

29. Grunkemeier GL, Li HH, Naftel DC, Starr A, Rahimtoola SH. Long-term performance of heart valve prostheses. *Curr Probl Cardiol* 2000; 25:73–156.

30. Turpie AGG, Gunstensen J, Hirsh J, Nelson H, Gent M. Randomised comparison of two intensities of oral anticoagulant therapy after tissue heart valve replacement. *Lancet* 1988; 1:1242–1245.

31. Saour JN, Sieck JO, Mamo LAR, Gallus AS. Trial of different intensities of anticoagulation in patients with prosthetic heart valves. *N Engl J Med* 1990; 322:428–432.

32. Altman R, Rouvier G, Gurfinkel E *et al*. Comparison of two levels of anticoagulant therapy in patients with substitute heart valves. *J Thorac Cardiovasc Surg* 1991; 101:427–431.

33. Acar J, Iung Boissel JP *et al*. AREVA: Multicenter randomized comparison of low-dose versus standard-dose anticoagulation in patients with mechanical prosthetic heart valves. *Circulation* 1996; 94:2107–2112.

34. Huth C, Friedl A, Rost A. Intensity of oral anticoagulation after implantation of St. Jude Medical aortic prosthesis: analysis of GELIA database. *Eur Heart J* 2001; 3(suppl Q):Q33–Q38.

35. Butchart EG, Ionescu A, Payne N, Giddings J, Grunkemeier GL, Fraser AG. A new scoring system to determine thromboembolic risk after heart valve replacement. *Circulation* 2003; 108(suppl II):68–74.

36. Butchart EG. Thrombogenesis and its management. In: Acar J, Bodnar E (eds). *Textbook of Acquired Heart Valve Disease*. ICR Publishers, London, 1995, pp 1048–1120.

37. Blood Pressure Lowering Treatment Trialists' Collaboration. Effects of different blood-pressure-lowering regimens on major cardiovascular events: results of prospectively-designed overviews of randomised trials. *Lancet* 2003; 362:1527–1535.

38. Ambrose JA, Barua RS. The pathophysiology of cigarette smoking and cardiovascular disease. *JACC* 2004; 43:1731–1737.

39. Kuusisto J, Mykkanen L, Pyorala K, Laakso M. Non-insulin-dependent diabetes and its metabolic control are important predictors of stroke in elderly subjects. *Stroke* 1994; 25:1157–1164.

40. Sacco RL. Reducing the risk of stroke in diabetes: what have we learned that is new? *Diabetes Obes Metab* 2002; 4(suppl 1):S27–S34.

41. Stroke Prevention in Atrial Fibrillation Investigators. Prediction of thromboembolism in atrial fibrillation. II Echocardiographic features of patients at risk. *Ann Intern Med* 1992; 116:6–12.

42. Rosito GA, D'Agostino RB, Massaro J *et al*. Association between obesity and a prothrombotic state: the Framingham Offspring Study. *Thromb Haemost* 2004; 91:683–689.

43. Kurth T, Gaziano M, Berger K *et al*. Body mass index and the risk of stroke in men. *Arch Intern Med* 2002; 162:2557–2562.

44. Jood K, Jern C, Wilhelmsen L, Rosengren A. Body mass index in mid-life is associated with a first stroke in men. *Stroke* 2004; 35:2764–2769.

45. Rexrode KM, Hennekens CH, Willett WC *et al*. A prospective study of body mass index, weight change and risk of stroke in women. *JAMA* 1997; 277:1539–1545.

46. Bath P, Algert C, Chapman N *et al*. Association of mean platelet volume with risk of stroke among 3134 individuals with history of cerebrovascular disease. *Stroke* 2004; 35:622–626.

47. Sharpe PC, Trinick T. Mean platelet volume in diabetes mellitus. *Q J Med* 1993; 86:739–742.

48. Warkentin TE, Kelton JG. Acquired platelet disorders. In: Bloom AL, Forbes CD, Thomas DP, Tuddenham EGD (eds). *Haemostasis and Thrombosis*. Churchill Livingstone, Edinburgh, 1994; 767–818.

49. Martin JF, Trowbridge EA, Salmon G *et al*. The biological significance of platelet volume: its relationship to bleeding time, platelet thromboxane B_2 production and megakaryocyte nuclear DNA concentration. *Thromb Res* 1983; 32:443–460.

50. Ernst E, Resch KL. Therapeutic interventions to lower plasma fibrinogen concentration. *Eur Heart J* 1995; 16(suppl A):47–53.

51. Cook PJ, Honeybourne D, Lip GYH *et al*. Chlamydia pneumoniae antibody titres are significantly associated with acute stroke and transient cerebral ischaemia. *Stroke* 1998; 29:404–410.

52. Elkind MSV, Lin IF, Grayston JT *et al*. Chlamydia pneumoniae and the risk of first ischaemic stroke. *Stroke* 2000; 31:1521–1525.

53. Gieffers J, Fullgraf H, Jahn J *et al*. Chlamydia pneumoniae infection in circulating human monocytes is refractory to antibiotic treatment. *Circulation* 2001; 103:351–356.

54. Bosch J, Yusuf S, Pogue J *et al*. Use of ramipril in preventing stroke: double blind randomised trial. *BMJ* 2002; 324:699–702.

55. Di Napoli P, Taccardi AA, Oliver M, De Caterina R. Statins and stroke: evidence for cholesterol-independent effects. *Eur Heart J* 2002; 23:1908–1921.

56. MRC Asymptomatic Carotid Surgery Trial Collaborative Group. Prevention of disabling and fatal strokes by successful carotid endarterectomy in patients without recent neurological symptoms: randomised controlled trial. *Lancet* 2004; 363:1491–1502.

57. Thijssen HHW, Hamulyak K, Willigers H. 4-hydroxycoumarin oral anticoagulants: pharmacokinetics-response relationship. *Thromb Haemost* 1988; 60:35–38.

58. Weinstock DM, Chang P, Aronson DL *et al*. Comparison of plasma prothrombin and factor VII and urine prothrombin F1 concentrations in patients on long-term warfarin therapy and those in the initial phase. *Am J Hematol* 1998; 57:193–199.

59. van den Besselaar AMHP. Oral anticoagulant therapy. In: Bloom AL, Forbes CD, Thomas DP, Tuddenham EGD (eds). *Haemostasis and Thrombosis*. Churchill Livingstone, Edinburgh, 1994, pp 1439–1458.

60. Miller GJ, Meade TW. Hypercoagulability. In: Butchart EG, Bodnar E (eds). *Current Issues in Heart Valve Disease: Thrombosis, Embolism and Bleeding*. ICR Publishers, London, 1992, pp 81–92.

61. Meade TW, Mellows S, Brozovic M *et al*. Haemostatic function and ischaemic heart disease: principal results of the Northwick Park Heart Study. *Lancet* 1986; 2:533–537.

62. Eriksson-Berg M, Deguchi H, Hawe E *et al*. Influence of factor VII gene polymorphisms and environmental factors on plasma factor VII concentrations in middle aged women with and without manifest coronary heart disease. *Thromb Haemost* 2005; 93:351–358.

63. Syrjanen J, Valtonen VV, Ivanainen M *et al*. Preceding infection as an important risk factor for ischaemic brain infarction in young and middle-aged patients. *BMJ* 1988; 296:1156–1160.

64. Grau AJ, Buggle F, Heindl S *et al*. Recent infection as a risk factor for cerebrovascular ischaemia. *Stroke* 1995; 26:373–379.

65. Gohlke-Bärwolf C, Acar J, Oakley C *et al*. Guidelines for the prevention of thromboembolic events in valvular heart disease. *Eur Heart J* 1995; 16:1320–1330.

66. Hammermeister K, Sethi GK, Henderson WG, Grover FL, Oprian C, Rahimtoola SH. Outcomes 15 years after valve replacement with a mechanical valve versus a bioprosthetic valve: final report of the Veterans Affairs randomized trial. *JACC* 2000; 36:1152–1158.

67. Butchart EG. Thrombogenicity, thrombosis and embolism. In: Butchart EG, Bodnar E (eds). *Current Issues in Heart Valve Disease: Thrombosis, Embolism and Bleeding*. ICR Publishers, London, 1992, pp 172–205.

68. Stein PD, Riddle JM, Kemp SR, Lee MW, Lewis JW, Magilligan DJ. Effect of warfarin on calcification of spontaneously degenerated porcine bioprosthetic valves. *J Thorac Cardiovasc Surg* 1985; 90:119–125.

69. Antonini-Canterin F, Zuppiroli A, Popescu BA *et al*. Effect of statins on the progression of bioprosthetic aortic valve degeneration. *Am J Cardiol* 2003; 92:1479–1482.

70. Undas A, Brummel KE, Musial J, Mann KG, Szczeklik A. Simvastatin depresses blood clotting by inhibiting activation of prothrombin, factor V and factor XIII and by enhancing factor Va inactivation. *Circulation* 2001; 103:2248–2253.

71. Palinski W. Immunomodulation: a new role for statins? *Nature Med* 2000; 6:1311–1312.

72. Blair KL, Hatton AC, White WD *et al*. Comparison of anticoagulation regimens after Carpentier-Edwards aortic or mitral valve replacement. *Circulation* 1994; 90(suppl II):214–219.

73. Heras M, Chesebro JH, Fuster V *et al*. High risk of thromboemboli early after bioprosthetic cardiac valve replacement. *JACC* 1995; 25:1111–1119.

74. Moinuddeen K, Quin J, Shaw R *et al*. Anticoagulation is unnecessary after biological aortic valve replacement. *Circulation* 1998; 98(suppl II):95–99.

75. Silverton NP, Abdulali SA, Yakirevich VS, Tandon AP, Ionescu MI. Embolism, thrombosis and anticoagulant haemorrhage in mitral valve disease. A prospective study of patients having valve replacement with the pericardial xenograft. *Eur Heart J* 1984; 5(suppl D):19–25.

76. Hill JD, LaFollette L, Szarnicki RJ *et al*. Risk-benefit analysis of warfarin therapy in Hancock mitral valve replacement. *J Thorac Cardiovasc Surg* 1982; 83:718–723.

77. Hirsh J, Levine M. Confusion over the therapeutic range for monitoring oral anticoagulation therapy in North America. *Thromb Haemost* 1988; 59:129–132.

78. Gherli T, Colli A, Fragnito C *et al*. Comparing warfarin with aspirin after biological aortic valve replacement: a prospective study. *Circulation* 2004; 110:496–500.

79. CTSNet Editors. Anticoagulation therapy after aortic tissue valve replacement: final results. *www.CTSNet.org* 2004.

80. Nunez L, Aguado ML, Larrea JL, Celemin D, Oliver J. Prevention of thromboembolism using aspirin after mitral valve replacement with porcine bioprostheses. *Ann Thorac Surg* 1984; 37:84–87.

81. David TE, Ho WIC, Christakis GT. Thromboembolism in patients with aortic porcine bioprostheses. *Ann Thorac Surg* 1985; 40:229–233.

82. Goldsmith I, Lip GYH, Mukundan S, Rosin MD. Experience with lose-dose aspirin as thrombo-prophylaxis for the Tissuemed porcine aortic bioprosthesis: a survey of five years' experience. *J Heart Valve Dis* 1998; 7:574–579.

83. Jamieson WRE. Discussion of David TE *et al*. (ref. 79). *Ann Thorac Surg* 1985; 40:232–233.

84. Petersen P, Boysen G, Godtfredsen J, Andersen ED, Andersen B. Placebo-controlled, randomised trial of warfarin and aspirin for prevention of thromboembolic complications in chronic atrial fibrillation. *Lancet* 1989; 1:175–179.

85. SPAF Study Group Investigators. Preliminary report of the stroke prevention in atrial fibrillation study. *N Engl J Med* 1990; 322:863–868.
86. Miller VT, Rothrick JF, Pearce LA, Feinberg WM, Hart RG, Anderson DC. Ischaemic stroke in patients with atrial fibrillation: effect of aspirin according to stroke mechanism. *Neurology* 1993; 43:32–36.
87. Oxenham H, Bloomfield P, Wheatley DJ *et al*. Twenty year comparison of a Bjork-Shiley mechanical heart valve with porcine prostheses. *Heart* 2003; 89:715–721.
88. Kannel WB, Wolf PA, Benjamin EJ, Levy D. Prevalence, incidence, prognosis and predisposing conditions for atrial fibrillation: population-based estimates. *Am J Cardiol* 1998; 82:2N–9N.
89. Oliver JM, Gallego P, Gonzalez A, Dominguez FJ, Gamallo C, Mesa JM. Bioprosthetic mitral valve thrombosis: clinical profile, transesophageal echocardiographic features and follow-up after anticoagulant therapy. *J Am Soc Echocardiogr* 1996; 9:691–699.
90. Fasol R, Lakew F. Early failure of bioprosthesis by preserved mitral leaflets. *Ann Thorac Surg* 2000; 70:653–654.
91. Korkolis DP, Passik CS, Marshalko SJ, Koullias GJ. Early bioprosthetic mitral valve 'pseudostenosis' after complete preservation of the native mitral apparatus. *Ann Thorac Surg* 2002; 74:1689–1691.
92. Unger P, Plein D, Pradier O, LeClerc JL. Thrombosis of aortic valve homograft associated with lupus anticoagulant antibodies. *Ann Thorac Surg* 2004; 77:312–314.
93. Davies H, Missen GAK, Blandford G, Roberts CI, Lessof MH, Ross DN. Homograft replacement of the aortic valve. A clinical and pathological study. *Am J Cardiol* 1968; 22:195–217.
94. Doty DB. Aortic valve replacement with homograft and autograft. *Semin Thorac Cardiovasc Surg* 1996; 8:249–258.
95. Medtronic Inc. Freestyle aortic root bioprosthesis. Clinical compendium. Data on file at Medtronic.
96. van Nooten G, Ozaki S, Herijgers P, Segers P, Verdonck P, Flameng W. Distortion of the stentless porcine valve induces accelerated leaflet fibrosis and calcification in juvenile sheep. *J Heart Valve Dis* 1999; 8:34–41.
97. Bach DS. Echocardiographic assessment of stentless aortic bioprosthetic valves. *J Am Soc Echocardiogr* 2000; 13:941–948.
98. Fraser AG. Ultrasonic detection of increased embolic risk. In: Butchart EG, Bodnar E (eds). *Current Issues in Heart Valve Disease: Thrombosis, Embolism and Bleeding*. ICR Publishers, London, 1992, pp 223–244.
99. Adams JE, Jaffe AS. Scintigraphic and haematological detection of thrombosis and increased embolic risk. In: Butchart EG, Bodnar E (eds). *Current Issues in Heart Valve Disease: Thrombosis, Embolism and Bleeding*. ICR Publishers, London, 1992, pp 206–222.
100. Yamamoto K, Ikeda U, Fukazawa H, Shimada K. Effects of aspirin on status of thrombin generation in atrial fibrillation. *Am J Cardiol* 1996; 77:528–530.
101. Kamath S, Blann AD, Chin BSP, Lip GYH. A prospective randomized trial of aspirin-clopidogrel combination therapy and dose-adjusted warfarin on indices of thrombogenesis and platelet activation in atrial fibrillation. *JACC* 2002; 40:484–490.
102. SPAF Investigators. Adjusted-dose warfarin versus low-intensity, fixed dose warfarin plus aspirin for high risk patients with atrial fibrillation: Stroke Prevention in Atrial Fibrillation III randomised clinical trial. *Lancet* 1996; 348:633–638.
103. Iung B, Baron G, Butchart EG *et al*. A prospective survey of patients with valvular heart disease in Europe: the Euro Heart Survey on Valvular Heart Disease. *Eur Heart J* 2003; 24:1231–1243.
104. Gohlke-Bärwolf C, Iung B, Butchart EG *et al*. Unexpected findings in anticoagulation management in patients with valvular heart disease after valve surgery. *Eur Heart J* 2003; 24(suppl):A 2278.
105. Ng FS, Camm AJ. Catheter ablation of atrial fibrillation. *Clin Cardiol* 2002; 25:384–394.
106. Viola N, Williams MR, Oz MC, Ad N. The technology in use for surgical ablation of atrial fibrillation. *Semin Thorac Cardiovasc Surg* 2002; 14:198–205.
107. Ad N, Cox JW. The significance of atrial fibrillation ablation in patients undergoing mitral valve surgery. *Semin Thorac Cardiovasc Surg* 2002; 14:193–197.
108. Lip GY. The prothrombotic state in atrial fibrillation: the atrium, the endothelium . . . and tissue factor? *Thromb Res* 2003; 111:133–135.
109. Marin F, Roldan V, Climent V, Garcia A, Marco P, Lip GYH. Is thrombogenesis in atrial fibrillation related to matrix metalloproteinase-1 and its inhibitor, TIMP-1? *Stroke* 2003; 34:1181–1186.
110. Pacifico A, Henry PD. Ablation for atrial fibrillation: are cures really achieved? *JACC* 2004; 43:1940–1942.
111. Woodman RC, Harker LA. Bleeding complications associated with cardiopulmonary bypass. *Blood* 1990; 76:1680–1697.

112. Kouchoukos NT, Blackstone EH, Doty DB, Hanley FL, Karp RB. Hypothermia, circulatory arrest and cardiopulmonary bypass. In: Kirklin JW, Barratt-Boyes B. *Cardiac Surgery,* 3rd edition. Churchill Livingstone, Philadelphia, 2003, pp 66–130.

113. Anderson JM, Schoen FH. Interactions of blood with artificial surfaces. In: Butchart EG, Bodnar E (eds). *Current Issues in Heart Valve Disease: Thrombosis, Embolism and Bleeding*, ICR Publishers, London, 1992, pp 160–171.

114. Laplace G, Lafitte S, Labèque JN *et al.* Clinical significance of early thrombosis after prosthetic mitral valve replacement. *JACC* 2004; 43:1283–1290.

115. Beppu S. Hypercoagulability in the left atrium: part I: echocardiography. *J Heart Valve Dis* 1993; 2:18–24.

116. Butchart EG. Prosthesis-specific and patient-specific anticoagulation. In: Butchart EG, Bodnar E (eds). *Current Issues in Heart Valve Disease: Thrombosis, Embolism and Bleeding*, ICR Publishers, London, 1992, pp 293–317.

117. Ernofsson M, Thelin S, Siegbahn A. Monocyte tissue factor expression, cell activation and thrombin formation during cardiopulmonary bypass: a clinical study. *J Thorac Cardiovasc Surg* 1997; 113:576–584.

118. Thulin LI, Olin CL. Initiation and long-term anticoagulation after heart valve replacements. *Arq Bras Cardiol* 1987; 49:265–268.

119. Fanikos J, Tsilimingras K, Kucher N, Rosen AB, Hieblinger MD, Goldhaber SZ. Comparison of efficacy, safety and cost of low-molecular-weight heparin with continuous infusion unfractionated heparin for initiation of anticoagulation after mechanical prosthetic valve implantation. *Am J Cardiol* 2004; 93:247–250.

120. Montalescot G, Polle V, Collet JP *et al.* Low molecular weight heparin after mechanical heart valve replacement. *Circulation* 2000; 101:1083–1086.

121. Hirsh J, Warkentin TE, Shaughnessy SG *et al.* Heparin and low-molecular-weight heparin. Mechanisms of action, pharmacokinetics, dosing, monitoring, efficacy and safety. *Chest* 2001; 119(suppl):64S–94S.

122. Russman S, Gohlke-Bärwolf C, Jähnchen E, Trenk D, Roskamm H. Age-dependent differences in the anticoagulant effect of phenprocoumon in patients after heart valve surgery. *Eur J Clin Pharmacol* 1997; 52:31–35.

123. Ansell J, Hirsh J, Dalen J *et al.* Managing oral anticoagulant therapy. *Chest* 2001; 119(suppl):22S–38S.

124. Ageno W, Turpie AGG. Exaggerated initial response to warfarin following heart valve replacement. *Am J Cardiol* 1999; 84:905–908.

125. Gurewich V. Ximelagatran – promises and concerns. *JAMA* 2005; 293:736–739.

126. McKernan A, Thomson JM, Poller L. The reliability of international normalised ratios during short-term oral anticoagulant treatment. *Clin Lab Haematol* 1988; 10:63–71.

127. Murray D, Pennell B, Olson J. Variability of prothrombin time and activated partial thromboplastin time in the diagnosis of increased surgical bleeding. *Transfusion* 1999; 39:56–62.

128. Arnsten JH, Gelfand JM, Singer DE. Determinants of compliance with anticoagulation: a case-control study. *Am J Med* 1977; 103:11–17.

129. Huber KC, Gersh BJ, Bailey KR *et al.* Variability in anticoagulation control predicts thromboembolism after mechanical cardiac valve replacement: a 23 year population-based study. *Mayo Clin Proc* 1997; 72:1103–1110.

130. Butchart EG, Payne N, Li HH, Buchan K, Mandana K, Grunkemeier GL. Better anticoagulation control improves survival after valve replacement. *J Thorac Cardiovasc Surg* 2002; 123:715–723.

131. Sixty Plus Reinfarction Study Research Group. Risks of long-term oral anticoagulant therapy in elderly patients after myocardial infarction: second report of the Sixty Plus Reinfarction Study Research Group. *Lancet* 1982; 1:64–68.

132. van der Meer FJM, Rosendaal FR, Vandenbroucke JP, Briet E. Bleeding complications in oral anticoagulant therapy. *Arch Intern Med* 1993; 153:1557–1562.

133. Feinberg WM, Cornell ES, Nightingale SD *et al.* Relationship between prothrombin activation fragment F1.2 and International Normalized Ratio in patients with atrial fibrillation. *Stroke* 1997; 28:1101–1106.

134. Koefoed BG, Feddersen C, Gullov AL, Petersen P. Effect of minidose warfarin, conventional dose warfarin and aspirin on INR and prothrombin fragment 1 + 2 in patients with atrial fibrillation. *Thomb Haemost* 1997; 77:845–848.

135. van Wersch JWJ, van Mourik-Alderliesten CH, Coremans A. Determination of markers of coagulation activation and reactive fibrinolysis in patients with mechanical heart valve prosthesis at different intensities of oral anticoagularion. *Blood Coag Fibrinol* 1992; 3:183–186.

136. Tientadakul P, Opartkiattikul N, Sangtawesin W *et al.* Effect of different oral anticoagulant intensities on prothrombin fragment 1 + 2 in Thai patients with mechanical heart valve prostheses. *J Med Assoc Thai* 1997; 80:81–86.

137. Cannegieter SC, Rosendaal FR, Wintzen AR *et al*. Optimal oral anticoagulant therapy in patients with mechanical heart valves. *N Engl J Med* 1995; 333:11–17.

138. Vink R, Kraaijenhagen RA, Hutten BA *et al*. The optimal intensity of vitamin K antagonists in patients with mechanical heart valves. A meta-analysis. *JACC* 2003; 42:2042–2048.

139. Butchart EG, Gohlke-Bärwolf C. Anticoagulation management of patients with prosthetic heart valves. *JACC* 2004; 44:1143–1144.

140. Pruefer D, Dahm M, Dohmen G, Horstkotte D, Bergemann R, Oelert H. Intensity of oral anticoagulation after implantation of St. Jude Medical mitral or multiple valve replacement: lessons learned from GELIA. *Eur Heart J* 2001; 3(suppl Q):Q39–Q43.

141. Butchart EG, Lewis PA, Bethel JA, Breckenridge IM. Adjusting anticoagulation to prosthesis thrombogenicity and patient risk factors. Recommendations for the Medtronic Hall valve. *Circulation* 1991; 84(suppl III):61–69.

142. Yasaka M, Yamaguchi T, Miyashita T, Tsuchiya T. Regression of intracardiac thrombus after embolic stroke. *Stroke* 1990; 21:1540–1544.

143. Grunkemeier GL, Wu YX. 'Our complication rates are lower than theirs': statistical critique of heart valve comparisons. *J Thorac Cardiovasc Surg* 2003; 125:290–300.

144. Aoyagi S, Nishimi M, Kawano H *et al*. Obstruction of St. Jude Medical valves in the aortic position: significance of a combination of cineradiography and echocardiography. *J Thorac Cardiovasc Surg* 2000; 120:142–147.

145. Palareti G, Leali N, Manotti C *et al*. Bleeding complications of oral anticoagulant treatment: an inception-cohort, prospective collaborative study (ISCOAT). *Lancet* 1996; 348:423–428.

146. Landefeld CS, Goldman L. Major bleeding in outpatients treated with warfarin: incidence and prediction by factors known at the start of outpatient therapy. *Am J Med* 1989; 87:144–152.

147. Launbjerg J, Egeblad H, Heaf J, Nielsen NH, Fugleholm AM, Ladefoged K. Bleeding complications to oral anticoagulant therapy: multivariate analysis of 1,010 treatment years in 551 outpatients. *J Intern Med* 1991; 229:351–355.

148. Hart RG, Boop BS, Anderson DC. Oral anticoagulants and intracranial haemorrhage: facts and hypotheses. *Stroke* 1995; 26:1471–1477.

149. Beyth RJ, Quinn LM, Landefeld S. Prospective evaluation of an index for predicting the risk of major bleeding in outpatients treated with warfarin. *Am J Med* 1998; 105:91–99.

150. Butchart EG, Li HH, Payne N, Buchan K, Grunkemeier GL. Twenty years' experience with the Medtronic Hall valve. *J Thorac Cardiovasc Surg* 2001; 121:1090–1100.

151. Hylek EM, Singer DE. Risk factors for intracranial hemorrhage in outpatients taking warfarin. *Ann Intern Med* 1994; 120:897–902.

152. Radberg JA, Olsson JE, Radberg CT. Prognostic parameters in spontaneous intracerebral hematomas with special reference to anticoagulant treatment. *Stroke* 1991; 22:571–576.

153. Hylek EM, Heiman H, Skates SJ *et al*. Acetaminophen and other risk factors for excessive warfarin anticoagulation. *JAMA* 1998; 279:657–662.

154. Crowther MA, Julian J, McCarty D *et al*. Treatment of warfarin-associated coagulopathy with oral vitamin K: a randomised controlled trial. *Lancet* 2000; 356:1551–1553.

155. Makris M, Watson HG. The management of coumarin-induced over-anticoagulation. *Br J Haematol* 2001; 114:271–280.

156. Penning-van Beest FJA, Rosendaal FR, Grobbee DE, van Meegan E, Stricker BHC. Course of the International Normalized Radio in response to oral vitamin K_1 in patients overanticoagulated with phenprocoumon. *Br Haematol* 1999; 104:241–245.

157. Llewellyn CA, Hewitt PE, Knight RS *et al*. Possible transmission of variant Creutzfeldt-Jakob disease by blood transfusion. *Lancet* 2004; 363:417–421.

158. Wollowitz S. Fundamentals of the psoralen-based Helinx technology for inactivation of infectious pathogens and leukocytes in platelets and plasma. *Semin Hematol* 2001; 38(suppl 11):4–11.

159. Hambleton J, Wages D, Radu-Radulescu L *et al*. Pharmacokinetic study of FFP photochemically treated with amotosalen (S-59) and UV light compared to FFP in healthy volunteers anticoagulated with warfarin. *Transfusion* 2002; 42:1302–1307.

160. Butler AC, Tait RC. Management of oral anticoagulant-induced intracranial haemorrhage. *Blood Rev* 1998; 12:35–44.

161. Butler AC, Tait RC. Restarting anticoagulation in prosthetic heart valve patients after intracranial haemorrhage: a 2-year follow-up. *Br J Haematol* 1998; 103:1064–1066.

162. Wijdicks EFM, Schievink WI, Brown RD, Mullany CJ. The dilemma of discontinuation of anticoagulation therapy for patients with intracranial hemorrhage and mechanical heart valves. *Neurosurgery* 1998; 42:769–773.

163. Sharma R, Gorbien MJ. Angiodysplasia and lower gastrointestinal tract bleeding in elderly patients. *Arch Intern Med* 1995; 155:807–812.

164. Warkentin TE, Moore JC, Anand SS, Lonn EM, Morgan DG. Gastrointestinal bleeding, angiodysplasia, cardiovascular disease and acquired von Willebrand syndrome. *Transfus Med Rev* 2003; 17:272–286.

165. Blich M, Fruchter O, Edelstein S, Edoute Y. Somatostatin therapy ameliorates chronic and refractory gastrointestinal bleeding caused by diffuse angiodysplasia in a patient on anticoagulation therapy. *Scand J Gastroenterol* 2003; 38:801–803.

166. Lafata JE, Martin SA, Kaatz S, Ward RE. The cost-effectiveness of different management strategies for patients on chronic warfarin therapy. *J Gen Intern Med* 2000; 15:31–37.

167. Rosengart TK. Anticoagulation self-testing after heart valve replacement. *J Heart Valve Dis* 2001; 11(suppl 1):S61–S65.

168. Rose P. Audit of anticoagulant therapy. *J Clin Pathol* 1996; 40:5–9.

169. Fitzmaurice DA, Machin SJ, on behalf of the British Society of Haematology Task Force for Haemostasis and Thrombosis: Recommendations for patients undertaking self management of oral anticoagulation. *BMJ* 2001; 323:985–989.

170. Halhuber C. Quick test self-determination by patients. Adequate long-term anticoagulation can often only be performed with great difficulty. *Fortschr Med* 1988; 106:615–617.

171. Bernardo A, Halhuber C, Horstkotte D. Home prothrombin time estimation. In: Butchart EG, Bodnar E (eds). *Current Issues in Heart Valve Disease: Thrombosis, Embolism and Bleeding*. ICR Publishers, London, 1992, pp 325–330.

172. Lucas FV, Duncan A, Jay R *et al.* A novel whole blood capillary technique for measuring the prothrombin time. *Am J Clin Pathol* 1987; 88:442–446.

173. White R, McCurdy SY, von Marensdorff H, Woodruff DE, Leftgoff PA. Home prothrombin time monitoring after the initiation of warfarin therapy. *Ann Intern Med* 1989; 111:730–736.

174. Ansell JE, Holden A, Knapic N. Patient self-management of oral anticoagulation guided by capillary (fingerstick) whole-blood prothrombin times. *Arch Intern Med* 1989; 149:2509–2511.

175. White RH, McKittrick T, Hutchinson R, Twitchell J. Temporary discontinuation of warfarin therapy: changes in the international normalized ratio. *Ann Intern Med* 1995; 122:40–42.

176. Jacobson AK. Patient self-management of oral anticoagulant therapy: an international update. *J Thromb Thrombolys* 1998; 5:S25–S28.

177. Taborski VWE, Wittstamm FJ, Bernado A. Cost-effectiveness of self-management anticoagulant therapy in Germany. *Semin Thromb Haemost* 1999; 25:103–107.

178. Körtke H, Gohlke-Bärwolf C, Heik SCW, Horstkotte D. Empfehlungen zum INR-Selbstmanagement bei oraler Antikoagulation. *Z Kardiol* 1998; 87:983–985.

179. Bernardo A, Völler H. Leitlinien 'Gerinnungsselbstmanagement'. *Medizinische Wochenzeitschrift* 2001; 126:346–351.

180. Ansell JE, Hughes R. Evolving models of warfarin management: anticoagulation clinics, patient self-monitoring, and patient self-management. *Am Heart J* 1996; 132:1095–1100.

181. Hasenkam JM, Knudsen L, Kimose HH *et al.* Practicability of patient self-testing of oral anticoagulant therapy by the International Normalized Ratio (INR) using a portable whole blood monitor. A pilot investigation. *Thromb Res* 1997; 85:77–82.

182. Beyth RJ, Quinn L, Landefeld CS. A multicomponent intervention to prevent major bleeding complications in older patients receiving warfarin. A randomised controlled trial. *Ann Intern Med* 2000; 133:687–695.

183. Sawicki PT. A structured teaching and self-management program for patients receiving oral anticoagulation: a randomised controlled trial. *JAMA* 1999; 281:145–150.

184. Watzke HH, Forberg E, Svolba G, Jimenez-Boj E, Krinninger B. A prospective controlled trial comparing weekly self-testing and self-dosing with the standard management of patients on stable oral anticoagulant. *Thromb Haemost* 2000; 83:661–665.

185. Körtke H, Körfer R. International normalized ratio self-management after mechanical heart valve replacement: is an early start advantageous? *Ann Thorac Surg* 2001; 72:44–48.

186. Horstkotte D, Piper C, Wiemer M. Optimal frequency of patient monitoring and intensity of oral anticoagulation therapy in valvular heart disease. *J Thromb Thrombolys* 1998; 5:19–24.

187. Engelberger L, Carrel T, Schaff HV, Kennard ED, Holubkov R. Differences in heart valve procedures between North American and European centres: a report from the Artificial Valve Endocarditis Reduction Trial (AVERT). *J Heart Valve Dis* 2001; 10:562–571.

188. Moake JL, Turner NA, Stathopoulos NA, Nolasko L, Hellums JD. Shear-induced platelet aggregation can be mediated by vWF released from platelets, as well as by exogenous large or unusually large vWF multimers, requires adenosine diphosphate, and is resistant to aspirin. *Blood* 1988; 71:1366–1374.

189. Harker LA, Hanson SR, Kirkman TR. Experimental arterial thromboembolism in baboons: mechanisms, quantitation and pharmacologic prevention. *J Clin Invest* 1979; 64:559–569.

190. The PEP Trial Investigators. Prevention of pulmonary embolism and deep vein thrombosis with low dose aspirin: Pulmonary Embolism Prevention (PEP) trial. *Lancet* 2000; 355:1295–1302.

191. Hart RG, Benavente O, McBride R, Pearce LA. Antithrombotic therapy to prevent stroke in patients with atrial fibrillation: A meta-analysis. *Ann Intern Med* 1999; 131:492–501.

192. Butchart EG. Rationalising antithrombotic management for patients with prosthetic heart valves. *J Heart Valve Dis* 1995; 4:106–113.

193. Da Silva MS, Sobel M. Anticoagulants: to bleed or not to bleed, that is the question. *Semin Vasc Surg* 2002; 15:256–267.

194. Hurlen M, Abdelnoor M, Smith P, Erikssen J, Arnesen H. Warfarin, aspirin, or both after myocardial infarction. *N Engl J Med* 2002; 347:969–974.

195. Antithrombotic Trialists' Collaboration. Collaborative meta-analysis of randomised trials of antiplatelet therapy for prevention of death, myocardial infarction, and stroke in high risk patients. *BMJ* 2002; 324:71–86.

196. Kelly JP, Kaufman DW, Jurgelon JM, Sheehan J, Koff RS, Shapiro S. Risk of aspirin-associated major upper-gastrointestinal bleeding with enteric-coated or buffered product. *Lancet* 1996; 348:1413–1416.

197. Hart RG, Pearce LA. In vivo antithrombotic effect of aspirin: dose versus nongastrointestinal bleeding. *Stroke* 1993; 24:138–139.

198. He J, Whelton PK, Vu B, Klag MJ. Aspirin and risk of hemorrhagic stroke: a meta-analysis of randomised controlled trials. *JAMA* 1998; 238:1930–1935.

199. FitzGerald GA. Dipyridamole. *N Eng J Med* 1987; 316:1247–1257.

200. Bult H, Fret HR, Jordaens FH, Herman AG. Dipyridamole potentiates platelet inhibition by nitric oxide. *Thromb Haemost* 1991; 66:343–349.

201. Fuster V, Israel DH. Platelet inhibitor drugs after prosthetic heart valve replacement. In: Butchart EG, Bodnar E (eds). *Current Issues of Heart Valve Disease: Thrombosis, Embolism and Bleeding*. ICR Publishers, London, 1992, pp 247–262.

202. European Stroke Prevention Study 2. Efficacy and safety data. *J Neurol Sci* 1997; 151(suppl):S1–S77.

203. Forbes CD. Secondary stroke prevention with low-dose aspirin, sustained release dipyridamole alone and in combination. ESPS Investigators. European Stroke Prevention Study. *Thromb Res* 1998; 92:S1–S6.

204. Pouleur H, Buyse M. Effects of dipyridamole in combination with anticoagulant therapy on survival and thromboembolic events in patients with prosthetic heart valves. A meta-analysis of the randomized trials. *J Thorac Cardiovasc Surg* 1995; 110:463–472.

205. Chesebro J, Fuster V, Elveback LR. Trial of combined warfarin plus dipyridamole or aspirin therapy in prosthetic heart valve replacement: danger of aspirin compared with dipyridamole. *Am J Cardiol* 1983; 51:1537–1541.

206. Leonardi-Bee J, Bath PMW, Bousser MG *et al.* Dipyridamole for preventing recurrent ischemic stroke and other vascular events. *Stroke* 2005; 36:162–168.

207. CAPRIE Steering Committee. A randomised, blinded, trial of clopidogrel versus aspirin in patients at risk of ischaemic events (CAPRIE). *Lancet* 1996; 348:1329–1339.

208. Altman R, Boullon F, Rouvier J, de la Fuente L, Favaloro R. Aspirin and prophylaxis of thromboembolic complications in patients with substitute heart valves. *J Thorac Cardiovasc Surg* 1976; 72:127–129.

209. Dale J, Myhre E, Storstein O, Stormorken H, Efskind L. Prevention of arterial thromboembolism with acetylsalicylic acid. A controlled clinical study in patients with aortic ball valves. *Am Heart J* 1977; 94:101–111.

210. Turpie AG, Gent M, Laupacis A *et al.* A comparison of aspirin with placebo in patients treated with warfarin after heart valve replacement. *N Engl J Med* 1993; 329:524–529.

211. Cappelleri JC, Fiore LD, Brophy MT, Deykin D, Lau J. Efficacy and safety of combined anticoagulant and antiplatelet therapy versus anticoagulant monotherapy after mechanical heart valve replacement: a meta-analysis. *Am Heart J* 1995; 130:547–552.

212. Sullivan JM, Harken DE, Gorlin R. Pharmacologic control of thromboembolic complications of cardiac valve replacement. *N Engl J Med* 1971; 284:1391–1394.

213. Dale J, Myhre E, Loew D. Bleeding during acetylsalicylic acid and anticoagulant therapy in patients with reduced platelet reactivity after aortic valve replacement. *Am Heart J* 1980; 99:746–752.

214. Taylor TN, Davis PH, Torner JC *et al*. Lifetime cost of stroke in the United States. *Stroke* 1996; 27:1459–1466.

215. Massel D, Little SH. Risks and benefits of adding antiplatelet therapy to warfarin among patients with prosthetic heart valves: a meta-analysis. *JACC* 2001; 37:569–578.

216. Meschengieser S, Fondevila C, Frontroth J *et al*. Low-intensity oral anticoagulation plus low-dose aspirin versus high-intensity oral anticoagulation alone: a randomized trial in patients with mechanical prosthetic heart valves. *J Thorac Cardiovasc Surg* 1997; 113:910–916.

217. Rumack CM, Guggenheim MA, Rumack BH, Peterson RG, Johnson ML, Braithwaite WR. Neonatal intracranial hemorrhage and maternal use of aspirin. *Obstet Gynecol* 1981; 58:52S–56S.

218. Stuart MJ, Gross SJ, Elrad H, Graeber JE. Effects of acetylsalicylic acid ingestion on maternal and neonatal hemostasis. *N Engl J Med* 1982; 307:909–912.

219. Chesebro JH, Fuster V. Valvular heart disease and prosthetic valves. In: Verstraete M, Fuster V, Topol EJ (eds). *Cardiovascular Thrombosis*. Lippincott-Raven, Philadelphia, 1998; 365–394.

220. Hansson L, Zanchetti A, Carruthers SG *et al*. Effects of intensive blood-pressure lowering and low-dose aspirin in patients with hypertension: principal results of the Hypertension Optimal Treatment (HOT) randomised trial. *Lancet* 1998; 351:1755–1762.

221. Hart RG, Pearce LA, McBride R, Rothbart RM, Asinger RW. Factors associated with ischemic stroke during aspirin therapy in atrial fibrillation. Analysis of 2012 participants in the SPAF I-III clinical trials. *Stroke* 1999; 30:1223–1229.

222. Meade TW, Brennan PJ. Determination of who may derive most benefit from aspirin in primary prevention: subgroup results from a randomised controlled trial. *BMJ* 2000; 321:13–17.

223 Silber H, Khan SS, Matloff JM *et al*. The St. Jude valve. Thrombolysis as the first line of therapy for cardiac valve thrombosis. *Circulation* 1993; 87:30–37.

224. Lengyel M, Fuster V, Keltai M *et al*. Guidelines for management of left-sided prosthetic valve thrombosis: a role for thrombolytic therapy. *JACC* 1997; 30:1521–1526.

225. Renzulli A, De Luca L, Caruso A *et al*. Acute thrombosis of prosthetic valves: a multivariate analysis of the risk factors for a life-threatening event. *Eur J Cardiothorac Surg* 1992; 6:412–442.

226. Barbetseas J, Nagueh SF, Pitsavos C *et al*. Differentiating thrombus from pannus formation in obstructed mechanical prosthetic valves: an evaluation of clinical, transthoracic and transesophageal echocardiographic parameters. *JACC* 1998; 32:1410–1417.

227. Shiran A, Weissman NJ, Merdler A *et al*. Transesophageal echocardiographic findings in patients with nonobstructed prosthetic valves and suspected cardiac source of embolism. *Am J Cardiol* 2001; 88:1441–1444.

228. Montorsi P, De Bernardi F, Muratori M *et al*. Rose of cinefluoroscopy, transthoracic, and transesophageal echocardiography in patients with suspected prosthetic heart valve fibrinolysis. *Am J Cardiol* 2000; 85:58–64.

229. Shapira Y, Herz I, Sagie A. Fluoroscopy of prosthetic heart valves: does it have a place in the echocardiography era? *J Heart Valve Dis* 2000; 9:594–599.

230. Peterffy A *et al*. Late thrombosis of the Björk-Shiley tilting disc valve in the tricuspid position. *Scand J Thorac Cardiovasc Surg* 1980; 14:33.

231. Roudaut R, Lafitte S, Roudaut M *et al*. Fibrinolysis of mechanical prosthetic valve thrombosis: a single-center study of 127 cases. *JACC* 2003; 41:653–658.

232. Roudaut R, Labbé T, Lorient-Roudaut MF *et al*. Mechanical cardiac valve thrombosis. Is fibrinolysis justified? *Circulation* 1992; 86(suppl):II-8–II-15.

233. Lengyel M, Vandor L. The role of thrombolysis in the management of left-sided prosthetic valve thrombosis: a study of 85 cases diagnosed by transesophageal echocardiography. *J Heart Valve Dis* 2001; 10:636–649.

234. Edmunds LH, Jr, Clark RE, Cohn LH *et al*. Guidelines for reporting morbidity and mortality after cardiac valvular operations. *J Thorac Cardiovasc Surg* 1996; 112:708–711.

15

Stroke: thrombolysis and antithrombotic therapy

A. G. Vaishnav, L. C. Pettigrew

INTRODUCTION

'Stroke' may be defined as any physical disorder that alters global or regional blood flow to the brain resulting in hemorrhage, infarction, vasospasm, or inflammation. It is the third most common cause of adult mortality in the United States, accounting for 6.9% of total deaths in 1996 [1]. Every year, as many as 730 000 new cases of stroke occur in the American population [2]. With nearly 4.5 million surviving victims, stroke remains the most frequently encountered source of long-term disability in our society. Estimates of the national cost of this disease vary by the reference, but most authorities agree that at least $30 billion are spent annually to cover all expenses associated with the care of stroke victims [3]. The average direct cost per case, including all illness-related expenses, is approximately $50 000 [4]. Over a lifetime, the cost of ischaemic stroke is estimated to be more than $100 000 per person, as calculated for a stroke occurring in 1990 [4].

This chapter will review antithrombotic therapy for secondary stroke prevention and thrombolytic treatment of acute ischaemic stroke within the arterial circulation of the brain. Ischaemic stroke is a consequence of spontaneous thrombosis occurring within the intra- or extracranial arteries, inflammatory disorders of the macro- or microcirculation in the brain, or embolic particles arising from within the heart or the extracranial vessels (Figure 15.1). Large-artery atherosclerotic infarction results from impairment of normal perfusion, usually caused by severe stenosis or occlusion of the common or internal carotid or vertebral artery, and may include intra-arterial thrombosis or artery–artery emboli. Microatheromata, lipo-hyalinosis, and other occlusive diseases of the small penetrating arteries constitute the underlying pathology of small, subcortical 'lacunar' infarcts observed in hypertensive or diabetic micro-arteriopathy of the brain. From 20 to 35% of all hospitalised cases of ischaemic stroke are caused by cardiogenic emboli, most frequently from atrial fibrillation (AF). Less common causes of cardioembolic stroke include dilated cardiomyopathy with suppressed ejection fraction of the left ventricle, septic endocarditis with valvular vegetations, mural thrombi associated with left ventricular aneurysms after myocardial infarction (MI), myxomatous valvular degeneration, mitral valve prolapse, and non-bacterial thrombotic endocarditis observed with mucin-secreting cancers. After arising from deep veins in

Anand G. Vaishnav, Associate Professor of Neurology, Department of Neurology, University of Kentucky Chandler Medical Center, Lexington, Kentucky, USA.

L. Creed Pettigrew, Professor of Neurology and Director, University of Kentucky Stroke Program, Department of Neurology, University of Kentucky Chandler Medical Center, Lexington, Kentucky, USA.

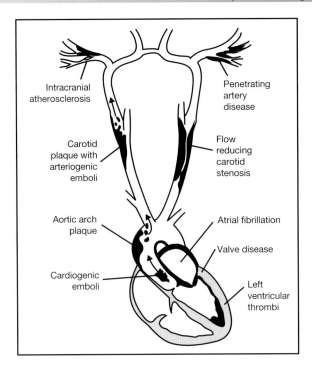

Figure 15.1 Diagram showing representative arterial and cardiac abnormalities causing ischaemic stroke. Reproduced with Permission [30].

the legs or the pelvis, 'paradoxical' venous emboli may enter the arterial circulation of the brain by traveling through a patent foramen ovale (PFO) in the heart. Prothrombotic disorders that include the antiphospholipid antibody syndrome, congenital micro-arteriopathies such as Fabry's disease, coagulopathies and haemoglobinopathies (haemoglobin SS or SC), and spontaneous carotid or vertebral arterial dissections arising from fibromuscular dysplasia account for fewer than 5% of hospitalised ischaemic stroke. Even after an extensive diagnostic evaluation, up to 30% of all hospitalised ischaemic strokes remain of unknown origin. Selection of optimal antithrombotic therapy for prevention of recurrent stroke should be based on elucidation of the underlying thromboembolic mechanism, rendered all the more challenging for patients with stroke of cryptogenic origin. For treatment of acute ischaemic stroke, the decision to employ systemic thrombolysis or an alternate approach to enhance cerebral reperfusion must be guided by careful patient selection under rigid time constraints.

ANTITHROMBOTIC THERAPY IN SECONDARY STROKE PROPHYLAXIS

Pharmaceutical agents shown to be effective for secondary stroke prophylaxis include aspirin, ticlopidine (Ticlid®), clopidogrel (Plavix®), and a combination of aspirin and extended-release dipyridamole (Aggrenox®). The role of each agent in secondary stroke prophylaxis will be considered individually in the succeeding paragraphs.

Several randomised, controlled trials have addressed the role of aspirin for the prevention of cerebral infarction following transient ischaemic attack (TIA) or stroke [5–15]. These trials gave conflicting results because of dissimilar study designs and a broad spectrum of aspirin doses selected for evaluation. In an attempt to gain consensus on the role of aspirin in treatment or prevention of stroke and other thrombotic disorders, the

Antithrombotic Trialists, known formerly as the Antiplatelet Trialists, conducted a meta-analysis of available randomised, controlled clinical trials of antiplatelet therapy. The most recent summary prepared by the Antithrombotic Trialists included all antiplatelet trials completed before 1997 and was published in 2002 [16]. This meta-analysis included 144 051 patients with previous MI, acute MI, previous TIA or stroke, and acute stroke. As in earlier reports from the former Antiplatelet Trialists, the meta-analysis emphasised the composite outcome of stroke, MI or vascular death. The Antithrombotic Trialists determined that antiplatelet therapy reduced the odds of this composite outcome by approximately 25% in high-risk patients. The odds reduction attributable to aspirin alone was 23%. Antiplatelet agents reduced the odds of a non-fatal stroke by 25%, non-fatal MI by 34%, and vascular death by 15%. In a smaller meta-analysis of ten trials enrolling only patients with prior stroke or TIA, Algra and van Gijn [17] concluded that aspirin reduced the odds for the cluster of stroke, MI, or vascular death by only 16% over placebo. In a meta-regression analysis of more than 5000 patients in eleven trials, Johnson and colleagues [18] also confirmed that aspirin therapy reduced the risk of secondary stroke and demonstrated that this reduction was uniform (approximately 15%) across doses of 50 to 1500 mg/day.

The efficacy of ticlopidine in stroke prevention was confirmed in two double-blind, randomised, prospective trials conducted in North America: the Ticlopidine Aspirin Stroke Study (TASS) [20] and the Canadian American Ticlopidine Study (CATS) [21]. In the TASS study, 3069 patients with TIA, transient monocular blindness, reversible ischaemic neurologic deficit, or minor ischaemic stroke were enrolled and treated with ticlopidine 250 mg or aspirin 650 mg, twice daily for as long as six years of follow-up observation. At one year, risk reduction for non-fatal and fatal stroke in patients treated with ticlopidine was 48% using on-treatment analysis and 46% using intention-to-treat analysis. However, this benefit was lost over time as the cumulative event rate for stroke in the two treatment groups became parallel after the first year. In the CATS study, 1053 patients with atherothrombotic stroke within the previous four months were enrolled and treated with ticlopidine 250 mg, twice daily, or matched placebo [21]. At the end of the trial, efficacy analysis showed a significant relative risk reduction of 30% in favour of ticlopidine for the primary outcome measure of stroke, MI, or vascular death.

In addition to TASS and CATS, ticlopidine was tested in one other clinical trial for prevention of symptomatic vascular disease after stroke in blacks, the African-American Antiplatelet Stroke Prevention Study (AAASPS) [22]. A total of 1809 patients in this trial were randomised to treatment with ticlopidine (500 mg/day) or aspirin (650 mg/day). The primary outcome measure was the familiar composite of recurrent stroke, MI, or vascular death. The trial was halted after just over six years of recruitment when interim futility analysis revealed less than 1% probability of ticlopidine being shown superior to aspirin in prevention of the primary outcome.

The Clopidogrel vs. Aspirin in Patients at Risk of Ischaemic Events (CAPRIE) study enrolled 19 185 patients with ischaemic stroke ($n = 6431$), MI ($n = 6302$), or atherosclerotic peripheral arterial disease ($n = 6452$) who were treated with clopidogrel 75 mg or aspirin 325 mg daily [23]. The composite endpoint of stroke, MI, or vascular death was used as the primary outcome measure. Within the entire CAPRIE population, those subjects enrolled with peripheral arterial disease experienced the greatest benefit from treatment with clopidogrel. These patients had a composite event rate of 3.71% per year, compared with 4.86% in aspirin-treated subjects with peripheral arterial disease (significant relative risk reduction of 23.8%). In contrast, MI patients in the clopidogrel group had an increase in relative risk of 3.7% for the composite outcome measure, suggesting that aspirin was of greater benefit for this condition. For the stroke patients, there was no significant difference in the composite outcome measure between the treatment groups indicating that the two drugs were equivalent in this population. The overall conclusion from CAPRIE was that clopidogrel is marginally more effective than aspirin for prevention of the composite endpoint of ischaemic stroke, MI, or vascular death, but ineffective in reducing the rate of recurrent stroke.

Clinical trials performed to evaluate clopidogrel as an antithrombotic agent in the wake of the CAPRIE study have been designed to optimise drug selection for specific atherothrombotic disorders. In the Clopidogrel in Unstable Angina to Prevent Recurrent Events (CURE) study [24], 12 562 patients with acute coronary syndromes (unstable angina 74.9%; MI 25.1%) less than 24 h in duration were randomised to a loading dose of clopidogrel 300 mg followed by 75 mg daily (6259 patients) or placebo (6303) in addition to open-label aspirin dosed between 75 and 325 mg per day. Patients with MI who had ST-segment elevation on an initial electrocardiogram were excluded. Follow-up was conducted for up to 12 months with a composite primary outcome of death from any cardiovascular cause, nonfatal MI (chest pain with doubling of cardiac enzymes or expected electrocardiographic changes), and stroke (ischaemic, haemorrhagic, or uncertain if brain imaging was not performed). The clopidogrel and aspirin group had significantly lower incidence of the primary outcome, 9.3%, compared to 11.4% in the aspirin-only group (relative risk with clopidogrel compared to placebo 0.8 [20% relative risk reduction]; 95% CI 0.72–0.90; $P < 0.001$). The proportion of patients who developed stroke after being randomised to clopidogrel/aspirin, 1.2%, was lower than 1.4% in the aspirin-only group but was not statistically significant. Major bleeding, defined as systemic or intracranial haemorrhages that were disabling, intra-ocular haemorrhages, and any haemorrhage requiring transfusion of two units of blood, was significantly higher in the clopidogrel/aspirin group, 3.7 vs. 2.7% (relative risk 1.38; $P = 0.001$), although event rates of life-threatening haemorrhages were similar in the two groups.

After CURE established that combined aspirin/clopidogrel was superior to aspirin alone for prevention of vascular endpoints following acutely symptomatic coronary insufficiency, the Clopidogrel for the Reduction of Events During Observation (CREDO) study was initiated to determine the optimal duration of combination therapy following percutaneous coronary intervention (PCI) [25]. A total of 2116 patients with symptomatic coronary artery disease (CAD) undergoing angiography with planned or expected PCI were treated with aspirin (81–325 mg) after the procedure and were randomised to concomitant therapy with clopidogrel 75 mg daily or placebo. As with CURE, the primary 1-year outcome was the composite of death, MI, and stroke (defined as a focal neurological deficit of vascular origin lasting 24 h) in the intent-to-treat population. For the entire study population, randomisation to long-term combination therapy was associated with 26.9% reduction in relative risk of the composite endpoint at 1 year (95% CI 3.9–44.4%; $P = 0.02$). Following the precedent observed in CURE, patients on combination therapy experienced a trend toward an increase in major bleeding (8.8% aspirin/clopidogrel vs. 6.7% aspirin only; $P = 0.07$).

As suggested in an editorial written by Albers and Amarenco [26], the results from CURE and, by extrapolation, CREDO, cannot be extended to patients with symptomatic cerebrovascular disease. First, the number of strokes that occurred in both CURE and CREDO were too small to assess the efficacy of clopidogrel and aspirin for primary stroke prevention. Second, although coronary and cerebral arterial diseases share the same pathogenic mechanism of atherothrombosis, each has its own recurrence rate that appears unique to the affected circulatory system [27]. CURE and CREDO focused only on symptomatic coronary atherothrombosis and were not designed to observe a robust effect in patients with cerebrovascular disease. Third, the risk of haemorrhagic complications associated with the use of drugs that affect platelet function is typically higher in patients with symptomatic cerebrovascular disease than in other vascular disorders. The most likely cause of this difference may be regional perturbation of the blood–brain barrier in many stroke patients that will increase the likelihood of drug-induced haemorrhage. When the risk of major haemorrhage was added to the apparent benefit of clopidogrel/aspirin in CURE, the relative risk reduction favouring the combination over aspirin fell from 20 to 8% [26].

Combined therapy with aspirin and clopidogrel has been tested specifically in patients with symptomatic cerebrovascular disease enrolled in MATCH (Management of Atherothrombosis with Clopidogrel in High-Risk Patients with Recent Transient Ischaemic Attack or Ischaemic Stroke) [28]. This randomised, controlled clinical trial recruited 7599 subjects with TIA or stroke and at least one vascular risk factor to treatment with clopidogrel 75 mg/day and random assignment to low-dose aspirin (75 mg/day) or placebo. The primary endpoint was the first occurrence of any event in the composite of ischaemic stroke, MI, vascular death, and re-hospitalisation for acute ischaemic disease in any circulatory system. The numbers of patients who incurred primary outcome events, 596 (16%) in the aspirin/clopidogrel combination (n = 3797 assigned to treatment) and 636 (17%) in the clopidogrel monotherapy group (n = 3802 assigned), were effectively identical, producing no reduction in absolute or relative risk. However, the number of patients with life-threatening bleeding events, most commonly gastrointestinal haemorrhage, almost doubled from 49 (1%) in the clopidogrel monotherapy group (n = 3781 assigned with complete safety profile) to 96 (3%) in the aspirin/clopidogrel combination (n = 3759 assigned; 95% CI 1.26 [0.64–1.88]; $P < 0.0001$). Addition of low-dose aspirin to clopidogrel in MATCH resulted in a significantly higher bleeding rate that offset any potential benefit.

Because of differences in subject population, study design, and selected outcome measures, the TASS, CATS, CAPRIE, AAASPS, and MATCH studies cannot be employed to rationalise the choice of one thienopyridine compound over the other for secondary stroke prevention. However, ticlopidine is recognised to have a less acceptable side-effect profile because of reversible neutropaenia observed in the TASS and CATS studies (0.9% of treated subjects) and for more than 60 reported cases of thrombocytopaenia, thrombotic thrombocytopaenic purpura (TTP), and aplastic anaemia resulting from prolonged exposure to this drug. [27, 30]. Clopidogrel has also been associated with higher than expected incidence of TTP during the first two weeks of drug administration [31], although the overall risk is clearly lower than with ticlopidine. Because of the more favourable safety margin of clopidogrel over ticlopidine, Albers and colleagues (2004) [19] representing the Seventh Consensus Conference on Antithrombotic Therapy of the American College of Chest Physicians, recommend clopidogrel exclusively for use in all cerebrovascular disorders for which a thienopyridine drug would be considered.

ASPIRIN AND DIPYRIDAMOLE

The anti-aggregatory mechanism of aspirin has been described. Dipyridamole exerts multiple actions on platelets and endothelial cells to prevent thrombosis. It inhibits cyclic nucleotide phosphodiesterase activity, thereby increasing the intracellular content of cyclic 3', 5'-guanosine monophosphate (cGMP) and cyclic 3', 5'-adenosine monophosphate (cAMP). These cyclic nucleotides serve as second messengers within the platelet. By increasing the levels of cGMP and cAMP, dipyridamole potentiates the natural anti-aggregatory effects of nitric oxide (NO) and prostacyclin (PGI$_2$) synthesised and released within the vascular lumen. Both NO and PGI$_2$ bind to receptors on the platelet membrane and smooth muscle cells in arterial vessels to stimulate the production of cyclic nucleotides, resulting in vasodilation and inhibition of platelet aggregation [32, 33]. The increase in vessel wall cAMP stimulated by dipyridamole contributes to the antithrombotic effect by decreasing the intrinsic thrombogenicity of the injured vascular surface [34, 35]. Dipyridamole also inhibits the cellular uptake of adenosine, a potent vasodilator and an inhibitor of both platelet activation and aggregation *via* its stimulation of adenylate cyclase [33]. In 1999, the Food and Drug Administration (FDA) approved Aggrenox®, a capsule containing a 25-mg tablet of aspirin and 200 mg of extended release (ER)-dipyridamole in granules, for secondary stroke prevention.

The combination of aspirin and dipyridamole fared poorly in early trials of secondary stroke prevention. A meta-analysis of three studies including 1574 patients with cerebrovascular disease as the dominant presentation of systemic atherosclerosis found an insignificant trend favouring prevention of recurrent, non-fatal stroke with various combinations of aspirin and instant release (IR)-dipyridamole (17% odds reduction compared to aspirin) [36]. However, in 1990, the final results of the first European Stroke Prevention Study (ESPS) were published [37]. In this trial, IR-dipyridamole at a daily dosage of 225 mg (75 mg, three times per day) was combined with aspirin 990 mg daily (330 mg, three times per day) for 2 years in patients with TIA or minor ischaemic stroke. The combination treatment showed a significant relative risk reduction in the incidence of stroke of 38% over placebo, although the contribution of each individual component remained unknown.

The relative risk reduction observed with aspirin and IR-dipyridamole in ESPS-1 was substantially greater than that found in trials using aspirin alone, in part forming the basis of ESPS-2. The objectives of ESPS-2 were to determine the individual efficacy of aspirin and dipyridamole for prophylaxis of secondary stroke, and to establish whether a combination of low-dose aspirin and high-dose, extended release (ER)-dipyridamole was superior to the use of either agent alone [38]. The results of ESPS-2 were published in 1996 and summarised with all supporting data in 1997 [15, 39]. Patients who experienced a stroke or TIA within the three months preceding enrolment were studied in a multicentre, randomised, prospective trial with two years of follow-up. ESPS-2 incorporated a 2×2 factorial study design with random allocation of patients into one of four twice-daily treatment groups: 25 mg aspirin ($n = 1649$), 200 mg ER-dipyridamole ($n = 1654$), 25 mg aspirin plus 200 mg ER-dipyridamole ($n = 1650$), and placebo ($n = 1649$). The combination of low-dose aspirin and ER-dipyridamole was identical to what has now been marketed as Aggrenox®. All randomised patients were included in the statistical analysis for outcome events of fatal or non-fatal stroke, stroke or death from any cause, and all-cause mortality. The investigators found that both dipyridamole and aspirin had an independent and statistically significant effect in reducing the risk of subsequent stroke (16 and 18%, respectively) when compared with placebo. However, the combination of ER-dipyridamole plus aspirin was additive and produced 37% reduction in stroke incidence relative to placebo ($P < 0.001$). Dipyridamole combined with aspirin reduced the risk of stroke by 23% more than aspirin alone ($P = 0.006$).

Aggrenox® is the only combination of aspirin and dipyridamole that has been shown to be effective for secondary stroke prevention. With the completion of the ESPS-2 study, it may be considered as a rational alternative to aspirin for stroke prophylaxis in patients who experience episodes of cerebral ischaemia. Its superiority to clopidogrel and ticlopidine has not been demonstrated in a prospective, comparative clinical trial. Three pivotal clinical trials, TASS, CAPRIE, and ESPS-2, compared individual antiplatelet agents with aspirin. The data from each trial show that, compared with aspirin, there was a greater reduction in the relative risk of the composite vascular outcome of stroke, MI or vascular death with the aspirin/ER-dipyridamole combination used in ESPS-2 than with thienopyridines used in TASS and CAPRIE. Now that physicians are able to choose from aspirin, the thienopyridines, and aspirin/ER-dipyridamole, they can tailor an approach to secondary stroke prevention for each individual patient. The thienopyridines and the aspirin/ER-dipyridamole combination may be particularly beneficial for patients who had their first stroke while taking aspirin and who are not candidates for long-term anticoagulation or a surgical procedure such as carotid endarterectomy. Bolstered by safety concerns associated with use of the thienopyridines, Aggrenox® has become the most attractive alternative to aspirin for prevention of recurrent stroke.

The use of warfarin for the primary prevention of stroke in patients with AF or high risk of cerebral embolisation associated with cardiac valvular prostheses is now established beyond question [40, 41]. The SPIRIT trial was the only large, randomised comparison of vigorous oral anticoagulation (international normalised ratio [INR] of 3.0–4.5) with 30 mg of aspirin per day for prevention of recurrent, non-cardioembolic stroke [42]. This study was stopped prematurely because of a significant increase in the number of major bleeding complications, including intracerebral haemorrhage (ICH), in the anticoagulation group. The Warfarin-Aspirin Recurrent Stroke Study (WARSS) was a prospective, randomised comparison of warfarin dosed to achieve an INR range of 1.4–2.8 with 325 mg of aspirin every day for secondary prophylaxis of non-cardioembolic stroke [43]. This well-designed trial enrolled 2206 patients no later than 30 days after onset of stroke symptoms. The primary endpoint was recurrent stroke or death from any cause within two years of randomisation. The last WARSS patient completed follow-up in 2000 and confirmation of endpoint status exceeded 98% in both treatment groups. With its results now published, WARSS found that there was no significant difference between aspirin and warfarin treatment in recurrent ischaemic stroke, death, or serious haemorrhage, with or without accommodation for patients lost to follow-up [44]. As concluded in an editorial that accompanied publication of the WARSS results [45], warfarin administered to achieve any INR level is more dangerous and costly than aspirin, with no added benefit in efficacy for stroke prophylaxis.

WARSS demonstrated that warfarin has no role in the prevention of recurrent stroke unrelated to AF or cardiac valvular prosthesis. Two substudies utilising the WARSS population, the Antiphospholipid Antibody Stroke Study (APASS) and the Patent Foramen Ovale in Cryptogenic Stroke Study (PICSS), focused on the potential effectiveness of warfarin therapy in specific cohorts of stroke patients. The APASS investigators hoped to determine if warfarin dosed to achieve the WARSS INR range of 2 was more effective than aspirin in preventing recurrent stroke associated with elevated titres of antiphospholipid antibodies. As published in 2004 [46], APASS showed that the presence of an antiphospholipid antibody (lupus anticoagulant or anti-cardiolipin antibody) in patients with ischaemic stroke did not predict either increased risk for subsequent vascular occlusive events over two years or a differential response to warfarin or aspirin therapy. In PICSS, the effectiveness of aspirin and warfarin therapy was examined in a cohort of the WARSS population who had PFO or other structural anomalies of the heart discovered on transoesophageal echocardiography (TEE). The PICSS study found that the presence of large or small PFO with or without atrial septal aneurysm had no effect on the rate of recurrent vascular thrombotic events and was not modified by patient exposure to warfarin or aspirin [47].

In another examination of the role of warfarin for secondary stroke prevention in a specific cohort of patients, the Warfarin Aspirin Symptomatic Intracranial Disease (WASID) study was performed as a retrospective trial in patients with 50–99% stenosis of an intracranial artery [48]. Sixty-three patients received 325 mg of aspirin and 88 were anticoagulated with warfarin. There was a significantly lower incidence of vascular events in the warfarin-treated group but an increased incidence of major haemorrhagic complications. A prospective clinical trial funded by the National Institute of Neurological Disorders and Stroke, also titled WASID, has been terminated prematurely in a futility analysis showing that warfarin is not superior to aspirin for prevention of recurrent stroke associated with intracranial arterial stenosis, when balanced against haemorrhagic complications [49].

In present-day stroke therapy, warfarin is of demonstrated value only as a primary prophylactic agent in patients with AF and mechanical cardiac prostheses. The WARSS trial clearly proved that it is not superior to antithrombotic therapy for prevention of recurrent, non-cardiogenic stroke. The ongoing European–Australian Stroke Prevention in Reversible Ischaemia Trial (ESPRIT) will compare an intermediate range of INR values (2.0–3.0) to two different antiplatelet regimens [50], but its impact on clinical practice after WARSS cannot be foreseen. Because of the risk of spontaneous haemorrhage from occult mycotic aneurysms in the brain, warfarin is not indicated for prophylaxis against cardiogenic emboli associated with acute or subacute bacterial endocarditis. As shown by APASS, it does not have demonstrated superiority to aspirin for prevention of stroke in patients with the prothrombotic disorder associated with the antiphospholipid antibody syndrome.

As demonstrated by PICSS, warfarin is no more effective than aspirin for prevention of paradoxical emboli to the brain in patients with PFO. As predicted by the WASID prospective study, warfarin is not superior to aspirin for prevention of recurrent ischaemic stroke associated with intracranial arterial stenosis.

THROMBOLYSIS IN ACUTE ISCHAEMIC STROKE

The most exciting advance that has emerged from the past 25 years of clinical research in acute stroke therapy is intravenous or intra-arterial thrombolysis. The first major trial reporting probable efficacy was the European Cooperative Acute Stroke Study (ECASS) [51] conducted in more than 70 centres distributed throughout 14 countries. ECASS I was a placebo-controlled, randomised, prospective trial designed to test the efficacy and safety of 1.1 mg/kg recombinant tissue plasminogen activator (rt-PA) given intravenously in acute ischaemic stroke. All patients were enrolled within 6 h of the onset of symptoms. At three months, primary endpoints were scored on the Barthel Index (BI), a 100-point instrument designed to test independence in activities of daily living, and the modified Rankin scale (mRS), an array of six levels varying from normal function to death. Cerebral angiography was not required for randomisation or confirmation of arterial occlusion. Patients were excluded if an initial CT scan showed haemorrhage, early signs of brain oedema, or a zone of decreased tissue density exceeding 33% of the projected distribution of the middle cerebral artery (MCA). The statistical analysis of ECASS was designed to detect a difference of 15 or more BI points or of at least one level on mRS. The ECASS investigators enrolled 620 patients, but only 511 patients remained eligible for statistical analysis after exclusion of protocol violations. The rate of symptomatic ICH was higher in the treated patients (19.8 vs. 6.5% in the placebo group), but there was no significant difference in the mortality rate at one month. Intention-to-treat analysis of data from all 620 patients showed no difference in outcome between the treatment and placebo groups. After exclusion of the 109 patients because of protocol violations pertaining to misinterpreted CT scans or entry criteria, the treatment group had an absolute increase of 11.7% in the number of patients with favourable mRS measured at 90 days.

The NINDS (National Institute of Neurological Disorders and Stroke) rt-PA Stroke Study Group published its historic findings in December of 1995, less than one year after the ECASS report. The NINDS investigators had also published two open-label, dose-escalation studies showing that administration of less than 0.95 mg/kg of rt-PA could be done in relative safety and resulted in early neurological improvement [52, 53]. Based upon the encouraging results of these open-label studies, the NINDS group proceeded with a randomised, double-blind, placebo-controlled, prospective trial that was conducted in two parts. Part 1 assessed changes in neurological deficits 24 h after the onset of stroke. Part 2 was conducted as a pivotal efficacy trial to determine whether treatment with rt-PA resulted in sustained clinical benefit at three months. To prevent bias, the investigators remained unaware of the results of Part 1 until Part 2 had been completed. The primary hypothesis for Part 2 was that there would be 'consistent and persuasive difference between the rt-PA and placebo groups in terms of the proportion of patients who recovered with minimal or no deficit three months after treatment'. Each patient was treated intravenously with placebo or rt-PA in a dose of 0.9 mg/kg, 10% of which was given as a bolus followed by delivery of the remaining 90% as a constant infusion over 60 min. All patients had to be enrolled and treated within three hours of the onset of symptoms. To detect intracranial haemorrhage, CT scans were performed at 24 h, between 7 and 10 days after the onset of stroke, and if neurological deterioration occurred at any time after treatment. Four outcome measures, including the BI, the mRS, the Glasgow outcome scale, and the NIH stroke scale (NIHSS), were fashioned into a global test statistic applied to the primary hypothesis of Part 2.

Eight centres in the United States enrolled 624 patients in the NINDS study between 1991 and 1994. In Part 1, there was no difference between the placebo and treatment groups in the primary outcome measure completed at 24 h (improvement by 4 or more points on the NIHSS or complete resolution of neurological deficit). In Part 2, the number of patients with favourable scores on each of the four outcome measures after three months was higher in the treatment group than in the placebo arm. As evaluated by the global test statistic, the odds ratio for a favourable outcome with administration of rt-PA was 1.7 (95% CI 1.2–2.6; $P = 0.008$), 30% higher than would be seen in placebo-treated patients. As compared with the placebo group, there was a 12% absolute increase in the number of patients with BI of 95 or 100 in the rt-PA group. There was also an 11% absolute increase in the number of treated patients with an NIHSS of 0 or 1. Similar results demonstrating the benefit of active treatment were seen with the mRS and Glasgow outcome scales. These beneficial effects were so robust that they occurred despite stratification of the patients according to age, stroke subtype or severity, and presymptomatic use of aspirin. Furthermore, the NINDS investigators published follow-up data showing that the 30% greater likelihood of favourable outcome noted three months after treatment persisted to six and 12 months [54]. They also conducted a cost–benefit analysis that demonstrated net savings and improved quality of life for patients treated with recombinant rt-PA [55].

Although patients treated with rt-PA fared better than those given placebo, there was no significant difference in mortality between the two groups at three, six, or 12 months [54, 56]. Symptomatic ICH occurred during the first 36 h in 6.4% of the rt-PA treated patients, compared to only 0.6% of patients in the placebo arm ($P < 0.001$). Of the 20 symptomatic haemorrhages that developed in the rt-PA patients during the first 36 h, nine were fatal. Minor external bleeding during the first 10 days was also more common with rt-PA than placebo (23 vs. 3%). Greater severity of the initial neurological deficit and evidence of oedema or mass effect on the baseline CT scan were associated with higher risk of symptomatic ICH in patients treated with rt-PA [57]. Considering the added burden of mortality and long-term morbidity associated with the ICH that affected patients given rt-PA, it is all the more remarkable that this treatment remained significantly effective over placebo up to 12 months later. After FDA approval of rt-PA in 1996, the Stroke Council of the American Stroke Association, a division of the American Heart Association (AHA), issued practice guidelines for its use in acute ischaemic stroke [58]. These guidelines recommend administering intravenous rt-PA at a dose of 0.9 mg/kg (maximum dose 90 mg) to ischaemic stroke patients who present within three hours of symptom onset. A loading bolus of 10% of the total dose should be given over one minute with the balance to be infused over one hour.

Adherence to the guidelines for thrombolytic therapy is mandatory, as shown by a report on community use of rt-PA from Cleveland-area hospitals. Katzan and colleagues [59] found an in-hospital mortality rate of 15.7% and ICH occurrence of 22% in 70 patients treated with rt-PA. These authors found deviations from the national guidelines in 50% of cases, including use of antithrombotic drugs within 24 h of rt-PA administration in 37.1% and treatment beyond three hours in 12.9%. Mortality and haemorrhage rates approximate those observed with the NINDS rt-PA Stroke Study when the drug is used by well-trained stroke therapists following the guidelines written in advisory statements published by the AHA and the American Academy of Neurology [60, 61].

Other trials of systemic thrombolytic therapy in acute ischaemic stroke have failed to meet the standard set by the NINDS rt-PA Stroke Study, possibly because treatment was delayed beyond three hours [62]. Three large, randomised, double-blind, placebo-controlled trials evaluating intravenous streptokinase given up to six hours after the onset of stroke symptoms showed no benefit before being terminated prematurely because of increased rates of ICH and mortality in treated patients [63–65]. Because of these drawbacks, streptokinase has been abandoned as therapy for acute ischaemic stroke. In the wake of the NINDS rt-PA Stroke Study, two groups of investigators attempted to determine if plasminogen activator could be effective even when administered more than three hours after the onset of stroke symptoms. In the European Cooperative Acute Stroke Study II (ECASS II), patients who presented within six hours of the onset of ischaemic stroke symptoms were treated using the NINDS rt-PA dosing regimen of 0.9 mg/kg [66]. To prevent the large number of protocol violations observed in ECASS I, the steering committee for ECASS II undertook more rigorous training of investigators to improve interpretation of CT scans and treat hypertension appropriately. The primary endpoint was a favourable outcome on the mRS, using the dichotomised method of analysis employed in the NINDS rt-PA Stroke Study. Eight hundred patients were enrolled in ECASS II, but only 158 (19.8%) were treated within three hours. A favourable outcome of no more then 1 point on the mRS was seen in 40.3% of patients in the rt-PA group and 36.6% in the placebo group, but was not statistically significant. *Post hoc* analysis based on a dichotomised mRS representing physical independence (0–2) uncovered a statistically significant benefit to treatment with rt-PA, with 54.3% of treated patients returning to independence compared to 46% of placebo patients ($P = 0.024$). Symptomatic ICH occurred more frequently in the rt-PA treated group (8.8%) compared to 3.4% in the placebo group, but there was no difference in mortality at 30 or 90 days. The ECASS investigators concluded that their data failed to support the use of rt-PA beyond three hours.

The second attempt to extend the time window of rt-PA administration was the Alteplase Thrombolysis for Acute Noninterventional Therapy in Ischemic Stroke (ATLANTIS) study [67]. Like ECASS II, ATLANTIS was originally designed to show if the benefits of systemic thrombolysis could extend up to six hours. After the publication of the NINDS rt-PA Stroke Study in 1995, the time window for enrolment was changed to encompass three to five hours. The primary endpoint for the modified study was good outcome defined as a score of 0 or 1 point on the NIHSS at 90 days. After 761 patients had been enrolled in ATLANTIS, the trial was terminated prematurely because of projected lack of benefit with active treatment. Again there was no difference in mortality between the two treatment groups, suggesting that 'delayed' administration of rt-PA was safe. The ATLANTIS investigators followed the precedent established by their counterparts in ECASS II by concluding that the use of rt-PA for acute ischaemic stroke should not be undertaken after three hours.

Several meta-analyses have been performed on pooled data from the accumulated thrombolytic treatment studies to determine a consensus on the use of rt-PA in acute ischaemic stroke. Hacke and colleagues [68] evaluated the data in the NINDS rt-PA Stroke Study and both ECASS trials, for an aggregate total of 2044 patients (1034 rt-PA-treated and 1010 placebo-treated subjects) who received 0.9 or 1.1 mg/kg rt-PA up to six hours after estimated stroke onset. To reconcile differences between definitions of clinically relevant ICH after thrombolysis, this meta-analysis included all cases of symptomatic ICH in the NINDS trial with both types of parenchymal haemorrhage (PH1 and PH2) in the ECASS trials. There was a modest differential effect on clinically relevant ICH in rt-PA-treated patients, driven by time to treatment ≤3 or 6 h (odds ratio [OR] 2.68; 95% CI 1.56–4.62 vs. OR 3.23; 95% CI 2.39–4.37, respectively), with no change in overall mortality. A similar differential supporting earlier treatment was observed in reduction of combined disability and death (mRS ≥3) with 45% reduction of unfavourable outcome after treatment ≤3 h and 37% reduction at ≤6 h. The Cochrane Library [69] analysed all randomised, placebo-controlled trials of any thrombolytic agent in patients with ischaemic stroke through completion of the PROACT studies (see below), resulting in an aggregate of 5216 patients (2889 in rt-PA trials). Although exposure to thrombolytic therapy increased the risk of death within the first 10 days after ischaemic stroke (OR 1.85; 95% CI 1.48–2.32), surviving patients were less likely to experience delayed death or severe disability (mRS ≥3) when treated ≤3 (OR 0.58; 95% CI 0.46–0.74) or 6 h (0.83; 95% CI 0.73–0.94) after stroke symptom onset. In the most recently published meta-analysis including only large, randomised trials in which rt-PA was compared to placebo [70], data from the NINDS rt-PA Stroke Study (Parts 1 and 2), both

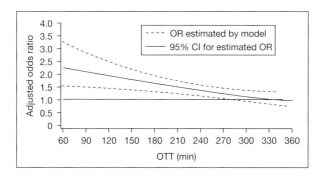

Figure 15.2   Model estimating odds ratio for favourable outcome at three months in rt-PA-treated patients compared with controls from a meta-analysis of ECASS I and II, NINDS rt-PA Stroke Study, and ATLANTIS (Reprinted with permission [70]).

ECASS trials, and ATLANTIS were considered together to derive an aggregate of 2775 patients. The odds of a favourable, 3-month outcome, defined as mRS ≤1, BI 95–100, and NIHSS ≤1, decreased as time to treatment increased. The OR for favourable outcome with rt-PA treatment within 0–90 min was 2.8 (95% CI 1.8–4.5), compared to 1.6 (95% CI 1.1–2.2) for 91–180 min, 1.4 (95% CI 1.1–1.9) for 181–270 min, and 1.2 (95% CI 0.9–1.5) for 271–360 min. Figure 15.2 is taken from the original publication of this meta-analysis and shows that the point estimate of the odds of a favourable outcome after rt-PA treatment, adjusted for age, baseline glucose level and various other factors, is close to 1.0 with rt-PA treatment at 360 min, suggesting reduced probability of benefit beyond this time. Higher risk of ICH (PH2 by ECASS criteria) was associated with exposure to rt-PA ($P = 0.0001$) and age ($P = 0.0002$) but not time to treatment, implying that the stepwise fall in OR for favourable outcome was driven by the diminishing life span of the ischaemic penumbra rather than by increasing risk of haemorrhage with delayed treatment.

UNANSWERED QUESTIONS IN STROKE THERAPY

What is the role of intra-arterial thrombolysis in the treatment of acute ischaemic stroke?
Direct intra-arterial infusion of a thrombolytic agent into a freshly occluded cerebral blood vessel may be an effective alternative to systemic thrombolysis. Intra-arterial thrombolysis has the theoretical advantage of delivering high concentrations of drug to the clot and minimising systemic complications. The tip of a micro-catheter used to administer the thrombolytic agent may also be employed to physically disrupt the clot in support of the chemical action of the drug. These potential advantages must be weighed against the longer time and highly specialised facilities required to perform diagnostic cerebral angiography that must precede intra-arterial thrombolysis. A geographic analysis of the United States showed that only 37% of the American population would have access to centres capable of performing intra-arterial thrombolysis [71], whereas most community hospitals should be capable of offering systemic rt-PA.

Several non-randomised studies of intra-arterial thrombolysis have shown impressive patency rates exceeding 50% with risk of ICH comparable to that observed in the NINDS rt-PA Stroke Study [62, 72–75]. Recombinant t-PA is the only drug that may be used off-label for intra-arterial thrombolysis in the United States, after problems in the industrial synthesis of urokinase caused its removal from the commercial market. Recombinant prourokinase (rpro-UK; Prolyse), the inactive single chain precursor of urokinase that has greater fibrin specificity, has been used in two randomised trials of intra-arterial thrombolysis in acute ischaemic stroke. The Prolyse in Acute Cerebral Thromboembolism Trial (PROACT) was a phase II study that enrolled patients who presented within six hours of symptom onset and had acute occlusion of the MCA on angiography [76]. Forty-six patients who displayed Thrombolysis in Acute Myocardial Infarction (TIMI) grade 0 or 1 of the M1 or M2 portions of the MCA were randomised 2:1 to receive intra-arterial rpro-UK (6 mg) or placebo over 120 min into the proximal face of the thrombus. All patients received intravenous heparin. Recanalisation efficacy was evaluated at the end of the 120-min infusion and ICH causing neurological deterioration was assessed at 24 h. Partial (TIMI 2) or complete (TIMI 3) reperfusion through the occluded MCA segment was observed in 58% of the rpro-UK group and in only 14% of the placebo-treated patients ($P = 0.017$). Haemorrhagic transformation causing neurological deterioration within 24 h of treatment occurred in 15.4% of the rpro-UK-treated patients and 7.1% of the placebo group, but was not significant due to the small numbers of subjects. Based upon the encouraging results of the original PROACT study, PROACT II was designed as a phase III trial and conducted in 54 university and community hospitals in the United States and Canada. One hundred and eighty patients with the same clinical and angiographic characteristics as those enrolled in the original PROACT study were randomised 2:1 to receive 9 mg of intra-arterial rpro-UK over 120 min plus intravenous heparin or heparin only. Recanalisation efficacy was again determined at the end of 120 min. The primary endpoint of PROACT II was the percentage of patients achieving an mRS of 2 or less at 90 days following the initial therapy. For this primary analysis, 40% of rpro-UK patients and 25% of control patients met the criteria showing benefit of intra-arterial rpro-UK ($P = 0.04$). There was no significant difference in mortality between the rpro-UK (25%) and control (27%) patients. The recanalisation rate was 66% for the rpro-UK group and 18% for controls ($P < 0.001$). Intracerebral haemorrhage with neurological deterioration within 24 h occurred in 10% of rpro-UK patients and 2% of control patients ($P = 0.06$).

The results of the PROACT studies indicate that intra-arterial thrombolysis can be performed effectively in patients with occlusion of major intracranial vessels. Although PROACT II showed clinical efficacy at 90 days, the high rate of ICH associated with intra-arterial clot lysis prevented FDA approval of rpro-UK. Notwithstanding the Herculean efforts required of the participating investigators in PROACT II (12 323 patients were screened clinically), a third PROACT study is being considered to provide additional support for FDA approval. The PROACT studies have shown that intra-arterial thrombolysis is feasible and will be available in a limited number of comprehensive stroke care centres in metropolitan areas.

In an attempt to make intra-arterial thrombolysis more accessible, the Emergency Management of Stroke (EMS) Investigators performed a small pilot study (EMS Bridging Trial) comparing this therapeutic strategy to its combination with intravenous (IV) thrombolysis begun in the community setting [77]. This study was initiated prior to the NINDS rt-PA Stroke Study and was terminated once that trial began. Thirty-five patients presenting within 3 h of the onset of stroke symptoms were randomised to receive either 0.6 mg/kg of IV rt-PA or placebo and were taken immediately to angiography upon arrival at a specialised centre. If thrombotic occlusion of an intracranial artery was identified, patients were given intra-arterial (IA) rt-PA. The dose of intra-arterial (IA) rt-PA was determined by the amount needed to establish vessel patency and did not exceed 20 mg. Mechanical disruption of the clot was permitted. In the group receiving combination therapy, 67% had partial or complete recanalisation at 2 h compared to 60% of patients undergoing intra-arterial thrombolysis. Three patients had life-threatening ICH, all in the combination therapy group. Although the small number of patients included in the EMS Bridging Trial did not afford a scientifically valid conclusion, it showed proof of concept for the 'drip [rt-PA] and ship' approach that is now used informally in several locations around the United States.

In the wake of the EMS Bridging Trial, several small pilot studies confirmed the feasibility of the IV–IA combination approach [78–80]. The latest development in combination thrombolytic therapy for acute stroke has been the Interventional Management of Stroke (IMS) study, funded by the NINDS, that was begun in 2001 and has now been published [81]. In the IMS trial, 80 subjects with median NIHSS of 18 were enrolled at 17 medical centres in the United States in an open-labeled, single-group investigation of IV rt-PA (0.6 mg/kg) administered within 3 h of stroke symptom onset, followed immediately by cerebral angiography to determine the presence of an intra-arterial thrombus. Once the thrombus was identified, a microcatheter was positioned to inject rt-PA beyond and within the clot and to facilitate continuous infusion for up to 2 h or until thrombolysis was achieved. Intra-arterial rt-PA infusion had to begin within 5 h of symptom onset. Of the 80 patients enrolled, 77 underwent angiography and 62 completed the combined IV–IA therapy. Within the 62 patients who underwent combined therapy, the rate of partial or complete (TIMI 2 or 3) recanalisation was 56% (35/62). Of these 35 subjects, 34% had favourable outcome with mRS 0 – 1 at 3 months, compared to only 12% of patients who did not recanalise ($P = 0.013$). The overall 3-month mortality rate was 16% (13/80 subjects), numerically lower but not statistically different from the placebo-treated (24%) and rt-PA-treated (21%) groups in the NINDS rt-PA Stroke Study [56]. The rate of post-procedural intracerebral haematomas occupying more than 30% of the infarcted tissue and causing local mass effect (ECASS PH2) was 7.5% (6/80 subjects), numerically higher than observed in the rt-PA-treated group (3.4%) in the NINDS rt-PA Stroke Study but not statistically different. Although the results of the IMS trial highlight the potential for combined IV–IA use of thrombolytics to treat acute thrombotic stroke, even more so in consideration of the severe neurological deficits in the enrolled patients, the relatively high rate of 3-month mortality and the allocation of dedicated resources required to achieve the modest gain of the trial demand confirmation in a randomised, placebo-controlled, efficacy trial.

Are there alternatives to intravenous rt-PA for acute ischaemic stroke?

Building upon the success of the NINDS rt-PA Stroke Study, groups of investigators have evaluated other pharmacological agents as alternatives to IV rt-PA. The defibrinogenating agent, ancrod, is extracted from the venom of the Malayan pit viper. A phase III trial of ancrod given within 6 h of stroke onset failed to show benefit, perhaps because fibrinogen levels remained higher than desired [82]. In the more recently completed Stroke Treatment with Ancrod (STAT) trial, 500 patients were randomly assigned to receive ancrod ($n = 248$) or placebo ($n = 252$) as a continuous 72-h intravenous infusion beginning within 3 h of stroke onset followed by 1-h infusions at 96 and 120 h [83]. The ancrod regimen was designed to reduce plasma fibrinogen levels to 1.18–2.03 μmol/l. The primary endpoint was functional status defined as survival to 90 days with a BI of 95 or more or at least the estimated premorbid value. A larger proportion of patients in the ancrod group finished the trial with the targeted BI, 42.2%, than in the placebo group, 34.4% ($P = 0.04$). There was no difference in mortality at 90 days (25.4% for ancrod and 23% for placebo). There was a trend toward a higher rate of symptomatic ICH in the ancrod group vs. placebo (5.2 vs. 2.0%; $P = 0.06$), as well as a significant increase in asymptomatic ICH (19.0 vs. 10.7%; $P = 0.01$). The authors concluded that ancrod could be administered effectively with an acceptable margin of safety. Clinical efficacy was enhanced by more rapid defibrogenation. However, the complexity of titrating the dose of ancrod to serial fibrogen levels makes this therapeutic approach more complex than what is already available with rt-PA at a similar level of haemorrhagic complications. Defibrogenation has also been studied in patients presenting more than six hours after the onset of ischaemic stroke through ESTAT, the European Stroke Treatment with Ancrod Trial, that has not yet been reported [84].

Table 15.1 Comparison of tissue plasminogen activator to desmoteplase

	Tissue plasminogen activator	*Desmoteplase*
Molecular weight	65,000 MW	52,000 MW
Chemical structure	Glycosylated	Non-glycosylated
Half-life	3–6 min	4.5 h
Method of administration	60 min front-loaded infusion	Single-bolus over 2 min
Weight adjustment	Required	Required
Specificity in presence of fibrin	105 000-fold increase	550-fold increase
Selectivity in presence of fibrin compared with fibrinogen	12 900-fold increase	72-fold increase
Defibrinogenation of whole blood	Yes	No
Activated by β-amyloid	Yes	No
Neuronal toxicity *in vitro*	Yes	No

Second-generation thrombolytic or antithrombotic agents are beginning to emerge in clinical trials. A dose-escalation study of E6010, a second-generation thrombolytic drug with a longer half-life than rt-PA, has been conducted in patients presenting within 6 h of symptom onset [85]. Pharmacological antagonists of the GPIIb/IIIa receptor are powerful new antithrombotic agents that may be as beneficial in ischaemic stroke as they are in acute coronary syndromes [86]. Abciximab, a chimeric monoclonal antibody that binds nonspecifically to the GPIIb/IIIa receptor, has been evaluated in the Abciximab in Emergent Stroke Treatment Trial (AbESTT) [87]. In this randomised, double-masked, placebo-controlled phase 2b study, abciximab was given within 6 h of ishaemic stroke onset by bolus (0.25 mg/kg), then by continuous infusion (0.125 mg/kg) over 12 h. More than 50% of the abciximab-treated group had good clinical outcome (mRS 0–1) compared to 40% in placebo-treated controls.

The most promising alternative to rt-PA in the thrombolytic treatment of stroke is desmoteplase, a novel thrombolytic protein isolated from the saliva of South American vampire bats and mass-produced by recombinant technology. As shown in Table 15.1, desmoteplase has several technical advantages over rt-PA in that it is highly specific and selective for fibrin, can be administered rapidly by bolus, minimises systemic and cerebral bleeding by preservation of whole-blood fibrinogen, and has no recognised neurotoxicity. Hacke and colleagues [88] reported the results of a novel phase II trial, Desmoteplase in Acute Stroke (DIAS), in which patients were selected for treatment with desmoteplase or placebo after magnetic resonance (MR) imaging to confirm the presence of a 'perfusion/diffusion' mismatch. In this approach, viable candidates for delayed reperfusional therapy are identified by imaging that will reveal a target volume of poorly perfused, but viable, tissue surrounding an infarct core. The trial was conducted at 44 centres located in 12 countries excluding the United States. The safety endpoint of DIAS was symptomatic ICH. Efficacy endpoints included the rate of reperfusion on MRI obtained 4–8 h after treatment and clinical outcome as assessed by NIHSS, mRS, and BI at 90 days. The first 47 patients were randomised to fixed doses of desmoteplase (25, 37.5, or 50 mg) or placebo without adjustment for body weight. Symptomatic ICH occurred within 24 h of drug administration in 8 of 30 desmoteplase-treated patients (26.7%), causing this dosing regimen to be abandoned in favour of a weight-adjusted strategy (62.5, 90, or 125 µg/kg vs. placebo). After the weight-adjusted regimen was implemented and another 57 patients were enrolled, the overall symptomatic ICH rate fell to 2.2%, the MRI reperfusion rate in the 125 µg/kg dose tier rose to 71.4% ($P = 0.0012$ in comparison to placebo), and favourable 90-day outcome observed with this dose climbed to 60% ($P = 0.009$ in comparison to placebo). At the 2005 International Stroke Conference held in New Orleans, Louisiana, the results of a companion trial conducted in the United States, Dose Escalation Study of Desmoteplase in Acute Ischaemic Stroke (DEDAS), was reported to show no symptomatic ICH in actively-treated patients and no growth of the ischaemic lesion on MRI after treatment with 125 µg/kg desmoteplase. In 2005, a phase III efficacy trial of desmoteplase vs. placebo will be inaugurated at over 100 international centres, using computed tomography (CT) or MRI perfusion studies to recruit patients who present within 3 and 9 h of ischaemic stroke onset.

What is the role of augmentative technology to enhance systemic or intra-arterial thrombolysis in acute stroke?

Despite the demonstrated benefit of systemic thrombolysis and the potential for successful intra-arterial clot lysis shown by the PROACT studies, there are physical barriers that limit the effectiveness of any thrombolytic drug against thrombus lodged within the cerebral circulation. Older thrombi lose intrinsically bound plasminogen, the substrate for the rate-limiting step of conversion to plasmin, and retract from the intimal surface while undergoing chemical changes that make them less receptive to thrombolysis [89]. In addition, the stump-like occlusions typically found in MCA trunk (M1) and carotid 'T' lesions provide only restricted surface area upon which a thrombolytic agent can be injected from an end-hole infusion catheter lodged within the arterial lumen. Most importantly, mechanical removal of the thrombus should minimise the risk of post-reperfusion haemorrhage associated with sole use of a systemic or intra-arterial thrombolytic drug. Among divergent endovascular approaches, the common goals are to achieve recanalisation of the occluded cerebral artery within or acceptably beyond the 3-h time limit for systemic thrombolysis, to control ICH and other periprocedural complications, and to enhance clinical recovery over natural history.

Alternative technology devices that have been developed to augment thrombolysis in acute stroke include catheter-deployed snares [90], intra-arterial lasers, the Angiojet catheter (Possis Medical, Inc., Minneapolis, MN) which dissolves the clot through mechanical disruption and local vortex suction [91], and the EKOS catheter (EKOS, Bothell, WA) which uses high-frequency ultrasound to achieve clot dissolution [see Kuether et al., 2002 for review] [92]. The effect of angioplasty to recanalise acutely occluded cerebral vessels has been reported [93]. Of these, the EKOS MicroLys US catheter (Figure 15.3) is the most promising and has been tested successfully in a recently published safety trial [94]. This device combines a micro-infusion conduit through its distal port for administration of thrombolytic drug with a 2.1-MHz ring sonography transducer that creates a circumferential pulse wave within the artery (see Figure 15.3). The EKOS catheter can be placed coaxially through a sheath-catheter system and navigated over a guidewire. Through activation of the ultrasound transducer, non-thermal micro-cavitation and dissolution of the thrombus can be achieved to expand clot surface area targeted by a thrombolytic drug injected through the distal port. In the safety trial of the EKOS catheter, 14 patients with angiographically demonstrated occlusion of intracranial vessels (five MCA, five carotid 'T', and four basilar artery occlusions) underwent treatment with combined use of the EKOS catheter, administration of rt-PA or reteplase (an alternate plasminogen activator), and intravenous heparin within 6 (anterior circulation occlusions) or 24 (posterior circulation occlusions) hours after symptom onset. Use of the catheter did not result in vessel perforation, dissection, or occlusion, although three of the 12 patients died within 24 h of ICH or brain oedema. Recanalisation rates observed at 60 and 90 min after activation of the EKOS catheter exceeded 60% and were directly comparable to the best angiographic results in PROACT II. After 3 months of follow-up, surviving patients had functional outcomes that were similar to those in the active treatment groups in PROACT II and the EMS trial. The clinical efficacy of augmented thrombolysis with the EKOS catheter awaits a randomised,

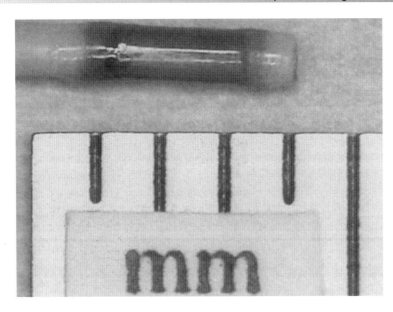

Figure 15.3   The EKOS MicroLys US catheter used to augment intra-arterial thrombolysis by emitting high-frequency, low-energy ultrasound Reproduced with permission [92].

prospective, placebo-controlled trial or an expedited medical device approval from the FDA, such as has been granted for the Merci Retriever device (see below).

Mechanical clot fragmentation using laser technology has been tested in a safety and feasibility study conducted with the endovascular photoacoustic recanalisation (EPAR) device (Endovasix Inc., Belmont, CA) [95]. The emulsification of thrombus achieved by the EPAR is produced by the conversion of photonic to acoustic energy, resulting in mechanical thrombolysis and not direct laser-induced ablation (Figure 15.4). The EPAR catheter is passed coaxially over a guidewire, navigated through the occlusive thrombus in the cerebral artery, activated to draw clot fragments through ports in the tip of the device, and is withdrawn back through the thrombus to achieve complete dissolution. In the EPAR safety trial, 34 patients (median NIHSS 19) were enrolled and treated within 6 or 24 h by location of the thrombus in the anterior or posterior circulation, respectively, as in the EKOS trial. The overall recanalisation rate was 41.1% (14/34 subjects). Complete EPAR treatment was achieved in 18 patients, with vessel recanalisation in 11 (61.1%). An adverse event directly resulting from use of the device caused the death of one patient. Symptomatic haemorrhages occurred in two patients (5.9%) for an overall mortality rate of 38.2%. Thirty days after treatment, five of 34 patients (14.7%) had recovered to mRS score 0–2. As with the EKOS catheter, approval of the EPAR laser device for removal of intra-arterial clot in acute ischaemic stroke must be validated in a properly designed and executed pivotal trial or by specialised device approval from the FDA.

The most spectacular success with an augmentative technology to enhance the effectiveness of thrombolysis for acute thrombotic stroke is the combination of transcranial Doppler (TCD) ultrasound with routine intravenous use of rt-PA. The potential for externally applied, high-frequency, low-energy ultrasound to accelerate clot fragmentation with IV rt-PA and ameliorate embolic stroke has been established in animal models [96]. In 2004, Alexandrov and colleagues [97] published the results of CLOTBUST (Combined Lysis of Thrombus in Brain Ischemia Using Transcranial Ultrasound and Systemic t-PA), a phase II, multicentre trial of standard IV rt-PA and randomisation to continuous or short-term

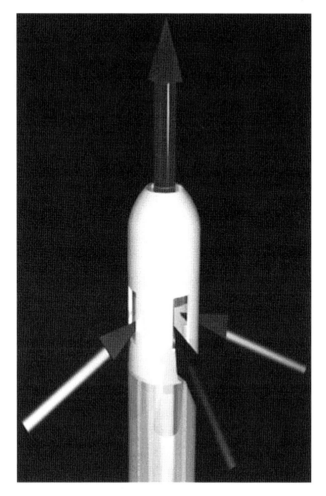

Figure 15.4 EPAR device used to augment intra-arterial thrombolysis by the conversion of photonic to acoustic energy, without direct laser-induced ablation Reproduced with permission [95].

monitoring with TCD. The CLOTBUST investigators enrolled 126 patients within 3 h of stroke onset involving the MCA, treated all with IV rt-PA (0.9 mg/kg total dose), and randomised each to two hours of continuous TCD or periodic, short assessments to evaluate MCA patency. Standard, 2-MHz, pulsed-wave diagnostic ultrasound transducers were used at all sites. Endovascular treatment to include IA thrombolysis was permitted after two hours of study participation, if the MCA remained occluded. The primary endpoint in CLOTBUST was complete recanalisation of the occluded MCA with early or dramatic recovery by prespecified intervals on the NIHSS. The median NIHSS at baseline was similar in the two groups (16 in continuous TCD and 17 in control; P = NS), there was no significant delay with incorporation of TCD into IV rt-PA treatment (150 min in continuous TCD and 130 min in control; P = NS), and the rate of symptomatic ICH within 72 h of treatment was exactly the same (4.8%). Within two hours of rt-PA administration, the combined primary endpoint was reached by 31 patients in the continuous TCD group (49%) vs. 19 (30%) in the control group (P = 0.03). At 3 months, there was a numerically larger proportion of patients

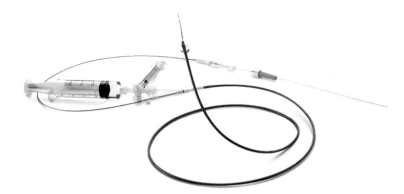

Figure 15.5   The Merci Retriever used to improve cerebral arterial flow by mechanical retraction of thrombus (courtesy of Concentric Medical Inc., Mountain View, CA).

in the continuous TCD group who had mRS of 0 or 1 (42%; 22/53) compared to the control group (29%; 14/49; P = NS) with no difference in mortality. CLOTBUST demonstrated that continuous TCD monitoring can safely augment systemic thrombolysis for acute ischaemic stroke, should be amenable to demonstration of clinical efficacy in a properly designed and executed phase III trial, and would reduce dependency on endovascular specialists to perform 'rescue' treatment of intra-arterial thrombosis. Although this approach successfully adapts an existing technology for a new and valuable purpose, widespread implementation of the technique would be limited by its application to only the small number of patients with major occlusions of the MCA or the basilar artery, the requirement for highly trained operators spending extended time at the patient bedside, and the addition of technical complexity to systemic thrombolysis that could further limit the already constrained number of rt-PA treatments.

Is mechanical clot removal an alternative to systemic or intra-arterial thrombolysis for acute stroke?
Presently, the only endovascular device approved by the FDA for removal of intra-arterial thrombus to reperfuse ischaemic brain is the Merci Retriever (Concentric Medical Inc., Mountain View, CA; Figure 15.5). In the open-label phase I trial of this device (Mechanical Embolus Removal in Cerebral Ischaemia; MERCI 1) [98], 28 patients with acute ischaemic stroke of less than 8-h onset underwent control angiography to demonstrate acute embolic occlusion of the internal carotid artery, the M1 segment of the MCA, the basilar artery, or the vertebral artery. The primary outcome measure in MERCI 1 was defined as TIMI grade 2 or 3 recanalisation without vessel perforation, arterial dissection, or embolisation in a previously uninvolved vascular territory. Successful recanalisation was achieved in 12 patients (43%) using only the Merci Retriever. An additional six patients were recanalised after ineffective deployment of the device followed by intra-arterial administration of rt-PA, for an overall recanalisation rate of 64%. Among the 18 patients who were revascularised, 50% (9/18) made a significant recovery defined as mRS ≤3 (ambulatory with assistance) at 30 days. Of the 10 patients in whom revascularisation failed, none made a significant recovery. There were no cases of symptomatic ICH. Ten patients, 5 of whom achieved TIMI 2 or 3 status after treatment, died from complications of their stroke.

   MERCI 1 was designed as a phase 1 trial with the limited goal of demonstrating safe utilisation of the Merci Retriever in acute ischaemic stroke. A phase 2 study (MERCI 2) [99] has now been completed and showed achievement of recanalisation in comparison to historical controls, the placebo group of PROACT II. Patient selection criteria were the same in the two MERCI trials. In MERCI 2, 114 patients with acute ischaemic stroke due to embolic arterial occlusion underwent deployment of the Merci Retriever and were followed for 90 days afterwards. In the 114 patients, recanalisation was achieved in 61 (54%; 95% CI 44–63%) compared to only 18% in the PROACT II placebo group. Four of the 114 patients (3.5%) experienced device-related complications: two had embolic infarctions during clot retrieval and two developed arterial dissection or vessel perforation. Nine of the 114 patients (8%) experienced symptomatic ICH. Although MERCI 2 was not designed as a clinical efficacy study, it was encouraging to note that 53% of the successfully recanalised patients completed 90-day follow-up with mRS of 0–2 compared to only 6% in the unrecanalised group. Based on the consideration of an advisory panel, the Center for Devices and Radiological Health within the FDA approved the Merci Retriever '. . . to restore blood flow in the neurovasculature by removing thrombus . . .,' although the clinical efficacy of the device has yet to be established in comparison to placebo-treated controls [100]. A placebo-controlled trial of mechanical embolectomy using the Merci Retriever (Magnetic Resonance and REcanalisation of Stroke Clots Using Embolectomy; MR-RESCUE) is presently underway. Patients with anterior circulation infarcts who present within 8 h of stroke onset will be randomised to mechanical embolectomy or medical therapy: the response to therapy will be stratified by the MR pattern at randomisation ('penumbral' vs. 'non-penumbral'). Once completed and if successful, MR-RESCUE could provide a pivotal test of clinical efficacy for use of the Merci Retriever in reperfusion of ischaemic brain that has not yet been accomplished with the MERCI I and II trials.

ACKNOWLEDGEMENTS

Financial support was provided by NIH M01 RR02602 (University of Kentucky General Clinical Research Center). The authors would also like to thank Sherry Chandler Williams, E.L.S., for preparation and editing of the chapter.

REFERENCES

1. Peters KD, Kochanek KD, Murphy SL. Deaths: final data for 1996. *Natl Vital Stat Rep* 1998; 47:1–100.
2. Broderick J, Brott T, Kothari R *et al*. The Greater Cincinnati/Northern Kentucky Stroke Study: preliminary first-ever and total incidence rates of stroke among blacks. *Stroke* 1998; 29:415–421.
3. Matchar DB, Samsa GP, Matthews JR *et al*. The Stroke Prevention Policy Model: linking evidence and clinical decisions. *Ann Intern Med* 1997; 127:704–711.
4. Taylor TN, Davis PH, Torner JC, Holmes J, Meyer JW, Jacobson MF. Lifetime cost of stroke in the United States. *Stroke* 1996; 27:1459–1466.
5. Fields WS, Lemak NA, Frankowski RF, Hardy RJ. Controlled trial of aspirin in cerebral ischemia. *Stroke* 1977; 8:301–314.
6. A randomized trial of aspirin and sulfinpyrazone in threatened stroke. The Canadian Cooperative Study Group. *New Engl J Med* 1978; 299:53–59.
7. Reuther R, Dorndorf W. Aspirin in patients with cerebral ischemia and normal angiograms or non-surgical lesions: the results of a double-blind trial. In: Breddin K, Dorndorf W, Loew D, Marx R (eds). Acetylsalicylic acid in cerebral ischemia and coronary heart disease: IV: Colfarit-Symposion, Berlin, 30.9.–1.10.1977. FK Schattauer Verlag, Stuttgart, Germany, 1978, pp 97–106.
8. Guiraud-Chaumeil B, Rascol A, David J, Boneu B, Clanet M, Bierme R. Prévention des récidives des accidents vasculaires cérébraux ischémiques par les anti-agrégants plaquettaires: Résultats d'un essai thérapeutique contrôlé de 3 ans. *Revue Neurologique (Paris)* 1982; 138:367–385.
9. Bousser MG, Eschwege E, Haguenau M *et al*. 'AICLA' controlled trial of aspirin and dipyridamole in the secondary prevention of athero-thrombotic cerebral ischemia. *Stroke* 1983; 14:5–14.
10. Sorensen PS, Pedersen H, Marquardsen J *et al*. Acetylsalicylic acid in prevention of stroke in patients with reversible cerebral ishaemic attacks: a Danish Cooperative Study. *Stroke* 1983; 14:15–22.
11. Britton M, Helmers C, Samuelsson K. High-dose acetylsalicylic acid after cerebral infarction: A Swedish Cooperative Study. *Stroke* 1987; 18:325–334.

12. A comparison of two doses of aspirin (30 mg vs. 283 mg a day) in patients after a transient ischemic attack or minor ischemic stroke. The Dutch TIA Trial Study Group. *N Engl J Med* 1991; 325:1261–1266.

13. Swedish Aspirin Low-Dose Trial (SALT) of 75 mg aspirin as secondary prophylaxis after cerebrovascular ischaemic events. The SALT Collaborative Group. *Lancet* 1991; 338:1345–1349.

14. The United Kingdom transient ischaemic attack (UK-TIA) aspirin trial: Final results. UK-TIA Study Group. *J Neurol Neurosurg Psychiatry* 1991; 54:1044–1054.

15. Diener HC, Cunha L, Forbes C, Sivenius J, Smets P, Lowenthal A. European Stroke Prevention Study. 2. Dipyridamole and acetylsalicylic acid in the secondary prevention of stroke. *J Neurol Sci* 1996; 143:1–13.

16. Collaborative meta-analysis of randomised trials of antiplatelet therapy for prevention of death, myocardial infarction, and stroke in high risk patients. *Br Med J* 2002; 324:71–86.

17. Algra A, van Gijn J. Aspirin at any dose above 30 mg offers only modest protection after cerebral ischemia. *J Neurol Neurosurg Psychiatry* 1996; 60:197–199.

18. Johnson ES, Lanes SF, Wentworth CEI, Satterfield MH, Abebe BL, Dicker LW. A metaregression analysis of the dose-response effect of aspirin on stroke. *Arch Int Med* 1999; 159:1248–1253.

19. Albers GW, Amarenco P, Easton JD, Sacco RL, Teal P. Antithrombotic and thrombolytic therapy for ischemic stroke: the Seventh ACCP Conference on Antithrombotic and Thrombolytic Therapy. *Chest* 2004; 126:483S–512S.

20. Hass WK, Easton JD, Adams HP, Jr et al. A randomized trial comparing ticlopidine hydrochloride with aspirin for the prevention of stroke in high-risk patients. Ticlopidine Aspirin Stroke Study Group. *N Engl J Med* 1989; 321:501–507.

21. Gent M, Blakely JA, Easton JD et al. The Canadian American Ticlopidine Study (CATS) in thromboembolic stroke. *Lancet* 1989; 1:1215–1220.

22. Gorelick PB, Richardson D, Kelly M et al. Aspirin and ticlopidine for prevention of recurrent stroke in black patients: a randomized trial. *JAMA* 2003; 289:2947–2957.

23. A randomised, blinded, trial of clopidogrel versus aspirin in patients at risk of ischaemic events (CAPRIE). CAPRIE Steering Committee. *Lancet* 1996; 348:1329–1339.

24. Yusuf S, Zhao F, Mehta SR, Chrolavicius S, Tognoni G, Fox KK. Effects of clopidogrel in addition to aspirin in patients with acute coronary syndromes without ST-segment elevation. *N Engl J Med* 2001; 345:494–502.

25. Steinhubl SR, Berger PB, Mann JT, 3rd et al. Early and sustained dual oral antiplatelet therapy following percutaneous coronary intervention: a randomized controlled trial. *JAMA* 2002; 288: 2411–2420.

26. Albers GW, Amarenco P. Combination therapy with clopidogrel and aspirin: can the CURE results be extrapolated to cerebrovascular patients? *Stroke* 2001; 32:2948.

27. Albers GW. Choice of end points in antiplatelet trials: which outcomes are most relevant to stroke patients? *Neurology* 2000; 54:1022–1028.

28. Diener HC, Bogousslavsky J, Brass LM et al. Aspirin and clopidogrel compared with clopidogrel alone after recent ischaemic stroke or transient ischaemic attack in high-risk patients (MATCH): randomised, double-blind, placebo-controlled trial. *Lancet* 2004; 364:331–337.

29. Bennett CL, Weinberg PD, Rozenberg-Ben-Dror K, Yarnold PR, Kwaan HC, Green D. Thrombotic thrombocytopenic purpura associated with ticlopidine. A review of 60 cases. *Ann Intern Med* 1998; 128:541–544.

30. Love BB, Biller J, Gent M. Adverse haematological effects of ticlopidine. Prevention, recognition and management. *Drug Safety* 1998; 19:89–98.

31. Bennett CL, Connors JM, Carwile JM et al. Thrombotic thrombocytopenic purpura associated with clopidogrel. *N Engl J Med* 2000; 342:1773–1777.

32. Moncada S, Korbut R. Dipyridamole and other phosphodiesterase inhibitors act as antithrombotic agents by potentiating endogenous prostacyclin. *Lancet* 1978; 1:1286–1289.

33. Müller TH, Binder K, Guth BD. Pharmacology of current and future antithrombotic therapies. *Cardiol Clin* 1994; 12:411–442.

34. Weber E, Haas TA, Müller TH et al. Relationship between vessel wall 13-HODE synthesis and vessel wall thrombogenicity following injury: influence of salicylate and dipyridamole treatment. *Thromb Res* 1990; 57:383–392.

35. Buchanan MR, Brister SJ. A rationale for targeting antithrombotic therapy at the vessel wall: improved antithrombotic effect and decreased risk of bleeding. *Wiener Klinische Wochenschrift* 1999; 111:81–89.

36. Wilterdink JL, Easton JD. Dipyridamole plus aspirin in cerebrovascular disease. *Arch Neurol* 1999; 56:1087–1092.
37. European Stroke Prevention Study. European Stroke Prevention Study Group. *Stroke* 1990; 221:1122–1130.
38. Diener HC. Dipyridamole trials in stroke prevention. *Neurology* 1998; 51:S17–S19.
39. European Stroke Prevention Study 2. Efficacy and safety data. *J Neurol Sci* 1997; 151(suppl):S1–S77.
40. Barnett HJ, Eliasziw M, Meldrum HE. Drugs and surgery in the prevention of ischemic stroke. *N Engl J Med* 1995; 332:238–248.
41. Ezekowitz MD, Levine JA. Preventing stroke in patients with atrial fibrillation. *JAMA* 1999; 281:1830–1835.
42. A randomized trial of anticoagulants versus aspirin after cerebral ischemia of presumed arterial origin. The Stroke Prevention in Reversible Ischemia Trial (SPIRIT) Study Group. *Ann Neurol* 1997; 42:857–865.
43. The feasibility of a collaborative double-blind study using an anticoagulant. The Warfarin-Aspirin Recurrent Stroke Study (WARSS), The Antiphospholipid Antibodies and Stroke Study (APASS), The Patent Foramen Ovale in Cryptogenic Stroke Study, The Hemostatic Activation Study (HAS), The Genes for Stroke Study (GENESIS). *Cerebrovasc Dis* 1997; 7:100–112.
44. Mohr JP, Thompson JLP, Lazar RM *et al*. A comparison of warfarin and aspirin for the prevention of recurrent ischemic stroke. *N Engl J Med* 2001; 345:1444–1451.
45. Powers WJ. Oral anticoagulant therapy for the prevention of stroke [Editorial]. *N Engl J Med* 2001; 345:1493–1495.
46. Levine SR, Brey RL, Tilley BC *et al*. Antiphospholipid antibodies and subsequent thrombo-occlusive events in patients with ischemic stroke. *JAMA* 2004; 291:576–584.
47. Homma S, Sacco RL, Di Tullio MR, Sciacca RR, Mohr JP. Effect of medical treatment in stroke patients with patent foramen ovale: patent foramen ovale in Cryptogenic Stroke Study. *Circulation* 2002; 105:2625–2631.
48. Chimowitz MI, Kokkinos J, Strong J *et al*. The Warfarin-Aspirin Symptomatic Intracranial Disease Study. *Neurology* 1995; 45:1488–1493.
49. Chimowitz MI, Lynn MJ, Howlett-Smith H *et al*. Comparison of warfarin and aspirin for symptomatic intracranial arterial stenosis. *N Engl J Med* 2005; 352:1305–1316.
50. Major ongoing stroke trials. *Stroke* 2001; 32:2448–2449.
51. Thrombolyse bei Schlaganfall–Ergebnisse der ECASS-Studie (European Cooperative Acute Stroke Study). *Nervenarzt* 1995; 66:1–8.
52. Brott TG, Haley ECJ, Levy DE *et al*. Urgent therapy for stroke. Part I. Pilot study of tissue plasminogen activator administered within 90 minutes. *Stroke* 1992; 23:632–640.
53. Haley EC, Jr, Levy DE, Brott TG *et al*. Urgent therapy for stroke. Part II. Pilot study of tissue plasminogen activator administered 91–180 minutes from onset. *Stroke* 1992; 23:641–645.
54. Kwiatkowski TG, Libman RB, Frankel M *et al*. Effects of tissue plasminogen activator for acute ischemic stroke at one year. National Institute of Neurological Disorders and Stroke Recombinant Tissue Plasminogen Activator Stroke Study Group. *N Engl J Med* 1999; 340:1781–1787.
55. Fagan SC, Morgenstern LB, Petitta A *et al*. Cost-effectiveness of tissue plasminogen activator for acute ischemic stroke. NINDS rt-PA Stroke Study Group. *Neurology* 1998; 50:883–890.
56. Tissue plasminogen activator for acute ischemic stroke. The National Institute of Neurological Disorders and Stroke rt-PA Stroke Study Group. *N Engl J Med* 1995; 333:1581–1587.
57. Intracerebral hemorrhage after intravenous t-PA therapy for ischemic stroke. The NINDS t-PA Stroke Study Group. *Stroke* 1997; 28:2109–2118.
58. Adams HP, Jr, Adams RJ, Brott T *et al*. Guidelines for the early management of patients with ischemic stroke: A scientific statement from the Stroke Council of the American Stroke Association. *Stroke* 2003; 34:1056–1083.
59. Katzan IL, Furlan AJ, Lloyd LE *et al*. Use of tissue-type plasminogen activator for acute ischemic stroke: the Cleveland area experience. *JAMA* 2000; 283:1151–1158.
60. Albers GW, Bates VE, Clark WM, Bell R, Verro P, Hamilton SA. Intravenous tissue-type plasminogen activator for treatment of acute stroke: the Standard Treatment with Alteplase to Reverse Stroke (STARS) study. *JAMA* 2000; 283:1145–1150.
61. Buchan AM, Barber PA, Newcommon N *et al*. Effectiveness of t-PA in acute ischemic stroke: outcome relates to appropriateness. *Neurology* 2000; 54:679–684.
62. del Zoppo GJ, Ferbert A, Otis S *et al*. Local intra-arterial fibrinolytic therapy in acute carotid territory stroke. A pilot study. *Stroke* 1988; 19:307–313.

63. Randomised controlled trial of streptokinase, aspirin, and combination of both in treatment of acute ischaemic stroke. Multicentre Acute Stroke Trial–Italy (MAST-I) Group. *Lancet* 1995; 346:1509–1514.

64. Donnan GA, Davis SM, Chambers BR *et al*. Streptokinase for acute ischemic stroke with relationship to time of administration: Australian Streptokinase (ASK) Trial Study Group. *JAMA* 1996; 271:961–966.

65. Thrombolytic therapy with streptokinase in acute ischemic stroke. The Multicenter Acute Stroke Trial–Europe Study Group. *N Engl J Med* 1996; 334:145–150.

66. Hacke W, Kaste M, Fieschi C *et al*. Randomised double-blind placebo-controlled trial of thrombolytic therapy with intravenous alteplase in acute ischaemic stroke (ECASS II). Second European-Australasian Acute Stroke Study Investigators. *Lancet* 1998; 352:1245–1251.

67. Clark WM, Wissman S, Albers GW, Jhamandas JH, Madden KP, Hamilton S. Recombinant tissue-type plasminogen activator (Alteplase) for ischemic stroke 3 to 5 h after symptom onset. The ATLANTIS Study: a randomized controlled trial. Alteplase Thrombolysis for Acute Noninterventional Therapy in Ishaemic Stroke. *JAMA* 1999; 282:2019–2026.

68. Hacke W, Brott T, Caplan L *et al*. Thrombolysis in acute ischemic stroke: controlled trials and clinical experience. *Neurology* 1999; 53:S3–S14.

69. Wardlaw JM, del Zoppo G, Yamaguchi T, Berge E. Thrombolysis for acute ischaemic stroke. *Cochrane Database of Systematic Reviews* 2003:Art. No.: CD000213. DOI: 10.1002/14651858. CD000213.

70. Hacke W, Donnan G, Fieschi C *et al*. Association of outcome with early stroke treatment: pooled analysis of ATLANTIS, ECASS, and NINDS rt-PA stroke trials. *Lancet* 2004; 363:768–774.

71. Scott PA, Lowell MJ, Longstreth K. Analysis of U.S. population with geographic access to interventional neuroradiology and intra-arterial thrombolysis for acute ischemic stroke. *Stroke* 1997; 28:266(abstract).

72. Mori E, Tabuchi M, Yoshida T, Yamadori A. Intracarotid urokinase with thromboembolic occlusion of the middle cerebral artery. *Stroke* 1988; 19:802–812.

73. Zeumer H, Freitag HJ, Zanella F, Thie A, Arning C. Local intra-arterial fibrinolytic therapy in patients with stroke: urokinase versus recombinant tissue plasminogen activator (r-TPA). *Neuroradiology* 1993; 35:159–162.

74. Barnwell SL, Clark WM, Nguyen TT, O'Neill OR, Wynn ML, Coull BM. Safety and efficacy of delayed intraarterial urokinase therapy with mechanical clot disruption for thromboembolic stroke. *AJNR Am J Neuroradiol* 1994; 15:1817–1822.

75. Sasaki O, Takeuchi S, Koike T, Koizumi T, Tanaka R. Fibrinolytic therapy for acute embolic stroke: intravenous, intracarotid, and intra-arterial local approaches. *Neurosurgery* 1995; 36:246–252.

76. del Zoppo GJ, Higashida RT, Furlan AJ, Pessin MS, Rowley HA, Gent M. PROACT: a phase II randomized trial of recombinant pro-urokinase by direct arterial delivery in acute middle cerebral artery stroke. PROACT Investigators. Prolyse in Acute Cerebral Thromboembolism. *Stroke* 1998; 29:4–11.

77. Lewandowski CA, Frankel M, Tomsick TA *et al*. Combined intravenous and intra-arterial r-TPA versus intra-arterial therapy of acute ischemic stroke: Emergency Management of Stroke (EMS) Bridging Trial. *Stroke* 1999; 30:2598–2605.

78. Ernst R, Pancioli A, Tomsick T *et al*. Combined intravenous and intra-arterial recombinant tissue plasminogen activator in acute ischemic stroke. *Stroke* 2000; 31:2552–2557.

79. Hill MD, Barber PA, Demchuk AM *et al*. Acute intravenous–intra-arterial revascularization therapy for severe ischemic stroke. *Stroke* 2002; 33:279–282.

80. Suarez JI, Zaidat OO, Sunshine JL, Tarr R, Selman WR, Landis DM. Endovascular administration after intravenous infusion of thrombolytic agents for the treatment of patients with acute ischemic strokes. *Neurosurgery* 2002; 50:251–9; discussion 259–260.

81. Combined intravenous and intra-arterial recanalization for acute ischemic stroke: the Interventional Management of Stroke Study. *Stroke* 2004; 35:904–11.

82. Ancrod for the treatment of acute ischemic brain infarction. The Ancrod Stroke Study Investigators. *Stroke* 1994; 25:1755–1759.

83. Sherman DG, Atkinson RP, Chippendale T *et al*. Intravenous ancrod for treatment of acute ischemic stroke: the STAT study: a randomized controlled trial. Stroke Treatment with Ancrod Trial. *Stroke* 2000; 283:2395–2403.

84. Orgogozo JM, Verstraete M, Kay R, Hennerici M, Lenzi GL. Outcomes of ancrod in acute ischemic stroke. *JAMA* 2000; 284:1926–1927.

85. Mori E, Takakura K, Yamaguchi T *et al*. Multicenter trial of a novel modified t-PA, E6010, by IV bolus injection in patients with acute carotid territory stroke. EAST Study Group. *Cerebrovasc Dis* 1996; 6:191(abstract).

86. Bhatt DL, Topol EJ. Current role of platelet glycoprotein IIb/IIIa inhibitors in acute coronary syndromes. *JAMA* 2000; 284:1549–1558.
87. Mitsias PD, Lu M, Morris D *et al*. Treatment of acute supratentorial ischemic stroke with abciximab is safe and may result in early neurological improvement. A preliminary report. *Cerebrovasc Dis* 2004; 18:249–250.
88. Hacke W, Albers G, Al-Rawi Y *et al*. The Desmoteplase in Acute Ischemic Stroke Trial (DIAS): a phase II MRI-based 9-h window acute stroke thrombolysis trial with intravenous desmoteplase. *Stroke* 2005; 36:66–73.
89. Blinc A, Francis CW, Trudnowski JL, Carstensen EL. Characterization of ultrasound-potentiated fibrinolysis in vitro. *Blood* 1993; 81:2636–2643.
90. Kerber CW, Barr JD, Berger RM, Chopko BW. Snare retrieval of intracranial thrombus in patients with acute stroke. *J Vasc Interv Radiol* 2002; 13:1269–1274.
91. Lutsep HL, Clark WM, Nesbit GM, Kuether TA, Barnwell SL. Intraarterial suction thrombectomy in acute stroke. *AJNR Am J Neuroradiol* 2002; 23:783–786.
92. Keuther TA, Nesbit GM, Barnwell SL. Mechanical thrombolysis of acute ischemic stroke. *Stroke Cerebrovasc Dis* 2002; 11:162–173.
93. Balousek PA, Knowles HJ, Higashida RT, del Zoppo GJ. New interventions in cerebrovascular disease: the role of thrombolytic therapy and balloon angioplasty. *Curr Opin Cardiol* 1996; 11:550–557.
94. Mahon BR, Nesbit GM, Barnwell SL *et al*. North American clinical experience with the EKOS MicroLysUS infusion catheter for the treatment of embolic stroke. *AJNR Am J Neuroradiol* 2003; 24:534–538.
95. Berlis A, Lutsep H, Barnwell S *et al*. Mechanical thrombolysis in acute ischemic stroke with endovascular photoacoustic recanalization. *Stroke* 2004; 35:1112–1116.
96. Daffertshofer M, Huang Z, Fatar M *et al*. Efficacy of sonothrombolysis in a rat model of embolic ischemic stroke. *Neurosci Lett* 2004; 361:115–119.
97. Alexandrov AV, Molina CA, Grotta JC *et al*. Ultrasound-enhanced systemic thrombolysis for acute ischemic stroke. *N Engl J Med* 2004; 351:2170–2178.
98. Gobin YP, Starkman S, Duckwiler GR *et al*. MERCI 1: a phase 1 study of Mechanical Embolus Removal in Cerebral Ischemia. *Stroke* 2004; 35:2848–2854.
99. Smith WS. Comparison of MERCI mortality with NINDS, for the MERCI Study Investigators. *Stroke* 2005; 36:490 (abstract).
100. Felten RP, Ogden NR, Pena C, Provost MC, Schlosser MJ, Witten CM. The Food and Drug Administration medical device review process: clearance of a clot retriever for use in ischemic stroke. *Stroke* 2005; 36:404–406.

16

Atrial fibrillation: antithrombotic therapy

R. De Caterina, G. Renda

INTRODUCTION – ATRIAL FIBRILLATION REVISITED

DEFINITION

Atrial fibrillation (AF) is a supraventricular tachyarrhythmia characterised by uncoordinated atrial activation with consequent deterioration of atrial mechanical function. Atrial fibrillation features atrial wavelets propagating in different directions, causing disorganised atrial depolarization without effective atrial contraction [1, 2].

On the electrocardiogram, atrial fibrillation is described by the replacement of consistent P waves by rapid oscillations (fibrillatory 'f' waves) that vary in size, shape and timing, at a rate of 350 to 600 beats/min, associated with an irregular, frequently rapid ventricular response when atrio-ventricular (AV) conduction is intact [3]. The ventricular response to atrial fibrillation depends on the electrophysiological properties of the AV node, the level of vagal and sympathetic tone, and the action of drugs [4].

PATHOPHYSIOLOGICAL MECHANISMS

The atria of patients with atrial fibrillation display structural abnormalities beyond changes caused by the underlying heart disease [5]. Histological examinations have shown patchy fibrosis with juxtaposition of normal and diseased atrial fibres, which may account for the non-homogeneity of atrial refractoriness [6, 7]. Fibrosis or fatty infiltration may also affect the sinus node, and may be a reaction to inflammatory or degenerative processes that are difficult to detect. The role of inflammation in the pathogenesis of atrial fibrillation has not yet been evaluated, but histological changes consistent with myocarditis were reported in 66% of atrial biopsy specimens from patients with lone atrial fibrillation [7]. Atrial fibre hypertrophy has been described as a major feature in atrial fibrillation patients [6]. Atrial hypertrophy and dilatation may be either a cause or a consequence of persistent atrial fibrillation, because progressive atrial enlargement has been demonstrated echocardiographically [8]. A recent experimental study showed that heart failure facilitates the induction of sustained atrial fibrillation, mediated by extensive interstitial fibrosis [9]. In most patients, however, it is not possible to identify the underlying anatomic process responsible for the arrhythmia.

Raffaele De Caterina, Professor of Cardiology, Institute of Cardiology, "G. d'Annunzio" University – Chieti, Ospedale San Camillo de Lellis, Chieti, Italy.

Giulia Renda, Associate in Cardiology, "G. d'Annunzio" University – Chieti, Ospedale San Camillo de Lellis, Chieti, Italy.

CLASSIFICATION

The pattern of atrial fibrillation may be defined in terms of the number of episodes, duration, frequency, mode of onset and possible triggers, and response to therapy, although these features are difficult to discern when atrial fibrillation is first encountered in an individual patient.

Different labels have been used to describe the pattern of atrial fibrillation, including acute, chronic, paroxysmal, intermittent, constant, persistent, and permanent, but the classification scheme recommended by the latest Guidelines for the Management of Patients with Atrial Fibrillation of the American College of Cardiology (ACC), American Heart Association (AHA) and European Society of Cardiology (ESC) [10] is the following:

Paroxysmal: when a patient has two or more episodes, atrial fibrillation is considered recurrent and if the arrhythmia terminates spontaneously, recurrent atrial fibrillation is designated paroxysmal;

Persistent: atrial fibrillation episodes do not terminate spontaneously, but do convert with either electrical or pharmacological cardioversion;

Permanent: atrial fibrillation does not terminate either spontaneously or with electrical or pharmacological cardioversion, or cardioversion has not been attempted (i.e., chronic atrial fibrillation).

This terminology applies to episodes of atrial fibrillation that last more than 30 seconds and that are unrelated to a reversible cause. Secondary atrial fibrillation occurring in the setting of acute myocardial infarction (MI), cardiac surgery, pericarditis, myocarditis, hyperthyroidism, pulmonary embolism, pneumonia, or acute pulmonary disease is considered separately, because it is less likely to recur once the precipitating condition is resolved.

EPIDEMIOLOGY

Atrial fibrillation is the most common arrhythmia encountered in clinical practice, accounting for approximately one-third of hospitalisations for cardiac rhythm disturbances.

The prevalence of atrial fibrillation is estimated at 0.4% of the general population, increasing with age [11]: it is observed to be less than 1% in people under 60 years of age and greater than 6% in those over 80 years [12–14]. The age-adjusted prevalence is higher in men [14, 15]. Atrial fibrillation is most common in patients with congestive heart failure or valvular heart disease, and increases in prevalence with the severity of these conditions. The frequency of atrial fibrillation in patients with no history of cardiopulmonary disease ('lone' atrial fibrillation) varies from less than 12% of all cases of atrial fibrillation [14, 16–18] to over 30% in some series [19, 20].

In prospective studies, the incidence of atrial fibrillation increases from less than 0.1% per year in people under 40 years of age to greater than 1.5 and 2% per year, respectively, in women and in men over 80 years of age [21–23]. The age-adjusted incidence increased over a 30-year period in the Framingham Study [21], and this may have implications for the future impact of atrial fibrillation on the population. During 38 years of follow-up in the Framingham Study, 20.6% of men who developed atrial fibrillation had congestive heart failure at enrolment, compared with 3.2% of those without atrial fibrillation; the corresponding incidences in women were 26.0 and 2.9% [24].

Secular trends of atrial fibrillation prevalence are informative of the epidemiology of this arrhythmia. A recent study evaluated the prevalence rates of atrial fibrillation in patients with incident stroke and in age- and gender-matched controls over a 30-year period in a population of Rochester, Minnesota [25]. Consistent with other studies [14, 24, 26, 27], the authors observed that age is a potent risk factor for the development of atrial fibrillation: each decade of age was associated with a doubling of the odds for atrial fibrillation. However, even after adjustment for age, the prevalence of atrial fibrillation increased significantly during a 22-year period among men in the Framingham study [28] and during a 30-year period among men and women in this Rochester study [25]. The authors suggest that changes over time in the prevalence of comorbid conditions, such as hypertension, coronary artery disease, diabetes mellitus and heart failure, may play an important role in the origin and propagation of this epidemic. Therefore, on the one hand an increasing number of people now reach the age at which the risk of atrial fibrillation becomes common; on the other hand, a significantly higher proportion of the elderly population have comorbidities, which in themselves are risk factors for the development of atrial fibrillation. A possible pathophysiological link between these conditions and the development of atrial fibrillation is diastolic dysfunction, recently identified as a predictor of non-valvular atrial fibrillation [29]. Another explanation of the increasing prevalence of atrial fibrillation may be the increasing prevalence of valvular heart disease over time. Such an increasing prevalence is not only due to increased diagnosis, with a more widespread use of echocardiography, but also to an actual increase in the number of older individuals developing degenerative valve disease [30]. Finally, other factors, such as alcohol consumption, sleep apnoea, thyroid disorders, infection, or pulmonary disease, which themselves undoubtedly have multiple causes, can also affect secular trends in the prevalence of atrial fibrillation.

ATRIAL FIBRILLATION AS A MARKER OF UNDERLYING CONDITIONS

The association between atrial fibrillation and other pathologic conditions has suggested the role of atrial fibrillation as a 'marker' of these other diseases. According to this hypothesis, the increase in mortality associated with atrial fibrillation might not be directly caused by the arrhythmia, but by the underlying condition. Several elements support this hypothesis. Lone atrial fibrillation, which affects patients without structural heart disease, does not appear to have an adverse effect on survival. Although the association between atrial fibrillation and stroke is undisputed [13, 31–34], and although blood stasis with thrombus formation in the atria and atrial appendages has long been considered the mechanisms connecting atrial fibrillation and stroke, increasing evidence now suggests that a hypercoagulable state is often present. Endothelial or endocardial changes, as well as a prothrombotic tendency, may affect the development of thrombus and stroke [35]. Abnormalities in haemostasis and platelet function have been described not only in patients with atrial fibrillation, but also in those with conventional cardiovascular risk factors of atrial fibrillation [36–38]. Cognitive impairment, configuring a pathologic condition named 'vascular dementia', occurs in association with atrial fibrillation even in the absence of stroke [39–43]. Atrial fibrillation also contributes to the development and exacerbation of heart failure [44], although the underlying mechanisms are not fully understood. There is some evidence that tachycardia-induced cardiomyopathy may play a role [45–47]. In turn, heart failure is a risk factor for atrial fibrillation [48], and diastolic dysfunction, which might occur because of a structural remodelling of the left atrium [49] and distension of the pulmonary veins [50], may represent the link between these two conditions [29], which together influence morbidity and mortality in the affected patients. Finally, the overlapping pattern of risk factors for atrial fibrillation and atherosclerosis, and the non-cardioembolic nature of stroke in as many as >25% of cases in patients with atrial fibrillation, due to intrinsic cerebrovascular disease (present in about 12% of such patients [51]), other cardio-embolic sources, or athero-embolism from the proximal aorta [52, 53], highlight the possibility that atrial fibrillation may be a marker of a non-compliant atherosclerotic circulation, and that this last is the final transducer of the increased prevalence of cardiovascular events and increased mortality in patients with this condition [54, 55].

THE THROMBOEMBOLIC RISK IN ATRIAL FIBRILLATION

Atrial fibrillation is an independent risk factor for stroke. In general, it confers a four- to five-fold higher risk to affected patients compared with the unaffected population [13, 21,

31, 32], and is probably the major cause of embolic stroke [56]. The annualised stroke rate is about 3.2–3.3%, and is considered similar in patients with paroxysmal atrial fibrillation and in patients with permanent atrial fibrillation [57]. The rate of stroke is higher in patients with prior stroke or transient ischaemic attack (10–12% per year) [58, 59] and in patients with mitral stenosis [60].

The frequency of stroke related to atrial fibrillation increases with age [13]. The effect of ageing in increasing the risk of stroke in atrial fibrillation is multifactorial. In such patients, ageing is associated with left atrial enlargement, reduced flow velocity in the left atrial appendage and the presence of spontaneous echo-contrast [8, 61, 62]. Moreover, age is a risk factor for atherosclerosis, including the presence of complex aortic arch plaques, and is associated with stroke also independent of atrial fibrillation [63]; an age-related prothrombotic diathesis was shown by elevated levels of prothrombin activation fragment F 1 + 2, in the general population [64–66] and in patients with atrial fibrillation [67, 68]. In the Stroke Prevention in Atrial Fibrillation (SPAF) studies, age was a more potent risk factor when combined with other risk factors such as hypertension [68]: about half of all elderly patients with atrial fibrillation have chronic hypertension [69] (a major risk factor for cerebrovascular disease), and approximately 12% harbour cervical carotid artery stenoses [51].

Hypertension is a powerful independent predictor of stroke in patients with non-rheumatic atrial fibrillation [69, 70]. In a recent large trial, a history of hypertension was strongly associated with findings of left atrial stasis and the presence of thrombi at trans-oesophageal echocardiography (TEE) and of complex aortic plaques [71], which all determine a high risk of thromboembolism. The strong association between hypertension and stroke in patients with non-rheumatic atrial fibrillation needs further clarification. In addition to its own potential implication in generating atheroembolic cerebrovascular disease, hypertension – especially systolic hypertension – might be a sign of a non-compliant atherosclerotic aorta, which increases the impedance to left atrial and left ventricular emptying, promoting chamber dilatation and stasis. Diabetes emerged as a risk factor for stroke in some studies [72], but this has not been a consistent observation.

In subjects with lone atrial fibrillation, in the absence of structural heart disease, the risk of stroke is largely governed by the presence and extent of additional risk factors. In the Framingham study, over a mean follow-up period of 11 years, an approximately four-fold risk of stroke was demonstrated in subjects with lone atrial fibrillation (28.2%), but having one or more risk factors for stroke, compared with an age- and gender-matched population (6.8%) [17]. In a subsequent study from Olmsted County, Minnesota, including subjects with no risk factors and younger than 60 years, the 15-year cumulative stroke rate was, conversely, very low (1.3%) [18]. In a more recent experience from the same population, patients with one risk factor (i.e., age >60 years) had a combined risk of stroke and transient ischaemic attack (TIA) higher than control subjects (without risk factors), but substantially lower than the Framingham population [73]. Another difference between younger and older patients was in the proportion at which chronic atrial fibrillation developed during the follow-up. Therefore, the mere presence of lone atrial fibrillation does not appear to confer by itself increased risk for stroke.

Chronicity may be a risk factor for stroke in the population with lone atrial fibrillation. In a recent study of patients younger than 50 years from Trieste, Italy, patients (66%) remaining in paroxysmal atrial fibrillation during a 10-year follow-up experienced a low thromboembolism rate (0.36/100 patient-years), while patients (34%) with chronic atrial fibrillation had a significantly higher rate of thromboembolism (1.3/100 patient-years) [74]. Moreover, although until now the stroke rate is considered similar in patients with paroxysmal atrial fibrillation and those with permanent atrial fibrillation, recent data suggest that patients with paroxysmal atrial fibrillation do not have increased mortality, with the exception of the subgroup converting to chronic atrial fibrillation, in whom a small increase in risk was present [75]. An explanation for chronicity being a risk factor may be in the increased left atrial dimensions occurring in this group [76].

PATHOPHYSIOLOGICAL MECHANISMS OF STROKE IN ATRIAL FIBRILLATION

Traditional concepts on the pathophysiology of stroke in atrial fibrillation implicate stasis and thrombus formation in a structurally abnormal and dilated atrium because of the contribution of the three factors of Virchow's triad: blood stasis, parietal abnormalities (endothelial dysfunction), and blood hypercoagulability [77]. The occlusion of a cerebral artery would be thus due to an embolus dislodged from the left atrium. Thrombi arise most frequently in the left atrial appendage, the morphology and function of which can be assessed by transoesophageal Doppler echocardiography [78]. This technique demonstrates reduced flow velocities (stasis) in the left atrial appendage related to the loss of organised mechanical contractions and associated with the presence of spontaneous echo-contrast [79–83]. Endothelial dysfunction has been difficult to demonstrate as a distinct mechanism contributing to thrombus formation in patients with atrial fibrillation. The increase of von Willebrand factor in the systemic circulation and the atrial tissue in some patients [84–86] may prove the existence of this mechanism. Biochemical markers of coagulation and platelet activation may reflect a systemic hypercoagulable state associated with atrial fibrillation. Systemic fibrinogen degradation products and fibrin D-dimer levels, indicating active intravascular thrombogenesis, are increased in both permanent and paroxysmal atrial fibrillation [84, 85, 87–90]; elevated beta-thromboglobulin and platelet factor 4 in selected patients indicate platelet activation [84, 89, 91], but these data are relatively weak. Such biochemical markers of coagulation and platelet activation do not distinguish between a reactive process secondary to intravascular coagulation and a primary hypercoagulable state. Recent investigations suggest that atrial fibrillation may itself cause a hypercoagulable state [91, 92] and, as described above, be a marker for other conditions predisposing to stroke. The complex pathogenesis of thromboembolism in patients with atrial fibrillation, involving the coexistence of many factors, some of which are incompletely defined, may have important consequences for therapy (see below).

PREVENTION OF THROMBOEMBOLISM

According to the latest guidelines of the ACC/AHA/ESC [10] and the recently issued Seventh American College of Chest Physicians (ACCP) Consensus Conference on Antithrombotic Therapy [93], antithrombotic strategies in atrial fibrillation include anticoagulants, antiplatelet drugs, or their combination. Such guidelines are summarised below.

ANTICOAGULANT THERAPY

Oral anticoagulants
Warfarin and related coumarin derivatives are inhibitors of vitamin K, depressing the synthesis of four vitamin K-dependent coagulation factors, II, VII, IX and X, and of two inhibitory proteins, protein C and protein S. All such factors are inactive until they are carboxylated by an enzymatic system using reduced vitamin K as a cofactor. Reduction of vitamin K is performed by numerous and different enzymes which are inhibited by oral anticoagulants: the deficiency of reduced vitamin K causes decreased synthesis of all the above-mentioned coagulation factors and inhibitory proteins [94]. The intensity of oral anticoagulants' effects on the synthesis of coagulation factors differs among patients and in the same patient over time. This variability explains the need for close monitoring. The test universally used to monitor the effect of oral anticoagulants is the prothrombin time (PT). For its inter-laboratory standardisation, the international normalised ratio (INR) is now universally recommended [95]. Table 16.1 shows a practical nomogram constructed by the Hamilton group [96], for the management of warfarin therapy in atrial fibrillation based on INR values.

Table 16.1   INR management nomogram [96]

INR value	Suggested warfarin adjustment	INR recheck date
≤1.3	Increase dose by 50%	5 to 7 days
1.4	Increase dose by 33%	5 to 7 days
1.5 to 1.8	Increase dose by 25%	5 to 7 days
1.9	Increase dose by 10%	7 to 14 days
2.0 to 2.8	No change	14 to 28 days
2.9 to 3.1	Reduce dose by 10%	7 to 14 days
3.2 to 3.5	Reduce dose by 25%	7 to 10 days
3.6 to 3.7	Reduce dose by 33%	5 to 7 days
3.8 to 3.9	Hold for 1 day, reduce dose by 33%	5 to 7 days
4.0 to 4.4	Hold for 1 day, reduce dose by 33%	3 to 7 days
4.5 to 5.0	Hold for 2 days, reduce dose by 33%	3 to 7 days
5.1 to 6.0	Hold for 3 days, reduce dose by 33%	3 to 7 days
≥6.1	To be determined by attending physician	3 to 5 days

This nomogram assumes patients are not initiating warfarin. Patients initiating warfarin should be started on 4 mg/day (weight <80 kg) or 6 mg/day (weight >80 kg) and their INR checked in one week. The nomogram should then be consulted for dose adjustments.

Before 1990, antithrombotic therapy for prevention of thromboembolism in patients with atrial fibrillation was mainly limited to those with rheumatic heart disease and prosthetic heart valves [13], in which the high risk of thromboembolism has long been appreciated. Between 1989 and 1992, five large randomised trials using INR ranges of approximately 1.8 to 4.2, evaluated oral anticoagulation in patients with non-valvular atrial fibrillation [95, 97–100], and a sixth trial focused on secondary prevention in patients who had survived a non-disabling stroke or transient cerebral ischaemic attack [58]. A meta-analysis of these trials showed that adjusted-dose oral anticoagulation is highly efficacious for the prevention of all strokes (both ischaemic and haemorrhagic strokes), with a risk reduction of 61% compared with placebo [101]. The maximum protection against ischaemic stroke in atrial fibrillation is probably already achieved with an INR range of 2.0 to 3.0 [59, 102, 103].

The incremental risk of serious bleeding was <1% per year among patients participating in these clinical trials, and an INR range between 2.0 and 3.0 clearly conferred the best risk/benefit ratio [69, 95]. However, all these trials excluded patients considered at high risk of bleeding and, since patients' age and the intensity of anticoagulation are the two most powerful predictors of major bleeding [104–107], trial participants, having an average age of 69 years, were carefully selected and managed. It is thus unclear whether the relatively low rates of major haemorrhage also apply to patients with atrial fibrillation encountered in clinical practice, who have a mean age of about 75 years and whose anticoagulation therapy is less closely controlled [26]. The only placebo-controlled trial involving patients with a mean age of 75 years reported a 38% withdrawal rate from anticoagulation after 1 year [69], and another trial comparing anticoagulation in patients with atrial fibrillation under and over 75 years, all with an INR range 2.0–4.5, and a mean INR 2.7, found an increased risk of major haemorrhage in patients over 75 years compared with younger ones [69, 97]. The problem of the very elderly patients is that they have a higher risk of stroke, but the benefit of anticoagulation therapy is offset by an elevated risk of bleeding. Therefore, targeting the lowest adequate intensity of anticoagulation to minimise the risk of bleeding is particularly important for these patients: low-intensity anticoagulation (target INR 2.0) may be as effective and safer in patients over 75 years [95], at least until results of ongoing clinical trials will become available. In the Italian Study on Complications of Oral Anticoagulant Therapy (ISCOAT), the rate of bleeding was higher in older patients (10.5 per 100 patient-years in those aged 70 or over, 6.0 in those aged under 70; relative risk 1.75) and much higher as INR values increased [108]. The authors suggested caution in the treatment of elderly patients, and they underlined the importance of close monitoring of anticoagulation intensity to reduce periods of overdosing.

A particular condition predisposing to systemic embolism is electrical or pharmacological cardioversion to sinus rhythm. There have been no randomised, prospective clinical trials evaluating the usefulness of anticoagulant therapy in preventing systemic embolization in this setting, and current recommendations are therefore based on published, but not controlled, observations [109, 110]. In patients with atrial fibrillation with unknown duration or having lasted for more than 48 h, oral anticoagulation should be given for 3 weeks before and 3–4 weeks after cardioversion [109, 111, 112]. In atrial fibrillation of short duration, i.e., <48 h, anticoagulation before cardioversion may not be required, but it would anyway appear safer first to exclude the presence of left atrial thrombi by TEE. The role of TEE has become increasingly important in evaluating thromboembolic risk in patients with atrial fibrillation, particularly those undergoing cardioversion [78, 113]. Detection of left atrial or left atrial appendage thrombus stands as a contraindication to elective cardioversion of atrial fibrillation. The absence of detectable thrombus, however, does not preclude thromboembolism after cardioversion if patients do not receive anticoagulation therapy [112, 114]. A TEE-guided strategy for elective cardioversion of atrial fibrillation has been reported to result in comparable outcomes for thromboembolism and death compared with conventional anticoagulation for 3 weeks before and 4 weeks after cardioversion [115]. Manning et al. suggested that TEE might be used to identify patients without thrombi in the left atrial appendage, who would not require anticoagulation [116], but a subsequent investigation [112] and a meta-analysis of several clinical studies [110] found this approach to be unreliable.

The role of TEE in thromboembolic risk stratification of patients with atrial fibrillation beyond cardioversion is discussed below.

In Table 16.2 the latest ACC/AHA/ESC recommendations for antithrombotic therapy in patients with atrial fibrillation undergoing cardioversion are reported.

Heparins

The term heparin refers to a family of mucopolysaccharide chains of varying length and composition, with a mean molecular weight of 15 000 Daltons (range 3000–30 000 Daltons). Heparin contains a unique pentasaccharide unit with a high affinity binding sequence for antithrombin (AT)III, which is an inhibitor of coagulation serine proteases, i.e., thrombin and activated factor X, IX, XI and XII. Heparins form a complex with this ATIII, accelerating its inhibitory action. Unfractionated heparin (UFH) binds to endothelial cells, macrophages, numerous plasma proteins and platelet factor (PF)4: this fact explains the highly variable individual dose requirements to obtain the same antithrombotic effect, the need of therapeutic monitoring and some collateral effects [117]. The most commonly used test for therapeutic monitoring is the activated partial thromboplastin time (aPTT). The range of aPTT relating to clinical efficacy of heparin is 1.5–2 times the basal value [117]. The most common and major side-effect of heparin is bleeding. Another, less common, but severe side-effect is heparin-induced thrombocytopaenia (HIT), two types of which are known [117]: early HIT, occurring during the first five days of treatment, with unknown aetiology, not severe and reversible; and late HIT, occurring between the fifth and the fifteenth day of treatment, due to antibodies against the heparin–PF4 complex, interacting with the CD32 receptor and causing abnormal platelet activation and the formation of prothrombotic platelet particles [118]. This latest type of HIT is frequently associated with venous and arterial thrombotic complications.

Table 16.2   Recommendations for antithrombotic therapy in patients with AF undergoing cardioversion [10]

Class I:
1) Administer anticoagulation therapy regardless of the method (electrical or pharmacological) used to restore sinus rhythm. (Level of evidence: B)
2) Anticoagulate patients with AF lasting more than 48 h or of unknown duration, for at least 3 to 4 weeks before and after cardioversion (INR 2 to 3). (Level of evidence: B)
3) Perform immediate cardioversion in patients with acute (recent onset) AF accompanied by symptoms or signs of haemodynamic instability resulting in angina pectoris, MI, shock, or pulmonary oedema, without waiting for prior anticoagulation. (Level of evidence: C)
    a. If not contraindicated, administer heparin concurrently by an initial intravenous bolus injection followed by a continuous infusion in a dose adjusted to prolong the activated partial thromboplastin time at 1.5 to two times the reference control value. (Level of evidence: C)
    b. Next, provide oral anticoagulation (INR 2 to 3) for a period of at least 3 to 4 weeks, as for patients undergoing elective cardioversion. (Level of evidence: C)
    c. Limited data from recent studies support subcutaneous administration of low-molecular-weight heparin in this indication. (Level of evidence: C)
4) Screening for the presence of thrombus in the LA or LAA by TEE is an alternative for routine pre-anticoagulation in candidates for cardioversion of AF. (Level of evidence: B)
    a. Anticoagulate patients in whom no thrombus is identified in the form of intravenous unfractionated heparin by an initial bolus injection before cardioversion, followed by a continuous infusion in a dose adjusted to prolong the activated partial thromboplastin time at 1.5 to two times the reference control value. (Level of evidence: B)
    b. Next, provide oral anticoagulation (INR 2 to 3) for a period of at least 3 to 4 weeks, as for patients undergoing elective cardioversion. (Level of evidence: B)
    c. Limited data are available to support the subcutaneous administration of low-molecular-weight heparin in this indication. (Level of evidence: C)
    d. Treat patients in whom thrombus is identified by TEE with oral anticoagulation (INR 2 to 3) for at least 3 to 4 weeks before and after restoration of sinus rhythm. (Level of evidence: B)

Class IIb:
1) Cardioversion without TEE guidance during the first 48 h after the onset of AF. (Level of evidence: C)
    a. In these cases, anticoagulation before and after cardioversion is optional, depending on assessment of risk. (Level of evidence: C)
2) Anticoagulate patients with atrial flutter undergoing cardioversion in the same way as for patients with AF. (Level of evidence: C)

Low-molecular-weight heparins (LMWH) are fractions of the heparin molecules, obtained by chemical or enzymatic depolymerization, with lesser dimensions (mean molecular weight of 5000 Daltons, range 1000–10 000 Daltons), lesser capacity to inactivate thrombin compared with factor Xa (antifactor Xa to antithrombin III ratio between 4:1 and 2:1; this ratio is 1:1 for UFH), and lesser capacity to bind plasma proteins, PF4 and endothelial cells. These characteristics result in a higher bioavailability (after subcutaneous injection: >90 vs. 30% for UFH), reduced plasma clearance, longer half-life (anti-Xa activity 3–4 h vs. 30–150 min for UFH), less interindividual variability of the anticoagulant response, and reduced risk of thrombocytopaenia [119]. Therefore, LMWH are more practical, cause less complications compared with UFH, and – to a large extent – they do not need monitoring [119].

The use of heparins in atrial fibrillation is limited to the patients in whom it is necessary to interrupt oral anticoagulant therapy in preparation for elective surgical procedures. In patients with mechanical prostheses, it is generally appropriate to substitute oral anticoagulants with UFH or LMWH to prevent thrombosis [120, 121]. In patients with atrial fibrillation without mechanical prostheses, anticoagulation may be interrupted for a period of up to 1 week for surgical or diagnostic procedures carrying a risk of bleeding, without substituting oral anticoagulants with heparins [10]. In high-risk patients, or when a series of procedures requires the interruption of oral anticoagulation for a period longer than 1 week, UFH or LMWH may be administered [10]. The use of LMWH instead of UFH in patients with atrial fibrillation is based largely on extrapolations from data in trials of prevention of venous thromboembolism, in which LMWH have proven as effective and safe as UFH. The practice of 'bridging' with LMWH in patients awaiting major surgery has been recently evaluated in a large prospective study to assess its efficacy and safety when initiated out of hospital in patients at high risk of arterial embolism, including patients with prosthetic valves and atrial fibrillation with a major risk factor. Here warfarin was held for 5 days pre-operatively, with LMWH given 3 days pre-operatively and at least 4 days postoperatively [122]. The conclusions of this study were that such bridging therapy with subcutaneous LMWH is feasible; however, the optimal approach for the management of patients who require temporary interruption of warfarin to have invasive procedures is uncertain [122].

The latest ACC/AHA/ESC guidelines [10] also suggest the use of UFH in patients with acute (recent onset) atrial fibrillation accompanied by symptoms or signs of haemodynamic instability, without waiting for prior anticoagulation (Table 16.2): it is possible to administer heparin concurrently by an initial intravenous bolus injection followed by a continuous infusion in a dose adjusted to prolong the activated partial thromboplastin time at 1.5 to 2 times the reference control value.

Limited data from recent studies support the subcutaneous administration of LMWH in this setting, as well as in patients with atrial fibrillation attempting a TEE-guided cardioversion as an alternative to the recommended strategy of at least 3-week prophylaxis with oral anticoagulants (at doses similar to those for treatment of deep vein thrombosis [93].

ANTIPLATELET THERAPY

Aspirin
The best characterised mechanism of action of aspirin is mainly related to its capacity to permanently inactivate the cyclooxygenase (COX) activity of prostaglandin (PG)H synthase-1 and PGH synthase-2 (also referred to as COX-1 and COX-2) in various tissues. These isozymes catalyse the first step in prostanoid biosynthesis. COX-1 is a predominantly constitutive enzyme, COX-2 is predominantly induced by inflammatory and mitogenic stimuli. The antiplatelet effect of aspirin is due to the inhibition of platelet COX-1-dependent synthesis, from arachidonic acid, of thromboxane (TX)A_2, a powerful inducer of vasoconstriction and of platelet aggregation [123]. The molecular mechanism for the permanent inactivation of COX activity by aspirin is related to the acetylation of a strategically located serine residue (i.e., Ser529 in the human COX-1 and Ser516 in the human COX-2) that prevents substrate access to the catalytic site of the enzyme [124]. Aspirin has a short half-life in the human circulation and is much more potent in inhibiting platelet COX-1 than monocyte COX-2 [125], so that it appears to be ideally suited to act on anucleate platelets, inducing a permanent defect in TXA$_2$-dependent platelet function. Moreover, since aspirin probably also inactivates

COX-1 in relatively mature megakaryocytes, and since only about 10% of the platelet pool is replenished each day, once-a-day dosing of aspirin is able to maintain a virtually complete inhibition of platelet TXA_2 production. On the contrary, inhibition of COX-2 needs higher doses of aspirin, due to a lesser sensitivity (about 170 times less) of COX-2 to aspirin, compared with COX-1 [126], and a shorter between-dose interval, because nucleated cells rapidly resynthesise the enzyme. (See also the specific chapter on Aspirin in this book.)

Aspirin is by far the most widely used antiplatelet drug, and has been tested in patients across the entire spectrum of severity of atherosclerotic vascular disease, from healthy low-risk individuals to patients presenting with acute MI or acute ischaemic stroke. The most recently completed review of the Antithrombotic Trialists' Collaboration has reported a meta-analysis of 65 trials using aspirin in high-risk patients, and found a 23% odds reduction in vascular events in the aspirin-treated groups [127]. The risk of vascular complications is the major determinant of the absolute benefit of aspirin therapy, with the greatest benefit in patients with unstable angina (50 subjects in whom a vascular event is prevented by aspirin per 1000 treated for 1 year) and the lowest benefit in healthy subjects (about 1 subject in whom a vascular event is prevented by aspirin per 1000 treated for 1 year) [128].

In patients with atrial fibrillation, aspirin offers only modest protection against stroke. A meta-analysis of randomised trials on patients with non-valvular atrial fibrillation showed a stroke reduction of 19% in those treated with aspirin compared with those receiving placebo [101]. The effect of aspirin on stroke in these trials was less consistent than that of oral anticoagulants, with a stroke reduction of 33% in patient treated with anticoagulants compared with those receiving aspirin [101, 129]. Differences in patient features may influence aspirin efficacy: aspirin reduced the occurrence of stroke with higher efficacy in primary compared with secondary prevention trials, in which patients had a higher rate of stroke [101]. Aspirin may be more efficacious for patients with atrial fibrillation and hypertension or diabetes [129, 130], and for the reduction of non-cardioembolic vs. cardioembolic ischaemic strokes [53]. Patients with high-risk atrial fibrillation (stroke risk >6% per year) seem to be better protected against stroke by adjusted-dose oral anticoagulation compared with aspirin, while the relative risk reduction is smaller in patients with lower stroke risk [101]. Therefore, oral anticoagulants may be most beneficial for atrial fibrillation patients at higher intrinsic thromboembolic risk, offering only modest reductions over aspirin for patients at low risk.

The combination of aspirin with low-dose oral anticoagulation (INR <1.5) adds little protection against stroke compared with aspirin alone in patients with atrial fibrillation [59], while combining aspirin with an oral anticoagulant at higher anticoagulation intensities may accentuate intracranial haemorrhage (ICH), particularly in elderly patients [131].

Indobufen

Indobufen, a reversible inhibitor of platelet cyclooxygenase, is another antiplatelet drug which has been studied as an alternative to aspirin and compared with warfarin in the secondary prevention of major vascular events in non-rheumatic atrial fibrillation. The Studio Italiano sulla Fibrillazione Atriale (SIFA) compared indobufen (100 or 200 mg twice daily) with warfarin (INR 2.5–3.5) for 12 months in patients with non-rheumatic atrial fibrillation having experienced a recent TIA or ischaemic stroke. The primary outcome in this study was the combined incidence of non-fatal stroke (including intracerebral bleeding), pulmonary or systemic embolism, non-fatal MI, and vascular death. At the end of the follow-up, no statistically significant difference between treatments on the incidence of primary outcome events was observed. The frequency of non-cerebral major bleeding complications was low, and the few cases of gastrointestinal bleeding were all observed in the warfarin group [132]. However the small number of patients recruited in this study limits the clinical applicability of these results, and further investigation, in larger sample sizes, is necessary to confirm the efficacy of indobufen compared with warfarin in the prevention of stroke in non-rheumatic atrial fibrillation. Thus, indobufen is not recommended for the prevention of thromboembolism in patients with atrial fibrillation in the latest ACC/AHA/ESC guidelines [10].

HOW TO CHOOSE ANTITHROMBOTIC THERAPY

Criteria for the selection of an antithrombotic regimen in atrial fibrillation should be guided by the patient's overall risk profile, which is defined by the patient's thromboembolic profile and the patient's haemorrhagic profile. Other important elements in the selection however also include the feasibility of adequate monitoring of oral anticoagulants and the patient's preferences.

RISK FACTORS FOR THROMBOEMBOLISM

Risk factors for thromboembolism in atrial fibrillation are currently divided into high- and moderate-risk factors, according to the Sixth ACCP Consensus Conference on Antithrombotic Therapy [133]:

High-risk factors include:
- Age >75 years
- Previous stroke/TIA or systemic embolism
- Hypertension
- Heart failure or left ventricular (LV) dysfunction
- Rheumatic mitral disease
- Mechanical valve prostheses

Moderate-risk factors include:
- Age 65–75 years
- Diabetes
- Coronary artery disease (CAD) with preserved LV function

Based on these risk factors, the ACCP Consensus Conference issued recommendations about the choice of antithrombotic therapy in atrial fibrillation, which are similar to those of the latest ACC/AHA/ESC guidelines (Table 16.3).

RISK FACTORS FOR BLEEDING

Factors implying a high haemorrhagic risk in patients being treated with oral anticoagulants are:

- Age >85 years
- Previous major bleeding
- Tendency to falls
- Difficulty in maintaining an adequate INR range
- Low compliance
- Difficulty in patient follow-up for logistic reasons

ACC/AHA/ESC GUIDELINES

The latest guidelines for antithrombotic therapy in patients with atrial fibrillation [10] are described and commented upon in this section. The recommendations are evidence-based

Table 16.3 Risk-based approach to antithrombotic therapy in patients with atrial fibrillation [10]

Patient features	Antithrombotic therapy	Grade of recommendation
Age <60 years, no heart disease (lone AF)	Aspirin (325 mg per day) or no therapy	I
Age <60 years, heart disease but no risk factors*	Aspirin (325 mg per day)	I
Age ≥60 years, no risk factors*	Aspirin (325 mg per day)	I
Age ≥60 years with diabetes mellitus	Oral anticoagulation (INR 2.0–3.0)	I
or coronary artery disease	Addition of aspirin, 81–162 mg/day is optional	IIb
Age ≥75 years, especially women	Oral anticoagulation (INR 2.0)	I
Heart failure Left ventricular ejection fraction ≤35% Thyrotoxicosis, hypertension	Oral anticoagulation (INR 2.0–3.0)	I
Rheumatic heart disease (mitral stenosis) Prosthetic heart valves Prior thromboembolism Persistent atrial thrombus on TEE	Oral anticoagulation (INR 2.5–3.5 or higher)	I

and derived primarily from published data. The weight of evidence was ranked highest (A) when the data were derived from multiple randomised clinical trials, and intermediate (B) when based on a limited number of randomised trials, non-randomised studies, or observational registries. The lowest rank (C) was given when the primary basis for the recommendation was expert consensus.

Recommendations summarise both the evidence and expert opinion:

Class I: Conditions for which there is evidence for and/or general agreement that the procedure or treatment is useful and effective;

Class II: Conditions for which there is conflicting evidence and/or a divergence of opinion about the usefulness/efficacy of a procedure or treatment;

Class IIa: The weight of evidence or opinion is in favour of the procedure or treatment;

Class IIb: Usefulness/efficacy is less well established by evidence or opinion;

Class III: Conditions for which there is evidence and/or general agreement that the procedure or treatment is not useful/effective and in some cases may be harmful.

CLASS I:

1) Administer antithrombotic therapy (oral anticoagulation or aspirin) for thromboembolic prevention to all patients with atrial fibrillation, except those with lone atrial fibrillation. (Level of evidence: A)

2) Individualise the selection of the antithrombotic agent, based upon assessment of the absolute risks of stroke, the risk of bleeding, and the relative risk/benefit ratio for a particular patient. (Level of evidence: A)

3) Administer chronic oral anticoagulant therapy in a dose adjusted to achieve a target INR of 2 to 3 in patients at high risk of stroke, unless contraindicated. (Level of evidence: A)

   a. The need for anticoagulation should be re-evaluated at regular intervals. (Level of evidence: A)

b. The INR should be determined at least weekly during the initiation of oral anti-coagulation therapy, and monthly when the patient is stable. (Level of evidence: A) (See also the specific chapter in this book.)

4) Aspirin in a dose of 325 mg daily is an alternative in low-risk patients or in those with certain contraindications to oral anticoagulation. (Level of evidence: A). *Our comment: although not based on experience in trials for atrial fibrillation, lower doses, in the range of 80–150 mg daily, may be as effective and possibly safer* [127].

5) Oral anticoagulation for patients with atrial fibrillation who have rheumatic mitral valve disease or prosthetic heart valves (mechanical or tissue valves). (Level of evidence: B)

a. Base the target intensity of anticoagulation on the particular type of prosthesis, but not less than INR 2 to 3. (Level of evidence: B)

CLASS IIA:

1) Target a lower INR of 2 (range 1.6 to 2.5) for primary prevention of ischaemic stroke and systemic embolism in patients over 75 years old considered at increased risk of bleeding complications, but without frank contraindications to oral anticoagulant therapy. (Level of evidence: C)

2) Manage antithrombotic therapy for patients with atrial flutter, in general, similarly as for those with atrial fibrillation. (Level of evidence: C)

3) Select antithrombotic therapy using the same criteria irrespective of the pattern of atrial fibrillation (i.e., for patients with paroxysmal, persistent, or permanent atrial fibrillation). (Level of evidence: B). *Our Comment: In patients who experience brief or minimally symptomatic recurrences of paroxysmal atrial fibrillation (two or more episodes) prevention of thromboembolism is appropriate* [10].

CLASS IIB:

1) Interrupt anticoagulation for a period of up to 1 week for surgical or diagnostic procedures that carry a risk of bleeding, without substituting heparin in patients with atrial fibrillation who do not have mechanical prosthetic heart valves. (Level of evidence: C)

2) Administer unfractionated or low-molecular-weight heparin intravenously or subcutaneously, respectively, in selected high-risk patients or when a series of procedures requires interruption of oral anticoagulant therapy for a period longer than 1 week. (Level of evidence: C)

3) Manage patients with CAD with anticoagulation (INR 2 to 3) based on the same criteria used for patients without CAD. (Level of evidence: C)

a. A low dose of aspirin (less than 100 mg/day) or clopidogrel (75 mg/day) may be given concurrently with anticoagulation, but these strategies have not been evaluated sufficiently and may be associated with an increased risk of bleeding. (Level of evidence: C). *Our comment: new data from the Warfarin-Aspirin Reinfarction Study II (WARIS II) indicate the superiority of adding aspirin to oral anticoagulants (INR 2.0–3.0) compared with aspirin alone in patients after an acute MI. Therefore, for such CAD patients with atrial fibrillation, it seems that there is now a full rationale and literature supporting the recommendation of adding low-dose aspirin to oral anticoagulation* [134].

4) Treatment with aspirin is optional for primary prevention of stroke in patients under 60 years of age without heart disease or risk factors for thromboembolism (lone atrial fibrillation). (Level of evidence: C)

CLASS III:

Long-term anticoagulation for stroke prevention in patients under 60 years of age without heart disease (lone atrial fibrillation) and without risk factors for thromboembolism. (Level of evidence: C)

THE ROLE OF TRANSOESOPHAGEAL ECHOCARDIOGRAPHY

Transoesophageal echocardiography is the most sensitive and specific imaging technique for the detection of thrombi in the left atrium or the left atrial appendage, by far surpassing transthoracic echocardiography [135]. Beside its usefulness in the detection of thrombi before cardioversion, TEE may be helpful in risk stratification of atrial fibrillation patients. The following echocardiographic findings have been associated with a higher risk of thromboembolism: presence of thrombus; dense spontaneous echo-contrast; or reduced velocity of blood flow in the left atrial appendage; and complex atheromatous plaque in the thoracic aorta [71]. Other echocardiographic signs, such as the diameter of the left atrium and fibrocalcific endocardial abnormalities, have been variably associated with thromboembolism and may interact with other factors. However, whether the absence of these abnormalities identifies a low-risk group of patients with other clinical risk factors who could safely avoid anticoagulation, while being suggested [61, 62] has not been established. Therefore, although TEE can provide additional information for stratifying thromboembolic risk, at present there is no clear evidence that TEE findings add independently to risk stratification when clinical and transthoracic echocardiographic risk factors are considered [136].

NEW ANTICOAGULANTS

LIMITATIONS OF COUMARIN DERIVATIVES

Although warfarin and similar coumarin derivatives clearly have the greatest efficacy in preventing stroke in atrial fibrillation among treatments commonly available, they carry a substantial risk of major bleedings (approximately 1.2% per year), and have a narrow therapeutic window, necessitating frequent coagulation monitoring to ensure appropriate dosing [133]. The marked variability in the dose–response relationship of oral anticoagulants makes it is unusually difficult to remain within the ideal INR range. Absorption from the gastrointestinal tract of the various coumarin derivatives is generally quite good, but their dose response is influenced by many other factors, including: (1) numerous drug interactions; (2) the dietary intake of vitamin K; (3) hepatic dysfunction; (4) changes in the gut flora; (5) patient compliance; and (6) alcohol intake. These factors are common, so that even within the controlled setting of a clinical trial it has not been possible to stay within the therapeutic window more than 50% of the time [100]. This creates the necessity of unpleasant, frequent and assiduous monitoring of the prothrombin time in every patient treated with oral anticoagulants in order to reduce the risk of serious bleedings on the one hand, and of undertreatment on the other. Even with careful monitoring, patient selection is required to screen out patients who might be at increased risk of haemorrhage [68, 106, 108, 137]. Several trials used some criteria to exclude patients from enrolment: dementia, elevated creatinine, anaemia with haemoglobin below 100 g/l, blood pressure >180/100 mmHg despite treatment, severe chronic alcoholism, previous intracranial haemorrhage, severe bleeding with a therapeutic INR while receiving a vitamin K antagonist, predisposition to head trauma and requirement for non-steroidal anti-inflammatory drugs [95, 97–99].

Other reasons vitamin K antagonists for atrial fibrillation are so poorly tolerated and actually impractical for many patients include the clear disadvantages of having to be tied to the medical system for life-long anticoagulation monitoring, with restriction of travelling, anxiety, cost and loss of freedom, the need to avoid most non-steroidal anti-inflammatory drugs and to carefully control alcohol consumption, and for caution in the use of other drugs and in changing dietary patterns because of potential drug interactions. In summary, therapy with vitamin K antagonists is complex, potentially dangerous and unpleasant, and this has resulted in considerable difficulty in convincing physicians and patients to adhere to current practice guidelines, with a resulting undertreatment in a considerable proportion of patients at risk [138]. This is ample justification for the need for safer, more convenient alternatives to coumarin derivatives for stroke prevention.

XIMELAGATRAN

Ximelagatran is an oral direct thrombin inhibitor currently under investigation as an anti-coagulant for prevention and treatment of thromboembolism. Its pharmacokinetic profile is predictable and stable over time [139], and unaffected by body weight, age, sex, or ethnic origin [140–142]. After ingestion, ximelagatran is absorbed from the small intestine and undergoes rapid biotransformation to melagatran, the active agent [143]. Ximelagatran has stable and highly predictable pharmacokinetics, with rapid onset of action and metabolism independent of the hepatic cytochrome P450 enzyme system and elimination by the kidneys. It has a plasma half-life of 4 to 5 h and is therefore administered orally twice daily [143]. It has a low potential for drug interactions and no known food interactions, making coagulation monitoring and dose adjustments unnecessary [139–141].

Ximelagatran has been evaluated for venous thromboprophylaxis in high-risk orthopaedic patients in six phase III trials. In three of these studies [144–146] it has been compared with enoxaparin and in the other three [147–149] with warfarin. Data from the first three studies are not completely concordant. In the METHRO III trial [146] ximelagatran showed efficacy and safety similar to pre-operative enoxaparin, in the Platinum Hip study [144], postoperative enoxaparin was more effective and showed an incidence of bleeding similar to the postoperative ximelagatran regimen, whereas in the EXPRESS trial [145] the combination of pre-operative melagatran and postoperative ximelagatran was more effective than pre-operative enoxaparin, but at the cost of more bleeding. In all three trials in which it has been compared with warfarin [147–149] ximelagatran showed greater efficacy.

In the treatment of venous thromboembolism, ximelagatran has been evaluated in two phase III trials [150, 151], where it has been shown to be an effective and safe alternative to treatment with LMWH followed by warfarin for the acute treatment. In acute coronary syndromes (ACS), ximelagatran appears to reduce all-cause mortality, non-fatal MI, and severe recurrent ischaemia in the ESTEEM study [152].

Two phase III trials have compared ximelagatran 36 mg twice daily with warfarin (targeted to an INR of 2.0–3.0) for the prevention of cardioembolic events in high-risk patients with non-valvular atrial fibrillation [153, 154]. The SPORTIF III study [153] randomised 3407 such subjects in an open-label fashion to receive either ximelagatran or adjusted-dose warfarin. Ximelagatran was proven here to be at least as effective as (and possibly better than) well-controlled, dose-adjusted warfarin in preventing stroke and systemic embolic events (1.6 events/year in the ximelagatran group vs. 2.3% in the warfarin group; $P = 0.10$, at the intention-to-treat analysis; 1.3 events/year in the ximelagatran group vs. 2.2% in the warfarin group; $P = 0.018$, at the on-treatment analysis). Ximelagatran also caused less bleeding than warfarin (major + minor bleeding: 25.8 events/year in the ximelagatran group vs. 29.8% in the warfarin group; $P = 0.007$) and offered fixed oral dosing without coagulation monitoring [153]. The trend of efficacy and the net clinical benefit (deaths + primary events + major bleeding: 4.6 events/year in the ximelagatran group vs. 6.1% events/year in the warfarin group; relative risk reduction 25%; $P = 0.022$) was in favour of ximelagatran.

The SPORTIF V trial randomised 3922 participants with non-valvular atrial fibrillation (and more than one additional vascular risk factor) to receive either ximelagratran or adjusted-dose warfarin [154]. Contrary to SPORTIF III, SPORTIF V was a double-blind, double-dummy trial. The results showed a comparable efficacy and safety between the two drugs but, differently from SPORTIF III, with a trend towards a greater efficacy for warfarin (1.6 events/year in the ximelagatran group vs. 1.2% in the warfarin group). When the results of SPORTIF III and V were combined, ximelagatran was associated with a 16% relative risk reduction in the composite outcome measure of all strokes (ischaemic or haemorrhagic), systemic embolic events, major bleeding and death. In both trials transient elevation of liver enzymes was reported in a small proportion of patients (incidence of about 6%), similarly to previous clinical experience with the drug. Although the problem appears to be self-limited and reversible in most cases, there is a need for further scrutiny of this side-effect of the drug.

FACTOR Xa INHIBITORS

Factor Xa inhibitors act indirectly or directly. New indirect inhibitors, fondaparinux and idraparinux, are synthetic analogs of the unique pentasaccharide sequence that mediates the interaction of heparin with antithrombin [155]. Once the pentasaccharide/antithrombin (ATIII) complex binds factor Xa, the pentasaccharide dissociates from antithrombin/Xa complex and can be re-utilised to catalyse other similar types of reactions.

Fondaparinux binds antithrombin with high affinity, has excellent bioavailability after subcutaneous injection, and has a plasma half-life of 17 h, permitting once-daily administration [156]. The drug is excreted unchanged in the urine and is contraindicated in patients with severe renal impairment (creatinine clearance <30 ml/min). There is no antidote for fondaparinux. Fondaparinux has been evaluated for the prevention and treatment of venous thromboembolism. It has been shown to be more effective than enoxaparin in four large phase III trials for thromboprophylaxis: PENTATHLON, PENTHIFRA, PENTAMAKS and EPHESUS [157–160] in patients undergoing surgery for hip fracture or elective hip or knee arthroplasty, for which indications it is now licensed. In a meta-analysis of these studies, fondaparinux reduced the risk of venous thromboembolism by 55% compared with enoxaparin [161]. Major bleeding occurred more frequently in the fondaparinux-treated group, but the incidence of bleeding leading to death, re-operation or occurring in a critical organ was not significantly different between the two groups [161].

Fondaparinux has also been evaluated in general surgery patients, compared to dalteparin, in the PEGASUS study [162], and in acutely-ill, hospitalised, medical patients, compared to placebo, in the ARTEMIS study [163]. In the first of such studies, both the efficacy of the two drugs in the prevention of thromboembolism and the incidence of major bleeding were not statistically different. In the second study, fondaparinux showed superiority compared with placebo.

Fondaparinux has been evaluated for the initial treatment of venous thromboembolism in two double-blind, non-inferiority, randomised, phase III clinical trials. The MATISSE-DVT trial [164], in which fondaparinux has been compared with enoxaparin in patients with deep venous thrombosis, and the MATISSE-PE trial [165], in which fondaparinux has been compared with UFH in patients with pulmonary embolism. In these studies fondaparinux was at least as effective and safe as enoxaparin or UFH for the initial treatment of venous thromboembolism.

Fondaparinux has also been evaluated for the treatment of acute coronary syndromes in two phase II studies [166, 167], where bleeding was similar in all treatment groups. Based on these results, phase III trials with fondaparinux in patients with non-ST-elevation (MICHELANGELO: OASIS 5) and ST-elevation myocardial infarction (MICHELANGELO: OASIS 6) have been initiated.

Idraparinux is a derivate of fondaparinux. It has 100% bioavailability *via* the subcutaneous route, is excreted mainly in the urine, has a linear, dose-dependent pharmacokinetic profile, reaches peak concentration in 1–3 h, has a plasma half-life of 130 h allowing a once-weekly administration, and has no significant binding to other blood, plasma or endothelial proteins [168]. Idraparinux was compared with warfarin in the PERSIST trial, a phase II trial of 659 patients with proximal deep venous thrombosis. The primary outcomes were similar in all idraparinux groups and did not differ from those in the warfarin group, but there was a clear dose response for major bleeding in patients treated with idraparinux with less bleeding with 2.5 mg idraparinux than with warfarin [169].

One phase III study, the AMADEUS trial, is ongoing for the evaluation of idraparinux compared with warfarin in patients with atrial fibrillation.

CLOPIDOGREL PLUS ASPIRIN: AN ALTERNATIVE OPTION

Ticlopidine and clopidogrel are the two thienopyridines of clinical interest. They are both non-competitive but selective adenosine diphosphate (ADP) receptor antagonists (irreversibly blocking the $P2Y_{12}$ platelet receptor), but the use of ticlopidine is limited by the occurrence of bone marrow depression leading to leukopaenia with neutropaenia in about 1% of patients and occasionally to thrombocytopaenia and pancytopaenia [170]. Clopidogrel is chemically related to ticlopidine and has a similar mechanism of action, but is largely free of the risk of blood dyscrasia [171]. Because of its superior safety profile and tolerability, clopidogrel is now the thienopyridine of choice in clinical practice. The effectiveness and safety of clopidogrel, alone and in combination with aspirin, have been established in a large number of important randomised trials. A single large phase III trial, the CAPRIE study [172], tested its efficacy and safety at 75 mg daily compared with aspirin at 325 mg daily: clopidogrel was found to be slightly more effective than aspirin, and no excess neutropaenia was associated with its use.

The benefits of combining a thienopyridine with aspirin were first conclusively demonstrated in patients undergoing coronary artery stent placement procedures. Four randomised studies [173–176] have compared ticlopidine plus aspirin with warfarin plus aspirin, showing less stent thrombosis with ticlopidine plus aspirin with less bleeding. Two trials have compared ticlopidine plus aspirin with aspirin alone [175, 177], showing an even more impressive effect of the combination compared with aspirin alone. Moreover, two trials have reported that the combination of clopidogrel plus aspirin has similar efficacy against thrombotic events as ticlopidine plus aspirin, but with less toxicity [178, 179].

The CURE trial [180] has demonstrated the efficacy and safety of adding clopidogrel (a loading dose of 300 mg, followed by 75 mg daily) to aspirin in the long-term management of patients with ACS without ST-segment elevation. The PCI-CURE study [181] documented that pre-treatment with clopidogrel yielded a 1.5% absolute risk reduction when compared with standard aspirin in the 1-month composite of cardiovascular death or MI after stent-percutaneous coronary intervention (PCI) among patients with non-ST-segment elevation ACS, and the combination of aspirin and clopidogrel has become standard treatment for 1 month after coronary stent implantation. The more recent CREDO trial [182] has demonstrated that, following PCI, long-term (1-year) clopidogrel therapy significantly reduces the risk of adverse ischaemic events.

There is a rationale to evaluate the combination of clopidogrel plus aspirin for prevention of vascular complications associated with atrial fibrillation. The idea that antiplatelet agents are not effective against thrombotic events related to stasis is no longer tenable. Furthermore, the typical patient with atrial fibrillation who requires antithrombotic therapy also has multiple risk factors for vascular disease, as well as for left atrial thrombus.

Since the effect of adding clopidogrel to usual care with aspirin in CURE [180] involved an additional risk reduction of 20% in vascular events, and since the addition of ticlopidine to aspirin significantly reduced death or MI compared with aspirin alone after PCI, one can conclude that the effect of adding clopidogrel to aspirin in patients with atrial fibrillation will be a further reduction in vascular events compared to aspirin alone. Moreover, based on the results of the four trials comparing the combination of ticlopidine plus aspirin vs. warfarin plus aspirin in the prevention of stent thrombosis (discussed above), it is also possible that clopidogrel plus aspirin will be equivalent to warfarin in patients with atrial fibrillation. As discussed above, in patients with atrial fibrillation, the likely benefit of warfarin over aspirin for the outcome of total vascular events is a relative risk reduction of about 20%, which is similar to the additional benefit that one would expect from adding clopidogrel to aspirin. On these presumptions, the Atrial Fibrillation Clopidogrel Trial with Irbesartan for prevention of Vascular Events (ACTIVE) is now on its way. ACTIVE is a parallel randomised controlled evaluation of clopidogrel plus aspirin, with factorial evaluation of irbesartan, for the prevention of vascular events, in patients with atrial fibrillation. The aim of this trial is to demonstrate that the combination clopidogrel plus aspirin is truly equivalent to warfarin for prevention of vascular events in atrial fibrillation and is superior to aspirin alone. On the other hand, it is expected that antiplatelet therapy will be safer. Our preliminary experience in the Clopidogrel-Aspirin Atrial Fibrillation (CLAAF) Pilot Study, in a small number of non-high risk patients with persistent or permanent atrial fibrillation, randomised to warfarin or to the combination of clopidogrel and aspirin for three weeks, and undergoing TEE to search for variations in TEE parameters as surrogate endpoints for thromboembolism [183], testify to the feasibility of this approach and to the need of truly comparing its efficacy against warfarin.

CONCLUSIONS

The past 20 years have led to a considerable improvement in the antithrombotic prophylaxis of atrial fibrillation, through a proper stratification of the thromboembolic risk, the establishment of the proper ranges of anticoagulation with warfarin, and the demonstration of its superiority over treatment with single antiplatelet agents in high-risk patients. The years to come will likely see warfarin therapy being replaced with better tolerated and more manageable drugs.

In September 2004 the ACTIVE W Study was terminated due to the manifest superiority of the warfarin arm over the combination of aspirin and clopidogrel arm. The ACTIVE A Study continues.

REFERENCES

1. Konings KT, Kirchhof CJ, Smeets JR, Wellens HJ, Penn OC, Allessie MA. High-density mapping of electrically induced atrial fibrillation in humans. *Circulation* 1994; 89:1665–1680.
2. Ruffy R. Atrial Fibrillation. In: Zipes D, Jalife J (eds). *Cardiac Electrophysiology: From Cell to Bedside*. WB Saunders Company, Philadelphia, 1994, p. 682.
3. Bellet S (ed). *Clinical Disorders of the Heart Beat*. Lea & Febiger, Philadelphia, 1971.
4. Prystowsky E, Katz A. Atrial fibrillation. In: Topol E (ed). *Textbook of Cardiovascular Medicine*. Lippincott-Raven, Philadelphia, 1998, pp. 1827–1861.
5. Bharti S, Lev M. Histology of the normal and diseased atrium. In: Falk R, Podrid P (eds). *Atrial Fibrillation: Mechanism and Management*. Raven Press, New York, 1992, pp 15–39.
6. Guiraudon C, Ernst N, Yee R, Lein G. The pathology of drug resistant lone atrial fibrillation in eleven surgically treated patients. In: Kingma J, Van Hernel N, Lie K (eds). *Atrial Fibrillation: A Treatable Disease?* Kluwer Academic Publ, Dordrecht, 1992, pp 41–57.
7. Frustaci A, Chimenti C, Bellocci F, Morgante E, Russo MA, Maseri A. Histological substrate of atrial biopsies in patients with lone atrial fibrillation. *Circulation* 1997; 96:1180–1184.
8. Dittrich HC, Pearce LA, Asinger RW *et al.* Left atrial diameter in nonvalvular atrial fibrillation: An echocardiographic study. Stroke Prevention in Atrial Fibrillation Investigators. *Am Heart J* 1999; 137:494–499.
9. Li D, Fareh S, Leung TK, Nattel S. Promotion of atrial fibrillation by heart failure in dogs: atrial remodeling of a different sort. *Circulation* 1999; 100:87–95.

10. Fuster V, Ryden LE, Asinger RW *et al*. ACC/AHA/ESC guidelines for the management of patients with atrial fibrillation: executive summary. A Report of the American College of Cardiology/ American Heart Association Task Force on Practice Guidelines and the European Society of Cardiology Committee for Practice Guidelines and Policy Conferences (Committee to Develop Guidelines for the Management of Patients With Atrial Fibrillation): developed in Collaboration With the North American Society of Pacing and Electrophysiology. *J Am Coll Cardiol* 2001; 38:1231–1266.

11. Ostranderld J, Brandt R, Kjelsberg M, Epstein F. Electrocardiographic findings among the adult population of a total natural community, Tecumseh, Michigan. *Circulation* 1965; 31:888–898.

12. Flegel KM, Shipley MJ, Rose G. Risk of stroke in non-rheumatic atrial fibrillation. *Lancet* 1987; 1:526–529.

13. Wolf PA, Abbott RD, Kannel WB. Atrial fibrillation as an independent risk factor for stroke: the Framingham Study. *Stroke* 1991; 22:983–988.

14. Furberg CD, Psaty BM, Manolio TA, Gardin JM, Smith VE, Rautaharju PM. Prevalence of atrial fibrillation in elderly subjects (the Cardiovascular Health Study). *Am J Cardiol* 1994; 74:236–241.

15. Kannel WB, Abbott RD, Savage DD, McNamara PM. Coronary heart disease and atrial fibrillation: the Framingham Study. *Am Heart J* 1983; 106:389–396.

16. Evans W, Swann P. Lone auricular fibrillation. *Br Heart J* 1954; 16:189–194.

17. Brand FN, Abbott RD, Kannel WB, Wolf PA. Characteristics and prognosis of lone atrial fibrillation. 30-year follow-up in the Framingham Study. *JAMA* 1985; 254:3449–3453.

18. Kopecky SL, Gersh BJ, McGoon MD *et al*. The natural history of lone atrial fibrillation. A population-based study over three decades. *N Engl J Med* 1987; 317:669–674.

19. Levy S, Maarek M, Coumel P *et al*. Characterization of different subsets of atrial fibrillation in general practice in France: the ALFA study. The College of French Cardiologists. *Circulation* 1999; 99:3028–3035.

20. Murgatroyd FD, Gibson SM, Baiyan XH *et al*. Double-blind placebo-controlled trial of digoxin in symptomatic paroxysmal atrial fibrillation. *Circulation* 1999; 99:2765–2770.

21. Wolf PA, Abbott RD, Kannel WB. Atrial fibrillation: a major contributor to stroke in the elderly. The Framingham Study. *Arch Intern Med* 1987; 147:1561–1564.

22. Krahn AD, Manfreda J, Tate RB, Mathewson FA, Cuddy TE. The natural history of atrial fibrillation: incidence, risk factors, and prognosis in the Manitoba Follow-Up Study. *Am J Med* 1995; 98:476–484.

23. Psaty BM, Manolio TA, Kuller LH *et al*. Incidence of and risk factors for atrial fibrillation in older adults. *Circulation* 1997; 96:2455–2461.

24. Benjamin EJ, Levy D, Vaziri SM, D'Agostino RB, Belanger AJ, Wolf PA. Independent risk factors for atrial fibrillation in a population-based cohort. The Framingham Heart Study. *JAMA* 1994; 271:840–844.

25. Tsang TS, Petty GW, Barnes ME *et al*. The prevalence of atrial fibrillation in incident stroke cases and matched population controls in Rochester, Minnesota: changes over three decades. *J Am Coll Cardiol* 2003; 42:93–100.

26. Feinberg WM, Blackshear JL, Laupacis A, Kronmal R, Hart RG. Prevalence, age distribution, and gender of patients with atrial fibrillation. Analysis and implications. *Arch Intern Med* 1995; 155:469–473.

27. Sudlow M, Thomson R, Thwaites B, Rodgers H, Kenny RA. Prevalence of atrial fibrillation and eligibility for anticoagulants in the community. *Lancet* 1998; 352:1167–1171.

28. Wolf PA, Benjamin EJ, Belanger AJ, Kannel WB, Levy D, D'Agostino RB. Secular trends in the prevalence of atrial fibrillation: The Framingham Study. *Am Heart J* 1996; 131:790–795.

29. Tsang TS, Gersh BJ, Appleton CP *et al*. Left ventricular diastolic dysfunction as a predictor of the first diagnosed nonvalvular atrial fibrillation in 840 elderly men and women. *J Am Coll Cardiol* 2002; 40:1636–1644.

30. Lindroos M, Kupari M, Heikkila J, Tilvis R. Prevalence of aortic valve abnormalities in the elderly: an echocardiographic study of a random population sample. *J Am Coll Cardiol* 1993; 21:1220–1225.

31. Wolf PA, Dawber TR, Thomas HE, Jr., Kannel WB. Epidemiologic assessment of chronic atrial fibrillation and risk of stroke: the Framingham Study. *Neurology* 1978; 28:973–977.

32. Cairns JA, Connolly SJ. Nonrheumatic atrial fibrillation. Risk of stroke and role of antithrombotic therapy. *Circulation* 1991; 84:469–481.

33. Whisnant JP, Wiebers DO, O'Fallon WM, Sicks JD, Frye RL. A population-based model of risk factors for ischemic stroke: Rochester, Minnesota. *Neurology* 1996; 47:1420–1428.

34. Simons LA, McCallum J, Friedlander Y, Simons J. Risk factors for ischemic stroke: Dubbo Study of the elderly. *Stroke* 1998; 29:1341–1346.

35. Lip GY. The prothrombotic state in atrial fibrillation: new insights, more questions, and clear answers needed. *Am Heart J* 2000; 140:348–350.

36. Kumagai K, Fukunami M, Ohmori M, Kitabatake A, Kamada T, Hoki N. Increased intracardiovascular clotting in patients with chronic atrial fibrillation. *J Am Coll Cardiol* 1990; 16:377–380.

37. Lip GY. Does atrial fibrillation confer a hypercoagulable state? *Lancet* 1995; 346:1313–1314.

38. Poli KA, Tofler GH, Larson MG et al. Association of blood pressure with fibrinolytic potential in the Framingham offspring population. *Circulation* 2000; 101:264–269.

39. Ott A, Breteler MM, de Bruyne MC, van Harskamp F, Grobbee DE, Hofman A. Atrial fibrillation and dementia in a population-based study. The Rotterdam Study. *Stroke* 1997; 28:316–321.

40. O'Connell JE, Gray CS, French JM, Robertson IH. Atrial fibrillation and cognitive function: case-control study. *J Neurol Neurosurg Psychiatry* 1998; 65:386–389.

41. Kilander L, Andren B, Nyman H, Lind L, Boberg M, Lithell H. Atrial fibrillation is an independent determinant of low cognitive function: a cross-sectional study in elderly men. *Stroke* 1998; 29:1816–1820.

42. Breteler MM. Vascular involvement in cognitive decline and dementia. Epidemiologic evidence from the Rotterdam Study and the Rotterdam Scan Study. *Ann N Y Acad Sci* 2000; 903:457–465.

43. Sabatini T, Frisoni GB, Barbisoni P, Bellelli G, Rozzini R, Trabucchi M. Atrial fibrillation and cognitive disorders in older people. *J Am Geriatr Soc* 2000; 48:387–390.

44. Scheinman MM. Atrial fibrillation and congestive heart failure: the intersection of two common diseases. *Circulation* 1998; 98:941–942.

45. Shinbane JS, Wood MA, Jensen DN, Ellenbogen KA, Fitzpatrick AP, Scheinman MM. Tachycardia-induced cardiomyopathy: a review of animal models and clinical studies. *J Am Coll Cardiol* 1997; 29:709–715.

46. Stevenson WG, Stevenson LW. Atrial fibrillation in heart failure. *N Engl J Med* 1999; 341:910–911.

47. Redfield MM, Kay GN, Jenkins LS, Mianulli M, Jensen DN, Ellenbogen KA. Tachycardia-related cardiomyopathy: a common cause of ventricular dysfunction in patients with atrial fibrillation referred for atrioventricular ablation. *Mayo Clin Proc* 2000; 75:790–795.

48. Pozzoli M, Cioffi G, Traversi E, Pinna GD, Cobelli F, Tavazzi L. Predictors of primary atrial fibrillation and concomitant clinical and hemodynamic changes in patients with chronic heart failure: a prospective study in 344 patients with baseline sinus rhythm. *J Am Coll Cardiol* 1998; 32:197–204.

49. Tsang TS, Barnes ME, Bailey KR et al. Left atrial volume: important risk marker of incident atrial fibrillation in 1655 older men and women. *Mayo Clin Proc* 2001; 76:467–475.

50. Jais P, Shah DC, Takahashi A, Hocini M, Haissaguerre M, Clementy J. Long-term follow-up after right atrial radiofrequency catheter treatment of paroxysmal atrial fibrillation. *Pacing Clin Electrophysiol* 1998; 21(11 Pt 2):2533–2538.

51. Kanter MC, Tegeler CH, Pearce LA et al. Carotid stenosis in patients with atrial fibrillation. Prevalence, risk factors, and relationship to stroke in the Stroke Prevention in Atrial Fibrillation Study. *Arch Intern Med* 1994; 154:1372–1377.

52. Bogousslavsky J, Van Melle G, Regli F, Kappenberger L. Pathogenesis of anterior circulation stroke in patients with nonvalvular atrial fibrillation: the Lausanne Stroke Registry. *Neurology* 1990; 40:1046–1050.

53. Miller VT, Rothrock JF, Pearce LA, Feinberg WM, Hart RG, Anderson DC. Ischemic stroke in patients with atrial fibrillation: effect of aspirin according to stroke mechanism. Stroke Prevention in Atrial Fibrillation Investigators. *Neurology* 1993; 43:32–36.

54. Wyse DG, Gersh BJ. Atrial fibrillation: a perspective: thinking inside and outside the box. *Circulation* 2004; 109:3089–3095.

55. Cha YM, Redfield MM, Shen WK, Gersh BJ. Atrial fibrillation and ventricular dysfunction: a vicious electromechanical cycle. *Circulation* 2004; 109:2839–2843.

56. Wolf PA, D'Agostino RB, Belanger AJ, Kannel WB. Probability of stroke: a risk profile from the Framingham Study. *Stroke* 1991; 22:312–318.

57. Hart RG, Pearce LA, Rothbart RM, McAnulty JH, Asinger RW, Halperin JL. Stroke with intermittent atrial fibrillation: incidence and predictors during aspirin therapy. Stroke Prevention in Atrial Fibrillation Investigators. *J Am Coll Cardiol* 2000; 35:183–187.

58. Secondary prevention in non-rheumatic atrial fibrillation after transient ischaemic attack or minor stroke. EAFT (European Atrial Fibrillation Trial) Study Group. *Lancet* 1993; 342:1255–1262.

59. Adjusted-dose warfarin versus low-intensity, fixed-dose warfarin plus aspirin for high-risk patients with atrial fibrillation: Stroke Prevention in Atrial Fibrillation III randomised clinical trial. *Lancet* 1996; 348:633–638.

60. Chimowitz MI, DeGeorgia MA, Poole RM, Hepner A, Armstrong WM. Left atrial spontaneous echo contrast is highly associated with previous stroke in patients with atrial fibrillation or mitral stenosis. *Stroke* 1993; 24:1015–1019.

61. Goldman ME, Pearce LA Hart RG *et al.* Pathophysiologic correlates of thromboembolism in nonvalvular atrial fibrillation: I. Reduced flow velocity in the left atrial appendage (The Stroke Prevention in Atrial Fibrillation [SPAF-III] study). *J Am Soc Echocardiogr* 1999; 12:1080–1087.

62. Asinger RW, Koehler J, Pearce LA *et al.* Pathophysiologic correlates of thromboembolism in nonvalvular atrial fibrillation: II. Dense spontaneous echocardiographic contrast (The Stroke Prevention in Atrial Fibrillation [SPAF-III] study). *J Am Soc Echocardiogr* 1999; 12:1088–1096.

63. Blackshear JL, Pearce LA, Hart RG *et al.* Aortic plaque in atrial fibrillation: prevalence, predictors, and thromboembolic implications. *Stroke* 1999; 30:834–840.

64. Hursting MJ, Stead AG, Crout FV, Horvath BZ, Moore BM. Effects of age, race, sex, and smoking on prothrombin fragment 1.2 in a healthy population. *Clin Chem* 1993; 39:683–686.

65. Cushman M, Psaty BM, Macy E *et al.* Correlates of thrombin markers in an elderly cohort free of clinical cardiovascular disease. *Arterioscler Thromb Vasc Biol* 1996; 16:1163–1169.

66. Lowe GD, Rumley A, Woodward M *et al.* Epidemiology of coagulation factors, inhibitors and activation markers: the Third Glasgow MONICA Survey. I. Illustrative reference ranges by age, sex and hormone use. *Br J Haematol* 1997; 97:775–784.

67. Feinberg WM, Cornell ES, Nightingale SD *et al.* Relationship between prothrombin activation fragment F1.2 and international normalized ratio in patients with atrial fibrillation. Stroke Prevention in Atrial Fibrillation Investigators. *Stroke* 1997; 28:1101–1106.

68. Hart RG, Pearce LA, McBride R, Rothbart RM, Asinger RW. Factors associated with ischemic stroke during aspirin therapy in atrial fibrillation: analysis of 2012 participants in the SPAF I-III clinical trials. The Stroke Prevention in Atrial Fibrillation (SPAF) Investigators. *Stroke* 1999; 30:1223–1229.

69. Risk factors for stroke and efficacy of antithrombotic therapy in atrial fibrillation. Analysis of pooled data from five randomized controlled trials. *Arch Intern Med* 1994; 154:1449–1457.

70. Patients with nonvalvular atrial fibrillation at low risk of stroke during treatment with aspirin: Stroke Prevention in Atrial Fibrillation III Study. The SPAF III Writing Committee for the Stroke Prevention in Atrial Fibrillation Investigators. *JAMA* 1998; 279:1273–1277.

71. Zabalgoitia M, Halperin JL, Pearce LA, Blackshear JL, Asinger RW, Hart RG. Transesophageal echocardiographic correlates of clinical risk of thromboembolism in nonvalvular atrial fibrillation. Stroke Prevention in Atrial Fibrillation III Investigators. *J Am Coll Cardiol* 1998; 31:1622–1626.

72. Predictors of thromboembolism in atrial fibrillation: I. Clinical features of patients at risk. The Stroke Prevention in Atrial Fibrillation Investigators. *Ann Intern Med* 1992; 116:1–5.

73. Kopecky SL, Gersh BJ, McGoon MD *et al.* Lone atrial fibrillation in elderly persons: a marker for cardiovascular risk. *Arch Intern Med* 1999; 159:1118–1122.

74. Scardi S, Mazzone C, Pandullo C, Goldstein D, Poletti A, Humar F. Lone atrial fibrillation: prognostic differences between paroxysmal and chronic forms after 10 years of follow-up. *Am Heart J* 1999; 137(4 Pt 1):686–691.

75. Ruigómez A, Johansson S, Wallander M, García Rodríguez L. Predictors and prognosis of paroxysmal atrial fibrillation in general practice. In press.

76. Predictors of thromboembolism in atrial fibrillation: II. Echocardiographic features of patients at risk. The Stroke Prevention in Atrial Fibrillation Investigators. *Ann Intern Med* 1992; 116:6–12.

77. Bogousslavsky J, Cachin C, Regli F, Despland PA, Van Melle G, Kappenberger L. Cardiac sources of embolism and cerebral infarction – clinical consequences and vascular concomitants: the Lausanne Stroke Registry. *Neurology* 1991; 41:855–859.

78. Mugge A, Kuhn H, Nikutta P, Grote J, Lopez JA, Daniel WG. Assessment of left atrial appendage function by biplane transesophageal echocardiography in patients with nonrheumatic atrial fibrillation: identification of a subgroup of patients at increased embolic risk. *J Am Coll Cardiol* 1994; 23:599–607.

79. Daniel WG, Nellessen U, Schroder E *et al.* Left atrial spontaneous echo contrast in mitral valve disease: an indicator for an increased thromboembolic risk. *J Am Coll Cardiol* 1988; 11:1204–1211.

80. Black IW, Chesterman CN, Hopkins AP, Lee LC, Chong BH, Walsh WF. Hematologic correlates of left atrial spontaneous echo contrast and thromboembolism in nonvalvular atrial fibrillation. *J Am Coll Cardiol* 1993; 21:451–457.

81. Pop GA, Meeder HJ, Roelandt JR *et al.* Transthoracic echo/Doppler in the identification of patients with chronic non-valvular atrial fibrillation at risk for thromboembolic events. *Eur Heart J* 1994; 15:1545–1551.

82. Fatkin D, Kelly RP, Feneley MP. Relations between left atrial appendage blood flow velocity, spontaneous echocardiographic contrast and thromboembolic risk *in vivo*. *J Am Coll Cardiol* 1994; 23:961–969.

83. Li YH, Lai LP, Shyu KG, Hwang JJ, Kuan P, Lien WP. Clinical implications of left atrial appendage flow patterns in nonrheumatic atrial fibrillation. *Chest* 1994; 105:748–752.

84. Gustafsson C, Blomback M, Britton M, Hamsten A, Svensson J. Coagulation factors and the increased risk of stroke in nonvalvular atrial fibrillation. *Stroke* 1990; 21:47–51.

85. Heppell RM, Berkin KE, McLenachan JM, Davies JA. Haemostatic and haemodynamic abnormalities associated with left atrial thrombosis in non-rheumatic atrial fibrillation. *Heart* 1997; 77:407–411.

86. Lip GY. Hypercoagulability and haemodynamic abnormalities in atrial fibrillation. *Heart* 1997; 77:395–396.

87. Asakura H, Hifumi S, Jokaji H et al. Prothrombin fragment F1 + 2 and thrombin-antithrombin III complex are useful markers of the hypercoagulable state in atrial fibrillation. *Blood Coagul Fibrinolysis* 1992; 3:469–473.

88. Lip GY, Lowe GD, Rumley A, Dunn FG. Fibrinogen and fibrin D-dimer levels in paroxysmal atrial fibrillation: evidence for intermediate elevated levels of intravascular thrombogenesis. *Am Heart J* 1996; 131:724–730.

89. Lip GY, Lip PL, Zarifis J et al. Fibrin D-dimer and beta-thromboglobulin as markers of thrombogenesis and platelet activation in atrial fibrillation. Effects of introducing ultra-low-dose warfarin and aspirin. *Circulation* 1996; 94:425–431.

90. Mitusch R, Siemens HJ, Garbe M, Wagner T, Sheikhzadeh A, Diederich KW. Detection of a hypercoagulable state in nonvalvular atrial fibrillation and the effect of anticoagulant therapy. *Thromb Haemost* 1996;75:219–223.

91. Sohara H, Amitani S, Kurose M, Miyahara K. Atrial fibrillation activates platelets and coagulation in a time-dependent manner: a study in patients with paroxysmal atrial fibrillation. *J Am Coll Cardiol* 1997; 29:106–112.

92. Tsai LM, Chen JH, Tsao CJ. Relation of left atrial spontaneous echo contrast with prethrombotic state in atrial fibrillation associated with systemic hypertension, idiopathic dilated cardiomyopathy, or no identifiable cause (lone). *Am J Cardiol* 1998; 81:1249–1252.

93. Singer DE, Albers GW, Dalen JE, Go AS, Halperin JL, Manning WJ. Antithrombotic Therapy in Atrial Fibrillation: The Seventh ACCP Conference on Antithrombotic and Thrombolytic Therapy. *Chest* 2004; 126(3 suppl):429S–456S.

94. Suttie JW. The biochemical basis of warfarin therapy. *Adv Exp Med Biol* 1987; 214:3–16.

95. Ezekowitz MD, Bridgers SL, James KE et al. Warfarin in the prevention of stroke associated with nonrheumatic atrial fibrillation. Veterans Affairs Stroke Prevention in Nonrheumatic Atrial Fibrillation Investigators. *N Engl J Med* 1992; 327:1406–1412.

96. Wilson S, Crowther MA, Costantini L. An interim analysis to improve precision of warfarin anticoagulation in a randomized clinical trial. *Blood* 1999; 94:115b.

97. Petersen P, Boysen G, Godtfredsen J, Andersen ED, Andersen B. Placebo-controlled, randomised trial of warfarin and aspirin for prevention of thromboembolic complications in chronic atrial fibrillation. The Copenhagen AFASAK study. *Lancet* 1989; 1:175–179.

98. The effect of low-dose warfarin on the risk of stroke in patients with nonrheumatic atrial fibrillation. The Boston Area Anticoagulation Trial for Atrial Fibrillation Investigators. *N Engl J Med* 1990; 323:1505–1511.

99. Stroke Prevention in Atrial Fibrillation Study. Final results. *Circulation* 1991; 84:527–539.

100. Connolly SJ, Laupacis A, Gent M, Roberts RS, Cairns JA, Joyner C. Canadian Atrial Fibrillation Anticoagulation (CAFA) Study. *J Am Coll Cardiol* 1991; 18:349–355.

101. Hart RG, Benavente O, McBride R, Pearce LA. Antithrombotic therapy to prevent stroke in patients with atrial fibrillation: a meta-analysis. *Ann Intern Med* 1999; 131:492–501.

102. Optimal oral anticoagulant therapy in patients with nonrheumatic atrial fibrillation and recent cerebral ischemia. The European Atrial Fibrillation Trial Study Group. *N Engl J Med* 1995; 333:5–10.

103. Hylek EM, Skates SJ, Sheehan MA, Singer DE. An analysis of the lowest effective intensity of prophylactic anticoagulation for patients with nonrheumatic atrial fibrillation. *N Engl J Med* 1996; 335:540–546.

104. Hylek EM, Singer DE. Risk factors for intracranial hemorrhage in outpatients taking warfarin. *Ann Intern Med* 1994; 120:897–902.

105. Fihn SD, Callahan CM, Martin DC, McDonell MB, Henikoff JG, White RH. The risk for and severity of bleeding complications in elderly patients treated with warfarin. The National Consortium of Anticoagulation Clinics. *Ann Intern Med* 1996; 124:970–979.

106. Bleeding during antithrombotic therapy in patients with atrial fibrillation. The Stroke Prevention in Atrial Fibrillation Investigators. *Arch Intern Med* 1996; 156:409–416.

107. Gorter JW. Major bleeding during anticoagulation after cerebral ischemia: patterns and risk factors. Stroke Prevention In Reversible Ischemia Trial (SPIRIT). European Atrial Fibrillation Trial (EAFT) study groups. *Neurology* 1999; 53:1319–1327.

108. Palareti G, Leali N, Coccheri S *et al.* Bleeding complications of oral anticoagulant treatment: an inception-cohort, prospective collaborative study (ISCOAT). Italian Study on Complications of Oral Anticoagulant Therapy. *Lancet* 1996; 348:423–428.

109. Stein B, Halperin JL, Fuster V. Should patients with atrial fibrillation be anticoagulated prior to and chronically following cardioversion? *Cardiovasc Clin* 1990; 21:231–247; discussion 48–49.

110. Moreyra E, Finkelhor RS, Cebul RD. Limitations of transesophageal echocardiography in the risk assessment of patients before nonanticoagulated cardioversion from atrial fibrillation and flutter: an analysis of pooled trials. *Am Heart J* 1995; 129:71–75.

111. Manning WJ, Silverman DI, Katz SE *et al.* Impaired left atrial mechanical function after cardioversion: relation to the duration of atrial fibrillation. *J Am Coll Cardiol* 1994; 23:1535–1540.

112. Black IW, Fatkin D, Sagar KB *et al.* Exclusion of atrial thrombus by transesophageal echocardiography does not preclude embolism after cardioversion of atrial fibrillation. A multicenter study. *Circulation* 1994; 89:2509–2513.

113. Stoddard MF, Dawkins PR, Prince CR, Ammash NM. Left atrial appendage thrombus is not uncommon in patients with acute atrial fibrillation and a recent embolic event: a transesophageal echocardiographic study. *J Am Coll Cardiol* 1995; 25:452–459.

114. Fatkin D, Kuchar DL, Thorburn CW, Feneley MP. Transesophageal echocardiography before and during direct current cardioversion of atrial fibrillation: evidence for 'atrial stunning' as a mechanism of thromboembolic complications. *J Am Coll Cardiol* 1994; 23:307–316.

115. Klein AL, Grimm RA, Murray RD *et al.* Use of transesophageal echocardiography to guide cardioversion in patients with atrial fibrillation. *N Engl J Med* 2001; 344:1411–1420.

116. Manning WJ, Silverman DI, Gordon SP, Krumholz HM, Douglas PS. Cardioversion from atrial fibrillation without prolonged anticoagulation with use of transesophageal echocardiography to exclude the presence of atrial thrombi. *N Engl J Med* 1993; 328:750–755.

117. Hirsh J, Fuster V. Guide to anticoagulant therapy. Part 1: Heparin. American Heart Association. *Circulation* 1994; 89:1449–1468.

118. Warkentin TE, Hayward CP, Boshkov LK *et al.* Sera from patients with heparin-induced thrombocytopenia generate platelet-derived microparticles with procoagulant activity: an explanation for the thrombotic complications of heparin-induced thrombocytopenia. *Blood* 1994; 84:3691–3699.

119. Hirsh J, Levine MN. Low molecular weight heparin. *Blood* 1992; 79:1–17.

120. Bonow RO, Carabello B, de Leon AC, Jr *et al.* Guidelines for the management of patients with valvular heart disease: executive summary. A report of the American College of Cardiology/American Heart Association Task Force on Practice Guidelines (Committee on Management of Patients with Valvular Heart Disease). *Circulation* 1998; 98:1949–1984.

121. Stein PD, Alpert JS, Bussey HI, Dalen JE, Turpie AG. Antithrombotic therapy in patients with mechanical and biological prosthetic heart valves. *Chest* 2001; 119(1 suppl):220S–227S.

122. Kovacs MJ, Kearon C, Rodger M *et al.* Single-Arm Study of Bridging Therapy With Low-Molecular-Weight Heparin for Patients at Risk of Arterial Embolism Who Require Temporary Interruption of Warfarin. *Circulation* 2004; 110:1658–1663.

123. Bye A, Lewis Y, O'Grady J. Effect of a single oral dose of aspirin on the platelet aggregation response to arachidonic acid. *Br J Clin Pharmacol* 1979; 7:283–286.

124. Loll P, Picot D, Garavito R. The structural basis of aspirin activity inferred from the crystal structure of inactivated prostaglandin H2 synthase. *Nat Struct Biol* 1995; 2:637–643.

125. Cipollone F, Patrignani P, Greco A *et al.* Differential suppression of thromboxane biosynthesis by indobufen and aspirin in patients with unstable angina. *Circulation* 1997; 96:1109–1116.

126. Vane J, Bakhle Y, Botting R. Cyclooxygenase 1 and 2. *Ann Rev Pharmacol Toxicol* 1998; 38:97–120.

127. Antithrombotic Trialists' Collaboration. Collaborative meta-analysis of randomised trials of antiplatelet therapy for prevention of death, myocardial infarction, and stroke in high risk patients. *Br Med J* 2002; 324:71–86.

128. Patrono C, Coller B, Dalen JE *et al*. Platelet-active drugs : the relationships among dose, effectiveness, and side-effects. *Chest* 2001; 119(1 suppl):39S-63S.

129. The efficacy of aspirin in patients with atrial fibrillation. Analysis of pooled data from 3 randomized trials. The Atrial Fibrillation Investigators. *Arch Intern Med* 1997; 157:1237–1240.

130. Munger TM, Packer DL, Hammill SC *et al*. A population study of the natural history of Wolff-Parkinson-White syndrome in Olmsted County, Minnesota, 1953–1989. *Circulation* 1993; 87:866–873.

131. Hart RG, Benavente O, Pearce LA. Increased risk of intracranial hemorrhage when aspirin is combined with warfarin: A meta-analysis and hypothesis. *Cerebrovasc Dis* 1999; 9:215–217.

132. Morocutti C, Amabile G, Fattapposta F *et al*. Indobufen versus warfarin in the secondary prevention of major vascular events in nonrheumatic atrial fibrillation. SIFA (Studio Italiano Fibrillazione Atriale) Investigators. *Stroke* 1997; 28:1015–1021.

133. Albers GW, Dalen JE, Laupacis A, Manning WJ, Petersen P, Singer DE. Antithrombotic therapy in atrial fibrillation. *Chest* 2001; 119(1 suppl):194S–206S.

134. Hurlen M, Abdelnoor M, Smith P, Erikssen J, Arnesen H. Warfarin, aspirin, or both after myocardial infarction. *N Engl J Med* 2002; 347:969–974.

135. Aschenberg W, Schluter M, Kremer P, Schroder E, Siglow V, Bleifeld W. Transesophageal two-dimensional echocardiography for the detection of left atrial appendage thrombus. *J Am Coll Cardiol* 1986; 7:163–166.

136. Hirsh J, Dalen J, Guyatt G. The sixth (2000) ACCP guidelines for antithrombotic therapy for prevention and treatment of thrombosis. American College of Chest Physicians. *Chest* 2001; 119(1 suppl):1S–2S.

137. Levine MN, Raskob G, Landefeld S, Kearon C. Hemorrhagic complications of anticoagulant treatment. *Chest* 1998; 114(5 suppl):511S–523S.

138. Frykman V, Beerman B, Ryden L, Rosenqvist M. Management of atrial fibrillation: discrepancy between guideline recommendations and actual practice exposes patients to risk for complications. *Eur Heart J* 2001; 22:1954–1959.

139. Eriksson UG, Bredberg U, Gislen K *et al*. Pharmacokinetics and pharmacodynamics of ximelagatran, a novel oral direct thrombin inhibitor, in young healthy male subjects. *Eur J Clin Pharmacol* 2003; 59:35–43.

140. Johansson LC, Andersson M, Fager G, Gustafsson D, Eriksson UG. No influence of ethnic origin on the pharmacokinetics and pharmacodynamics of melagatran following oral administration of ximelagatran, a novel oral direct thrombin inhibitor, to healthy male volunteers. *Clin Pharmacokinet* 2003; 42:475–484.

141. Johansson LC, Frison L, Logren U, Fager G, Gustafsson D, Eriksson UG. Influence of age on the pharmacokinetics and pharmacodynamics of ximelagatran, an oral direct thrombin inhibitor. *Clin Pharmacokinet* 2003; 42:381–392.

142. Sarich TC, Teng R, Peters GR *et al*. No influence of obesity on the pharmacokinetics and pharmacodynamics of melagatran, the active form of the oral direct thrombin inhibitor ximelagatran. *Clin Pharmacokinet* 2003; 42:485–492.

143. Gustafsson D, Nystrom J, Carlsson S *et al*. The direct thrombin inhibitor melagatran and its oral prodrug H 376/95: intestinal absorption properties, biochemical and pharmacodynamic effects. *Thromb Res* 2001; 101:171–181.

144. Colwell CW, Jr, Berkowitz SD, Davidson BL *et al*. Comparison of ximelagatran, an oral direct thrombin inhibitor, with enoxaparin for the prevention of venous thromboembolism following total hip replacement. A randomized, double-blind study. *J Thromb Haemost* 2003; 1:2119–2130.

145. Eriksson BI, Agnelli G, Cohen AT *et al*. The direct thrombin inhibitor melagatran followed by oral ximelagatran compared with enoxaparin for the prevention of venous thromboembolism after total hip or knee replacement: the EXPRESS study. *J Thromb Haemost* 2003; 1:2490–2496.

146. Eriksson BI, Agnelli G, Cohen AT *et al*. Direct thrombin inhibitor melagatran followed by oral ximelagatran in comparison with enoxaparin for prevention of venous thromboembolism after total hip or knee replacement. *Thromb Haemost* 2003; 89:288–296.

147. Francis CW, Davidson BL, Berkowitz SD *et al*. Ximelagatran versus warfarin for the prevention of venous thromboembolism after total knee arthroplasty. A randomized, double-blind trial. *Ann Intern Med* 2002; 137:648–655.

148. Francis CW, Berkowitz SD, Comp PC *et al*. Comparison of ximelagatran with warfarin for the prevention of venous thromboembolism after total knee replacement. *N Engl J Med* 2003; 349:1703–1712.

149. Colwell C, Berkowitz S, Comp P *et al*. Randomized, double-blind comparison of ximelagatran, an oral direct thrombin inhibitor, and warfarin to prevent venous thromboembolism (VTE) after Total knee replacement (TKR) EXULT-b. *Blood* 2003; 102:11(abstract 39).

150. Fiessinger JN, Huisman M, Davidson BL *et al.* THRIVE Treatment Study Investigators. Ximelagatran vs. low-molecular-weight heparin and warfarin for the treatment of deep vein thrombosis: a randomised trial. *JAMA* 2005; 293:681–689.

151. Schulman S, Wahlander K, Lundstrom T, Clason SB, Eriksson H. Secondary prevention of venous thromboembolism with the oral direct thrombin inhibitor ximelagatran. *N Engl J Med* 2003; 349:1713–1721.

152. Wallentin L, Wilcox RG, Weaver WD *et al.* Oral ximelagatran for secondary prophylaxis after myocardial infarction: the ESTEEM randomised controlled trial. *Lancet* 2003; 362:789–797.

153. Olsson SB. Stroke prevention with the oral direct thrombin inhibitor ximelagatran compared with warfarin in patients with non-valvular atrial fibrillation (SPORTIF III): randomised controlled trial. *Lancet* 2003; 362:1691–1698.

154. Albers GW, Diener HC, Frison L *et al.*; SPORTIF Executive Steering Committee for the SPORTIF V Investigators. Ximelagatran vs. warfarin for stroke prevention in patients with nonvalvular atrial fibrillation: a randomized trial. *JAMA* 2005; 293:690–698.

155. Rezaie AR. Prothrombin protects factor Xa in the prothrombinase complex from inhibition by the heparin-antithrombin complex. *Blood* 2001; 97:2308–2313.

156. Samama MM, Gerotziafas GT. Evaluation of the pharmacological properties and clinical results of the synthetic pentasaccharide (fondaparinux). *Thromb Res* 2003; 109:1–11.

157. Eriksson BI, Bauer KA, Lassen MR, Turpie AG. Fondaparinux compared with enoxaparin for the prevention of venous thromboembolism after hip-fracture surgery. *N Engl J Med* 2001; 345:1298–1304.

158. Bauer KA, Eriksson BI, Lassen MR, Turpie AG. Fondaparinux compared with enoxaparin for the prevention of venous thromboembolism after elective major knee surgery. *N Engl J Med* 2001; 345:1305–1310.

159. Lassen MR, Bauer KA, Eriksson BI, Turpie AG. Postoperative fondaparinux versus preoperative enoxaparin for prevention of venous thromboembolism in elective hip-replacement surgery: a randomised double-blind comparison. *Lancet* 2002; 359:1715–1720.

160. Turpie AG, Bauer KA, Eriksson BI, Lassen MR. Postoperative fondaparinux versus postoperative enoxaparin for prevention of venous thromboembolism after elective hip-replacement surgery: a randomised double-blind trial. *Lancet* 2002; 359:1721–1726.

161. Turpie AG, Bauer KA, Eriksson BI, Lassen MR. Fondaparinux vs. enoxaparin for the prevention of venous thromboembolism in major orthopedic surgery: a meta-analysis of 4 randomized double-blind studies. *Arch Intern Med* 2002; 162:1833–1840.

162. Bauersachs RM. Fondaparinux: an update on new study results. *Eur J Clin Invest* 2005; (suppl 1):27–32 (review).

163. Cohen A, Gallus A, Lassen M *et al.* Fondaparinux vs. placebo for the prevention of venous thromboembolism in acutely ill medical patients (ARTEMIS). *J Thromb Haemost* 2003; (suppl P2406).

164. Buller HR, Davidson BL, Decousus H *et al.* Fondaparinux or enoxaparin for the initial treatment of symptomatic deep venous thrombosis: a randomized trial. *Ann Intern Med* 2004; 140:867–873.

165. Buller HR, Davidson BL, Decousus H *et al.* Subcutaneous fondaparinux versus intravenous unfractionated heparin in the initial treatment of pulmonary embolism. *N Engl J Med* 2003; 349:1695–1702.

166. Coussement PK, Bassand JP, Convens C *et al.* A synthetic factor-Xa inhibitor (ORG31540/SR9017A) as an adjunct to fibrinolysis in acute myocardial infarction. The PENTALYSE study. *Eur Heart J* 2001; 22:1716–1724.

167. Ferguson JJ. Meeting highlights: highlights of the 51st annual scientific sessions of the American College of Cardiology. Atlanta, Georgia, USA. March 17–20, 2002. *Circulation* 2002; 106:E24–E30.

168. Herbert JM, Herault JP, Bernat A *et al.* Biochemical and pharmacological properties of SANORG 34006, a potent and long-acting synthetic pentasaccharide. *Blood* 1998; 91:4197–4205.

169. PERSIST Investigators. A novel long-acting synthetic factor Xa inhibitor (idraparinux sodium) to replace warfarin for secondary prevention in DVT: a phase II evaluation. *Blood* 2002; 100: 301 (abstract).

170. McTavish D, Faulds D, Goa KL. Ticlopidine. An updated review of its pharmacology and therapeutic use in platelet-dependent disorders. *Drugs* 1990; 40:238–259.

171. Schrör K. The basic pharmacology of ticlopidine and clopidogrel. *Platelets* 1993; 4:252.

172. A randomised, blinded, trial of clopidogrel versus aspirin in patients at risk of ischaemic events (CAPRIE). CAPRIE Steering Committee. *Lancet* 1996; 348:1329–1339.

173. Schomig A, Neumann FJ, Kastrati A *et al.* A randomized comparison of antiplatelet and anticoagulant therapy after the placement of coronary-artery stents. *N Engl J Med* 1996; 334:1084–1089.

174. Bertrand ME, Legrand V, Boland J et al. Randomized multicenter comparison of conventional anticoagulation versus antiplatelet therapy in unplanned and elective coronary stenting. The full anticoagulation versus aspirin and ticlopidine (FANTASTIC) study. Circulation 1998; 98:1597–1603.

175. Leon MB, Baim DS, Popma JJ et al. A clinical trial comparing three antithrombotic-drug regimens after coronary-artery stenting. Stent Anticoagulation Restenosis Study Investigators. N Engl J Med 1998; 339:1665–1671.

176. Urban P, Macaya C, Rupprecht HJ et al. Randomized evaluation of anticoagulation versus antiplatelet therapy after coronary stent implantation in high-risk patients: the multicenter aspirin and ticlopidine trial after intracoronary stenting (MATTIS). Circulation 1998; 98:2126–2132.

177. Hall P, Nakamura S, Maiello L et al. A randomized comparison of combined ticlopidine and aspirin therapy versus aspirin therapy alone after successful intravascular ultrasound-guided stent implantation. Circulation 1996; 93:215–222.

178. Muller C, Buttner HJ, Petersen J, Roskamm H. A randomized comparison of clopidogrel and aspirin versus ticlopidine and aspirin after the placement of coronary-artery stents. Circulation 2000; 101:590–593.

179. Bertrand ME, Rupprecht HJ, Urban P, Gershlick AH, Investigators FT. Double-blind study of the safety of clopidogrel with and without a loading dose in combination with aspirin compared with ticlopidine in combination with aspirin after coronary stenting: the clopidogrel aspirin stent international cooperative study (CLASSICS). Circulation 2000; 102:624–629.

180. Yusuf S, Zhao F, Mehta SR, Chrolavicius S, Tognoni G, Fox KK. Effects of clopidogrel in addition to aspirin in patients with acute coronary syndromes without ST-segment elevation. N Engl J Med 2001; 345:494–502.

181. Mehta SR, Yusuf S, Peters RJ et al. Effects of pretreatment with clopidogrel and aspirin followed by long-term therapy in patients undergoing percutaneous coronary intervention: the PCI-CURE study. Lancet 2001; 358:527–533.

182. Steinhubl SR, Berger PB, Mann JT, 3rd et al. Early and sustained dual oral antiplatelet therapy following percutaneous coronary intervention: a randomized controlled trial. JAMA 2002; 288:2411–2420.

183. Lorenzoni R, Lazzerini G, Cocci F, De Caterina R. Short-term prevention of thromboembolic complications in patients with atrial fibrillation with aspirin plus clopidogrel: the Clopidogrel-Aspirin Atrial Fibrillation (CLAAF) pilot study. Am Heart J 2004; 148:e6.

17

Venous thromboembolism: pathophysiology and diagnosis

W. Ageno, A. G. G. Turpie

EPIDEMIOLOGY OF VENOUS THROMBOEMBOLISM

Pulmonary embolism (PE) and deep vein thrombosis (DVT) represent a spectrum of a single disease defined as venous thromboembolism (VTE). It has been estimated that approximately 30% of apparently isolated episodes of PE are associated with silent DVT [1], and that the frequency of silent PE ranges between 40% and 50% in patients affected by DVT [2]. VTE is a common cause of morbidity and mortality, with approximately 200 000 first-in-life cases reported each year in the United States [3]. However, the real incidence, prevalence, and mortality rates of VTE are likely to be underestimated because the disease is often clinically silent and because autopsy data are limited. Where autopsy data were available and PE identified as the cause of death, it was often observed that the preceding thrombosis was not clinically recognised [4]. Failure to recognise VTE reflects the unreliability of the clinical diagnosis and the poor sensitivity of screening tests [5] (Table 17.1). Furthermore, for as many as 22% of all patients with VTE, death is sudden and there is no time for any intervention [4]. Mortality after VTE diagnosis, i.e., within 7 days of VTE onset, was reported to occur in as many as 25% of patients in an unselected population [6] (Table 17.2). The results of a large international registry of PE patients carried out in 52 experienced centres [7] revealed a 17.4% mortality rate at 3 months. VTE is also associated with a high likelihood of recurrence. Prandoni and colleagues [8] reported a 17% recurrence rate of VTE two years after a first episode of DVT, 24% after 5 years, and 30% after 8 years. Very similar rates were subsequently reported by Heit and colleagues [9] (Table 17.3).

PATHOPHYSIOLOGY OF VENOUS THROMBOEMBOLISM

Patients may present with symptomatic VTE or develop VTE as a complication of hospitalisation for medical illness or in the postoperative period. The individual risk of VTE varies as a result of the interaction between two main predisposing factors: intrinsic risk factors and clinical risk factors. Approximately one-half of symptomatic ambulant patients will have no predisposing VTE cause; so called idiopathic or unprovoked VTE, whereas the remainder will have readily identifiable risk factors which may be permanent or transient. Permanent risk factors can be either genetic such as inherited thrombophilia, or acquired such as cancer

Walter Ageno, Associate Professor of Internal Medicine, Department of Clinical Medicine, University of Insubria University of Insubria, Varese, Italy.

Alexander G. G. Turpie, Professor of Medicine, McMaster University, HHS-General Hospital, Hamilton, Ontario, Canada.

Table 17.1 Annual incidence of venous thromboembolism [5]

Incidence of VTE	17/100 000
New cases of VTE/year/USA	201 000
New cases of DVT/year/USA	107 000
New cases of PE/year/USA	94 000

Table 17.2 Survival after venous thromboembolism [6]

Time from index event	DVT (%)	PE (%)	VTE (%)
7 days	96.2	59.1	74.8
30 days	94.5	55.6	72.0
90 days	91.9	52.1	68.9
1 year	85.4	47.7	63.6
5 years	72.6	39.4	53.5
8 years	65.2	34.5	47.5

Table 17.3 Long-term recurrences after venous thromboembolism [9]

Time from index event	Cumulative incidence (%)
7 days	1.6
30 days	5.2
90 days	8.3
180 days	10.1
1 year	12.9
2 years	16.6
5 years	22.8
10 years	30.4

or a previous episode of VTE. Predisposing factors for VTE were summarised two centuries ago by the German pathologist Virchow [10]. In his famous triad, Virchow identified hyper-coagulability, venous stasis, and endothelial damage as the main factors underlying venous thrombosis (Tables 17.4 and 17.5). Stasis predisposes to venous thrombosis by preventing activated coagulation factors from being diluted by non-activated blood, by preventing clearance of activated coagulation factors, and by preventing mixing of activated coagulation factors with inhibitors. Vessel wall damage is probably less important in the pathogenesis of DVT than in arterial thrombosis, but plays a major role in instances of vascular trauma, as in patients undergoing orthopaedic surgery. Venous damage is accompanied by endothelial cell detachment, which results in the exposure of blood to subendothelium.

Venous thrombi usually occur at regions of slow or disturbed flow and often begin as small deposits in large venous sinuses in the calf, in valve cusp pockets either in the deep vein of the calf or thigh, in venous segments that are subject to extrinsic compression, or in venous segments that have been exposed to direct trauma. Subsequent thrombus growth depends on the balance between the effects of thrombogenic stimuli and various protective mechanisms. Thus, extension of thrombosis is more likely to occur if the original thrombogenic stimulus persists or if marked endothelial damage or stasis occurs as a consequence of the original acute venous thrombosis.

When symptoms or signs of acute VTE occur, they are caused either by obstruction to venous outflow, by inflammation of the vein wall or perivascular tissue, by embolisation of

Table 17.4   Risk factors for VTE related to venous stasis

- Age
- Obesity
- Immobility (bed rest >4 days)
- Plaster cast
- Varicose veins
- Trauma

Table 17.5   Risk factors for VTE related to hypercoagulability

- Age
- Inherited or acquired thrombophilia (tendency to thrombosis)
- Active cancer
- High-dose oestrogen therapy
- Pregnancy
- Puerperium
- Increased blood viscosity
- Inflammatory disorders

the thrombus into the pulmonary circulation, or by a combination of these. Emboli to the pulmonary arterial circulation can lodge at the bifurcation of the pulmonary artery, but more frequently they affect pulmonary vessels of second, third, or fourth order. Subsequent pathophysiological effects vary accordingly from increased pulmonary vascular resistance to impaired gas exchange, alveolar hyperventilation, increased airway resistance, and decreased pulmonary compliance.

INDIVIDUAL RISK FACTORS FOR VENOUS THROMBOEMBOLISM

AGE

Advanced age has consistently been found to be associated with an increased risk of VTE. In the Study of Men Born in 1913 [11], 855 men were followed up prospectively from the age of 50 years to the age of 80 years. The cumulative probability of having experienced a first thromboembolic event was 0.5% at age 50 years, 2.0% at age 60 years, 8.2% at age 75 years, and 10.7% at age 80 years.

OBESITY

Obesity, and in particular abdominal obesity, has been shown to be an independent risk factor for venous thromboembolic events. In the Nurses' Health Study [12], a study aimed to identify risk factors for PE among a cohort of initially healthy female nurses, a body mass index of greater than $25.0 \, \text{g/m}^2$ was associated with a 1.7 relative risk of PE (95% CI 1.1–2.7) and a body mass index of greater than $29.0 \, \text{g/m}^2$ was associated with a 3.2 relative risk of PE (95% CI 1.7–6.0). Similarly, in a study by Tsai and colleagues [13] the incidence rate of VTE was 1.35 (95% CI 1.09–1.67) for patients with a body mass index between 25 and $30 \, \text{g/m}^2$, and 2.01 (95% CI 1.60–2.52) for patients with a body mass index of greater than $30 \, \text{g/m}^2$. Finally, abdominal obesity predicted VTE in the Study of Men Born in 1913 [14]. Men in the highest decile of waist circumference (≥ 100 cm) had an adjusted relative risk of 3.92 (95% CI 2.10–7.29) compared with men with a waist circumference of less than 100 cm.

Table 17.6   Inherited and acquired thrombophilic abnormalities

Inherited	Effect of abnormality
Antithrombin deficiency	Reduced inhibition of factors IIa, Xa, and others
Protein C deficiency	Reduced inhibition of factors Va and VIIIa
Protein S deficiency	Cofactor of protein C
Mut. R506Q (FV Leiden)	Causes resistance to activated protein C
Mut. G20210A (FII)	Causes increased levels of prothrombin
Acquired	
Antiphospholipid antibodies	
Inherited or acquired	
Hyperhomocysteinaemia	

Disturbed flow and impaired fibrinolytic activity, which have been consistently reported in obese patients, might be the underlying mechanism predisposing to venous thrombosis in such patients.

THROMBOPHILIA

Major hereditary prothrombotic conditions include those associated with reduced levels of inhibitors of the coagulation cascade and those associated with increased levels or function of the procoagulant factors (Table 17.6).

Inhibitors of the coagulation cascade include antithrombin, protein C, and protein S. Antithrombin deficiency is rare, occurring in about 0.2% of the general population and in 0.5% to 7.5% of patients presenting with VTE [15–17]. Antithrombin deficiency causes an important prothrombotic state. It has been estimated that approximately 60% of patients with antithrombin deficiency will have an episode of VTE by age 60 years [18].

Protein C deficiency is also found in approximately 0.2% of the normal population [19]. Among patients with venous thrombosis, protein C deficiency is detected in 2.5% to 6% [16, 20].

The frequency of protein S deficiency in the general population is unknown. It has been estimated that about one-third of patients with protein S deficiency will have venous thrombosis by age 60 years [21].

Prothrombotic conditions associated with increased levels or function of the coagulation factors include activated protein C resistance and factor V Leiden mutation, prothrombin gene mutation, and increased concentrations of factors VIII, IX, and XI.

Factor V Leiden is a relatively common mutation and is by far the most common cause of activated protein C resistance. It is present in approximately 5% of the normal population of northern European ethnicity, and in 10% of patients with VTE [22, 23]. Thus, patients with factor V Leiden have a relatively low risk for thrombosis, and in most cases VTE occurs in the presence of concomitant risk factors [24].

A similar prevalence is reported for prothrombin gene mutation, which is found in approximately 4% of the general population and in 5% to 10% of patients with VTE [23, 25]. Thus, for this mutation, the risk of VTE is also relatively low [21].

An association between increased levels of coagulation factors VIII, IX, and XI and an increased risk of VTE has also been reported. The mechanism underlying such association is still unclear [21].

High levels of homocysteine that can be either congenital or acquired may also be associated with a prothrombotic state. Congenital hyperhomocysteinaemia is most commonly caused by the mutation of genes cystathione β-synthase and methylenetetrahydrafolate

Table 17.7 Incidence of venous thromboembolism in surgical patients without prophylaxis

Total knee replacement	60–88%
Total hip replacement	29–68%
Arthroscopy	18%
General surgery	19–29%
Malignant disease	30–35%
Non-malignant disease	25–29%
Gynaecologic surgery	14–22%
Urologic surgery	10–35%

reductase [26, 27]. This latter mutation is very common in the general population [28]. Acquired forms are caused by dietary deficiencies of folate, vitamin B_{12}, or vitamin B_6.

Finally, the antiphospholipid antibody syndrome is an acquired, potentially severe prothrombotic condition. Clinical presentation includes VTE, arterial thrombosis that is generally less common than venous thrombosis, pregnancy, recurrent fetal loss, and premature deliveries [29].

HISTORY OF VTE

Previous venous thrombosis is an important independent risk factor for VTE. The results of an epidemiologic study of risk factors for DVT found history of VTE as the most important risk factor, with an odds ratio of 15.6 [30]. Patients with two or more episodes of VTE carry a very high risk of further recurrences if they are not adequately treated [31]. The rate of recurrent VTE is higher in patients without a readily identifiable risk factor than in patients with a definite, transitory risk factor such as a postoperative DVT.

DISEASE-RELATED RISK FACTORS FOR VENOUS THROMBOEMBOLISM

SURGERY

Surgical procedures, and in particular orthopaedic surgery, surgery for cancer, and neurosurgery are commonly complicated by VTE. The risk of VTE following surgical procedures in the absence of prophylactic strategies is well defined and is summarised in Table 17.7. The risk of VTE following minimally invasive joint surgery or following laparoscopic surgery is still poorly defined. The reported risk of VTE following knee arthroscopy varies from 0.6% to 17.9% [32–36], with the variation in rates attributable to study design and to diagnostic techniques. Laparoscopic surgery has gained wide acceptance and has replaced conventional open surgery in many settings. On the one hand, the reduction in tissue damage and the possibility to mobilise patients more quickly than is possible with open procedures may suggest that laparoscopic surgery is associated with a lower risk of thromboembolic complications. On the other hand, laparoscopic surgery has been shown to induce a hypercoagulable state similar to that of open surgery, based on markers of activation of coagulation, such as levels of thrombin–antithrombin complex, prothrombin fragment 1+2, and D-dimer among others [37, 38]. Moreover, patients undergoing laparoscopic procedures are prone to increased venous stasis as a result of the induction of pneumoperitoneum and prolonged use of the Trendelemburg position [39–41].

MEDICAL DISORDERS

The risk of VTE in medical patients can be as high as in surgical patients, but the issue of prevention of VTE has been less extensively studied in medical patients than in surgical patients

Table 17.8 Incidence of venous thromboembolism in medical patients without prophylaxis

Ischaemic stroke	11–75%
Myocardial infarction	17–34%
Congestive heart failure	20–40%
Intensive care	25–42%
General medicine	10–26%

(Table 17.8). However, autopsy studies have consistently indicated that 70% to 80% of all in-hospital deaths related to PE are not associated with surgical procedures, but actually occurred in medical patients [42–46]. Others have reported that 50% to 70% of symptomatic venous thromboembolic events related to hospitalisation occur in medical patients [47, 48]. Medical disorders with increased risk of VTE include ischaemic stroke, heart failure, acute respiratory failure, sepsis, acute rheumatic disease, and inflammatory bowel disease. In association with the underlying condition, prolonged immobilisation, an independent risk factor for VTE, plays a major role in a development of a thrombotic event [30].

CANCER

The prevalence of known cancer in patients with a new diagnosis of VTE ranges between 10% and 20% [49]. The prevalence of occult cancer in patients with idiopathic VTE varies between 4% and 10% [49]. Frequently, cancer diagnosed at the same time as or within one year after an episode of VTE is associated with an advanced stage of the disease and a poor prognosis [50]. The role of cancer arises from systematic hypercoagulability, but also results from external compression or from direct vascular invasion of tumour cells. The use of chemotherapy further increases the risk of VTE in patients with malignancy. A 10.9% annual incidence of VTE has been reported recently in cancer patients treated with chemotherapy [51].

PREGNANCY AND PUERPERIUM

The true incidence of VTE associated with pregnancy is still unknown, but there is evidence that the risk is increased compared with the incidence in non-pregnant individuals [52]. Fatal PE remains the most common cause of maternal mortality in many western countries [53, 54]. Data from retrospective studies suggest that the prevalence of VTE during pregnancy is approximately 1 per 1000–2000 pregnancies [55]. The risk of VTE spans all three trimesters of pregnancy, but DVT seems to occur more frequently antenatally, and in particular in the first trimester [56], whereas the risk of PE is greatest in the last 4 to 6 weeks of pregnancy and in the puerperium [57]. The principal risk factors for VTE during pregnancy are previous VTE and thrombophilia, but obesity, strict bed rest, advanced maternal age, infections, pre-eclampsia, and intercurrent diseases also contribute [58].

ORAL CONTRACEPTIVES AND HORMONE REPLACEMENT THERAPY

Oral contraceptives increase the risk of VTE. In particular, third generation oral contraceptives, which contain newer prostagens, cause adverse haemostatic changes including acquired resistance to activated protein C, and increase the risk of VTE more than second generation pills. Although the absolute risk of VTE in women taking oral contraceptives is very low, this risk is 2 to 4 times higher in women taking second generation oral contraceptives than in age-matched women not taking oral contraceptives, and 3 to 8 times higher in women taking third generation pills.

Postmenopausal hormone replacement therapy also increases the risk of VTE. In a meta-analysis of 12 studies, the relative risk of VTE was 2.1 among current users and was highest (3.5) during the first year of use [59].

CLASSIFICATION OF PATIENTS AT RISK FOR VENOUS THROMBOEMBOLISM

Knowledge of specific risk factors forms the basis for appropriate use of prophylaxis. Risk factors are often present in combination in a high proportion of hospitalised patients, and the risks are cumulative. Formal risk assessment models for DVT have been proposed for surgical patients and, more recently, for medical patients. In general, any disease leading to a prolonged immobilisation is of major importance in the formation of venous thrombi, likely as a result of venous stasis. The risk of VTE is highest in patients undergoing major orthopaedic surgery, in whom besides postoperative immobilisation, manipulation of the leg and torsion of the veins during the surgical procedure cause local vessel wall damage and stasis. For surgical patients, factors predisposing to thrombosis are mainly related to the procedure itself and include the site, technique, and duration of the procedure. The type of anaesthesia, in particular whether this is general or regional, also plays an important role. The concomitant presence of cancer or infection increases the likelihood of thrombosis. Medical patients also commonly present with multiple risk factors.

DIAGNOSIS OF VENOUS THROMBOEMBOLISM

Several studies have assessed different diagnostic approaches in patients with signs and/or symptoms suggesting VTE. Since no single test is ideal, a correct diagnosis is often accomplished by the appropriate combination of two or more tests.

PRE-TEST PROBABILITY

The assessment of pre-test probability is an essential step in the current diagnosis and management of patients with suspected VTE. Pre-test probability can be assessed either empirically or by using various decision rules or scoring systems. A correct evaluation of pre-test probability has been shown to optimise the positive and negative predictive values, and thus the clinical utility of non-invasive diagnostic tests [60]. Currently, the best known scoring system is the one proposed by Wells and colleagues for the diagnosis of DVT [61]. This scoring system incorporates typical signs, symptoms, risk factors, and the likelihood of an alternative diagnosis (Table 17.9). A similar score was also developed and validated for the diagnosis of PE [62] (Table 17.10).

COMPRESSION ULTRASOUND

Compression ultrasound (C-US) is a simple, non-invasive, widely used diagnostic test. Veins are compressed under gentle pressure with the ultrasound transducer. The inability to compress a vein indicates the presence of venous thrombosis. After extensive evaluation, C-US has shown an average sensitivity for symptomatic proximal DVT of 97%, and an average specificity of 98% [63]. Doppler studies do not add significant diagnostic accuracy. C-US has a low sensitivity for distal DVT. For this reason, C-US is usually restricted to compression of the proximal veins only and it is recommended that, in case of negative ultrasound result, the examination should be repeated within 7 days (serial C-US). The safety of this approach has been objectively validated [64, 65]. However, the serial C-US approach has limitations, the most relevant being that all patients with a negative test (approximately 75% to 80%) must come back to the hospital, with the attendant inconveniences and costs.

Table 17.9   Wells' simplified clinical probability score for suspected deep vein thrombosis [61]

Variable	Points
Active cancer (ongoing treatment or within last 6 months, or palliative)	1
Paralysis, paresis or recent plaster immobilisation of lower extremities	1
Recently bedridden for >3 days and/or major surgery within 4 weeks	1
Local tenderness	1
Thigh and calf swollen	1
Calf swelling 3 m > asymptomatic side (measured 10 m below tibial tuberosity)	1
Pitting oedema: symptomatic leg only	1
Dilated superficial veins (non varicose) in symptomatic leg only	1
Alternative diagnosis as or more likely than DVT	−2
Low probability ≤0	
Moderate probability 1–2	
High probability ≥3	

Table 17.10   Wells' simplified clinical probability score for suspected pulmonary embolism [62]

Variable	Points
Clinical signs and symptoms of DVT	3
PE as likely or more likely than an alternative diagnosis	3
Immobilisation (≥3 consecutive days) or surgery in previous 4 weeks	1.5
Previous DVT or PE	1.5
Heart rate >100 bpm	1.5
Haemoptysis	1
Active cancer (ongoing treatment or within the last 6 months, or palliative)	1
Low probability <2	
Moderate probability 2–6	
High probability >6	

To reduce these limitations, additional approaches have been developed. Recently, complete C-US of the lower limbs as a single test for the diagnosis of DVT has been proposed [66]. Complete C-US requires ultrasound examination of the entire venous system of the leg based on compression. This approach has been suggested as safe in the exclusion of DVT without the need for serial tests [66].

D-DIMER

D-dimer, a specific product of degradation of cross-linked fibrin, is a useful negative predictor to rule out VTE in patients with suspected VTE. Several D-dimer assays are now available in many clinical settings for rapid emergency testing [67]. The best D-dimer assays, quantitative enzyme linked immunoabsorbant assay (ELISA) or ELISA-derived methods, have a very high sensitivity, but usually have a low specificity which results in a high frequency of false-positive results [67]. Traditional latex tests have a low sensitivity and negative predictive value [68].

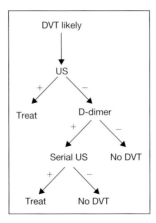

Figure 17.1 Dignosis of deep vein thrombosis

LUNG SCAN

Ventilation/perfusion (V/Q) lung scan is the traditional non-invasive test for suspected PE. However, pulmonary hypoperfusion is not highly specific for an embolus. The specificity of the test is increased by the presence of large perfusion defects or several segmental defects. High probability lung scans, defined by the presence of one or more mismatched segmental defects or two or more large mismatched subsegmental defects [62], are well validated for the diagnosis of PE. Similarly, a normal lung scan is well validated for the exclusion of PE. Unfortunately, most scans will result in intermediate or indeterminate probability and additional testing is required to make a definitive diagnosis.

HELICAL COMPUTED TOMOGRAPHY

Helical computed tomography (CT) is rapidly replacing V/Q lung scanning as the primary imaging test for suspected acute PE. Computer tomography allows direct visualisation of the thrombus or identifies an alternative diagnosis [69]. The major limitation of CT has been failure to detect PE beyond third-order pulmonary arterial branches, thus making the sensitivity of the test inadequate [70]. However, the newer generation CT scans have increased the sensitivity of the test from approximately 70% to more than 90% [71]. The safety of excluding PE after negative CT scan results is supported by the findings of recent studies [72].

DIAGNOSTIC STRATEGIES

The combination of D-dimer, pre-test clinical probability, and imaging tests has been evaluated in several diagnostic algorithms for both suspected DVT and PE. The goals of such algorithms are to improve the accuracy of the diagnostic approach to suspected VTE, to reduce the need for serial tests, additional imaging tests, or invasive tests, and to reduce the overall costs. The safety of excluding VTE without imaging tests when D-dimer is negative and clinical probability is low has been evaluated [73]. However, the predictive value of locally available laboratory and imaging tests should be evaluated before such algorithms are widely applied. A clinically useful approach to the diagnosis of DVT and stroke is provided in Figure 17.1 and for diagnosis of PE in Figure 17.2.

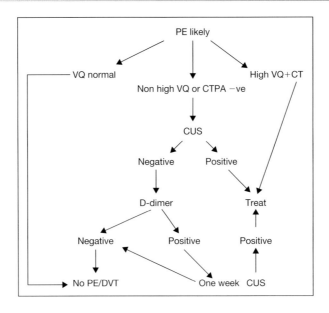

Figure 17.2 Diagnosis of pulmonary embolism

REFERENCES

1. Turkstra F, Kuijer PMM, van Beek EJR *et al*. Diagnostic utility of ultrasonography of leg veins in patients suspected of having pulmonary embolism. *Ann Intern Med* 1997; 12:775–781.
2. Meignan M, Rosso J, Gauthier H *et al*. Systematic lung scans reveal a high frequency of silent pulmonary embolism in patients with proximal deep venous thrombosis. *Arch Intern Med* 2000; 160:159–164.
3. Silverstein MD, Heit JA, Mohr DN, Petterson TM, O'Fallon WM, Melton III LJ. Trends in the incidence of deep vein thrombosis and pulmonary embolism: a 25-year population-based study. *Arch Intern Med* 1998; 158:585–593.
4. Anderson FA, Wheeler HB, Goldberg RJ *et al*. A population-based perspective of the hospital incidence and case-fatality rates of deep vein thrombosis and pulmonary embolism. The Worcester DVT study. *Arch Intern Med* 1991; 151:933–938.
5. Heit JA, Silverstein MD, Mohr DN *et al*. The epidemiology of venous thromboembolism in the community. *Thromb Haemost* 2001; 86:452–463.
6. Heit JA, Silverstein MD, Mohr DN, Petterson TM, O'Fallon WM, Melton III LJ. Predictors of survival after deep vein thrombosis and pulmonary embolism: a population-based, cohort study. *Arch Intern Med* 1999; 159:445–453.
7. Goldhaber SZ, Visani L, De Rosa M, for ICOPER. Acute pulmonary embolism: clinical outcomes in the International Cooperative Pulmonary Embolism Registry (ICOPER). *Lancet* 1999; 353:1386–1389.
8. Prandoni P, Lensing AWA, Cogo A *et al*. The long-term clinical course of acute deep venous thrombosis. *Ann Intern Med* 1996; 125:1–7.
9. Heit JA, Mohr DN, Silverstein MD, Petterson TM, O'Fallon WM, Melton III LJ. Predictors of recurrence after deep vein thrombosis and pulmonary embolism. *Arch Intern Med* 2000; 160:761–768.
10. Virchow R. *Gessamalte Abhandlungen zur wissenshaftlichen Medzin*. Medinger Sohn, Frankfurt, Germany, 1856: pp 219–732.
11. Hansson PO, Welin L, Tibblin G, Eriksson H. Deep vein thrombosis and pulmonary embolism in the general population. The Study of Men Born in 1913. *Arch Intern Med* 1997; 157:1665–1670.
12. Goldhaber SZ, Grodstein F, Stampfer MJ *et al*. A prospective study of risk factors for pulmonary embolism in women. *JAMA* 1997; 277:642–645.
13. Tsai AW, Cushman M, Rosamond WD, Heckbert SR, Polak JF, Folsom AR. Cardiovascular risk factors and venous thromboembolism incidence. *Arch Intern Med* 2002; 162:1182–1189.

14. Hansson PO, Eriksson H, Welin L, Svardsudd K, Wilhelmsen L. Smoking and abdominal obesity. Risk factors for venous thromboembolism among middle-aged men: The Study of Men Born in 1913. *Arch Intern Med* 1999; 159:1886–1890.

15. Mateo J, Oliver A, Borrell M, Sala N, Fontcuberta J. Laboratory evaluation and clinical characteristics of 2,132 consecutive unselected patients with venous thromboembolism – results of the Spanish Multicentric Study on Thrombophilia. *Thromb Haemost* 1997; 77:444–451.

16. Wells PS, Blajchman MA, Henderson P *et al.* Prevalence of antithrombin deficiency in healthy blood donors: a cross sectional study. *Am J Hematol* 1994; 45:321–324.

17. Tait RC, Walker ID, Perry DJ *et al.* Prevalence of antithrombin deficiency in the healthy population. *Br J Haematol* 1994; 87:106–112.

18. Martinelli I, Mannucci PM, De Stefano V *et al.* Different risks of thrombosis in four coagulation defects associated with inherited thrombophilia: a study of 150 families. *Blood* 1998; 92:2353–3258.

19. Tait RC, Walker ID, Reitsma PH *et al.* Prevalence of protein C deficiency in the healthy population. *Thromb Haemost* 1995; 73:87–93.

20. Ben-Tal O, Zivelin A, Selighson U. The relative frequency of hereditary thrombotic disorders among 107 patients with thrombophilia in Israel. *Thromb Haemost* 1989; 61:50–54.

21. Crowther MA, Kelton JG. Congenital thrombophilic states associated with venous thrombosis: a qualitative overview and proposed classification system. *Ann Intern Med* 2003; 138:128–134.

22. Lee DH, Henderson PA, Blajchman MA. Prevalence of factor V Leiden in a Canadian blood donor population. *CMAJ* 1996; 155:285–289.

23. Salomon O, Steinberg DM, Zivelin A *et al.* Single and combined prothrombotic factors in patients with idiopathic venous thromboembolism: prevalence and risk assessment. *Arterioscler Thromb Vasc Biol* 1999; 19:511–518.

24. Rodeghiero F, Tosetto A. Activated protein C resistance and factor V Leiden mutations are independent risk factors for venous thromboembolism. *Ann Intern Med* 1999; 130:643–650.

25. Rosendaal FR, Doggen CJ, Zivelin A *et al.* Geographic distribution of the 20210 G to A prothrombin variant. *Thromb Haemost* 1998; 79:706–708.

26. Goyette P, Frosst P, Rosenblatt DS, Rozen R. Seven novel mutations in the methylenetetrahydrofolate reductase gene and genotype/phenotype correlations in severe methylenetetrahydrofolate reductase deficiency. *Am J Hum Genet* 1995; 56:1052–1059.

27. Mudd SH, Skovby F, Levy HL *et al.* The natural history of homocystinuria due to cystathionine beta-synthase deficiency. *Am J Hum Genet* 1985; 37:1–31.

28. Kluijtmans LA, van den Heuvel LP, Boers GH *et al.* Molecular genetic analysis in mild hyperhomo-cysteinemia: a common mutation in the methylenetetrahydrofolate reductase gene is a genetic risk factor for cardiovascular disease. *Am J Hum Genet* 1996; 58:35–41.

29. Levine JS, Branch DW, Rauch J. The antiphospholipid syndrome. *N Engl J Med* 2002; 346:752–763.

30. Samama MM. An epidemiologic study of risk factors for deep vein thrombosis in medical outpatients. The Sirius Study. *Arch Intern Med* 2000; 160:3415–3420.

31. Schulman S, Granqvist S, Holmström M *et al.* The duration of oral anticoagulant therapy after a second episode of venous thromboembolism. *N Engl J Med* 1997; 336:393–398.

32. Dahl OE, Gudmundsen TE, Haukeland L. Late occurring clinical deep vein thrombosis in joint-operated patients. *Acta Orthop Scand* 2000; 71:47–50.

33. Demers C, Marcoux S, Ginsberg JS *et al.* Incidence of venographically proved deep vein thrombosis after knee arthroscopy. *Arch Intern Med* 1998; 158:47–50.

34. Jaureguito JW, Greenwald AE, Wilcox JF *et al.* The incidence of deep venous thrombosis after arthroscopic knee surgery. *Am J Sports Med* 1999; 27:707–710.

35. Delis KT, Hunt N, Strachan RK *et al.* Incidence, natural history and risk factors of deep vein thrombosis in elective knee arthroscopy. *Thromb Haemost* 2001; 86:817–821.

36. Stringer MD, Steadman CA, Hedges AR *et al.* Deep vein thrombosis after elective knee surgery: an incidence study in 312 patients. *J Bone Joint Surg Br* 1989; 71:492–497.

37. Nguyen NT, Owings JT, Gosselin R *et al.* Systemic coagulation and fibrinolysis after laparoscopic and open gastric bypass. *Arch Surg* 2001; 136:909–916.

38. Rahr HB, Fabrin K, Larsen JL, Thorlacius-Ussing O. Coagulation and fibrinolysis during laparoscopic cholecystectomy. *Thromb Res* 1999; 93:121–127.

39. Jorgensen JO, Lalak NJ, North L, Hanel K, Hunt DR, Morris DL. Venous stasis during laparoscopic cholecystectomy. *Surg Laparosc Endosc* 1994; 4:128–133.

40. Sobolewski AP, Deshmukh RM, Brunson BL *et al.* Venous hemodynamic changes during laparoscopic cholecystectomy. *J Laparoendosc Surg* 1995; 5:363–369.

41. Beebe DS, McNevin MP, Crain JM *et al.* Evidence of venous stasis after abdominal insufflation for laparoscopic cholecystectomy. *Surg Gynecol Obstet* 1993; 176:443–447.

42. Sandler DA, Martin JF. Autopsy proven pulmonary embolism in hospital patients: are we detecting enough deep vein thrombosis? *J R Soc Med* 1989; 82:203–205.

43. Goldhaber SZ, Savage DD, Garrison RJ *et al.* Risk factors for pulmonary embolism: the Framingham study. *Am J Med* 1983; 74:1023–1028.

44. Anderson FA, Wheeler HB, Goldberg RJ *et al.* A population-based perspective of the hospital incidence and case-fatality rates of deep vein thrombosis and pulmonary embolism. The Worcester DVT study. *Arch Intern Med* 1991; 151:933–938.

45. Lindblad B, Sternby NH, Bergqvist D. Incidence of venous thromboembolism verified by necropsy over 30 years. *Br Med J* 1991; 302:709–711.

46. Baglin TP, White K, Charles A. Fatal pulmonary embolism in hospitalised medical patients. *J Clin Pathol* 1997; 50:609–610.

47. Bouthier J. The venous thrombotic risk in nonsurgical patients. *Drugs* 1996; 52(suppl):16–29.

48. Goldhaber SZ, Dunn K, MacDougall RC. New onset of venous thromboembolism among hospitalized patients at Brigham and Women's Hospital is caused more often by prophylaxis failure than by withholding treatment. *Chest* 2000; 118:1680–1684.

49. Otten HM, Prins MH. Venous thromboembolism and occult malignancy. *Throm Res* 2001; 102:V187–V194.

50. Sorensen HT, Mellemkjaer L, Olsen JH, Baron JA. Prognosis of cancers associated with venous thromboembolism. *N Engl J Med* 2000; 343:1846–1850.

51. Otten HM, Mathijssen J, ten Cate H *et al.* Symptomatic venous thromboembolism in cancer patients treated with chemotherapy. An underestimated phenomenon. *Arch Intern Med* 2004; 164:190–194.

52. Macklon NS, Greer IA. Venous thromboembolic disease in obstetrics and gynaecology: the Scottish experience. *Scot Med J* 1996; 41:83–86.

53. Athrash HK, Koonin LM, Lawson HW, Franks AL, Smith JC. Maternal morbidity in the United States 1979–1986. *Obstet Gynaecol* 1990; 76:1055–1060.

54. Hogberg U, Innala E, Sandstrom A. Maternal mortality in Sweden. *Obstet Gynaecol* 1995; 84:240–244.

55. James K, Lohr J, Deshmukh R. Venous thrombotic complications of pregnancy. *Cardiovasc Surg* 1997; 4:777–782.

56. Rutherford S, Montoro M, McGehee W, Strong T. Thromboembolic disease associated with pregnancy: an 11 year review. *Am J Obstet Gynecol* 1991; 164:286(abstract).

57. Eldor A. The use of low molecular weight heparin for the management of venous thromboembolism in pregnancy. *Eur J Obstet Gynecol and Reproductive Biology* 2002; 104:3–13.

58. Bazzan M, Donvito V. Low molecular weight heparin during pregnancy. *Thromb Res* 2001; 101:V175-V186.

59. Nelson HD, Humphrey LL, Nygren P, Teutsch SM, Allan JD. Postmenopausal hormone replacement therapy: scientific review. *JAMA* 2002; 288:872–881.

60. Kelly J, Hunt J. The utility of pretest probability assessment in patients with clinically suspected venous thromboembolism. *J Thromb Haemost* 2003; 1:1888–1896.

61. Wells PS, Anderson DR, Bormani J *et al.* Value of assessment of pretest probability of deep vein thrombosis in clinical management. *Lancet* 1997; 350:1795–1798.

62. Wells PS, Ginsberg JS, Anderson DR *et al.* Use of a clinical model for safe management of patients with suspected pulmonary embolism. *Ann Intern Med* 1998; 129:997–1005.

63. Kearon C, Ginsberg JS, Hirsh J. The role of venous ultrasonography in the diagnosis of suspected deep venous thrombosis and pulmonary embolism. *Ann Intern Med* 1998; 129:1044–1049.

64. Birdwell BG, Raskob GE, Whitsett TL *et al.* The clinical validity of normal compression ultrasonography in outpatients suspected of having deep venous thrombosis. *Ann Intern Med* 1998; 128:1–7.

65. Cogo A, Lensing AWA, Koopman MM *et al.* Compression ultrasonography for diagnostic management fo patients with clinically suspected deep vein thrombosis: prospective cohort study. *Br Med J* 1998; 316:17–20.

66. Schellong SM, Schwarz T, Halbritter K *et al.* Complete compression ultrasonography of the leg veins as a single test for the diagnosis of deep vein thrombosis. *Thromb Haemost* 2003; 89:228–234.

67. Kelly J, Rudd A, Lewis RR, Hunt BJ. Plasma D-dimers in the diagnosis of venous thromboembolism. *Arch Intern Med* 2002; 162:747–756.

68. Perrier A, Bounameaux H. Cost-effective diagnosis of deep vein thrombosis and pulmonary embolism. *Thromb Haemost* 2001; 86:475–487.
69. Goldhaber SZ. Pulmonary embolism. *Lancet* 2004; 363:1295–1305.
70. Perrier A, Howarth N, Didier D *et al.* Performance of helical computed tomography in unselected outpatients with suspected pulmonary embolism. *Ann Intern Med* 2001; 135:88–97.
71. Qanadli SD, Hajjam ME, Mesurolle B *et al.* Pulmonary embolism detection: prospective evaluation of dual section helical CT versus selective pulmonary arteriography in 157 patients. *Radiology* 2000; 217:447–455.
72. Donato AA, Scheirer JJ, Atwell MS, Gramp J, Duszak R. Clinical outcomes in patients with suspected acute pulmonary embolism and negative helical computed tomographic results in whom anticoagulation was withheld. *Arch Intern Med* 2003; 163:2033–2038.
73. Anderson DR, Kovacs MJ, Kovacs G *et al.* Combined use of clinical assessment and d-dimer to improve the management of patients presenting to the emergency department with suspected deep vein thrombosis (the EDITED Study). *J Thromb Haemost* 2003; 1:645–651.

18

Antithrombotic therapy in venous thrombosis and pulmonary embolism

S. M. Bates, M. J. O'Donnell, J. Hirsh

INTRODUCTION

The annual incidence of venous thromboembolism (VTE), which consists of deep venous thrombosis (DVT) and pulmonary embolism (PE), is approximately 0.1%, increasing from 0.01% in early adulthood to nearly 1% in old age [1–3]. To minimise the risk of fatal pulmonary embolism, accurate diagnosis and prompt therapy are crucial [4]. Long-term complications include post-thrombotic syndrome [5–7], recurrent thromboembolism [8–13], and thromboembolic pulmonary hypertension [14]. Once venous thromboembolism is diagnosed, the goals of treatment are symptom relief and prevention of thrombus extension, embolisation, and recurrence. This chapter will review the antithrombotic therapy of venous thromboembolism, with an emphasis on treatment advances within the past five years.

ANTICOAGULANT THERAPY

Anticoagulant therapy has been the mainstay of treatment for venous thromboembolism since the landmark trial of Barritt and Jordan provided the first convincing evidence for its effectiveness [4]. In this randomised trial of 35 patients with clinically diagnosed pulmonary embolism, 25% of those who received no treatment died of autopsy-proven pulmonary embolism. In contrast, none of the patients who received intravenous unfractionated heparin (UFH) died. Treatment of patients with pulmonary embolism or deep venous thrombosis involves similar anticoagulant regimens; in part, because both conditions are manifestations of the same disorder (venous thromboembolism) with pulmonary embolism occurring frequently in patients with proximal deep venous thrombosis [15–17] and *vice versa* [18, 19].

INITIAL THERAPY

Unfractionated or low-molecular-weight heparin (LMWH) followed by oral anticoagulation is the cornerstone of initial therapy [4, 20–22]. Table 18.1 lists anticoagulant options for initial treatment of venous thromboembolism.

Shannon M. Bates, Associate Professor, Department of Medicine, McMaster University Medical Centre, Hamilton, Ontario, Canada.

Martin James O'Donnell, Assistant Professor, Department of Medicine, Henderson Research Centre, Hamilton, Ontario, Canada.

Jack Hirsh, Professor Emeritus, McMaster University, Henderson Research Centre, Hamilton, Ontario, Canada.

Table 18.1 Anticoagulant options for the acute treatment of venous thromboembolism

Drug	Dose
Unfractionated heparin	Intravenously: loading dose of 5000 units or 80 units/kg with infusion adjusted to maintain activated partial thromboplastin time within the therapeutic range*
Low-molecular-weight heparin**	
Dalteparin (Fragmin)	Subcutaneously: 100 units/kg every 12 h or 200 units/kg daily (Used in other countries but not FDA approved for this indication)
Enoxaparin (Lovenox)	Subcutaneously: 1 mg/kg every 12 h or 1.5 mg/kg daily[†] (FDA approved for acute treatment of deep venous thrombosis)
Tinzaparin (Innohep)	Subcutaneously: 175 units/kg daily[‡] (FDA approved for acute treatment of deep venous thrombosis)
Nadroparin (Fraxiparin)	Subcutaneously: 86 units/kg every 12 h or 171 units/kg daily[§] (Used in other countries but not FDA approved for this indication)
Fondaparinux (Arixtra)	Subcutaneously: 5 mg daily (<50 kg), 7.5 mg daily (50–100 kg), 10 mg daily (>100 kg) (FDA approved for acute treatment of deep venous thrombosis and pulmonary embolism)

*Activated partial thromboplastin time therapeutic range: corresponds to heparin levels of 0.35 to 0.70 units/ml by anti-factor Xa assay. High levels of heparin-binding proteins and factor VIII may result in 'heparin resistance'. In patients requiring greater than 35 000 units per day to attain a therapeutic activated partial thromboplastin time, the dosage can be titrated according to plasma heparin levels [24]; **Doses are variable in patients who are obese or who have renal dysfunction, and monitoring of anti-factor Xa levels has been suggested in these patients, with dose adjustment to target a range four hours post-injection of 0.6 to 1.0 units/ml for twice-daily dosing or 1.0 to 2.0 unit/ml for once-daily dosing. Despite little supporting data, most manufacturers recommend capping the dose for obese patients at that for a 90-kg patient. [†]Recommended maximum of 180 mg per day; [‡]Recommended maximum of 18 000 units per day; [§] Recommended maximum of 17 100 units per day.

UNFRACTIONATED HEPARIN

Unfractionated heparin is a sulfated glycosaminoglycan that exerts its anticoagulant effect primarily by binding to antithrombin and inducing conformational changes that accelerate the speed at which antithrombin inhibits coagulation enzymes [23]. Because UFH binds non-specifically to plasma and cellular proteins and, consequently, has a variable anticoagulant response among patients [23], laboratory monitoring using the activated partial thromboplastin time (aPTT) is recommended, with dose adjustment to target a therapeutic range [23]. The 'therapeutic range' differs depending on the aPTT reagent and coagulometer used to measure the aPTT [23]. Although a fixed ratio of 1.5 to 2.5 times control is commonly suggested, this results in variable (and usually subtherapeutic) anticoagulation because of the differing responsiveness of available reagents. Ideally, the therapeutic aPTT range for each reagent should correspond to ex-vivo plasma anti-factor Xa heparin levels of 0.3 to 0.7 units/ml [23].

Approximately 25% of patients require doses of UFH of more than 35 000 units per day to prolong the aPTT above the lower limit of the therapeutic range. These patients are termed 'heparin resistant' [23, 24]. Most of these patients have therapeutic heparin levels when measured by the anti-factor Xa assay and the discrepancy between the two tests is the result of high concentrations of procoagulants such as factor VIII, which shorten the aPTT [25]. These patients can be safely managed according to their anti-factor Xa heparin levels [25]. Less often, patients may fail to show elevations of both aPTT and measured heparin levels despite receiving large doses of UFH. This is usually the result of a combination of increased non-specific heparin binding to heparin-binding plasma proteins and increased heparin clearance [26]. Rarely, heparin resistance is caused by low levels of antithrombin.

Although evidence from a retrospective subgroup analysis of cohort studies suggested that patients who fail to achieve therapeutic heparin levels, as measured by aPTT, have a higher rate of subsequent recurrent venous thromboembolism [27], with modern dosage regimens the relationship between the prolongation of the aPTT with heparin and clinical efficacy and safety is not at all clear-cut. Neither a meta-analysis [28] nor a subgroup analysis of three randomised trials [29] demonstrated a relationship between 'subtherapeutic' aPTT and the risk of recurrent venous thromboembolism in patients who received adequate starting doses of UFH. Thus, it is likely that the initial dose of UFH is a better determinant of efficacy than the aPTT [23, 30, 31]. From a practical point of view, provided that patients are treated with an initial bolus followed by a continuous intravenous infusion of at least 30 000 units per day and warfarin is started soon after initiating heparin therapy, the efficacy of UFH is excellent.

During the initial treatment of venous thromboembolism, UFH is usually given intravenously by continuous infusion (initially 1200 to 1300 units/hour or 18 units/kg/h), after a loading dose of 5000 units or 80 units/kg [23]. Weight-based heparin nomograms with dosage adjustments to achieve a target aPTT facilitate achieving a therapeutic anticoagulant effect [23, 31]. This method has been shown to reduce mortality in patents with pulmonary embolism, as well as reduce the extension and recurrence of symptomatic proximal [30] and calf deep venous thrombosis [20]. Major haemorrhage occurs in up to 2% of patients with venous thromboembolism during initial intravenous UFH therapy, depending on heparin dose, patient age, and concomitant use or non-use of thrombolytic and antiplatelet agents [23].

A meta-analysis of randomised trials has shown that subcutaneous UFH is at least as effective and safe as intravenous heparin for the initial treatment of deep venous thrombosis, when given in adequate doses [32]. Because the bioavailability of UFH is less when given subcutaneously than by the intravenous route, larger initial doses of subcutaneous UFH are needed to achieve a therapeutic anticoagulant effect [23]. This point is highlighted by the results of a randomised trial in which recurrent venous thromboembolism occurred in 19.3% of patients given 15 000 units subcutaneously twice daily, compared with 5.2% of patients given the same total dose by continuous intravenous infusion [30]. The usual regimen for subcutaneous therapy includes an initial intravenous bolus of 5000 units, followed by an initial subcutaneous dose of 17 500 units twice daily adjusted to attain a therapeutic aPTT when drawn six hours after the morning dose [24].

Large, appropriately designed trials of subcutaneous UFH have not been conducted in patients with symptomatic pulmonary embolism. However, a recently published open-label, multicentre randomised trial of 720 consecutive patients with acute symptomatic venous thromboembolism which compared initial therapy, consisting of a bolus of UFH followed by a weight-based subcutaneous dosing regimen with adjustments to achieve a therapeutic aPTT with subcutaneous LMWH, did include a sizeable subgroup of patients with submassive pulmonary embolism [33]. During initial therapy, major bleeding occurred in 1.1% of those receiving UFH and 0.8% of those treated with LMWH (absolute difference 0.3%; 95% confidence interval [CI] −1.2–1.7%). Among the total study population, 4.2% of patients treated with UFH developed an episode of objectively confirmed venous thromboembolism during the 3-month follow-up period, compared with 3.9% of those randomised to LMWH (3.9%; absolute difference 0.3%; 95% CI −2.5–3.1%). Of the 119 patients who presented with pulmonary embolism, three had symptomatic recurrent venous thromboembolism (1 of 59 patients allocated to UFH and 2 of the 60 LMWH recipients).

Long-term use of heparin (longer than one month) can cause osteoporosis [23, 34, 35]. Heparin-induced thrombocytopaenia is an immune-mediated adverse effect of heparin with a strong association with thromboembolism − 30 to 50% of cases are associated with venous or arterial thrombosis [23, 36]. Patients with previous heparin-induced thrombocytopaenia (HIT) should receive alternative anticoagulants, such as danaparoid, lepirudin, or argatroban [23].

LOW-MOLECULAR-WEIGHT HEPARINS

Low-molecular-weight heparin preparations are produced by controlled enzymatic or chemical depolymerisation of UFH. Although UFH and LMWH share some biochemical properties, they differ in their anti-Xa to anti-IIa activity, a reflection of the differences in their chain-length [23]. LMWHs, which demonstrate less non-specific binding, improved bioavailability, and elicit more predictable dose responses than UFH [23], are administered subcutaneously once or twice daily in weight-adjusted doses [23] (Table 18.1), generally without monitoring. Meta-analyses of methodologically strong studies that included patients with deep venous thrombosis [37, 38], as well as those with pulmonary embolism [39], demonstrate that unmonitored, fixed-dose subcutaneous LMWHs are as effective as adjusted-dose intravenous UFH in preventing recurrent venous thromboembolism and cause less bleeding.

Because the anticoagulant response to weight-based dosing is predictable, coagulation monitoring is generally unnecessary during treatment with LMWH [23]. However, monitoring is recommended if LMWH is used in patients with renal insufficiency, pregnant women, and in obese patients [23]. When monitoring is deemed necessary, the anti-factor Xa assay is commonly used; although concerns remain about the reliability and clinical relevance of anti-factor Xa levels [40]. Suggested anti-factor Xa levels, measured four hours after subcutaneous injection, are 0.6 to 1.0 units/ml for twice-daily dosing and 1.0 to 2.0 units/ml for once-daily administration [23].

Although heparin-induced thrombocytopaenia develops less frequently with LMWHs than UFH [23, 36], these agents often cross-react with the culprit antibody and, therefore, are contraindicated in patients with previous heparin-induced thrombocytopaenia [23]. LMWHs also cause less osteoporosis than UFH [34, 35].

Cohort studies have shown that outpatient therapy with LMWHs is safe and effective for the majority of patients with venous thromboembolism, including those with symptomatic submassive pulmonary embolism [41–49]. If there is a system in place for administering medication (or teaching patients or caregivers to administer it) and monitoring, over 80% of outpatients can be treated without hospitalisation [23]. However, those with massive thrombosis, high risk for haemorrhage (for e.g., the very elderly, and those with recent surgery, or a prior history of bleeding or renal or liver disease), or serious coexistent illnesses are unsuitable for out-of-hospital treatment. Although more expensive than UFH, LMWHs reduce costs by reducing hospital admissions and laboratory monitoring [50]. Reductions in nursing time also make LMWHs cost-effective for inpatients [50].

THROMBOLYTIC THERAPY

Thrombolytic agents dissolve fresh clots and restore vessel patency more rapidly than anticoagulants [51]. They are given systemically or by regional catheter-directed infusion, which results in higher local drug concentrations.

Although thrombolytic therapy has the potential to prevent morbidity from post-thrombotic syndrome in patients presenting with deep vein thrombosis, by preventing venous valvular damage and subsequent venous hypertension, outcome data supporting this hypothesis are lacking. Theoretically, catheter-directed infusion should result in improved efficacy compared to systemic therapy but this remains untested [51]. Both routes cause substantially more bleeding than does heparin alone [51] and, although a recent systematic review suggests that thrombolytic therapy is associated with increased rates of early vein patency, it is unclear whether either route reduces the incidence of post-thrombotic syndrome [51]. Further, a decision analysis suggests that patients are not willing to risk potential adverse outcomes associated with thrombolytic therapy to prevent post-thrombotic syndrome [52]. Consequently, thrombolytic therapy is generally reserved for patients who have limb-threatening thrombosis, who have had symptoms for less than one week, and who have a low bleeding risk [24].

Some have suggested that this approach is overly conservative and that thrombolytic therapy should be strongly considered in patients with iliofemoral deep venous thrombosis, a reasonable life expectancy, and no predisposition to bleeding [53]. This assertion is not backed up by solid data from appropriately designed clinical trials. Thus, although one trial reported that catheter-directed thrombolysis of iliofemoral deep vein thrombosis resulted in improved quality of life at 22 months, compared with that of patients treated with anticoagulants [54], this study had methodologic shortcomings. Specifically, it is not clear that consecutive patients were approached for participation, treatment assignment was not randomised, and patients treated with anticoagulants may have had more disease comorbidity and thus, a lower expected quality of life. Further, although it is stated that the treatment cohorts were matched, there was a significant difference in age, suggesting that patients in the two groups were not matched at baseline. Until properly-designed studies are performed showing benefit, thrombolytic therapy, which is more expensive and associated with a greater risk of serious complications, should be reserved for those most likely to benefit and least likely to be harmed by the intervention. While the decision should be made on an individual patient basis, all the risks, the potential lack of long-term benefits, and the acknowledgment of the absence of high-quality supportive data must be discussed with the patient.

The indications for thrombolytic therapy in patients with pulmonary embolism remain controversial. A number of recently published meta-analyses have come to conflicting conclusions about the benefits of thrombolysis compared with heparin for the initial treatment of pulmonary embolism [55–57]. The pooled estimates reported in the most recent of these reviews revealed that compared with heparin, thrombolytic therapy was associated with a non-statistically significant reduction in pulmonary embolism or death (6.7 vs. 9.6%; odds ratio [OR] 0.67; 95% CI 0.40–1.12) and a non-significant increase in major bleeding (9.1 vs. 6.1%; OR 1.42; 95% CI 0.81–2.46) [55]. Thrombolysis is associated with greater initial angiographic resolution of thrombus and lower residual pulmonary vascular resistance than treatment with UFH [24]. However, the risk of major haemorrhage is significantly increased, with one systematic review reporting an incidence of intracranial haemorrhage of 2% [58]. Given the increased rate of complications with thrombolytic therapy and the low mortality rate in most patients with pulmonary embolism treated with conventional anticoagulation, it is recommended that thrombolysis should be reserved for patients at greatest risk of fatal pulmonary embolism. Patients with pulmonary embolism who present in shock have a high fatality rate and the results of a small randomised trial suggest that thrombolytic therapy should be considered in this circumstance [59]. When the meta-analysis described above specifically examined trials that enrolled patients with major (haemodynamically unstable) pulmonary embolism, thrombolytic therapy was associated with a significant reduction in recurrent pulmonary embolism or death compared with heparin (9.4 vs. 19.0%; OR 0.45; 95% CI 0.22–0.92) [55]. It has also been suggested that thrombolytic therapy should be used in patients with submassive pulmonary embolism who have echocardiographic evidence of right ventricular dysfunction at presentation [60]. Reported mortality rates with conventional therapy in these patients are conflicting [58]. In a recent randomised trial of 256 patients with submassive pulmonary embolism (pulmonary hypertension or right ventricular dysfunction) comparing alteplase (100 mg over 2 h) plus heparin with heparin alone, thrombolytic therapy reduced the primary endpoint, a combination of death or need to escalate therapy in-hospital with measures such as mechanical ventilation, pressor agents, or rescue thrombolysis because of clinical deterioration (11.0 vs. 24.6%; $P = 0.006$) [60]. However, most of this difference in favour of thrombolysis was driven by a reduction in clinical deterioration alone and this study was underpowered to reliably demonstrate a modest but clinically important survival benefit with thrombolysis in this patient population [55]. At present, routine thrombolysis in all patients with pulmonary embolism and right ventricular dysfunction is not recommended and further evaluation is warranted. Similarly, although elevated troponin concentrations at the time of presentation may signify right ventricular microinfarction and, thus, identify patients at high risk of a complicated hospital course, it is not clear that these patients routinely require thrombolysis [61].

The role of thrombolysis in preventing long-term complications of pulmonary embolism has not been well studied. The perception that chronic thromboembolic pulmonary hypertension is a very uncommon complication of acute pulmonary embolism has been challenged by the results of a recent study. Thus, in a long-term follow-up study of 223 patients diagnosed with a first pulmonary embolism, the cumulative incidence of symptomatic chronic thromboembolic pulmonary hypertension was 1.0% (95% CI 0–2.4%) at 6 months, 3.1% (95% CI 0.7–5.5%) at 1 year, and 3.8% (95% CI 1.1%–6.5%) at 2 years [14]. If confirmed, these findings would argue for a more liberal use of fibrinolytic therapy in patients with acute pulmonary embolism given that compared with standard anticoagulation, this intervention has been associated with more rapid resolution of radiologic and haemodynamic abnormalities associated with acute pulmonary embolism [62], as well as with superior capillary perfusion and diffusion at one year [63] and improved preservation of normal haemodynamic response to exercise at seven years [64]. However, data showing a reduction in the development of chronic thromboembolic pulmonary hypertension in patients receiving thrombolytic therapy compared with those treated with anticoagulation are lacking. Further, although some risk factors for the development of chronic thromboembolic pulmonary hypertension have been elucidated (recurrent pulmonary embolism, larger perfusion defects, younger age, and idiopathic pulmonary embolism at presentation) [14], we are still unable to clearly predict which patients are most likely to develop this complication and, hence, potentially benefit from more aggressive therapeutic strategies.

LONG-TERM THERAPY

After an initial course of treatment with UFH or LMWH, extended anticoagulation is required to prevent recurrent venous thromboembolism [24]. Warfarin (or other coumarins) at a dose titrated to achieve an international normalised ratio (INR) of 2.0 to 3.0 is commonly used for secondary prophylaxis and, as compared to placebo, reduces the risk of recurrence by 90% compared to placebo [24, 65]. Because the antithrombotic effect of warfarin, which probably best parallels the reduction in prothrombin levels, is delayed for 72 to 96 h, an initial period of overlap with UFH or LMWH is required [24, 66, 67]. By starting warfarin the same day as heparin, heparin therapy can be discontinued after about five days [24], provided the INR has been therapeutic for two consecutive days. Patients with massive thrombosis often receive an extended course of heparin (7 to 14 days).

There is conflicting evidence as to the optimal dose with which to initiate warfarin therapy. An initial randomised trial found a 5 mg initial daily dose of warfarin as effective as 10 mg daily, in achieving a therapeutic INR within five days, with less tendency toward excess anticoagulation [68]. However, a more recent trial that included only outpatients with venous thromboembolism found that patients randomised to the 10 mg initial dose group achieved a therapeutic INR 1.4 days earlier than patients in the 5 mg group and were more likely to have a therapeutic INR at day five than were patients in the 5 mg initial dose group (83 and 46%, respectively; $P < 0.001$) [69]. The groups did not differ with respect to rates of recurrent venous thromboembolism, major bleeding, number of INR measurements greater than 5.0, or death. Thus, there is certainly room for flexibility in selecting a starting warfarin dose. An initial dose of 10 mg daily is likely to be appropriate in otherwise healthy outpatients. However, a lower starting dose (5 mg daily or less) should be considered in inpatients and in patients with a baseline INR greater than 1.4.

Because of multiple drug and dietary interactions with warfarin, therapy must be frequently monitored and the dose adjusted to maintain an INR of between 2.0 and 3.0 [24]. Strategies to improve the safety of oral anticoagulation include management by a central anticoagulation clinic [70] or training patients to undertake point-of-care fingerstick INR testing with a point-of-care device and self-adjustment of the anticoagulant dose [71]. Potential advantages of self-management include improved patient convenience, with enhanced patient compliance, and more frequent monitoring, which may improve the quality of oral anticoagulant therapy [72, 73]. However, patient self-management requires that a training system be developed, and point-of-care devices and test strips are expensive [74, 75]. A number of studies have suggested that patient self-management is feasible and safe [71, 72, 76, 77] and, in terms of time spent within the therapeutic INR range, selected patients are capable of delivering at least the same quality of oral anticoagulant therapy as specialised anticoagulation clinics [71, 72, 76, 77]. Although a recent single-centre randomised trial of 737 patients did not demonstrate a statistically significant difference in the time spent within the target INR range between self-managed patients and those managed by a university hospital affiliated anticoagulation clinic, self-management appeared superior in terms of reduction in the number of major complications (severe haemorrhage or thromboembolism) with these type of events occurring in 7.3% of the clinic-managed patients and 2.2% of the self-managed patients (absolute difference 5.1%; 95% CI 1.7–8.5%) [78]. Although these results are promising, it is important to note that this was an unblinded single-centre trial and the drop-out rate in the patient self-management group was 21%.

INTENSITY OF WARFARIN THERAPY

It has been hypothesised that lowering the intensity of oral anticoagulation to an INR of 1.5 to 1.9 in patients receiving long-term therapy would lead to a decreased risk of major haemorrhage, without significantly compromising efficacy with respect to prevention of recurrent venous thromboembolism. The role of reduced intensity anticoagulation (INR 1.5 to 1.9) following three months of conventional therapy has been examined in two randomised controlled trials (Table 18.2). The results of the PREVENT study suggest that compared with placebo, low-intensity warfarin is highly effective and safe in preventing recurrence [79]. On the other hand, the ELATE study found that low-intensity warfarin was somewhat less effective and no safer than conventional-intensity warfarin for extended treatment of unprovoked venous thromboembolism [80].

In both studies, the small number of major bleeding events likely precludes a truly accurate assessment of the true risk of major haemorrhage with either regimen. However, the major haemorrhage rates for the low-intensity arms in both studies were essentially identical. The results of the two studies together suggest that although low-intensity warfarin is much more effective than placebo in preventing recurrent venous thromboembolism, it is less effective than conventional-intensity warfarin and does not reduce the risk of major haemorrhage compared to standard therapy. As such, warfarin targeted to an INR of 2.0 to 3.0 remains the best therapy for patients receiving long-term anticoagulation for prevention of recurrent venous thromboembolism.

Table 18.2 Results of randomised trials examining reduced intensity warfarin therapy

Outcome	Study	Placebo %/person yr	Low-intensity* %/person year	Standard-intensity %/person year	Hazard ratio (95% CI)
Recurrent VTE	PREVENT [79]	7.2	2.6		0.36 (0.19–0.67)
	ELATE [80]		1.9	0.7	2.8 (1.1–7.0)
Major Bleeding	PREVENT [79]	0.4	0.9		2.53 (0.49–13.03)
	ELATE [80]		1.1	0.9	1.2 (0.4–3.0)

VTE = Venous thromboembolism; CI = confidence interval; *low intensity PREVENT [79] – warfarin adjusted to INR of 1.5–2.0; ELATE [80] – warfarin adjusted to INR of 1.5–1.9

Results of retrospective studies in tertiary care centres suggested that high-intensity warfarin (maintenance of a target INR of 3.1 to 4.0) is more effective than standard-intensity warfarin (maintenance of a target INR of 2.0 to 3.0) in preventing recurrent venous thromboembolism in patients with antiphospholipid antibodies. However, in a recent double-blind multicentre randomised trial of 114 patients with antiphospholipid antibody syndrome and a history of arterial or venous thromboembolism, the incidence of recurrent thrombosis was not lower in patients receiving high-intensity warfarin therapy [81]. During a mean follow-up of 2.7 years, recurrent thrombosis occurred in 6 (10.7%) of 56 patients in the high-intensity group and 2 (3.4%) of 58 patients in the moderate-intensity group (hazard ratio [HR] 3.1; 95% CI 0.6–15.0). Three patients in the high-intensity group and four in the moderate-intensity group had major bleeding (HR 1.0; 95% CI 0.2–4.8). Similar results were obtained in another recently published randomised trial of similar size and design [82].

USE OF LONG-TERM LOW-MOLECULAR-WEIGHT HEPARIN

Patients with cancer who have venous thromboembolism have a two- to three-fold higher risk of recurrence and a two- to six-fold increase in the risk of haemorrhagic complications when treated with warfarin, compared with those without cancer [83–85]. A randomised study of such patients showed that after standard initial LMWH therapy, long-term LMWH reduced the recurrence rate seen with coumarin derivatives by one-half [86]. In this trial, cancer patients with acute symptomatic venous thromboembolism received dalteparin at a dose of 200 IU/kg subcutaneously once daily for five to seven days and then either a warfarin derivative for six months targeted to an INR of 2.5 or dalteparin alone for six months (200 IU/kg once daily for one month, followed by a daily dose of approximately 150 IU/kg for five months). Recurrent venous thromboembolism occurred in 27 of 338 patients (9%) in the dalteparin group and in 53 of 338 patients (17%) in the warfarin group (HR 0.48; $P = 0.002$; number needed to treat [NNT] to prevent one episode of recurrence = 13). The INR was at least 2.0 for 70% of the total treatment time in the patients randomised to oral anticoagulant therapy and 25 of the 53 recurrences occurred while the INR was 2.0 or above. Major bleeding rates were similar with both medications (6% in those receiving dalteparin vs. 4% of patients treated with oral anticoagulants), and daily injections were acceptable to patients. Therefore, this therapy should be considered in all patients with deep vein thrombosis and malignancy. The main practical limitation to the use of long-term LMWH is likely to be drug cost. Interestingly, one cost-effectiveness analysis has suggested that LMWH might be a cost-effective medication for the long-term treatment of venous thromboem-bolism, especially in patients at high risk of recurrence [87].

The role for long-term LMWH in other patients is less clear. Two systematic reviews of randomised controlled trials comparing LMWH to warfarin for secondary prophylaxis found statistically non-signficant reductions of approximately 30%, and over 25% in the rates of recurrent thrombosis and major bleeding, respectively [88, 89]. However, both meta-analyses share similar limitations in that the quality of oral anticoagulant control in many of the included studies was poor or poorly reported and a number of the studies were not blinded. Although LMWH has advantages over warfarin, the cost, need for daily injections and risk of osteoporosis with long-term therapy make it unsuitable for routine secondary prophylaxis.

DURATION OF ANTICOAGULANT THERAPY

The optimal duration of anticoagulant treatment should balance the risks of recurrence and bleeding. If the net benefit of continuing anticoagulant therapy is small or uncertain, then patient preference and cost of therapy become important factors.

In general, patients should receive at least three months of anticoagulants [24]. With an INR of 2.0 to 3.0, the annual major bleeding risk is approximately 3% [90]. In patients whose thrombosis was associated with a resolved major risk factor, the recurrence risk after three months of anticoagulation is approximately 3% per year [24]. Case-fatality rates of 5% for recurrence [91] and 10% for major bleeding [90] have been reported. Thus, after three months, the risk of fatal recurrence off treatment for these patients is lower than the risk of fatal haemorrhage with warfarin (approximately 0.15 vs. 0.3% per year) and three months of therapy suffices [24]. Although retrospective analyses have suggested that one month of anticoagulant therapy is adequate for patients whose venous thromboembolic event was provoked by a transient risk factor, the results of a recent double-blind trial in which 165 such patients were randomised to placebo or continuation of warfarin for a further two months suggest that the duration of anticoagulation should not be further reduced [92]. In this study, 6.0% of the patients assigned to placebo had recurrent venous thromboembolism during 11 months of follow-up, compared to 3.7% of those assigned to warfarin (absolute difference 2.3%; 95% CI −5.2%–10.0%). There were no major bleeds in either group. The authors concluded that decreasing the treatment duration in this patient population is likely to increase recurrent venous thromboembolism, without achieving a clinically important decrease in bleeding. When they combined the results of their study with subgroup analy-ses of four earlier studies [8, 93–95] that compared four or six weeks of anticoagulation with three or six months in patients with venous thromboembolism provoked by a transient risk factor, they concluded that shortening the duration of anticoagulation to four to six weeks doubles the frequency of recurrent thromboembolism within a year from diagnosis.

The optimal duration of therapy for patients with unprovoked (idiopathic) events or who have continuing risk factors remains controversial [8–13, 24, 96]. Patients with a first episode of unprovoked venous thromboembolism have an increased risk of recurrence after oral anti-coagulation is discontinued, compared with patients whose event occurred in the setting of a transient risk factor. Patients with unprovoked venous thromboembolism who are treated for approximately three months have a 10 to 27% risk of recurrence in the year after discon-tinuing anticoagulants [8, 9–12]. With six months of treatment, the recurrence risk is approx-imately 10% in the year after stopping anticoagulation [12, 13]; patients whose event occurred in association with a resolved minor risk factor (such as oestrogen-containing oral contra-ceptive use, history of travel, or non-specific transient illness) probably have a lower recur-rence risk (approximately 5% in the first year after stopping anticoagulation) [13]. Extending therapy beyond six months does not substantially reduce the recurrence risk following dis-

Table 18.3   Recommendations for duration of anticoagulant therapy [21, 24, 96]

Setting	Recurrence risk in the year after discontinuation	Duration
Major transient risk factor*	3%	3 months
Minor risk factor†, no thrombophilia	<10%, if risk factor avoided	6 months
	>10%, if risk factor persistent	At least 6 months or until factor resolves
Unprovoked, no or low risk thrombophilia‡	<10%	6 months§
Unprovoked, high risk thrombophilia¶	>10%	Indefinite
More than one unprovoked event	>10%	Indefinite
Malignancy, other ongoing risks	>10%	Indefinite

*Examples of major transient risk factors = major surgery, major medical illness, leg casting;
†Examples of minor transient risk factors = oral contraceptive or hormone replacement therapy;
‡Examples of low risk thrombophilias = heterozygosity for the factor V Leiden or prothrombin gene mutations; §Therapy may be prolonged if the patient prefers and/or the risk of bleeding is low; ¶Examples of high risk thrombophilias: antithrombin or protein C or protein S deficiency, homozygosity for the factor V Leiden mutation, homozygosity for the prothrombin gene mutation, double heterozygosity for these abnormalities, positivity for antiphospholipid antibodies.

continuation of treatment [11]. While continuing treatment prevents recurrence, it also exposes the patient to the risk of anticoagulant-induced bleeding. Based on estimated rates for recurrent venous thromboembolism and major bleeding above, extended anticoagulation should be considered for patients with unprovoked venous thromboembolism or a continuing risk factor whose estimated risk of major bleeding is less than 5% per year, whereas six months of therapy may be more appropriate for patients at higher risk of bleeding or those whose thrombosis occurred in association with a resolved minor risk factor (Table 18.3).

Clinical prediction rules have been developed to estimate the risk of major bleeding during anticoagulant therapy. Based on earlier data generated by Landefeld and colleagues [97], Beyth *et al.* developed and prospectively validated a modified Outpatient Bleeding Risk Index that includes four independent risk factors for major bleeding: age 65 years or greater, history of gastrointestinal bleeding, history of stroke, and one of four specific comorbid conditions (recent myocardial infarction, renal insufficiency, severe anaemia, or diabetes mellitus) [98]. Based on the number of risk factors present, this index classifies patients into three groups by predicted cumulative risk of major bleeding. Low-risk patients have no risk factors, patients with one or two risk factors are termed intermediate-risk, and patients deemed high-risk have three or four risk factors. In the validation study, low-, intermediate-, and high-risk patients had cumulative rates of major bleeding at 12 months of 3%, 8%, and 30%, respectively [92]. When the Outpatient Bleeding Risk Index was prospectively applied to 222 consecutive outpatients diagnosed with venous thromboembolism [99], the rates of major bleeding were lower than expected with annualised risks of 0% (95% CI 0–2.8%) and 4.3% (95% CI 1.1–11.1%) in the low- and intermediate-risk groups, respectively. The rate in the high-risk group could not be defined because only 2 patients fitted the criteria for this category. However, the index was able to discriminate between low- and intermediate-risk patients and could be used to guide decisions regarding treatment duration.

There are some data to suggest that patients with pulmonary embolism have a higher risk of recurrent venous thromboembolism after discontinuation of anticoagulant therapy than do those with deep vein thrombosis [48, 96, 100, 101]. In addition, after an initial pulmonary embolism, approximately 60% of recurrent episodes are also pulmonary embolism; whereas only 20% of recurrent episodes of venous thromboembolism are pulmonary embolism following an initial deep vein thrombosis [10, 91, 96, 101–103]. Finally, the risk of dying from pulmonary embolism is higher than that from deep vein thrombosis [5, 102–111]. As such, it has been suggested that patients presenting with pulmonary embolism may benefit from increasing the duration of therapy. However, more data are required before these findings can be incorporated into routine recommendations regarding duration of therapy. Similarly, the role that residual deep vein thrombosis [10, 11, 80, 112–113] and elevated D-dimer levels [96, 114–116] after stopping treatment should play in the determination of anticoagulant duration remains controversial.

Although it is assumed that the presence of a thrombophilic abnormality increases the risk of recurrence and, consequently, justifies prolonged therapy, the available data are inconsistent, and these assumptions remain unproven [44, 96, 117–119]. That said, indefinite therapy is generally recommended for patients with a high risk of thrombophilia (for example, a deficiency of antithrombin, protein C or protein S; persistently positive antiphospholipid antibodies; or homozygosity for factor V Leiden mutation or the prothrombin mutation or heterozygosity for both).

NEW ANTICOAGULANTS

The limitations of traditional anticoagulants have prompted development of new agents. Agents in advanced stage of development include parenteral synthetic analogs of the unique pentasaccharide sequence that mediates the interaction of heparin and antithrombin (fondaparinux and idraparinux) and oral direct thrombin inhibitors (ximelagatran) (Table 18.4).

In a large randomised non-inferiority trial comparing fondaparinux with enoxaparin for the acute treatment of deep vein thrombosis, rates of symptomatic recurrent venous thromboembolism and major bleeding were not statistically different between groups [120]. Similarly, in an open-label randomised trial of 2213 patients, fondaparinux was found to be at least as safe as intravenous UFH for the initial treatment of pulmonary embolism [121].

Idraparinux is a hyper-methylated derivative of fondaparinux. Its plasma half-life is 80 to 130 h [122]; consequently, idraparinux is given once weekly by subcutaneous injection. Idraparinux was evaluated in a phase II trial in which 659 patients with proximal deep vein thrombosis were randomised to receive one of four doses of idraparinux or warfarin (INR 2.0 to 3.0) for twelve weeks following five to seven days of enoxaparin treatment [123]. The rates of ultrasonographic and perfusion lung scanning normalization and deterioration were similar in all four idraparinux groups and did not differ from the warfarin group. There was a clear dose response for major bleeding in patients given idraparinux, with less bleeding at the 2.5 mg idraparinux dose than with warfarin. Phase III studies in patients with deep vein thrombosis and pulmonary embolism are underway.

Ximelagatran therapy was examined in a randomised trial of 2489 patients with acute deep vein thrombosis (with or without pulmonary embolism) that compared six months of ximelagatran monotherapy with six months of enoxaparin followed by warfarin; in this study, ximelagatran therapy was not inferior with respect to efficacy and safety [124]. A placebo controlled trial showed that ximelagatran reduced the risk of recurrent venous thromboembolism in patients who had already completed six months of standard treatment, without increasing the risk of major haemorrhage [125]. In contrast to warfarin, ximelagatran does not require anticoagulation monitoring. However, ximelagatran has potential limitations, including elevations of liver enzymes (specifically alanine aminotransferase) to more than 3 times the upper limit of normal in 5 to 10% of patients receiving long-term therapy. Typically, these findings are asymptomatic and reversible, even if the medication is

Table 18.4 Results of phase III trials examining new anticoagulants in the treatment of venous thromboembolism

Patient population (reference)	Patients enrolled (N)	Control	Treatment	Outcome
Ximelagatran				
Acute DVT (with or without symptomatic PE) [124]	2489	Ximelagatran: 36 mg orally twice daily	Enoxaparin/ warfarin: 1 mg/kg of enoxaparin SC twice daily for at least 5 days until INR therapeutic	Recurrence at 6 months Ximelagatran: 2.1% Enoxaparin/ warfarin: 2.0% AD 0.2% (95%CI −1.0–1.3%) Major bleeding Ximelagatran: 1.3% Enoxaparin/ warfarin: 2.2% AD −1.0% (95% CI −2.1–0.1%)
Symptomatic DVT or PE after 6 months of therapy [125]	1233	Ximelagatran: 24 mg orally twice daily for 18 months	Placebo	Symptomatic recurrence at 18 months Ximelagatran: 2.8% Placebo: 12.6% HR 0.16 (95% CI 0.09–0.3) Major bleeding Ximelagtran: 1.1% Placebo: 1.3% HR 1.16 (95% CI 0.35–3.8)
Fondaparinux				
Acute symptomatic DVT [120]	2205	Fondaparinux: weight-based dose SC once daily for at least 5 days, until INR therapeutic	Enoxaparin: 1 mg/kg SC twice-daily for at least 5 days, until INR therapeutic	Symptomatic recurrence at 3 months Fondaparinux: 3.9% Enoxaparin: 4.1% AD −0.15% (95% CI −1.8–1.5%) Major bleeding during initial therapy Fondaparinux: 1.1% Enoxaparin: 1.2% AD −0.1% (95% CI −1.0–0.8%)

Table 18.4 (Continued)

Patient population (reference)	Patients enrolled (N)	Control	Treatment	Outcome
Acute symptomatic PE [121]	2213	*Fondaparinux:* weight-based dose SC once daily for at least 5 days, until INR therapeutic	*Unfractionated heparin:* continuous intravenous infusion, adjusted to an aPTT of 1.5 to 2.5 × control for at least 5 days, until INR therapeutic	Symptomatic recurrence at 6 months *Fondaparinux:* 3.8% *Heparin:* 5.0% AD −1.2% (95% CI −3.0–0.5%) Major bleeding during initial therapy *Fondaparinux:* 1.3% *Heparin:* 1.1% AD 0.2% (95% CI −0.7–1.1%)

DVT = deep vein thrombosis; PE = pulmonary embolism; SC = subcutaneously; aPTT = activated partial thromboplastin time; CI = confidence interval; AD = absolute difference; HR = hazard ratio.

continued. In the acute treatment study, a retrospective analysis of locally reported adverse events showed a higher rate of serious coronary events with ximelagatran therapy (10/1240 patients compared with 1/1249 patients treatment with enoxaparin) [124].

The Food and Drug Administration has recently approved fondapariunux for the initial treatment of venous thromboembolism. However, they and the European regulatory agency have declined to similarly approve ximelgatran, citing concerns about hepatic toxicity [126].

INFERIOR VENA CAVAL FILTERS

Interruption of the inferior vena cava to prevent pulmonary embolism arising from lower extremity deep venous thrombosis has become widely used since inferior vena caval filters became available some 30 years ago. However, reliable data concerning their efficacy and safety are still limited. Inferior vena caval filters are felt to be useful in patients who fail or have a contraindication to anticoagulation [24]. In a randomised trial of 400 patients with proximal vein thrombosis who received at least three months of anticoagulants alone or with a filter, the incidence of early pulmonary embolism (by day 12) was significantly lower in patients with filters (1.1 vs. 4.8% in those with no filter, $P=0.03$) [127]. However, this difference did not persist; at two years, the reduction in symptomatic pulmonary embolism in the filter-treated patients was not significant and mortality was similar in both groups. The approximately two-fold increased risk of recurrent deep venous thrombosis in patients with filters (20.8% compared with 11.6%) suggests that anticoagulants should be started if and when it is safe to do so. The use of filters to prevent embolisation of 'free-floating' iliofemoral thrombosis, pulmonary embolism in patients with deep vein thrombosis and reduced cardiopulmonary reserve, and in the treatment of venous thromboembolism in cancer patients with primary or metastatic cerebral tumours remains controversial

[24]. Temporary filters are often used if anticoagulation is likely to be safe within 10 to 14 days.

CONCLUSIONS

Recent advances have enhanced treatment options for patients with deep vein thrombosis and pulmonary embolism. A number of issues, however, have yet to be resolved. The optimal duration of anticoagulant therapy in various subgroups of patients with venous thromboembolism has yet to be determined. The long-term clinical benefits and thrombolytic therapy in patients with submassive pulmonary embolism and in those with extensive deep vein thrombosis await clarification in well-designed clinical trials. Several promising new antithrombotic agents are under development, including a number of orally active direct factor Xa and direct thrombin inhibitors. However, these drugs are in the early stages of clinical development and further work is needed to establish their safety and efficacy. As yet, of the new anticoagulants, only fondaparinux has been approved for the treatment of venous thromboembolism.

REFERENCES

1. Nordstom M, Lindblad B, Bergqvist D, Kjellstrom T. A prospective study of the incidence of deep vein thrombosis within a defined urban population. *J Intern Med* 1992; 232:155–160.
2. White RH. The epidemiology of venous thromboembolism. *Circulation* 2003; 107(suppl 1):I-4–I-8.
3. Silverstein MD, Heit JA, Mohr DN, Petterson TM, O'Fallon WM, Melton III LJ. Trends in the incidence of deep vein thrombosis and pulmonary embolism: a 25-year population-based study. *Arch Intern Med* 1998; 158:585–593.
4. Barritt DW, Jordan SC. Anticoagulant drugs in the treatment of pulmonary embolism: a controlled trial. *Lancet* 1960; 1:309–312.
5. Prandoni P, Lensing AWA, Cogo A *et al*. The long-term clinical course of acute deep venous thrombosis. *Ann Intern Med* 1996; 125:1–7.
6. Brandjes DPM, Buller HR, Heijboer H, Huisman MV, de Rijk M, Jagt H. Randomized trial of effect of compression stockings in patients with symptomatic proximal-vein thrombosis. *Lancet* 1997; 349:759–762.
7. Ginsberg JS, Hirsh J, Julian J *et al*. Prevention and treatment of postphlebitic syndrome: results of a 3-part study. *Arch Intern Med* 2001; 161:2105–2109.
8. Shulman S, Rhedin AS, Lindmarker P *et al*. and the Duration of Anticoagulation Trial Study Group. A comparison of six weeks with six months of oral anticoagulant therapy after a first episode of venous thromboembolism. *N Engl J Med* 1995; 332:1661–1665.
9. Kearon C, Gent M, Hirsh J, Weitz J *et al*. A comparison of three months of anticoagulation with extended anticoagulation for a first episode of idiopathic venous thromboembolism. *N Engl J Med* 1999; 340:901–907.
10. Agnelli G, Prandoni P, Santamaria MG *et al*. for the Warfarin Optimal Duration Italian Trial Investigators. Three months versus one year of oral anticoagulant therapy for idiopathic deep venous thrombosis. *N Engl J Med* 2001; 19:165–169.
11. Kearon C for the LAFIT Investigators. Rate of recurrent venous thromboembolism (VTE) after completing two years of anticoagulation for a first episode of idiopathic VTE. *Thromb Haemost* (suppl) 2001 (ISSN 0340–6245) (abstract).
12. Pinede L, Ninet J, Duhaut P *et al*. for the Investigators of the 'Durée Optimale du Traitement AntiVitamines K' (DOTAVK) Study. Comparison of 3 and 6 months of oral anticoagulant therapy after a first episode of proximal deep vein thrombosis or pulmonary embolism and comparison of 6 and 12 weeks of therapy after isolated calf deep vein thrombosis. *Circulation* 2001; 103:2453–2460.
13. Baglin T, Luddington R, Brown K, Baglin C. Incidence of recurrent venous thromboembolism in relation to clinical and thrombophilic risk factors: prospective cohort study. *Lancet* 2003; 362:523–526.
14. Pengo V, Lensing AWA, Prins MH *et al*. for the Thromboembolic Pulmonary Hypertension Study Group. Incidence of chronic thromboembolic pulmonary hypertension after pulmonary embolism. *N Engl J Med* 2004; 350:2257–2264.

15. Doyle DJ, Turpie AG, Hirsh J *et al*. Adjusted subcutaneous heparin or continuous intravenous heparin in patients with acute deep vein thrombosis. *Ann Intern Med* 1987; 107: 441–445.

16. Huisman MV, Buller HR, ten Cate JW *et al*. Unexpected high prevalence of silent pulmonary embolism in patients with deep vein thrombosis. *Chest* 1998; 95:498–502.

17. Moser KM, Fedullo PF, LittleJohn JK, Crawford R. Frequent asymptomatic pulmonary embolism in patients with deep venous thrombosis. *JAMA* 1994; 27:223–225.

18. Hull RD, Hirsh J, Carter CJ *et al*. Pulmonary angiography, ventilation lung scanning, and venography for clinically suspected pulmonary embolism with abnormal perfusion lung scan. *Ann Intern Med* 1983; 98:891–898.

19. Girard P, Musset D, Parent F *et al*. High prevalence of detectable deep venous thrombosis in patients with acute pulmonary embolism. *Chest* 1999; 116:903–908.

20. Lagerstedt CI, Olsson CB, Fagher BO, Albrechtsson U, Oqvist BW. Need for long-term anticoagulant treatment in patients with symptomatic calf-vein thrombosis. *Lancet* 1985; 1:515–518.

21. Hirsh J, Hoak J. Management of deep vein thrombosis and pulmonary embolism. A statement for healthcare professionals. From the Council on Thrombosis (in Consultation with the Council on Cardiovascular Radiology), American Heart Association. *Circulation* 1996; 93:2212–2245.

22. Brandjes DPM, Heijboer H, Buller HR, de Rijk M, Jagt H, ten Cate JW. Acenocoumarol and heparin compared with acenocoumarol alone in the initial treatment of proximal-vein thrombosis. *N Engl J Med* 1992; 327:1485–1489.

23. Hirsh J, Raschke R. Heparin and low-molecular-weight heparin. The Seventh ACCP Conference on Antithrombotic and Thrombolytic Therapy. *Chest* 2004; 1269:1884S–2203S.

24. Buller HR, Hull RD, Hyers TM, Prins MH, Raskob GE. Antithrombotic therapy for venous thromboembolic disease. The Seventh ACCP Conference on Antithrombotic and Thrombolytic Therapy. *Chest* 2004; 126:401S–428S.

25. Levine MN, Hirsh J, Gent M *et al*. A randomized trial comparing activated thromboplastin time with heparin assay in patients with acute venous thromboembolism requiring large daily doses of heparin. *Arch Intern Med* 1994; 154:49–56.

26. Young E, Prins M, Levine MN, Hirsh J. Heparin binding to plasma proteins, an important mechanism for heparin resistance. *Thromb Haemost* 1992; 67:639–643.

27. Hull RD, Raskob GE, Brant RF, Pineo GF, Valentine KA. Relation between the time to achieve the lower limit of the APTT therapeutic range and recurrent venous thromboembolism during heparin treatment for deep vein thrombosis. *Arch Intern Med* 1997; 57:2562–2568.

28. Anand S, Ginsberg JS, Kearon C, Gent M, Hirsh J. The relation between the activated partial thromboplastin time response and recurrence in patients with venous thrombosis treated with intravenous heparin. *Arch Intern Med* 1996; 156:1667–1681.

29. Anand SS, Bates SM, Ginsberg JS *et al*. Recurrent venous thrombosis and heparin therapy. An evaluation of the importance of early activated partial thromboplastin times. *Arch Intern Med* 1999; 159:2029–2032.

30. Hull RD, Raskob GE, Hirsh J *et al*. Continuous intravenous heparin compared with intermittent subcutaneous heparin in the initial treatment of proximal vein thrombosis. *N Engl J Med* 1986; 315:1109–1114.

31. Raschke RA, Reilly BM, Guidry JR, Fonantana JR, Srinivas S. The weight-based heparin dosing nomogram compared with a 'standard care' nomogram. A randomized trial. *Ann Intern Med* 1993; 119:874–881.

32. Hommes DW, Bura A, Mazzolai L, Buller HR, ten Cate JW. Subcutaneous heparin compared with continuous intravenous heparin administration in the initial treatment of deep vein thrombosis. *Ann Intern Med* 1992; 116:279–284.

33. Writing Committee for the Galilei Investigators. Subcutaneous adjusted-dose unfractionated heparin vs. fixed-dose low-molecular-weight heparin in the initial treatment of venous thromboembolism. *Arch Intern Med* 2004; 164:1077–1083.

34. Pettila V, Leinonen P, Markkola A, Hiilesmaa V, Kaaja R. Postpartum bone mineral density in women treated for thromboprophylaxis with unfractionated heparin or LMW heparin. *Thromb Haemost* 2002; 87:182–186.

35. Monreal M, Lafoz E, Olive A, del Rio L, Vedia C. Comparison of subcutaneous unfractionated heparin with a low molecular weight heparin (Fragmin) in patients with venous thromboembolism and contraindications to coumarin. *Thromb Haemost* 1994; 71:7–11.

36. Warkentin TE, Levine MN, Hirsh J *et al*. Heparin-induced thrombocytopenia in patients treated with low-molecular-weight heparin or unfractionated heparin. *N Engl J Med* 1995; 332:1330–1335.

37. Gould MK, Dembitzer AD, Doyle RL, Hastie TJ, Garger AM. Low-molecular-weight heparins compared with unfractionated heparin for treatment of acute venous thrombosis. A meta-analysis of randomised, controlled trials. *Ann Intern Med* 1999; 130:800–809.

38. Dolovich LR, Ginsberg JS, Douketis JD, Holbrook AM, Cheah G. A meta-analysis comparing low-molecular-weight heparins with unfractionated heparin in the treatment of venous thromboembolism: examining some unanswered questions regarding location of treatment, product type, and dosing frequency. *Arch Intern Med*. 2000; 160:181–188.

39. Quinlan DJ, McQuillan A, Eikelboom JW. Low-molecular-weight heparin compared with intravenous unfractionated heparin for treatment of pulmonary embolism. A meta-analysis of randomized, controlled trials. *Ann Intern Med* 2004; 140:175–183.

40. Greaves M for the Control of Anticoagulation Subcommittee of the Scientific and Standardization Committee of the International Society of Thrombosis and Haemostasis. Limitations of the laboratory monitoring of heparin therapy. *Thromb Haemost* 2002; 87:163–164.

41. Levine M, Gent M, Hirsh J *et al*. A comparison of low-molecular-weight heparin administered primarily at home with unfractionated heparin administered in the hospital for proximal deep vein thrombosis. *N Engl J Med* 1996; 334:677–681.

42. Koopman MMW, Prandoni P, Piovella F *et al*. for the TASMAN Study Group. Treatment of venous thrombosis with intravenous unfractionated heparin administered in the hospital as compared with subcutaneous low-molecular-weight heparin administered at home. *N Engl J Med* 1996; 334:682–687.

43. Wells PS, Kovacs MJ, Bormannis J *et al*. Expanding eligibility for outpatient treatment of deep venous thrombosis and pulmonary embolism with low-molecular-weight heparin. *Arch Intern Med* 1998; 158:1809–1812.

44. Harrison L, McGinnis J, Crowther M, Ginsberg JS, Hirsh J. Assessment of outpatient treatment of deep vein thrombosis with low-moelcular-weight heparin. *Arch Intern Med* 1998; 158:2001–2003.

45. Kovacs MJ, Anderson D, Morrow B, Gray L, Touchie D, Wells PS. Outpatient treatment of pulmonary embolism with dalteparin. *Thromb Haemost* 2000; 83:209–211.

46. Belcaro G, Nicolaides AN, Cesarone MR *et al*. Comparison of low-molecular-weight heparin, administered primarily at home with unfractionated heparin, administered in hospital and subcutaneous heparin, administered at home for deep vein thrombosis. *Angiology* 1999; 50:781–787.

47. Bocclon H, Elias A, Chale JJ, Cadene A, Gabriel S. Clinical outcome and cost of hospital vs. home treatment of proximal deep vein thrombosis with a low-molecular-weight heparin: the Vascular Midi-Pyrenees study. *Arch Intern Med* 2000; 160:1769–1773.

48. Simoneau G, Sors H, Charbonnier B *et al*. for the THESEE Group. A comparison of low-molecular-weight heparin with unfractionated heparin for acute pulmonary embolism. *N Engl J Med* 1997; 337:6639–9.

49. The Columbus Investigators. Low-molecular-weight heparin in the treatment of patients with venous thromboembolism. *N Engl J Med* 1997; 337:657–662.

50. Rodger M, Bredeson C, Wells PS, Beck J, Kearon C, Huebsch LB. Cost-effectiveness of low-molecular-weight heparin and unfractionated heparin in treatment of deep vein thrombosis. *CMAJ* 1998; 159:931–938.

51. Forster AJ, Wells PS. The rationale and evidence for the treatment of lower-extremity deep venous thrombosis with thrombolytic agents. *Curr Opin Hematol* 2002; 9:437–442.

52. O'Meara JJ, McNutt RA, Evans AT, Moore SW, Downs SM. A decision analysis of streptokinase plus heparin compared with heparin alone for deep vein thrombosis. *N Engl J Med* 1994; 330:1865–1869.

53. Vedantham S, Khilnani N, Min R. Deep vein thrombosis. *N Engl J Med* 2004; 351:2133–2134 (letter).

54. Comerota AJ, Thromb RD, Mathias SD, Haughton S, Mewissen M. Catheter-directed thrombolysis for iliofemoral deep venous thrombosis improves health-related quality of life. *J Vasc Surg* 2000; 132:130–137.

55. Wan S, Quinlan DJ, Agnelli G, Eikelboom JW. Thrombolysis compared with heparin for the initial treatment of pulmonary embolism: a meta-analysis of the randomized controlled trials. *Circulation* 2004; 110:744–749.

56. Agnelli G, Becattini C, Kirschstein T. Thrombolysis vs. heparin in the treatment of pulmonary embolism. A clinical outcome-based meta-analysis. *Arch Intern Med* 2002; 162:2537–2541.

57. Thabut G, Thabut D, Myers RP *et al*. Thrombolytic therapy of pulmonary embolism: a meta-analysis. *J Am Coll Cardiol* 2002; 41:1660–1667.

58. Dalen JE, Alpert JS, Hirsh J. The uncertain role of thrombolytic therapy for pulmonary embolism: is it effective? Is it safe? When is it indicated? *Arch Intern Med* 1997; 157:2550–2556.

59. Jerjes-Sanchez C, Ramirez-Rivera A, de Lourdes Garcia M *et al.* Streptokinase and heparin versus heparin alone in massive pulmonary embolism: a randomized controlled trial. *J Thromb Thrombolysis* 1995; 2:227–229.

60. Konstantinides S, Giebel A, Heusel G, Heinrich F, Kasper W, for the Management Strategies and Prognosis of Pulmonary Embolism – 3 Trial Investigators. Heparin plus alteplase compared with heparin alone in patients with submassive pulmonary embolism. *N Engl J Med* 2002; 327:1143–1150.

61. Konstantinides S, Geibel A, Olschewski M *et al.* Importance of cardiac troponins I and T in risk stratification of patients with acute pulmonary embolism. *Circulation* 2002; 106:1263–1268.

62. Anderson DR, Levine MN. Thrombolytic therapy for the treatment of acute pulmonary embolism. *CMAJ.* 1992; 146:1317–1324.

63. Sharma GV, Buleson VA, Sasahara AA. Effect of thrombolytic therapy on pulmonary-capillary blood volume in patients with pulmonary embolism. *N Engl J Med* 1980; 303:842–845.

64. Sharma GV, Folland ED, McIntyre KM, Sasahara AA. Long-term benefit of thrombolytic therapy in patients with pulmonary embolism. *Vasc Med* 2000; 5:91–95.

65. Prins MN, Hutten BA, Koopman MMW, Buller HR. Long-term treatment of venous thromboembolic disease. *Thromb Haemost* 1999; 82:892–898.

66. Hull RD, Raskob GE, Rosenbloom D *et al.* Heparin for 5 days as compared with 10 days in the initial treatment of proximal venous thrombosis. *N Engl J Med* 1990; 332:1260–1264.

67. Gallus A, Jackaman J, Tillett J, Mills W, Wycherley A. Safety and efficacy of warfarin started early after submassive venous thrombosis or pulmonary embolism. *Lancet* 1986; 2:1293–1296.

68. Crowther MA, Ginsberg JS, Kearon C *et al.* A randomized trial comparing 5 mg and 10 mg warfarin loading doses. *Arch Intern Med* 1999; 159:46–48.

69 Kovacs MJ, Rodger M, Anderson DR *et al.* Comparison of 10 mg and 5 mg warfarin initiation nomograms together with low-molecular-weight heparin for outpatient treatment of acute venous thromboembolism. A randomized, double-blind, controlled trial. *Ann Intern Med* 2003; 138:714–719.

70. Pengo V, Legnani C, Noventa F, Palareti G. Oral anticoagulant therapy in patients with nonrheumatic atrial fibrillation and risk of bleeding: a multicenter inception cohort study. *Thromb Haemost* 2001; 85:418–422.

71. Cromheecke ME, Levi M, Colly LP *et al.* Oral anticoagulation self-management and management by a specialist anticoagulation clinic: a randomised cross-over comparison. *Lancet* 2000; 356:97–102.

72. Taborski U, Muller-Berghaus G. State of the art patient self-management for control of oral anticoagulation. *Semin Thromb Hemost* 1999; 25:43–47.

73. Siebenhofer A, Berghold A, Sawicki PT. Systematic review of studies of self-management of oral anticoagulation. *Thromb Haemost* 2004; 91:225–232.

74. Sawicki PT, for the Working Group for the Study of patient Self-management of Oral Anticoagulation. A structured teaching and self-management program for patients receiving oral anticoagulation: a randomized controlled trial. *JAMA* 1999; 281:145–150.

75. Morsdorf S, Erdelbruch W, Taborski U *et al.* Training of patients for self-management of oral anticoagulant therapy: standards, patient suitability, and clinical aspects. *Semin Thromb Hemost* 1999; 25:109–115.

76. Gadisseur APA, Breukink-Engbers WGM, van der Meer FJM, van den Besselaar AMH, Sturk A, Rosendaal FR. Comparison of the quality of oral anticoagulant therapy through patient self-management and management by specialized anticoagulation clinics in the Netherlands. A randomized clinical trial. *Arch Intern Med* 2003; 163:2639–2646.

77. Sunderji R, Gin K, Shalansky K *et al.* A randomized trial of patient self-managed versus physician managed oral anticoagulation. *Can J Cardiol* 2004; 20:1117–1123.

78. Menendez-Jandula B, Souto JC, Oliver A *et al.* Comparing self-management of oral anticoagulant therapy with clinic management. A randomized trial. *Ann Intern Med* 2005; 142:1–10.

79. Ridker PM, Goldhaber SZ, Danielson E *et al.* for the PREVENT Investigators. Long-term, low-intensity warfarin therapy for the prevention of recurrent venous thromboembolism. *N Engl J Med* 2003; 348:1425–1434.

80. Kearon C, Ginsberg JS, Kovacs MJ *et al.* for the ELATE Investigators. Comparison of low-intensity warfarin therapy with conventional-intensity warfarin therapy for long-term prevention of recurrent venous thromboembolism. *N Engl J Med* 2003; 239:631–639.

81. Crowther MA, Ginsberg JS, Gent M *et al.* A randomized trial of two intensities of warfarin (international normalized ratio of 2.0 to 3.0 versus 3.1 to 4.0) for the prevention of recurrent thrombosis in patients with antiphospholipid antibodies. *N Engl J Med* 2003; 349: 1133–1138.

82. Finazzi G, Marchioli R, Brancaccio *et al.* A randomized clinical trial of high intensity warfarin vs. conventional antithrombotic therapy for the prevention of recurrent thrombosis in patients with antiphospholipid syndrome (WAPS). *J Thromb Haemost* 2005; 3:848–853.

83. Prandoni P, Lensing AW, Piccioli A *et al.* Recurrent venous thromboembolism and bleeding complications during anticoagulant treatment in patients with cancer and venous thrombosis. *Blood* 2002; 100:3484–3488.

84. Hutten BA, Prins MH, Gent M, Ginsberg J, Tijssen JG, Buller HR. Incidence of recurrent thromboembolic and bleeding complications among patients with venous thromboembolism in relation to both malignancy and achieved international normalized ratio: a retrospective analysis. *J Clin Oncol* 2000; 18:3978–3983.

85. Palareti G, Legnani C, Lee A *et al.* A comparison of the safety and efficacy of oral anticoagulation for the treatment of vnous thromboembolic disease in patients with or without malignancy. *Thromb Haemost* 2000; 84:805–810.

86. Lee AYY, Levine MN, Baker RI *et al.* for the Randomized Comparison of Low-Molecular-Weight Heparin versus Oral Anticoagulant Therapy for the Prevention of Recurrent Venous Thromboembolism in Patients with Cancer (CLOT) Investigators. Low-molecular-weight heparin versus a coumarin for the prevention of recurrent venous thromboembolism in patients with cancer. *N Engl J Med* 2003; 349:146–153.

87. Marchetti M, Pistorio A, Barone M, Serafini S, Barosi G. Low-molecular-weight heparin versus warfarin for secondary prophylaxis of venous thromboembolism: a cost-effectiveness analysis. *Am J Med* 2001; 111:130–139.

88. Van der Jeijden JF, Hutten BA, Buller HR, Prins MH. Vitamin K antagonists or low-molecular-weight heparin for the long-term treatment of symptomatic venous thromboembolism. *Cochrane Database Syst Rev* 2000; CD002001.

89. Iori A, Guercini F, Pini M. Low-molecular-weight heparin for the long-term treatment of symptomatic venous thromboembolism: meta-analysis of the randomized comparisons with oral anticoagulants. *J Thromb Haemost* 2003; 1:1906–1913.

90. Linkins L, Choi PT, Douketis JD. Clinical impact of bleeding in patients taking oral anticoagulant therapy for venous thromboembolism: a meta-analysis. *Ann Intern Med* 2003; 139:893–900.

91. Douketis JD, Kearon C, Bates S, Duku EK, Ginsberg JS. Risk of fatal pulmonary embolism in patients with treated venous thromboembolism. *JAMA* 1998; 279:458–462.

92. Kearon C, Ginsberg JS, Anderson DR *et al.* for the SOFAST Investigators. Comparison of 1 month with 3 months of anticoagulation for a first episode of venous thromboembolism associated with a transient risk factor. *J Thromb Haemost* 2004; 2:743–749.

93. Schulman S, Lockner D, Juhlin-Dannfelt A. The duration of oral anticoagulation after deep vein thrombosis. *Acta Med Scand* 1985; 217:547–552.

94. Research Committee of the British Thoracic Society. Optimum duration of anticoagulation for deep vein thrombosis and pulmonary embolism. *Lancet* 1992; 340:873–876.

95. Levine MN, Hirsh J, Gent M *et al.* Optimal duration of oral anticoagulant therapy: randomized trial comparing four weeks with three months of warfarin in patients with proximal deep vein thrombosis. *Thromb Haemost* 1995; 74:606–611.

96. Kearon C. Long-term management of patients after venous thromboembolism. *Circulation* 2004; 110(suppl 1):I-10–I-18.

97. Landefeld CS, Goldman L. Major bleeding in outpatients treated with warfarin: incidence and prediction by factors known at the start of outpatient therapy. *Am J Med* 1989; 87:144–152.

98. Beyth RJ, Quinn LM, Landefeld S. Prospective evaluation of an index for predicting the risk of major bleeding in outpatients treated with warfarin. *Am J Med* 1998; 105:91–99.

99. Wells PS, Forgie MA, Simms M *et al.* The outpatient bleeding risk index. Validation of a tool for predicting bleeding rates in patients treated for deep venous thrombosis and pulmonary embolism. *Arch Intern Med* 2003; 163:917–920.

100. Agnelli G, Prandoni P, Becattini C *et al.* for the Warfarin Optimal Duration Italian Trial Investigators. Extended oral anticoagulant therapy after a first episode of pulmonary embolism. *Ann Intern Med* 2003; 139:19–25.

101. Eichinger S, Weltermann A, Minar E et al. Symptomatic pulmonary embolism and the risk of recurrent venous thromboembolism. *Arch Intern Med* 2004; 164:92–96.

102. Murin S, Romano PS, White RH. Comparison of outcomes after hospitalization for deep venous thrombosis or pulmonary embolism. *Thromb Haemost* 2002; 88:407–414.

103. Kniffin WE, Jr, Baron JA, Barrett J et al. The epidemiology of diagnosed pulmonary embolism and deep venous thrombosis in the elderly. *Arch Intern Med* 1994; 154:861–866.

104. Bell WR, Simon TL. Current status of pulmonary embolic disease: pathophysiology, diagnosis, prevention and treatment. *Am Heart J* 1982; 103:239–262.

105. Stein PD, Henry JW. Prevalence of acute pulmonary embolism among patients in a general hospital and at autopsy. *Chest* 1995; 108:978–981.

106. Kearon C. Natural history of venous thromboembolism. *Circulation* 2003; 107:122–130.

107. Goldhaber SZ, Visni L, De Rosa M. Acute pulmonary embolism: clinical outcomes in the International Cooperative Pulmonary Embolism Registry (ICOPER). *Lancet* 1999; 353:1386–1389.

108. Heit JA, Silverstein MD, Mohr DN et al. Predictors of survival after deep vein thrombosis and pulmonary embolism: a population-based, cohort study. *Arch Intern Med* 1999; 159:445–453.

109. Ribeiro A, Lindmarker P, Juhlin-Dannfelt A et al. Echocardiography Doppler in pulmonary embolism: right ventricular dysfunction as a predictor of mortality rate. *Am Heart J* 1997; 134:479–487.

110. Bell CM, Redelmeier DA. Mortality among patients admitted to hospitals on weekends as compared with weekdays. *N Engl J Med* 2001; 345:663–668.

111. Beyth RJ, Cohen AM, Landefeld CS. Long-term outcomes of deep vein thrombosis. *Arch Intern Med* 1995; 155:1031–1037.

112. Piovella F, Crippa L, Barone M et al. Normalization rates of compression ultrasonography in patients with a first episode of deep vein thrombosis of the lower limbs: association with recurrence and new thrombosis. *Haematologica* 2002; 87:515–522.

113. Prandoni P, Lensing AWA, Prins MH et al. Residual venous thrombosis as a predictive factor of recurrent venous thromboembolism. *Ann Intern Med* 2002; 137:955–960.

114. Palareti G, Lagnani C, Cosmi B et al. Predictive value of D-dimer test for recurrent venous thromboembolism after anticoagulation withdrawal in subjects with a previous idiopathic event and in carriers of congenital thrombophilia. *Circulation* 2003; 108:313–318.

115. Palareti G, Leganani C, Cosmi B, Guazzaloca G, Pancani C, Coccheri S. Risk of venous thromboembolism recurrence: high negative predictive value of D-dimer performed after oral anticoagulation is stopped. *Thromb Haemost* 2002; 87:7–12.

116. Eichinger S, Minar E, Bialonczyk C et al. D-dimer levels and risk of recurrent venous thromboembolism. *JAMA* 2003; 290:1071–1074.

117. Christiansen S, Koster T, Vandenbroucke JP, Rosendaal FR. Risk factors for recurrent venous thrombosis: a prospective follow-up of the Leiden thrombophilia study (LETS). *Suppl Thromb Haemost* 2003; (ISSN 1740–3340) (abstract).

118. Baglin T, Luddington R, Brown K, Baglin C. Incidence of recurrent venous thromboembolism in relation to clinical and thrombophilic risk factors. *Suppl Thromb Haemost* 2003; (ISSN 1740–3340) (abstract).

119 Margaglione M, D'Andrea G, Colaizzo D et al. Coexistence of factor V Leiden and factor II A20210 mutations and recurrent venous thromboembolism. *Thromb Haemost* 1999; 82:1583–1587.

120. Buller HR, Davidson BL, Decousus H et al. for the Matisse Investigators. Fondaparinux or enoxaparin for the initial treatment. *Ann Intern Med* 2004; 140:867–873.

121. The Matisse Investigators. Subcutaneous fondaparinux versus intravenous unfractionated heparin in the initial treatment of pulmonary embolism. *N Engl J Med* 2003; 349:1695–1702.

122. Herbert JM, Herault JP, Bernat A et al. Biochemical and pharmacological properties of SANORG 34006, a potent and long-acting synthetic pentasaccharide. *Blood* 1998; 91:4197–4205.

123. PERSIST Investigators. A novel long-acting synthetic factor Xa inhibitor (idraparinux sodium) to replace warfarin for secondary prevention in DVT: a phase II evaluation *Blood* 2002; 100:301 (Abstract).

124. Fiessinger J-N, Huisman MV, Davidson DL et al. for the THRIVE Treatment Study Investigators. *JAMA* 2005; 293:681–689.

125. Schulman S, Wahlander K, Lundstrom T, Clason SB, Eriksson H for the THRIVE III Investigators. Secondary prevention of venous thromboembolism with the oral direct thrombin inhibitor ximelagatran. *N Engl J Med* 2003; 349:1713–1721.

126. Gurewich V. Ximelagatran – promises and concerns. *JAMA* 2005; 293:736–739.
127. Decousus H, Leizorovicz A, Parent F *et al.* for the Prévention du Risque d'Embolic Pulmonaire par interruption Cave Study Group. A clinical trial of vena caval filters in the prevention of pulmonary embolism in patients with proximal deep vein thrombosis. *N Engl J Med* 1998; 338:409–415.

19

Prevention and treatment of venous and arterial thrombosis in patients with specific conditions: diabetes, hypercoagulable states, pregnancy and renal diseases

M. M. Samama, J. Conard

INTRODUCTION

In this chapter, we will review pertinent literature and present our personal expert opinion on issues related to prevention and treatment of venous or arterial thrombosis in four conditions where thrombosis plays a significant role: diabetes and the metabolic syndrome, hereditary or acquired thrombophilia (the 'hypercoagulable states'), pregnancy, and renal disease.

DIABETES

Diabetes affects 150 million people worldwide and 20 million in the United States. Its prevalence is regularly increasing especially in developing countries [1]. The worldwide prevalence of obesity is increasing at an alarming rate, and is likely the main cause for the increasing prevalence of type 2 diabetes.

VENOUS THROMBOEMBOLISM (VTE)

Although atherosclerosis, which is common in diabetes, may predispose to venous thrombosis (VTE), as shown by Prandoni *et al.* [2], the risk of VTE in this category of patients is not well-documented [3, 4, 5]. According to the rare epidemiologic studies, the relative risk ratio for VTE in diabetic patients can be estimated to range between 1 and 2. In fact, in a recent Scandinavian study, it was shown that diabetic patients are more than two-fold at higher risk than the general population [6]. However, the number of diabetic patients was small in this well-conducted study.

Diabetic patients hospitalised for an acute illness and who are immobilised should receive a prophylactic treatment against VTE similar to non-diabetic patients [7]. In critically ill hospitalised patients, including diabetics, the risk of VTE is increased and prophylactic treatment seems fully justified.

It is generally accepted that surgery in diabetics does not carry a significantly increased risk for postoperative VTE as compared to non-diabetics. Prophylactic treatment should be

Meyer Michel Samama, Professor Emeritus of Haematology, Hotel Dieu University Hospital, Paris Notre-Dame, Paris, France.

Jacqueline Conard, Unite Hemostase-Thrombose, Hotel Dieu University Hospital, Paris Notre-Dame, Paris, France.

utilised according to the American Consensus Conference of Chest Physicians (ACCP) guidelines [8]. Search for thrombophilia and treatment of deep vein thrombosis (DVT) and/or pulmonary embolism (PE) are performed according to the guidelines for non-diabetic patients. A stringent control of glycaemia is recommended.

ARTERIAL THROMBOEMBOLISM

Atherothrombotic disorders are common in diabetic patients. Atherothrombosis is responsible for macro- and micro-angiopathy, this latter including retinopathy and nephropathy which are common in type 2 diabetes. A considerable amount of work has been devoted to the understanding of the pathophysiology of atherothrombosis in patients with diabetes [9].

PATHOPHYSIOLOGY OF ATHEROTHROMBOSIS

Hereditary thrombophilia plays a minor role in the development of arterial thromboembolism in diabetic patients. Several authors have evaluated the role of antithrombin (AT), protein C (PC), protein S (PS) deficiencies, factor V Leiden mutation, or the G20210A mutation of factor II. The conclusion of these investigations is that it is difficult to prove a causal relationship between hereditary thrombophilia and arterial thrombosis, except in rare cases [10]. In a meta-analysis of more than 17 000 patients with coronary cerebrovascular or peripheral arterial thrombotic events, the three most common gene alterations (the methylene-tetrahydrofolate reductase (MTHFR) polymorphism in homocysteine metabolism, factor V Leiden and factor II gene mutation) were identified at a slightly increased rate compared with controls [11]. Previously, Conard *et al.* had explored the potential role of AT, PC or PS deficiency, and found that it was rarely responsible for atheroembolic episodes [12]. In total, hereditary thrombophilia plays a minor role, if any, in the aetiology of arterial thrombosis.

Homocystinuria with an extremely elevated plasma homocysteine level, $>100\,\mu mol/l$ (normal <12 or $15\,\mu mol/l$) is an exception to this rule, but is extremely rare (1 out of 150 000 subjects), although less rare in Ireland than in other countries. Homocystinuria, through a toxic effect of homocysteine on vascular endothelial cells demonstrated long ago by Harker *et al.* [13] and some other mechanisms, can be responsible for acute myocardial infarction (MI) in young adults. Autopsies of some young patients have shown advanced atherosclerotic lesions. It can also be responsible for venous thromboembolism. The deficiency in cystathionine-synthase is the less rare genetic alteration in this group of patients. The term hyperhomocysteinaemia is used for a much less severe condition, which is however much more frequent. The homocysteine plasma concentration here is moderately elevated, ranging from 15 to $30–100\,\mu mol/l$. It can be acquired in different conditions, such as smoking or kidney insufficiency, but may be of genetic origin [14].

Among inherited causes of hyperhomocysteinaemia, the most frequent gene alteration is that of MTHFR in the heterozygous or homozygous state [15, 16]. However a causal relationship with venous thrombosis is still doubtful. In contrast, a causal relationship with coronary artery disease or ischaemic stroke due to atherosclerosis is generally accepted [16].

Search for hyperhomocysteinaemia is recommended in unexplained venous thrombosis and in arterial thrombosis, especially in an individual younger than 50 years of age. This recommendation seems justified, since a simple treatment with folic acid – with or without combination with vitamin B6 and B12 – could reduce the risk of thrombosis. Measurement of vitamin B12 and folates in blood is indicated before such a treatment.

BLOOD ALTERATION IN TYPE 2 DIABETES

Hypercoagulation, platelet hyperactivity and hypofibrinolysis are common features of type 2 diabetes, and have recently been extensively reviewed [17, 18]. Most blood alterations are due to hyperglycaemia, which is responsible for a hyperglycation of proteins, including platelet membrane proteins.

Obesity, frequently associated with type 2 diabetes, is a cause of important increased levels of plasminogen activator inhibitor (PAI)-1, since adipocytes synthesise this antifibrinolytic (prothrombotic) variable.

Recent studies have also shown that the thromboresistance of the vascular wall can be reduced by depressed synthesis of nitric oxide (NO) [9].

THE METABOLIC SYNDROME

Type 1 diabetes is due to insulin deficiency, while type 2 diabetes is primarily associated with insulin resistance. The metabolic syndrome was previously known as the pre-diabetic state. It is presently characterised by the coexistence of at least two of five conditions: abdominal obesity, insulin resistance, hypertension, dyslipidaemia (increased triglycerides and decreased HDL cholesterol levels), and microalbuminuria [19, 20].

When the metabolic syndrome coexists with diabetes, the prevalence of coronary artery disease reaches about 19%, since atherogenesis occurs early in the course of the metabolic syndrome. In the last decade, an important increase in obesity has been observed and, in parallel, the incidence of the metabolic syndrome has greatly increased [20].

Factors which are likely to promote cardiovascular events in these patients are, according to the literature, hyperglycaemia, dyslipidaemia, endothelial dysfunction, inflammation, hypofibrinolysis [17,18].

THERAPEUTIC CONSIDERATIONS IN DIABETES AND IN THE METABOLIC SYNDROME

Patients with diabetes are at increased risk of death due to cardiovascular disease. A greater awareness of this danger is needed. According to the pathogenesis of thrombosis in diabetic patients, a stringent control of glycaemia through improved diet and antidiabetic drugs is generally considered essential. Diet and exercise, in order to reduce gain in body weight, and a tight glycaemic control can slow down diabetes progression. In addition, treatment of hypertension and dyslipidaemia are the best available strategies to indirectly reduce the risks of arterial thrombosis (acute MI, ischaemic, stroke, peripheral arterial disease). Control of hypertension in order to achieve a target of 120/80 mmHg is highly recommended. Peroxysomal proliferation activator receptor-(PPAR)-alpha (fibrates) and gamma (thiazolidine-diones, glitazones) may counterbalance blood alterations and endothelial dysfunction and reduce the incidence of vascular complications in diabetes and the metabolic syndrome [21, 22, 23]. Interestingly, controlling dyslipidaemia and especially hypertriglyceridaemia may result in lowering PAI-1, as has been shown in patients treated with glitazones. The use of angiotensin-converting enzyme (ACE) inhibitors and angiotensin II receptor blockers are cornerstones for the treatment of diabetic patients to reduce the cardiovascular risk after a MI [24]. The use of ACE inhibitors is recommended even in patients with asymptomatic diabetes.

Finally, the role of statins in plaque regression should be considered. The combination of simvastatins with PAAR-gamma agonists is capable of inducing a regression of the plaques and may increase plaque stability [24].

PRIMARY AND SECONDARY PREVENTION OF CARDIOVASCULAR EVENTS WITH ANTIPLATELET AGENTS

Arterial thromboembolic episodes are more frequent in diabetic than in non-diabetic patients. Aspirin is indicated in secondary prevention and in primary prevention in patients at high risk (ACCP recommendation), although threshold levels for the latter indications are still debated. The risk–benefit ratio of aspirin given routinely in primary prevention is variable from patient to patient, and no support from large trials in diabetic patients is available [24].

Clopidogrel has the same indications as aspirin in patients with a previous coronary episode. Similar considerations are valid for acute episodes of stroke or peripheral arterial disease.

Aspirin, alone or in combination with dipyridamole and ticlopidine, effective antithrombotic agents in arterial thrombosis, have been considered in diabetic patients. The first large trials in the 90s were designed with the aim of reducing the development of diabetic retinopathy. Our group contributed to the DAMAD trial [25], which was followed by the TIMAD trial [26]. Aspirin and/or dipyridamole were used in the first study, while ticlopidine was the drug tested in the latter. Both studies have shown encouraging results for efficacy and tolerability of these long-term treatments.

Since these first studies, a large amount of work has been devoted to the potential advantages of a long-term prophylactic treatment with low-dose aspirin. Moreover, a reduced platelet response to aspirin in type 2 diabetes has been reported [27].

National health authorities and the American Diabetes Association (ADA) have recommended the use of low-dose aspirin in diabetic patients with macrovascular disease, and also suggested starting treatment for primary prevention [28]. This recommendation is not frequently followed, since adherence rates to the ADA guidelines for routine aspirin prophylaxis are extremely low [29].

HYPERCOAGULABLE OR THROMBOPHILIC STATES

DEFINITIONS

Thrombophilia can be defined as a condition that predisposes to thrombosis. It can be congenital or acquired, and several authors consider that hypercoagulable or prothrombotic states are synonymous with thrombophilic states [30].

Hypercoagulation is one of the three variables of the Virchow triad if we consider that it corresponds to the blood alteration indicated by this famous pathologist [31]. Congenital and acquired hypercoagulable states or thrombophilias have been studied in several books [32–34] and numerous reviews [35–38].

In 1965, the description of antithrombin III (ATIII) deficiency, a constitutional and familial disease associated with a high risk of VTE, confirmed the Virchow concept. The term thrombophilia was used for the first time. It applies to various genetic blood alterations discovered in the following years, protein C and protein S deficiency, and factor V Leiden and factor II G20210A gene mutations.

In parallel, several major risk factors predisposing to VTE are well recognised (Table 19.1) [39]. Among them, the antiphospholipid syndrome, associated (or not) with a lupus anticoagulant, is responsible for a predisposition to both venous and arterial thromboembolic episodes [40]. Very rare patients have a congenital form of this disease, while it is acquired in almost every other patient. Fetal loss caused by placental microthrombosis is another characteristic of the antiphospholipid syndrome. The secondary antiphospholipid syndrome is associated with an autoimmune disease, while no aetiology can be identified in the primary syndrome. It has to be noted that some primary syndromes can be converted to secondary syndromes in the years following the diagnosis, with the appearance of new symptoms.

Cancer is another important acquired risk factor for VTE since the discovery, by Armand Trousseau, chairman at Hotel-Dieu hospital in Paris, of a relationship between cancer and phlebitis in 1867 [41]. This causal relationship has been investigated, and at least two procoagulant factors, tissue factor and a cancer-activating protein, play a role in the pathogenesis of thrombosis [42, 43]. This topic – cancer and thrombosis – has been extensively documented in several books and recent reviews [44–47].

Table 19.1   Classification of major risk factors predisposing to thrombosis

Major predisposing risk factors		
Genetic	*Acquired*	*Mixed*
Deficiency in AT	Age Immobilisation	Hyperhomocysteinemia Increased level of:
Deficiency in PC	Surgery Cancer	• Factor VIII • Fibrinogen
Deficiency in PS	Pregnancy/post-partum oral contraception	• Factor XI • Factor IX
Factor V Leiden	Hormone replacement therapy	• Factor XII
Prothrombin gene G20210A mutation	Antiphospholipid antibody syndrome	
Fibrinogen, plasminogen deficiency	Myeloproliferative syndromes Paroxysmal haemoglobinuria Behcet disease . . .	
AT antithrombin, antithrombin III; PC protein C; PS protein S. Adapted with permission from [39].		

Several other acquired thrombophilic syndromes are well identified: myeloproliferative disorders, paroxysmal nocturnal haemoglobinuria, Behcet disease, oral contraception, hormone replacement therapy (HRT), and iatrogenic syndromes, such as heparin-induced thrombocytopaenia, the mechanism of which has some similarity with the antiphospholipid syndrome [48].

Chemotherapy and treatment with tamoxifen, thalidomide and other drugs are also predisposing causes to thrombosis [49].

In this review, we will concentrate mainly on prevention and treatment of thrombosis in the most common clinical conditions: constitutional thrombophilias and acquired thrombophilias, especially in patients with the antiphospholipid syndrome, cancer or with a myeloproliferative disease.

PREVENTION OF VTE EPISODES IN THROMBOPHILIAS

In order to adjust prophylactic treatment to the level of risk, it is important to classify individuals as previously asymptomatic or symptomatic, and to differentiate those with or without a provoked VTE event. Major predisposing risk factors are classified as congenital, acquired or mixed [39, 49] (Table 19.1).

Prophylaxis should be considered in every previously asymptomatic patient with congenital or acquired thrombophilia especially when a clinical situation predisposing to thrombosis, such as surgery, immobilisation, trauma, etc., is encountered [50, 51].

In women with thrombophilia, oestrogen–progestin contraceptives, HRT with oral oestrogens, or pregnancy, increase the risk for VTE [52, 53]. The level of risk and the benefit/risk ratio should be analysed case by case, but this is frequently a difficult task. In our group, hereditary thrombophilias are classified in three main groups according to the level of the thrombotic risk: high, moderate or low (Table 19.2).

In rare studies the quantitative level of risk has been well determined. Thus, the risk of a first venous thrombotic event in carriers of a familial thrombophilic defect has been the aim of

Table 19.2   Grading of severity in patients with various hereditary thrombophilias

Grading of severity	

High	AT deficiency
	Homozygous factor V Leiden mutation or
	   factor II G20210A mutation
	   combined abnormalities
	Homozygous protein C or protein S deficiency

Moderate	PC and PS deficiency
Low	Heterozygous factor V Leiden mutation Heterozygous factor II G20210A mutation

the European Prospective Cohort On Thrombophilia (EPCOT study) [54]. In this prospective analysis, in which 575 asymptomatic carriers and 118 controls were included, 26 (4.5%) and 7 (0.6%) from the two groups, respectively, experienced a first VTE episode during a 5.7 year follow-up. The mean incidence of the first event per year was eight times higher (0.8%) in thrombophilic subjects than in controls (0.1%). The highest incidence was associated with AT deficiency or combined defects, and the lowest incidence with factor V Leiden mutation. Interestingly, the incidence of bleeding associated with long-term anticoagulant treatment, as evaluated from the literature, seems somewhat higher than the risk of a first VTE in these asymptomatic patients with thrombophilia. Thus, in previously asymptomatic patients, pro-phylactic treatment does not seem justified. In contrast, it can be indicated for short periods of time when a precipitating risk factor, such as immobilisation, pregnancy, acute illness, surgery, etc. occurs. Indeed, in this study, 134 out of the 575 asymptomatic thrombophilic individuals received short-term anticoagulants mainly during surgery and pregnancy.

The thrombotic risk in patients with AT congenital deficiency is considered to be higher than that of patients with Protein C deficiency, but a precise quantification is not available. The incidence of the first event per year in these asymptomatic patients was 1.7%, and it was as high as in patients with combined defects.

In this study, 96 patients had AT deficiency, and nine episodes of VTE occurred (9%) during the 5.7 years follow-up. Finally, it has be to be noted that, in this important study, the risk of VTE might have been underestimated, due to preventive measures implemented by the treating physicians, who were aware of the presence of a thrombophilia defect and were familiar with this category of disease.

In symptomatic patients, the reported annual incidence of VTE ranges in the literature from less than 1% to about 3% for protein C and for protein S deficiency. For factor V Leiden, it ranges from 0.1% to 0.7% [55, 56].

Evaluation of the risk of VTE recurrence was the aim of the prospective EPCOT study restricted to symptomatic patients [56]. The relative risk of objectively confirmed VTE events prior to entry was calculated for the relatives with thrombophilia and the controls (excluding probands). The incidence was 4.4 per 1000 persons/year as compared to 0.3 per 1000 persons/year in controls. The highest incidence was found in combined defects and in AT deficiency, and the lowest in subjects with factor Leiden mutation (8.4, 5 and 1.5 per 1000 persons/year, respectively [56].

The risk of VTE in thrombophilic patients undergoing surgery has been investigated in a small number of studies. It is generally considered that high-risk thrombophilia (such as AT deficiency, homozygous protein C or protein S deficiencies or combined thrombophilias) should routinely receive a higher dosage and/or a more prolonged thrombosis prophylaxis after surgery than individuals without thrombophilia. However, the supporting data for this strategy are limited since these subjects are rare and few randomised studies have been conducted.

We have reviewed the existing literature through Medline from 1966 to 2005 in order to evaluate the level of risk of surgery-associated VTE for specific thrombophilias (key words were AT, protein C, protein S, activated protein C resistance, factor V Leiden, prothrombin or factor II mutation, and surgery, postoperative complications, thrombosis, thrombophilia or thromboembolism [57]. We did not take into account hyperhomocysteinaemia, since its role as a predisposing factor for VTE is debated. Two different methods were used for this evaluation of the available studies; firstly, we reviewed retrospective studies as to the outcome of different thrombophilic patients in all types of surgery; secondly, we reviewed studies reporting the incidence of postoperative VTE in patients carrying only one thrombophilic abnormality. The results of these investigations are in general negative, since they were unable to prove a significant relationship between the existence of a thrombophilic state and an increased frequency of postoperative venous thromboembolic episodes [58–64]. Interestingly, an APC resistance test performed with the original Dahlbäck's method was found to have some positive predictive value of post-operative thromboembolic events in elective replacement of the hip or knee [60]. It has to be remarked that several anecdotal reports have described thrombophilic patients with a post-operative thrombosis or with immediate recurrences after vascular surgery, but no systematic prospective study has evaluated this issue.

In patients undergoing surgery, LMWH is used to prevent postoperative VTE at the dose recommended for high-risk patients by the ACCP [51]. A prolonged duration of anticoagulant treatment should be considered. A 4- to 6-week duration of treatment after surgery might be appropriate.

Thus, very limited information and no precise recommendation is available regarding prophylactic treatment duration in thrombophilic patients, especially after surgery [65, 66].

TREATMENT DURATION AFTER A FIRST EPISODE OF VTE

In previously symptomatic patients, an important consideration is the length of anticoagulant treatment after a first episode [65].

The optimal duration of anticoagulation is related to the estimated risk of VTE recurrence and the benefit/risk ratio of treatment. A high risk will warrant more prolonged therapy.

According to the recent ACCP recommendations, subjects with factor V Leiden and the G20210A prothrombin gene mutation should not be considered at higher risk of VTE than normal individuals (Tables 19.3 and 19.4). This is in contrast with patients with AT, protein C or protein S deficiency, and individuals with combined thrombophilias [65–67].

CONSTITUTIONAL THROMBOPHILIA AND PREGNANCY

This important topic is discussed below in a separate section (Pregnancy, p. 343).

ACQUIRED THROMBOPHILIAS

PATIENTS WITH ANTIPHOSPHOLIPID (APL) ANTIBODIES

A grade 1C+ recommendation of the ACCP indicates that patients with APL antibodies and a first VTE episode should be treated for 12 months, and the authors suggest that indefinite anticoagulant therapy should be administrated (grade 2C) [65].

There has been some debate regarding the target (international normalised ratio) INR in these patients. Some authors maintain that an INR higher than in patients without APL antibodies [68–70] is required, while more recently the usual target INR of 2.5 has been considered satisfactory [71].

PATIENTS WITH CANCER

Patients with malignancies have a seven-fold increase of VTE compared with persons without malignancies. The risk increases during chemotherapy and hormonal treatment [72, 73].

A recent study has shown that, in patients with a VTE episode, LMWH might be more efficacious than warfarin [74]. A previous clinical trial in France had shown the potential advantage of LMWH over warfarin in the secondary prevention of VTE in patients with cancer [75].

The ACCP recommendation is to use LMWH for the first 3 to 6 months of long-term anticoagulant therapy. The grade is 1A, and anticoagulant therapy should be used indefinitely or until the cancer is resolved (grade 1C).

Literature concerning the VTE risk in cancer patients undergoing surgery has been recently reviewed [76], and recommendations have been made that prolonged prophylactic treatment should be considered in such patients.

Table 19.3 Long-term treatment of acute DVT of the leg in thrombophilic patients according to the ACCP recommendations and suggestions [65]

- For patients with DVT and cancer, we recommend LMWH for the first 3 to 6 months of long-term anticoagulant therapy (grade 1A). For these patients we recommend anticoagulant therapy indefinitely or until the cancer is resolved (grade 1C).
- For patients with a first episode of DVT who have documented antiphospholipid antibodies or who have two or more thrombophilic conditions (e.g., combined factor V Leiden and prothrombin 20210A gene mutations), we recommend indefinite anticoagulant therapy in these patients (grade 2C).

Underlying values and preferences. This recommendation ascribes a relatively high value to preventing recurrent thromboembolic events and a relatively low value to bleeding and cost.

- For patients with a first episode of DVT who have documented deficiency of antithrombin, protein C or protein S, or the factor V Leiden or prothrombin 20210A gene mutation, hyperhomocysteinaemia, or high factor VIII levels (>90th percentile of normal), we recommend treatment for 6 to 12 months (grade 1A). We suggest indefinite therapy for patients with idiopathic thrombosis (grade 2C).

Table 19.4 Long-term treatment of acute pulmonary embolism (PE) in thrombophilic patients according to the ACCP recommendations and suggestions [65]

- For patients with PE and cancer, we recommend LMWH for the first 3 to 6 months of long-term anticoagulant therapy (grade 1A). These patients should then receive anticoagulant therapy indefinitely or until the cancer is resolved (grade 1C).
- For patients with a first episode of PE who have documented antiphospholipid antibodies or who have two or more thrombophilic conditions (e.g., combined factor V Leiden and prothrombin 20210A gene mutations), we recommend treatment for 12 months (grade 1C+). For these patients, we also suggest indefinite anticoagulant therapy (grade 2C).

Underlying values and preferences. This recommendation ascribes a relatively high value to preventing recurrent thromboembolic events and a relatively low value to bleeding and cost.

- For patients with a first episode of PE who have documented deficiency of antithrombin, deficiency of protein C or protein S, or the factor V Leiden or prothrombin 20210A gene mutation, hyperhomocysteinaemia, or high factor VIII levels (>90th percentile of normal), we recommend treatment for 6 to 12 months (grade 1A). We suggest indefinite therapy for patients with idiopathic PE (grade 2C).

OTHER ACQUIRED THROMBOPHILIAS

As mentioned above, several other causes of acquired thrombophilia have been identified, including the use of oral contraceptives and HRT, pregnancy, myeloproliferative syndromes, paroxysmal nocturnal haemoglobinuria, acute promyelocytic leukaemia, Behcet disease, and iatrogenic thrombosis induced by some drugs, such as heparin-induced thrombocytopaenia, the administration of thalidomide combined with corticosteroids in multiple myeloma, HIV infection, etc. [77]

Myeloproliferative syndromes

Myeloproliferative disorders are divided into three clinical groups: idiopathic myelofibrosis, myelogenous leukaemia and thrombocytaemia. They feature a variable predisposition to thrombosis, especially in the portal system, which requires an anticoagulant treatment, the duration of which varies according to different clinical conditions [78, 79].

A particular condition is erythromelalgia in patients with thrombocytaemia, which seems to be associated with particularly high platelet counts and usually responds favourably to aspirin. Treatment of the underlying disease is essential, and must take into account the malignant transformation, which is one major risk of cytoreductive therapy [80]. The efficacy and safety of low-dose aspirin in the prevention of thrombotic complications in patients with essential thrombocytaemia has been evaluated, and it has been demonstrated that this treatment is well tolerated. Its efficacy should now be investigated in a larger trial [81].

In a recent work, hydroxyurea was compared with anagrelide in patients with high-risk essential thrombocytaemia. Patients received low-dose aspirin plus either anagrelide or hydroxyurea. Anagrelide plus aspirin was found to be less effective than anagrelide + hydroxyurea, although an equivalent long-term control of the platelet counts was achieved in both groups [82]. Patients at high risk are those with a platelet count higher than $1.5 \times 10^9/\mu l$ associated with a history of major arterial thrombosis or the presence of vascular thrombosis.

In pregnant women, essential thrombocytaemia increases the risk of thromboembolic complications. A first trimester abortion is relatively frequent [83].

In acute promyelocytic leukaemia, prevention of thrombohaemorrhagic complications by heparin has been widely used, but with inconsistent results. The adoption of all-trans-retinoic acid (ATRA) as a routine treatment has transformed the thrombohaemorrhagic pattern of the disease, with a rapid correction of coagulation and fibrinolytic abnormalities. However, anecdotal reports of arterial or venous thrombosis during ATRA treatment have been published [83–85]. Thus, more recent work envisages the potential usefulness of heparin prophylactic treatment to reduced an otherwise increased thrombotic risk.

Paroxysmal nocturnal haemoglobinuria (PNH)

In patients with PNH, venous thrombosis at unusual sites (cerebral, mesenteric, renal etc.) is a common complication [86]. Prophylactic anticoagulant treatment should be considered in all patients with PNH [86], and is part of the supportive treatment. An increased severity of the disease is observed during pregnancy, and prophylactic treatment with LMWH seems appropriate [87].

PREGNANCY

Pregnancy is an important risk factor of venous thrombosis [88, 89]. Thus, an antithrombotic treatment may be required for prevention or treatment of thrombosis in pregnant women at risk of thrombosis (history of venous thrombosis and/or thrombophilia). Antithrombotic therapy has also been proposed for the prevention of thrombosis and of some complications of pregnancy, such as fetal loss, intra-uterine growth retardation, pre-eclampsia, and abruption [90].

ANTITHROMBOTIC DRUGS AND PREGNANCY

Vitamin K antagonists (VKA) cross the placenta and may be responsible for embryopathy (nasal hypoplasia and/or stippled epiphyses) when used between 6 and 12 weeks of gestation, as well as for fetal haemorrhages [89, 90]. It has been suggested that the risk of embryopathy is dose-dependent, and higher when warfarin is administered at doses above 5 mg/day [91]. VKA are in any case to be avoided between the 6th and 12th week of gestation to prevent embryopathy, but also after the 36th week to prevent excessive bleeding to the mother and the foetus in the peripartum time. They are less and less used during pregnancy, except in women with prosthetic heart valves. Warfarin may be administered to breast-feeding mothers.

Unfractionated heparin (UFH) has for a long time been considered the anticoagulant of choice during pregnancy because it does not cross the placenta. However, UFH may induce allergy, heparin-induced thrombocytopaenia, and also a decrease in antithrombin or osteoporosis when administered for a long time.

Low-molecular-weight heparins are now the most commonly used anticoagulants during pregnancy because they do not cross the placenta and have fewer side-effects than UFH, in particular, less osteoporosis and less thrombocytopaenia [90, 92]. In addition, they have the advantage of an easier administration: one injection per day for prevention, two injections per day for treatment, meaning more comfort for the patient and frequent self-administration. The safety of LMWH has been considered as satisfactory in two studies including 486 and 624 women, respectively, who received various LMWHs or enoxaparin only during pregnancy [93, 94]. Enoxaparin, dalteparin and nadroparin have been the most commonly used LMWHs during pregnancy. Tinzaparin has been administered in small series but there is some concern about the risk of osteoporosis with this LMWH [95].

A heparinoid, danaparoid sodium (Orgaran®), has been administered during pregnancy in some women with history of heparin-induced thrombocytopaenia, apparently with no recurrence of thrombosis or bleeding events [96].

Pentasaccharide, a new antithrombotic drug, does not induce thrombocytopaenia. No placental transfer was found in the dually perfused human cotyledon *in vitro* [97]. This supports further evaluation in pregnant women.

Hirudin, a direct thrombin inhibitor, crosses the placenta, and should not be used during pregnancy. Ximelagatran, a prodrug of an active site-directed thrombin inhibitor, melagatran, has not been evaluated during pregnancy.

Thrombolytic treatments have been administered to pregnant women with life-threatening thrombosis, but the experience is limited. The risk of major bleeding is high when the treatment is used close to delivery.

Aspirin, given at low doses (<150 mg/day) during the 2nd and 3rd trimesters of pregnancy in women at risk of pregnancy-induced hypertension or intra-uterine growth retardation, is safe for the mother and the foetus. The safety of higher doses or administration during the 1st trimester of pregnancy is currently uncertain [90]. An increased risk of miscarriage has recently been suspected [98].

TREATMENT OF AN ACUTE EPISODE OF VTE IN PREGNANT WOMEN

When a pregnant woman has symptoms of VTE, it is important to have an objective diagnosis. Indeed such a diagnosis will influence future pregnancies, contraception and, later, any decision for HRT. In the ACCP guidelines, the level of evidence for the treatment during pregnancy is 1C+, meaning that the risk/benefit ratio is evident even though there are no randomised clinical trials in this condition [90].

In women with pulmonary embolism or deep vein thrombosis, therapeutic doses of UFH are administered as intravenous infusion (bolus of 5000 IU followed by 1000–2000 IU/hour) for 5 days, followed by LMWH by subcutaneous route (dalteparin 100 IU or enoxaparin 1 mg/kg body weight twice-daily) and continued throughout pregnancy [90]. The dose is calculated on body weight, and it could be the basal body weight or the body weight at the time of thrombosis. The early pregnancy weight has been proposed because LMWH does not cross the placenta, so that foeto-placental weight is not relevant and anti-Xa levels were not reported to differ when pregnancy progresses [92]. As the half-life of LMWH is shorter in pregnancy, twice-daily dosing is preferable, at least in the initial treatment period [90].

In pregnant women with calf vein thrombosis, although there is no clear recommendation, LMWH is usually the only treatment, without previous administration of UFH. Although no laboratory monitoring is required in non-pregnant women, it can be proposed to measure anti-Xa plasma level 3 to 4 hours after injection, at the beginning of the treatment and about once a month. The target anti-Xa level is 0.5 to 1.2 U/ml. This therapeutic range may vary with the LMWH used. Platelet count is also required for the first three weeks and once a month until delivery.

The same degree of hypocoagulability is maintained during the rest of pregnancy according to ACCP recommendations [90]. However, it may be modulated depending on the type of thrombotic episode (calf or proximal deep vein thrombosis and/or pulmonary embolism) and the moment when thrombosis occurs (1st, 2nd or 3rd trimester). In some cases, after 3 months of full therapeutic dose, the dose is reduced to a high prophylactic dose (once-a-day 60 mg enoxaparin, for instance).

In women with antithrombin deficiency, antithrombin concentrates may be recommended together with UFH or LMWH during the acute phase of thrombosis at sufficient doses to obtain a plasma level above 80% (starting at 30 to 50 U/kg body weight and repeating injections once a day) [99, 100].

When the woman is in labour, LMWH injections are discontinued: a delay of more than 24 hours is generally required to allow epidural anaesthesia. If induction of labour is planned, LMWH is discontinued the day before and epidural anaesthesia is possible.

After delivery (6 to 8 hours later), the treatment is restarted with LMWH, followed by VKA started 3–5 days after delivery and continued for at least 3 months. Elastic compression stockings are recommended.

In women at risk of bleeding, LMWH may be replaced by intravenous infusion of UFH because UFH is associated with a more stable hypocoagulability and avoids peak levels of anticoagulation. The short duration of action of UFH is more convenient if the treatment needs to be interrupted because a bleeding occurs.

PROPHYLAXIS OF VTE DURING PREGNANCY

Recommendations for prevention published by the American College of Chest Physicians [90] and by the French ANAES (Agence Nationale d'Accréditation et d'Evaluation en Santé) [101] are all of low grade of evidence, with risk/benefit ratio not evident, and based only on observational studies. This means that these recommendations may change in the near future, when new information becomes available, although randomised studies are very difficult in pregnancy [102]. Because of the lack of evidence-based recommendations, the prophylaxis is often decided on an individual basis. As compared with the ACCP recommendations published in 2001, repeated screening with non-invasive tests for deep vein thrombosis, such as compression ultrasonography, is no longer justified. The higher risk of AT-deficient women is now recognised, and elastic compression stockings are recommended ante- and post-partum in all women with a history of deep vein thrombosis [90].

PATIENTS WITH HISTORY OF VTE AND/OR CONGENITAL THROMBOPHILIA

BEFORE PREGNANCY

Pre-pregnancy counselling is important. Patients must be informed of the risk of VTE related to pregnancy, which depends on the personal history of VTE and the presence of thrombophilia. Special attention should be given to AT-deficient women, because the risk of thrombosis is high and thrombosis may occur in the very first weeks of pregnancy in women with a personal history of thrombosis. These women must know that they should contact their gynaecologist and a specialised haematologist as soon as the pregnancy test is positive. This also applies to women who are on VKA when they become pregnant, since a rapid replacement of VKA by subcutaneous heparin is mandatory.

When patients have a history of VTE before pregnancy, the advice of an angiologist or a vascular physician is important to evaluate the possible sequelae, the need for a compression ultrasound that could serve as a reference, and to judge the opportunity of elastic stockings.

DURING PREGNANCY

The prophylaxis is often decided on an individual basis after a multidisciplinary evaluation of the patient's risk, depending on different risk factors, such as the presence of thrombophilia and its type, a history of thrombosis before pregnancy, age of the mother, immobilisation during pregnancy, twin pregnancy. Different grades of prophylaxis using LMWH (enoxaparin in mg or dalteparin in units) have been proposed in ACCP guidelines:

- LMWH prophylactic dose: 40 mg or 5000 U once daily.
- LMWH intermediate dose: 40 mg or 5000 U twice daily.
- LMWH adapted dose: therapeutic dose adapted on body weight, twice daily (1 mg/kg or 100 U/kg) or once daily after the initial phase of treatment (200 mg or tinzaparin 175 U/kg).
- Anticoagulants during post-partum: warfarin for 4 to 6 weeks with a target INR of 2.5, or UFH or LMWH followed by warfarin with an overlap until the INR is >2, or LMWH without switching to warfarin.

The term 'surveillance' corresponds to a clinical vigilance and aggressive investigation of women with symptoms suspicious of DVT or PE.

Women with history of VTE but no known thrombophilia

When the previous thrombosis was associated with a transient risk factor that is no longer present, no prophylactic treatment, but clinical surveillance, is recommended during pregnancy in ACCP recommendations (grade 1C) [90]. This is based on one small-sized study [103]. In another study, a high risk of recurrence was found in pregnant women with history of VTE, although the first episode was frequently associated with a temporary risk factor such as oral contraception, pregnancy, stillbirth, surgery, trauma, bed rest [104]. Antenatal prophylaxis was suggested when the previous thrombosis was pregnancy- orestrogen-related or when additional risk factors are present, such as obesity [90]. We tend to propose prophylaxis during the 3rd trimester of pregnancy in all women who had previous DVT or PE and no known thrombophilia.

Women with inherited thrombophilia

Women with inherited thrombophilia have an increased risk of thrombosis during pregnancy and post-partum, but the magnitude of the risk is not similar [104–109]. Three levels of risk have been differentiated:

- High risk: heterozygous AT deficiency (except type II HBS), homozygous (PC) or PS deficiency.
- Intermediate risk: heterozygous PC deficiency, homozygous factor V Leiden or factor II 20210A, combined heterozygous factor V Leiden and factor II 20210A.
- Moderate risk: heterozygous factor V Leiden or factor II 20210A mutations, heterozygous PS deficiency, heterozygous type II heparin binding site AT deficiency.

The following guidelines result from the ACCP recommendations and from the prophylactic treatments presently evaluated in our group.

In women without thrombosis before pregnancy, if they are:

- at high risk: a prophylaxis is recommended throughout pregnancy. The dose is not well-defined, but a moderate dose is generally administered (enoxaparin 40 to 60 mg, which is equivalent to 4000 to 6000 units, or dalteparin 5000 units once-a-day), with the usual control of platelet count during the first 3 weeks of treatment followed by a once-a-month control. Measurement of coagulation activation markers is not required, unless it is part of a prospective protocol of surveillance.

  Anti-Xa activity may be checked once a month 3 to 4 hours after injection, and a level close to 0.3 U/ml seems appropriate.

  When labour starts, the woman should be advised to stop injections to allow epidural anaesthesia if the delay is long enough (more than 12 hours after last injection). If induction of labour is planned, the prophylaxis is stopped the day before delivery.
- at intermediate risk: a prophylaxis is recommended during part or throughout pregnancy depending on the associated risk factors. The dose of LMWH is 40 mg or 5000 U per day and the monitoring is the same as in higher risk.
- at moderate risk: clinical surveillance only may be recommended unless risk factors are present during pregnancy (such as bed rest).

In women with history of thrombosis before pregnancy without anticoagulant treatment when pregnancy starts, if they are:

- at high risk: LMWH (enoxaparin 40 to 60 mg or dalteparin 5000 U) is administered throughout pregnancy every 12 hour, adjusted to target an anti-Xa level of 0.2 to 0.6 U/ml 3 to 4 hours after injection.

  In AT-deficient women, it is important to start the prophylaxis very rapidly as soon as the pregnancy is diagnosed. AT concentrates at doses of 30 to 50 U/kg body weight are recommended the morning of delivery and for 2 days after.
- at intermediate risk: LMWH (enoxaparin 40 mg or dalteparin 5000 U) is administered daily throughout or during part of pregnancy.
- at moderate risk: LMWH (enoxaparin 40 mg or dalteparin 5000 U) is administered daily during part of pregnancy (2nd and/or 3rd trimester only).

In women with history of thrombosis before pregnancy on long-term VKA when pregnancy starts:

- Since there is a risk of embryopathy between 6 and 12 weeks of gestation, and assuming there is no risk before the 6th week, women are counselled to perform a pregnancy test as soon as possible. If the test is positive, heparin is substituted to VKA.

Weight-adjusted therapeutic dose of LMWH is generally recommended (target peak anti-Xa below 1 U/ml).

Replacement of VKA by heparin had been proposed before conception, but the duration of exposure to heparin was prolonged and the risk of osteoporosis was consequently increased: this option is now abandoned.

POST-PARTUM PERIOD

There is a consensus for prophylaxis during the post-partum period. A prophylaxis is administered for 6 weeks or longer, depending on the long-term strategy defined for the patient. LMWH (enoxaparin 40 mg or dalteparin 5000 U daily) or VKA, aiming at a target INR of 2.5, are proposed, in association with elastic stockings.

In women not on long-term VKA before pregnancy, LMWH may be more convenient because VKA requires monitoring and repeated blood sampling.

Breast-feeding is compatible with LMWH and with warfarin treatments.

Oral contraception with combined oestrogen–progestins is contraindicated, but progestin-only contraception can be proposed [110].

WOMEN WITH MECHANICAL HEART VALVES

Women with mechanical heart valves are at high risk of valve thrombosis during pregnancy. The risk of embryopathy with VKA administered between the 6th and the 12th week of pregnancy has to be balanced with the risk of valve thrombosis in the mother. Different options have been proposed: replacement of VKA, as soon as pregnancy starts, by LMWH twice-daily at a dose to obtain an anti-Xa level of 1.0 to 1.2 U 4 hours after injection, or UFH at a dose to obtain an activated partial thromboplastin time (aPTT) twice the control between two injections, or VKA during the 2nd trimester and UFH or LMWH for the 1st and 3rd trimester [90]. For cardiologists, the use of vitamin K antagonists is the most efficacious treatment for the mother and there is an agreement to their use during the 2nd and 3rd trimesters [111]. In women at high risk, the addition of low doses of aspirin is recommended.

The risk of thrombosis in these women is difficult to evaluate because the dose of UFH used in older studies might have been too low to prevent thrombosis and the materials used for prosthetic valves have changed and are now less thrombogenic. In addition, the risk related to valves on a mitral position is higher than in the aortic position, as shown in a recent study where LMWH at appropriate doses was a suitable option and no thrombotic complication was observed in women who had a prosthetic aortic valve [112].

WOMEN WITH PREGNANCY COMPLICATIONS

Women with APL syndrome have a well-demonstrated high risk of thrombosis and miscarriage, but the optimal treatment is still debated. Fetal outcome is improved by the administration of aspirin in combination with heparin (low-dose UFH or prophylactic LMWH) during pregnancy [90, 113]. LMWH at adjusted dose is recommended for women with APL syndrome and previous thrombosis. Different clinical and biological criteria are required for the diagnosis of APL syndrome but one may wonder whether a woman with both lupus anticoagulant and APL antibodies has a similar risk of thrombosis and miscarriage as a woman with APL antibodies only.

An association between inherited thrombophilia and late pregnancy complications has been suggested [114–116], and several studies indicate LMWH may be beneficial, especially after the 10th week of pregnancy [117]. However, the requirement of antithrombotic therapy may still be questioned and randomised trials are needed.

RENAL DISEASES

Three main conditions, glomerulonephritis, thrombotic thrombocytopaenic purpura and nephrotic syndrome are associated with a risk of thrombosis [118]. They are reviewed here along with other renal conditions involving a risk for thrombosis.

GLOMERULONEPHRITIS

Glomerular fibrin deposition is an important feature of glomerulonephritis. In patients with systemic lupus erythematosus (SLE), glomerular capillary thrombi have been observed. The mechanism of hypercoagulation in SLE is still obscure, although several hypotheses have been formulated.

The most recent haemostatic alteration described in these patients is an increase in D-Dimer, an indicator of an increased fibrin breakdown [119]. Increased platelet function may play a role in the progression of renal disease in glomerulonephritis, although antiplatelet drugs were not found to be efficacious [120].

Defibrination with Arvin or Ancrod (extracted from a snake venom) was used about 20 years ago with some success in patients with rapidly progressing glomerulonephritis [121].

UFH and LMWH are not clinically beneficial.

THROMBOTIC THOMBOCYTOPAENIC PURPURA (TTP) AND HAEMOLYTIC URAEMIC SYNDROME (HUS)

Acute renal failure, microangiopathic haemolytic uraemia and thrombocytopaenia are constant clinical symptoms of TTP, which was first observed by Moschowitz.

In HUS, the clinical symptoms are similar, and fever is present in both. The main difference in these two syndromes is the frequent presence of neurologic symptoms in TTP and a severe renal failure in HUS [122]. Interestingly, in TTP intravascular hyperfunctioning of platelets has just received an explanation for its mechanism [123]. Alterations of the depolymerisation of the multimeric von Willebrand factor molecule are responsible for an important increase in platelet aggregation, a causal relation to thrombocytopaenia and the ischaemic lesions, constituted of widespread hyaline thrombi composed mainly of platelets. These thrombi are present in arteries and capillaries of several organs, in contrast to the fibrin-rich thrombi observed in disseminated intravascular coagulation (DIC).

More recently, the presence of unusually large polymers of von Willebrand factor has been discovered in TTP. The most likely cause is an acquired autoimmune deficiency of a plasma metallo-protease, ADAMTS 13 or caspase, which is responsible for many cases of TTP [124, 125].

Rare cases of congenital deficiency in ADAMTS 13 have been reported. Several subtypes of TTP have been described [122], and several degrees of severity of TTP exist among patients suffering from the disease.

Routine laboratory testing is not usually available, and the conventional method requires time and expertise to be performed. The measurement of ADAMTS 13 in plasma can be helpful in diagnosis and in monitoring the efficacy of treatment when genetic alteration of ADAMTS 13 may be identified.

Idiopathic TTP has a better prognosis since the use of plasma transfusion and plasma exchange. Remission is obtained in about 80% of patients. Precise diagnosis and immediate treatment are essential in increasing the rate of remissions.

In contrast to idiopathic TTP, forms associated with cancer, infections and certain drugs are associated with a worse prognosis. The support of an intensive care unit (ICU) is frequently required [126].

In a recent study, a high mortality (35%) in a cohort of 63 patients with thrombotic microangiopathies with severe organ dysfunctions leading to hospitalisation in ICU has been reported. Neurologic impairment appears to be the main adverse prognostic factor correlated with mortality [127, 128]. The benefit obtained with plasma exchange does not always correlate with the presence of a severe deficiency in ADAMTS 13. Thus, the absence of ADAMTS 13 severe deficiency should not be used as a basis for withholding exchange treatment [127]. Moreover, a severe decrease in ADAMTS 13 activity was far from being constant in TTP–HUS in this series of patients.

Management of HUS requires meticulous fluid, electrolyte and hypertension control, while plasma exchange has no clear proven benefit. Supportive haemodialysis can be indicated in both TTP and HUS, but platelet transfusions are contraindicated.

In conclusion, although plasma exchange treatment has greatly improved the outcome of TTP, more work is needed for a better classification of the different clinical forms of TTP and to further increase the efficacy of treatment in TTP-HUS.

RENAL TRANSPLANTATION

Alteration of blood coagulation, platelets and fibrinolysis are observed after kidney transplantation. Some, but not all, of these haemostatic changes are due to the use of immunosuppressive drugs [129]. Moreover, in cases of acute or chronic allograft rejection, fibrin deposition in the transplanted kidney is observed.

One of the mechanisms of thrombotic events can be of immunological origin, being responsible for damage to the vascular endothelium.

Patients undergoing renal transplantation are at a higher risk of postoperative deep vein thrombosis [130]. They are also at higher risk of acute MI.

RENAL DISEASES AND EXAGGERATED RESPONSE TO LMWH

Since LMWHs have an almost exclusive renal clearance, accumulation of the drug in patients with severe renal insufficiency might be responsible for an increased risk of bleeding. Several health authorities have contraindicated the use of LMWH when the Cockroft index (calculated creatinine clearance) is <30 ml/min [131]. There is some dispute, however, among specialists, since it might be preferable to decrease the dose of LMWH and/or to monitor anti-Xa activity and to adjust the dose in order to prevent an unusual response to the drug by the patient. Moreover, it has been advocated that tinzaparin, which has a clearance closer to that of UFH than to the other LMWHs, can be used in patients with renal insufficiency [132].

In summary, the use of subcutaneous UFH might be better tolerated, but is less convenient in patients with renal insufficiency than that of LMWH. This topic has been recently reviewed in the ACCP conference [131].

NEPHROTIC SYNDROME

Both arterial and venous complications attributed to a hypercoagulable state are a common complication of the nephrotic syndrome. A most feared complication is renal vein thrombosis (RVT), the prevalence of which can be as high as 22%, as observed in a large prospective study [133]. A multifactorial mechanism is involved: hypercoagulability due to protein loss in the urine, an increase in factor VIII and in platelet function are the most common blood alterations.

Deep vein thrombosis of the lower extremities occurs in up to 15%, and can be associated with RVT. DVT can extend to the inferior vena cava; symptomatic PE is observed in 10 to 20% of patients with nephrotic syndrome [133–135].

Acquired deficiency in AT through the loss of proteins in urine is considered an important cause of VTE. In some studies, hypoalbuminuria and AT deficiency have been found to be associated in patients with VTE, but this is not a constant finding. Moreover, severe prothrombotic alteration of haemostasis and fibrinolysis has been observed in these patients.

Finally, although VTE is a common complication in patients with nephrotic syndrome, arterial thrombosis (femoral, mesenteric, brachial, cerebral and at other sites), the aetiology of which is still obscure, occurs in a small number of patients [132].

Antithrombotic therapy includes treatment and prevention of DVT, PE, renal vein thrombosis, arterial thrombosis and any thrombotic event [135–137].

The nephrologist plays a major role in the treatment of patients with nephrotic syndrome, while the haematologist's intervention can be helpful in some situations and in the monitoring of the anticoagulant treatment.

RENAL VEIN THROMBOSIS

Renal vein thrombosis (RVT) is a well-known complication of nephrotic syndrome [138], but has been encountered in rare patients with thrombophilia and without nephrotic syndrome [139, 140]. Thrombectomy and fibrinolysis have been used, but the first-line treatment is heparin and VKA, the latters being found to be effective in secondary but also in primary prevention.

Treatment with UFH should be rigorously monitored, especially because the associated AT deficiency may reduce the response to treatment. However, infusions of AT concentrates are rarely required [133]. LMWH have been used, but the risk of drug accumulation due to renal insufficiency should be considered.

In patients with RVT, long-term prophylactic treatment seems indicated, although no large randomised trial has been performed. A favourable benefit/risk ratio of prolonged VKA treatment in patients with a prior history of VTE is not established. Prophylaxis seems justified in patients with membranous glomerulopathy who are at a higher risk of VTE [141, 142]. Thus, the decision has to be made case by case in the absence of clear recommendations or suggestions by the healthcare authorities.

VASCULAR ACCESS THROMBOSIS

Prevention of vascular access thrombosis is important for maintaining successful haemodialysis.

A thrombosed dialysis access often requires rescue procedures to extend the life of the graft. In a recent work, age, gender and homocysteine level were not correlated with the incidence of vascular access thrombosis [143]. No specific prophylactic treatment has been recommended.

In contrast, graft declotting mechanisms have been discussed, and thrombectomy has been compared with thrombolysis. However, no individual declotting modality has proven itself superior to standard anticoagulant treatments [144].

SUMMARY

A moderate increase in the risk of VTE has been documented in diabetic patients. A very high risk for accelerated atherosclerosis and arterial thrombosis (atherothrombosis) is well recognised. Secondary prevention is commonly used in diabetic patients. Primary prevention seems appropriate and is recommended in diabetic patients who are at higher risk of coronary accidents, stroke and peripheral arterial disease, but is not currently used. Familial thrombophilias have been extensively investigated and three levels of risk have been proposed according to the variety of thrombophilias. However, the heterogeneity of the clinical presentation is a limitation to the observation of recommendations and suggestions presented at consensus conferences.

Several acquired thrombophilias have been well identified. An appropriate treatment is available, and should be strongly considered in patients at high risk.

The clinical management is more difficult than in congenital thrombophilias because of the lack of large studies in most conditions. Moreover, the duration of anticoagulant treatment is usually determined case-by-case, on the basis of individualised considerations.

LMWH is the anticoagulant of choice during pregnancy. Recommendations are clear for the treatment of an acute episode of thrombosis, even though some details remain to be clarified concerning the duration of full-dose treatment. More data are needed for patients with mechanical heart valves and women with history of pregnancy complications. A prophylaxis may be required during pregnancy and post-partum in women with the antiphospholipid antibody syndrome, history of venous thrombosis and/or thrombophilia. A combination of aspirin and LMWH is administered in women with the antiphospholipid antibody syndrome. There is a consensus concerning the administration of a prophylaxis during pregnancy in women with AT deficiency or combined thrombophilias and in the 6 weeks post-partum in all women with a congenital deficiency in AT, PC, PS or a factor V Leiden or a prothrombin G20210A mutation and/or previous VTE. Information is missing concerning the prophylaxis during pregnancy in other thrombophilias with or without previous thrombosis, the dose of anticoagulant to be administered and its duration-throughout or during part of the pregnancy.

At present, the decisions concerning prophylaxis are often taken on an individual basis, taking into account the thrombophilia and the other associated risk factors of thrombosis during pregnancy. A score might be useful in this respect.

Renal diseases are associated with a high risk of thrombosis which requires specific treatment according to the condition considered: glomerulonephritis, thrombotic thrombocytopaenic purpura and haemolytic uraemic syndrome, renal transplantation, nephrotic syndrome, RVT and vascular access thrombosis. Last, but not least, the potential exaggerated response of LMWH in kidney insufficiency is a matter of concern that is attracting more and more attention.

REFERENCES

1. Moreno PR, Fuster V. New aspects in the pathogenesis of diabetic atherothrombosis. *J Am Coll Cardiol* 2004; 44:2293–2300.
2. Prandoni P, Marchiori A, Bernardi E *et al*. An association between atherosclerosis and venous thrombosis. *N Engl J Med* 2003; 348:1435–1441.
3. Jones EW, Mitchell JRA. Venous thrombosis in diabetes mellitus. *Diabetologica* 1983; 25:502–505.
4. Bergqvst D, Arnadottir M, Bergentz SE *et al*. Juvenile diabetes mellitus a risk factor for postoperative venous thromboembolism? *Acta Med Scand* 1985; 217:307–308.
5. Samama MM, Dahl OE, Quinlan DJ, Mismetti P, Rosencher N. Quantification of risk factors for venous thromboembolism: a preliminary study for the development of a risk assessment tool. *Haematologica* 2003; 88:1410–1421.
6. Petrauskiene V, Falk M, Waernbaum I, Norberg M, Eriksson JW. The risk of venous thromboembolism is markedly elevated in patients with diabetes. *Diabetologica* 2005; 48:1017–1021.
7. Samama MM, Cohen AT, Darmon JY *et al*. For the prophylaxis in medical patients with enoxaparin study group. A comparison of enoxaparin with placebo for the prevention of venous thromboembolism in acutely ill medical patient. *N Engl J Med* 1999; 341:793–800.

8. Geerts WH, Pineo GF, Heit JA *et al.* Prevention of venous thromboembolism: the seventh ACCP Conference on Antithrombolytic Therapy. *Chest* 2004; 126(suppl 3):338S–400S.

9. Sobel BE, Schneider DJ. Cardiovascular complications in diabetes mellitus. *Current opinion in Pharmacology* 2005; 5:143–148.

10. Andreotti F, Becker RC. Atherothrombotic disorders, new insights from Hematology. *Circulation* 2005; 111:1855–1863.

11. Burzotta F, Paciaroni K, De Stefano V *et al.* G20210A prothrombin gene polymorphism and coronary ischaemic syndromes: a phenotype specific meta-analysis of 12034 subjects. *Heart* 2004; 90:82–86.

12. Conard J, Samama MM. Inhibitors of coagulation, atherosclerosis and arterial thrombosis. *Semin Thromb Hemost* 1986; 12:87–90.

13. Wall RT, Harlan JM, Harker LA, Stricker GE. Homocysteine-induced endothelial cell injury in vitro: a model for the study of vascular injury. *Thromb Res* 1980; 18:113–121.

14. De Luis D, Fernandez N, Aller R. Homocysteine in patients with diabetes mellitus. *Med Clin (Barc)* 2004; 122:27–32.

15. Verhaege R, de Moerloose P, Eikenboom JC *et al.* Genetic and acquired risk factors of venous thromboembolism 2003; 27:1–14.

16. Cattaneo M. Hyperhomocysteinemia and thrombosis. *Lipids* 2001; 36(suppl):S13–S26.

17. Sobel BE, Schneider DJ. Pletelet function, coagulopathy, and impaired fibrinolysis in diabetes. *Cardiol Clin* 2004; 22:511–526.

18. Johnstone MT, Veves A (eds). *Diabetes and cardiovascular disease*. Humana Press, Totowa, NJ, 2001, p 458.

19. Park YW, Zhu S, Palaniappan L, Heshka S, Carnethon MR, Heymsfiels SB. The metabolic syndrome: prevalence and associated risk factor findings in the US population from the Third National Health and Nutrition Examination Survey, 1988–1994. *Arch Int Med* 2003; 163:427–436.

20. Haffner S, Taegtmeyer H. Epidemic obesity and the metabolic syndrome? *Circulation* 2003; 108:1541–1545.

21. Tenenbaum A, Motro M, Fisman EZ, Tanne D, Boyko V, Behar S. Bezafibrate for the secondary prevention of myocardial infarction in patients with metabolic syndrome. *Arch Int Med* 2005; 165:1154–1160.

22. Current Treatment Options for the Metabolic Syndrome. *Curr Treat Options Cardiovasc Med* 2005; 7:61–74.

23. Knowler WC, Hamman RF, Edelstein SL *et al.* Prevention of type 2 diabetes with troglitazone in the diabetes prevention program. *Diabetes* 2005; 54:1150–1156.

24. Hovens MM, Tamsma JT, Beishuizen ED, Huisman MV. Pharamacological strategies to reduce cardiovascular risk in type 2 diabetes mellitus: an update. *Drugs* 2005; 65:433–445.

25. The DAMAD Study Group. Effect of aspirin alone and aspirin plus dipyridamole in early diabetic retinopathy. A multicenter randomised controlled clinical trial. *Diabetes* 1989; 38:491–498.

26. The TIMAD Study Group. Ticlopidine treatment reduces the progression of nonproliferative diabetic retinopathy. *Arch Ophtalmol* 1990; 108:1577–1583.

27. Evangelista V, Totani L, Rotondo S *et al.* Prevention of cardiovascular disease in type-2 diabetes: how to improve the clinical efficacy of aspirin. *Thromb Haemost* 2005; 93:8–16.

28. Bruno A, Grassi G, Dani F, Degiovanni M, Maghenzani G, Pagano G. Use of antiplatelet therapy in a diabetic outpatient service of a large urban public hospital. *Nutr Metab Cardiovasc Dis* 2005; 15:42–46.

29. Nguyen KX, Marinac JS, Sun C. Aspirin for primary prevention in patients with diabetes mellitus. *Fam Med* 2005; 37:112–117.

30. Girolami A, Simioni P, Scarano L, Girolami B. Venous and arterial thrombophilia. *Haematologica* 1997; 82:96–100.

31. Virchow R. Phlogose und thrombose in Gefäßsystem. In: Virchow R (ed.). *Gesammelte Abhandlugen zur Wissenschaftlichen Medicin*. von Meidinger Sohn, Frankfurt, 1856, p 458.

32. Conard J. Thrombophilia: diagnosis and management. In: Poller L, Thomson JM (eds). *Thrombosis and its management*. Churchill Livingstone, Edinburgh, 1993, p 113a.

33. Comp PC. Congenital and acquired hypercoagulable states. In: Hull R, Pineo GF (eds). *Disorders of Thrombosis*. WB Saunders Company, Philadelphia, 1996, pp 339–347.

34. Seghatchian MJ, Samama MM. Hypercoagulable states: an overview. In: Seghatchian MJ, Samama MM, Hecker SP (eds). *Hypergoagulable States*. CRC Press, Boca-Raton, 1996, pp 2–17.

35. Lane DA, Mannucci PM, Bauer KA *et al.* Inherited thrombophilia: Part 1. *Thromb Haemost* 1996; 76:651–662.

36. Lane DA, Mannucci PM, Bauer KA et al. Inherited thrombophilia: Part 2. *Thromb Haemost* 1997; 77:1047.

37. Mannucci PM. Aspects of the clinical management of hereditary thrombophilia: a personal perspective. *Haemostasis* 2000; 30:11–15.

38. Seligsohn U, Lubetsky A. Genetic susceptibility to venous thrombosis. *N Engl J Med* 2001; 344:1222–1231.

39. Franco RF, Reitsma PH. Genetic risk factors of venous thrombosis. *Hum Genet* 2001; 109:36–84.

40. Arnout J, Jankowski M. Antiphospholipid antibodies: prothrombotic antiphospholipid and laboratory diagnosis (Chap 21) In: Arnout J, Gaetano G, Hoylaerts M et al. (eds). *Thrombosis Fundamental and Clinical Aspects*. Leuven University Press, 2003, pp 371–392.

41. Trousseau A. *Phlegmasia Alba Dolens: Lectures on Clinical Medicine*. The new Sydenham Society, London, England, 1868, 5, pp 281–331.

42. Andoh D, Kubota T, Takada M et al. Tissue factor activity in leukemia cells. Special reference to disseminated intravascular coagulation. *Cancer* 1987; 59:748–754.

43. Falanga A, Gordon SG. Isolation and characterization of cancer procoagulant: a cysteine proteinase from malignant tissue. *Biochemistry* 1985; 24:5558–5567.

44. Lugassy G, Falanga A, Kakkar AK, Rickles FR (eds). *Thrombosis and Cancer*. Martin Dunitz, 2004.

45. Falanga A. Thrombophilia in Cancer. *Thromb Hemost* 2005; 31:104–110.

46. Rickles FR, Levine MN. Epidemiology of thrombosis in cancer. *Acta Haematol* 2001; 106:6–12.

47. Gouin-Thibault I, Achkar A, Samama MM. The thrombophilic state in cancer patients. *Acta Haematol* 2001; 106:33–42.

48. Matei D, Brenner B, Marder VJ. Acquired thrombophilic syndrome. *Blood Reviews* 2001; 15:31–48.

49. Lee AYY, Levine MN. The thrombophilic state induced by therapeutic agents in the cancer patient. *Semin Thromb Hemost* 1999; 25:137–1946.

50. Kearon C. Risk factors for recurrent venous thromboembolism and their implications for treatment. In Hematology 2004 American Society of Antiphospholipid Education program Book; San Diego, California, December 4–7, 2004; 445–455.

51. Geerts WH, Pineo GF, Heit JA et al. Prevention of venous thromboembolism. The Seventh ACCP Conference on Antithrombotic and Thrombolytic Therapy. *Chest* 2004; 126:338S–400S.

52. Gomes MP, Deitcher SR. Risk of venous thromboembolic disease associated with hormonal contraceptives and hormone replacement therapy: a clinical review. *Arch Int Med* 2004; 164:1965–1975.

53. Conard J, Horellou MH, Samama MM. Inherited thrombophilia and gestational venous thrombo-embolism. *Semin Thromb Hemost* 2003; 29:131–142.

54. Vossen CY, Conard J, Fontcuberta J et al. Familial thrombophilia and lifetime risk of venous thrombosis. *J Thromb Haemost* 2004; 2:1526–1532.

55. Baglin T, Luddington R, Brown K, Baglin C. Incidence of recurrent venous thromboembolism in relation to clinical and thrombophilic risk factors: a prospective cohort study. *Lancet* 2003; 362: 523–526.

56. Vossen CY, Conard J, Fontcuberta J et al. Risk of a first venous thrombotic event in carriers of a familial thrombophilic defect. The European Prospective Cohort on Thrombophilia (EPCOT). *J Thromb Haemost* 2004; 3:459–464.

57. Samama MM, Horellou MH, Elalamy I et al. D-dimer levels, constitutional thrombopohilia and venous thrombosis prediction: clinical aspects and implications. *J Thrombos* 2005 (in press).

58. De Stefano V, Leone G, Mastrangelo S et al. Thrombosis during pregnancy and surgery in patients with congenital deficiency of antithrombin III, protein C, protein S. *Thromb Haemost* 1994; 71:799–800.

59. The Procare Group. Comparison of thrombotic risk between 85 homozygotes and 481 heterozygotes carriers of the factor V Leiden mutation: retrospective analysis from the Procare study. *Blood Coagul Fibrinolysis* 2000; 135:1410–1413.

60. Lindahl TL, Lundahl TH, Nilsson L, Andersson CA. APC-resistance is a risk factor for postoperative thromboembolism in elective replacement of the hip or the knee. A prospective study. *Thromb Haemost* 1999; 81:18–21.

61. Ryan DH, Crowther MA, Ginsberg JS, Francis CW. Relation of factor V Leiden genotype to risk for acute deep venous thrombosis after joint replacement surgery. *Ann Intern Med* 1998; 128:270–276.

62. Woolson ST, Zehnder JL, Maloney WJ. Factor V Leiden and the risk of proximal venous thrombosis after total hip arthroplasty. *J Arthroplasty* 1998; 13:207–210.

63. Donaldson MC, Belkin M, Whittemore AD et al. Impact of activated protein C resistance on general vascular surgical patients. *J Vasc Surg* 1997; 25:1054–1060.

64. Tengborn L, Bergqvist D. Surgery in patients with congenital antithrombin III deficiency. *Acta Chir Scand* 1988; 154:179–183.

65. Buller HR, Agenilli G, Hull RD *et al.* Antithrombotic therapy for venous thromboembolic disease. The seventh ACCP Conference on Antithrombotic anf thrombolytic Therapy. *Chest* 2004; 126(suppl 3): 401S–428S.

66. Christiansen SC, Cannegieter SC, Koster T, Vandenbroucke JP, Frits RR. Thrombophilia, clinical factors, and recurrent venous thrombotic events. *JAMA* 2005; 293:2352–2361.

67. Van Den Belt AGM, Hutten BA, Prins MH. Duration of oral anticoagulant treatment in patients with venous thromboembolism and a deficiency of antithrombin, protein C or protein S- A decision analysis. *Thromb Haemost* 2004; 84:758–763.

68. Rosove MH, Brewer PMC. Antiphospholipid thrombosis: clinical course after the first thrombotic event in 70 patients. *Ann Int Med* 1992; 177:303–308.

69. Khamashta MA, Cuadrado MJK, Mujic F *et al.* The management of thrombosis in antiphospholipide antibody syndrome. *N Engl J Med* 1995; 332:993–997.

70. Derksen RHWM, De Groot PHG, Kater L, Nieuwenhuis HK. Patients with antiphospholipide antibodies and venous thrombosis should receive long term anticoagulant treatment. *Ann Rheum Dis* 1993; 52:689–692.

71. Douketis JD, Crowther MA, Julian JA *et al.* The effects of low intensity warfarin on coagulation activation in patients with antiphospholipide antibodies and systemic lupus erythematous. *Thromb Haemost* 1999; 82:1028–1032.

72. Baron JA, Gridley G, Weiderpass E, Nyren O, Linnet M. Venous thromboembolism and cancer. *Lancet* 1998; 351:1077–1080.

73. Prandoni P, Falanga A, Piccioli A. Cancer and venous thromboembolism. *Lancet Oncol* 2005; 6:401–410.

74. Lee AY, Levine MN, Baker RI *et al.* Randomised comparison of low molecular weight heparin versus oral anticoagulant therapy for the prevention of recurrent venous thromboembolism in patients with cancer (CLOT) Investigators. Low molecular weight heparin versus a coumarin for the prevention of recurrent antiphosp venous thromboembolism in patients with cancer. *N Engl J Med* 2003; 349:146–153.

75. Meyer G, Majanovic Z, Valcke J *et al.* Comparison of low molecular weight heparin and warfarin for the secondary prevention of venous thromboembolism inpatients with cancer: a randomised controlled study. *Arch Int Med* 2002; 162:1729–1735.

76. Levine M. Prevention of cancer associated thrombosis-An overview. In: Lugassy G, Falanga A, Kakkar AK, Rickles FR (eds). *Thrombosis and cancer*. Martin Dunitz, London, 2004, pp 151–161.

77. Matei D, Brenner B, Marder VJ. Acquired thrombophilic syndromes. *Blood Reviews* 2001; 15:31–48.

78. Pearson TC. The risk of thrombosis in essential thrombocythemia and polycythemia vera. *Semin Oncol* 2002; 29:16–21.

79. Elliott MA, Tefferi A. Thrombosis and haemorrhage in polycythaemia vera and essential thrombocythaemia. *Br J Haematol* 2005; 128: 275–290.

80. Barbui T, Finazzi G. When and how to treat essential thrombocythemia. *N Engl J Med* 2005; 353:85–86.

81. Gruppo Italiano Studia Policiteia (GISP) Low-dose aspirin in polycythaemia vera: a pilot study. *Br J Haematol* 1997; 97:453–456.

82. Harrisson CN, Campbell PJ, Buck G *et al.* Hydroxyurea compared with anagrelide in high-risk essential thrombocythemia. *N Engl J Med* 2005; 353:33–45.

83. Griesshammer M, Grunewald M, Michiels JJ. Acquired thrombophilia in pregnancy: essential thrombocythemia. *Semin Thromb Hemost* 2003; 29:205–212.

84. Dally N, Hoffman R, Haddad N, Sarig G, Rowe JM, Brenner B. Predictive factors of bleeding and thrombosis during induction therapy in acute promyelocytic leukelia-a single center experience in 34 patients. *Thromb Res* 2005; 116:109–114.

85. Escudier SM, Kantarjian HM, Estey EH. Thrombosis in patients with acute promyelocytic leukaemia treated with and without all-trans retinoic acid. *Leuk Lymphoma* 1996; 20:435–439.

86. Smith JJ. Paroxysmal nocturnal hemoglobinuria. *Clin Lab Sci* 2004; 17:172–177.

87. Hall C, Richards S, Hillmen P. Primary prophylaxis with warfarin prevents thrombosis in paroxysmal nocturnal hemoglobinuria (PNH). *Blood* 2003; 102:3587–3591.

88. Lindqvist P, Dahlback B, Marsal K. Thrombotic risk during pregnancy: a population study. *Obstet Gynecol* 1999; 94:595–599.

89. Greer IA, Thomson AJ. Management of venous thromboembolism in pregnancy. *Best Practice Res Clin Obstet Gynaecol* 2001; 15:583–603.

90. Bates SM, Greer IA, Hirsh J, Ginsberg S. Use of antithrombotic agents during pregnancy: the Seventh ACCP conference on antithrombotic and thrombolytic therapy. *Chest* 2004; 126:627S–644S.
91. Vitale N, De Feo M, De Santo LS *et al.* Dose-dependent fetal complications of warfarin in pregnant women with mechanical heart valves. *J Am Coll Cardiol* 1999; 33:1642–1645.
92. Greer I, Hunt BJ. Low molecular weight heparin in pregnancy: current issues. *Br J Haematol* 2004; 128:593–601.
93. Sanson BJ, Lensing AWA, Prins MH *et al.* Safety of low-molecular-weight heparin in pregnancy: a systematic review. *Thromb Haemost* 1999; 81:668–672.
94. Lepercq J, Conard J, Borel-Derlon A *et al.* Venous thromboembolism during pregnancy: a retrospective study of enoxaparin safety in 624 pregnancies. *Br J Obstet Gynaecol* 2001; 108:1134–1140.
95. Smith MP, Norris LA, Steer PJ *et al.* Tinzaparin sodium for thrombosis treatment and prevention during pregnancy. *Am J Obstet Gynecol* 2004; 190:495–501.
96. Lindhoff-Last E, Kreutzenbeck HJ, Magnani HN. Treatment of 51 pregnancies with danaparoid because of heparin intolerance. *Thromb Haemost* 2005; 93:63–69.
97. Lagrange F, Vergnes C, Brun JL *et al.* Absence of placental transfer of pentasaccharide (Fondaparinux, Arixtra) in the dually perfused human cotyledon in vitro. *Thromb Haemost* 2002; 87:831–835.
98. Li DK, Liu L, Odouli R. Exposure to non-steroidal anti-inflammatory drugs during pregnancy and risk of miscarriage: population based cohort study. *BMJ* 2003; 327:368.
99. De Stefano V, Leone G, De Carolis S *et al.* Management of pregnancy in women with antithrombin III congenital defect: report of four cases. *Thromb Haemost* 1988; 8:193–196.
100. Lechner K, Kyrle PA. Antithrombin III concentrates—are they clinically useful? *Thromb Haemost* 1995; 73:340–348.
101. ANAES Conférence de Consensus. Thrombophilie et grossesse. Prévention des risques thrombotiques maternels et placentaires. *Ann Med Interne* 2003; 154:422–430.
102. Gates S, Brocklehurst, Ayers S, Bowler U; on behalf of the Thromboprophylaxis in Pregnancy Advisory Group. Thromboprophylaxis and pregnancy: two randomised controlled pilot trials that used low-molecular-weight heparin. *Am J Obstet Gynecol* 2004; 191:1296–1303.
103. Brill-Edwards P, Ginsberg JS; for the Recurrence of Clot in This Pregnancy (ROCIT) Study Group. Safety of withholding antepartum heparin in women with a previous episode of venous thromboembolism. *N Engl J Med* 2000; 343:1439–1444.
104. Pabinger I, Grafenhofer H, Kaider A *et al.* Risk of pregnancy-associated recurrent venous thromboembolism in women with a history of venous thrombosis. *J Thromb Haemost* 2005; 3:949–954.
105. Conard J, Horellou MH, van Dreden P *et al.* Thrombosis and pregnancy in congenital deficiencies in AT III, protein C or protein S. Study of 78 women. *Thromb Haemost* 1990; 63:319–320.
106. McColl MD, Ramsay JE, Tait RC *et al.* Risk factors for pregnancy-associated venous thromboembolism. *Thromb Haemost* 1997; 78:1183–1188.
107. Samama MM, Rached RA, Horellou MH *et al.* Pregnancy-associated venous thromboembolism (VTE) in combined heterozygous factor V Leiden (FVL) and prothrombin (FII) 20210A mutation and in heterozygous FII single gene mutation alone. *Br J Haematol* 2003; 123:327–334.
108. Procare Group. Risk of venous thromboembolism during pregnancy in homozygous carriers of the factor V Leiden mutation: are there any predictive factors. *J Throm Haemost* 2004; 2:359–360.
109. Vossen CY, Conard J, Fontcuberta J *et al.* Risk of first venous thrombotic event in carriers of a familial thrombophilic defect. The European Prospective Cohort on Thrombophilia (EPCOT). *J Thromb Haemost* 2005; 3:459–464.
110. Conard J, Plu-Bureau G, Bahi N *et al.* Progestogen-only contraception in women at high risk of venous thromboembolism. *Contraception* 2004; 70:437–441.
111. The task force on the management of cardiovascular diseases during pregnancy of the European Society of Cardiology. Expert consensus document on management of cardiovascular diseases during pregnancy. *Europ Heart J* 2003; 24:761–781.
112. Oran B, Lee-Parritz A, Ansell J. Low molecular weight heparin for the prophylaxis of thromboembolism in women with prosthetic mechanical heart valves during pregnancy. *Thromb Haemost* 2004; 92:747–751.
113. Tincani A, Branch W, Levy RA *et al.* Treatment of pregnant patients with antiphospholipid syndrome. *Lupus* 2003; 12:524–529.
114. Brenner B, Hoffman R, Carp H *et al.* Efficacy and safety of two doses of enoxaparin in women with thrombophilia and recurrent pregnancy loss: the LVE-ENOX study. *J Thromb Haemost* 2005; 3:227–229.

115. Kovalevsky G, Gracia CR, Berlin JA *et al*. Evaluation of the association between hereditary thrombophilias and recurrent pregnancy loss: a meta-analysis. *Arch Intern Med* 2004; 164:558–563.

116. Vossen CY, Preston FE, Conard J *et al*. Hereditary thrombophilia and fetal loss: a prospective follow-up study. *J Thromb Haemost* 2004; 2:592–596.

117. Gris JC, Mercier E, Quere I *et al*. Low molecular-weight heparin versus low-dose aspirin in women with one fetal loss and a constitutional thrombophilic disorder. *Blood* 2004; 103:3695–3699.

118. Saito H. Thrombosis and renal disease. In: Ratnoff OD, Forbes CD (eds). *Disorders of Hemostasis*, 3rd edition. W.B. Saunders Company Philadelphia, 1996, pp 450–453.

119. Arkel YS, Ku DH, Le P, Carr AM. Comparison of a test for soluble fibrin polymer (TpP) with a standard quantitative ELISA for D-dimer in patients, without current thrombosis, who have cancer or renal disease. *Thromb Haemost* 2001; 86:1127–1128.

120. Donadio JV, Anderson CF, Mitchell JC *et al*. Membranoproliferative glomerulonephritis: a prospective clinical trial of platelet-inhibitor therapy. *N Engl J Med* 1984; 310:1421–1426.

121. Pollak VE, Glueck HI, Weiss MA *et al*. Defibrination with ancrod in glomerulonephritis: effects on clinical and histologic findings and on blood coagulation. *Am J Nephrol* 1982; 2:195–207.

122. Allford SL, Hunt BJ, Rose P, Machin SJ. Haemostasis and Thrombosis Task Force, British Committee for Standards in Haematology. Guidelines on the diagnosis and management of the thrombotic microangiopathic haemolytic anaemias. *Br J Haematol* 2003; 120:556–573.

123. Tsai HM. Molecular mechanisms in thrombotic thrombocytopenic purpura. *Semin Thromb Hemost* 2004; 30:549–557.

124. Sadler JE, Moake JL, Miyata T, George JN. Recent advances in thrombotic thrombocytopenic purpura. *Hematology* (Am Soc Hematol Educ Program) 2004; 407–423.

125. Amoura Z, Costedoat-Chalumeau N, Veyradier A *et al*. Thrombotic thrombocytopenic purpura with severe ADAMT-13 deficiency in two patients with primary antihpispholipid syndrome. *Arthritis & rheumatism* 2004; 50:3260–3264.

126. Pene F, Vigneau C, Auburtin M *et al*. Outcome of severe adult thrombotic microangiopathies in the intensive care unit. *Intensive Care Med* 2005; 31:71–78.

127. Vesely SK, George JN, Lämmle B *et al*. ADAMTS13 activity in thrombotic thrombocytopenic purpura-hemolytic uremic syndrome: relation to presenting features and clinical outcomes in a prospective cohort of 142 patients. *Blood* 2003; 102:60–68.

128. Kremer Hovinga Ja, Studt JD, Lammle B. The von Willebrand factor-cleaving protease (ADAMTS-13) and the diagnosis of thrombotic thrombocytopenia purpura (TTP). *Pathophysiol Haemost Thromb* 2003; 33:417–421.

129. Irish A. Hypercoagulability in renal transplant recipients. *Am J Cardiovasc Drugs* 2004; 4:139–149.

130. Brunkwall J, Bergqvist D, Bergentz SE *et al*. Postoperative deep venous thrombosis after renal transplantation. Effects of cyclosporine. *Transplantation* 1987; 43:647–649.

131. Hirsh J. Heparin and low molecular weight heparin. The seventh ACCP Conference on Antithrombotic and Thrombolytic Therapy. *Chest* 2004; 126(3 suppl 1):188S–203S.

132. Gouin-Thibault I, Pautas E, Siguret V. Safety profile of different low molecular weight heparins used at therapeutic dose. *Drug Saf* 2005; 28:333–349.

133. Singhal R, Brimble KS. Thromboembolic complications in the nephrotic syndrome: pathophysiology and clinical management. *Thromb Res* 2005 (in press).

134. Llach F. Hypercoagulability, renal vein thrombosis, and other thrombotic complications of nephrotic syndrome. *Kidney Int* 1985; 287:429–439.

135. Orth SR, Ritz E. The nephrotic syndrome. *New Engl J Med* 1998; 338:1202–1211.

136. Garibotto G, Giannoni M, Salvatore F. Complications of the nephrotic syndrome. *Ital Nefrol* 2003; 20:49–60.

137. Crew RJ, Radhakrishnan J, Appel G. Complications of the nephrotic syndrome and their treatment. *Clin Nephrol* 2004; 62:245–259.

138. Mitarai T. Prevention and management of complications in nephrotic syndrome. *Nippon Rinsho* 2004; 62:1893–1897.

139. Girolami A, Fabris F, Girolami B. Clinicial aspects of venous thrombophilia. *Pathophysiol Haemost Thromb* 2002; 32:258–262.

140. Martinez A, Gomez Rioja R, Rinon C *et al*. Prevalence of genetic prothrombotic factors (factor V Leiden and II20210 prothrombin mutation) in glomerular nephropathies with or without thrombosis. *Nefrologia* 2000; 20:139–144.

141. Marks DS, Massicotte MP, Steele BT *et al*. Neonatal renal venous thrombosis: clinical outcomes and prevalence of prothrombotic disorders. *J Pediatr* 2005; 146:811–816.

142. Risler T, Braun N, Erley CM. Treatment of glomerulonephritis. *Internist* 2003; 44:1083–1089.
143. Bowden RG, Wyatt FB, Wilson R, Wilborn C, Gentile M. Homocysteine and vascular access thrombosis in a cohort of end-stage renal disease patients. *Ren Fail* 2004; 26:709–714.
144. Bush RL, Lin PH, Lumsden AB. Management of thrombosed dialysis access: thrombectomy versus thrombolysis. *Semin Vasc Surg* 2004; 17:32–39.

20

Monitoring of antithrombotic drugs

K. Y. Saraff, D. Mukherjee, D. J. Moliterno

BACKGROUND AND RATIONALE FOR MONITORING

The availability of potent antiplatelet, antithrombin, and fibrinolytic therapies for treatment of acute coronary syndromes (ACS) and during percutaneous coronary interventions (PCI) has made monitoring of these therapies an important clinical issue. The use of these agents in combination has led to improved antithrombotic efficacy, albeit at the cost of increased bleeding in some situations. Currently available and evolving technologies to monitor the extent of inhibition of platelet aggregation and activity of antithrombotic agents will be covered in this chapter. The clinically important questions to be considered are whether the results generated from monitoring will effect a change that will improve efficacy (prevention of thrombotic events) or reduce adverse events (bleeding) from these therapies. Since novel and increasingly potent agents continue to be developed, monitoring anticoagulation will continue to be of special interest.

MONITORING OF ANTIPLATELET THERAPY

Antiplatelet therapy is important in managing both acute events and long-term risk in vascular disease. Of the available antiplatelet agents, the roles of aspirin and thienopyridines are well established in managing coronary artery disease; however, the dosing and the patient response issues continue to be refined. Likewise, the role of glycoprotein (GP) IIb/IIIa agents is also well established in the management of ACS and during coronary interventions [1–5]. It is an established fact that the efficacy of GPIIb/IIIa agents is strongly influenced by the percent of platelets inhibited, with an odds ratio of 0.44 for patients achieving greater than 95% platelet inhibition ($P = 0.019$).

While very effective, the GPIIb/IIIa agents can be associated with excess bleeding complications [7, 8]. Prolonged concurrent heparin administration combined with delayed sheath removal were thought to be partially responsible for excessive bleeding complications seen in the earlier GPIIb/IIIa trials [2, 5, 9]; however, despite the use of weight-adjusted heparin and earlier sheath removal, there remains an increase in minor bleeding risk associated with these agents. As has been suggested in previous studies, greater than 80% IIb/IIIa receptors must be occupied for the antagonist to be effective while greater than 90% inhibition may increase the bleeding risk [10]. Similarly, the complication of thrombocytopaenia may also be reduced by optimal dosing of the drug.

Kiran Y. Saraff, Cardiovascular Medicine Fellow, Gill Heart Institute, University of Kentucky, Lexington, Kentucky, USA.

Debrabrata Mukherjee, Associate Professor of Medicine, Director of Peripheral Interventional Programs, Gill Heart Institute, University of Kentucky, Lexington, Kentucky, USA.

David J. Moliterno, Chief of Cardiovascular Medicine, Professor and Vice Chair of Medicine, Gill Heart Institute, University of Kentucky, Lexington, Kentucky, USA.

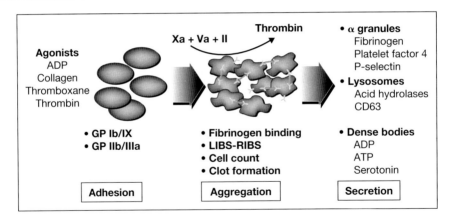

Figure 20.1 Platelets can respond to over 100 different agonists. When they do, they activate and may aggregate releasing vasoconstrictors, inhibitors of thrombolysis, and growth factors. Importantly, thrombin is generated on the platelet lipid-rich surface. (Reproduced with permission from: Mukherjee D, Moliterno DJ. Bedside platelet monitoring. In: Topol E (ed.). *Acute Coronary Syndromes*. Dekker Publishing, New York, NY, 2001, p. 566.)

During coronary interventions, monitoring of antiplatelet therapy may be necessary since the dosing regimen may not achieve a uniform receptor blockade in all patients, and hence may result in lack of efficacy or a higher incidence of complications. Similarly, assessment of receptor blockade after the discontinuation of IIb/IIIa therapy may help determine the return of normal platelet function. This information may help time the surgery or other invasive procedures. In long-term management of vascular disease, the role of aspirin and clopidogrel resistance may necessitate monitoring of platelet activity.

PLATELET ACTIVATION AND AGONISTS

Platelet activation can be induced by a variety of chemical and mechanical methods that work through several distinct intracellular pathways (Figure 20.1).

MONITORING OF ANTIPLATELET ACTIVITY

Usually a drug level in the plasma serves as a surrogate for drug effect, but because of variability, platelet count, receptor density, platelet functionality, and levels of platelet cofactors may influence the effect of IIb/IIIa antagonist. Therefore, whether the percentage of receptors blocked or the antagonism of final platelet function is a better parameter is not clear. For example, smaller doses of a IIb/IIIa antagonist may be excessive in patients with thrombocytopaenia or concurrent administration of other antiplatelet medications or in patients with illnesses that might affect platelet function.

Conventional turbidimetric platelet aggregometry using citrated platelet-rich plasma is the most accepted and widely used method of testing the platelet function. However, this test requires extensive sample preparation, quality control, operative experience, and expensive equipment. It is not clear whether platelet monitoring will affect the clinical outcomes.

PLATELET FUNCTION TESTS

Table 20.1 lists the currently available platelet function tests, their substrates, and principles of assessment.

Table 20.1 List of commonly available platelet function assays, their substrate, and principles of assessment

Test	Whole blood	Platelet-rich plasma (PRP)	Point-of-care test	Principle
Ivy bleeding time	Yes		Yes	Primary haemostasis
Light transmission aggregometry		Yes		Aggregation
Flow cytometry	Yes			Activation
Thromboelastograph	Yes			Clot strength
PFA-100	Yes		Yes	Primary haemostasis
Clot signature	Yes		Yes	Adhesion, analyser aggregation
Platelet works	Yes		Yes	Aggregation
Rapid platelet function	Yes		Yes	Aggregation

Ivy bleeding time

This test evaluates the primary haemostasis (which comprises platelet adhesion, release reaction, aggregation, and primary plug formation), and assesses an overall ability of platelets to form a thrombus. It is rapid, non-invasive, and can assess overall platelet function. However, the test requires a dedicated technologist and can take up to 30 minutes to perform. The accuracy, validity, and the predictability of this test is not proven. A normal range of bleeding time is 7 to 10 minutes.

Light transmission aggregometry

This test is the most commonly practised platelet function assay. This assay involves preparation of both platelet-rich plasma (PRP) and platelet-poor plasma (PPP) from a sample of citrated blood, then pipetting them into matched cuvettes at 37°C. The instrument is calibrated such that the amount of light transferred through PPP is defined as 100% aggregation and the light transmitted through unstimulated PRP is defined as 0% aggregation. Some laboratories use a standard platelet count in the PRP between 250 000–350 000/μl. Platelet agonists such as adenosine diphosphate (ADP), collagen, and epinephrine can be used to initiate aggregation. A magnetic bar is used to achieve stirring. The change in light transmission through the PRP is monitored. With the progression of aggregation, the turbidity of the PRP decreases and transmitted light is increased, which is then received and converted to an electrical signal, amplified, and recorded. Results are expressed as a percentage of aggregation.

Several instruments available such as Chrono-Log (Haverton, PA), Bio-Data (Hartboro, PA), Payton-Scientific (Buffalo, NY), and Helena Laboratories (Beaumont, TX) use this technique.

This test is widely available and has been used for more than three decades. It has the advantage of being able to be standardised, being well accepted, and being most widely used for clinical correlation. The disadvantages are that it is labour-intensive and time-consuming. Further, the process of centrifugation may result in loss of a subset of platelets. In addition, it is often difficult to compare results from one clinical site to the other. Preparation and centrifugation steps in preparation of PRP, cuvette size, speed of the stir bar, the agonist used, and concentration of the agonist can all result in variation in the test result. This assay has been used for phase 2 studies for the development of GPIIb/IIIa inhibitors and can be used clinically.

Flow cytometry

When the platelet agonist binds to the receptors, the number of activation dependent modifications of platelet surface antigens can be detected. Examples include increased numbers of

GPIIb/IIIa complexes and reduced numbers of GPIb-IX complexes, conformational changes of IIb/IIIa complexes with exposure of activation epitopes, and newer expression of alpha granule protein such as CD 62P or CD 63 occur. The expression of these new surface proteins can be detected easily by flow cytometry. Flow cytometry is currently used in research settings to study inherited and acquired platelet disorders. To perform this test, platelets are first labelled with a fluorescent conjugated monoclonal antibody and placed in a flow chamber where the cells are passed at a rate of 1000 to 10 000 cells per minute through a laser beam. When the labelled cells are exposed to laser they emit fluorescence, which is detected and processed along with the forward and sidelight scattering properties of a cell. Activation state of the circulating platelet is assessed with an activation dependent monoclonal antibody.

While the test involves a minimal amount of whole blood sample and handling, it requires expensive equipment and a dedicated technologist. Therefore, it is primarily used as research tool.

Rapid platelet function assay

The *Ultegra*-RPFA (Accumetrics, San Diego, CA) is an automated whole blood cartridge based point-of-care device, which allows for rapid and reproducible evaluation of platelet function in patients treated with GPIIb/IIIa agents. The principle used in this study is that activated platelets bind fibrinogen. The agglutination of fibrinogen-coated polystyrene micro particles in whole blood depends on the proportion of unblocked platelet GbIIb/IIIa receptors. Therefore GbIIb/IIIa agents prevent this interaction, resulting in decreased agglutination of the particles in proportion to the degree of receptor blockade achieved. This test uses the thrombin receptor activating peptide (iso-TRAP) as the speed of bead agglutination is more rapid and reproducible if the platelets are activated. A standard citrated tube, or if eptifibatide is the agent used, PPACK (phe-pro-arg chloromethyl ketone) is used as an anticoagulant to collect the whole blood. The tube is then inserted into a disposable plastic cartridge from where the blood is automatically drawn into two sample channels containing lyophilised isotrap and fibrinogen-coated beads. A steel ball driven by a microprocessor then mixes the sample for 70 seconds. An automated detector is used to measure the light absorbance of the sample 16 times per second. As more and more platelets interact with the fibrinogen-coated beads leading to agglutination, the amount of light transmitted increases. The rate of agglutination is noted as the slope of the change of absorbance over a fixed time interval and is reported as mV per 10 seconds. The individual patient's pre-IIb/IIIa therapy baseline slope is retained in memory and all additional specimens are reported as a raw slope as well as the percentage of the baseline slope. The advantages of *Ultegra*-RPFA over turbidimetric aggregometry are the use of whole blood, semi-automated format, rapidity of test completion, a digital readout, and duplicate analysis. The disadvantage is that it requires a baseline sample comparison and a specific agonist.

PFA 100 analyser

The platelet functional analyser (PFA 100; Dade Behring, Miami, FL) evaluates primary haemostasis through interplatelet interactions in high shear stress conditions using whole blood flow through an aperture [11]. This test utilises citrated whole blood, which is drawn through a capillary tube under vacuum resulting in high shear stress and has been directed through a precisely defined aperture in a membrane pre-treated with either collagen and epinephrine or collagen and ADP. Platelet adhesion and aggregation at the aperture results in occlusion, which is then reported as closure time. The whole testing process takes about 10 minutes. Occlusion of the aperture is blocked by antibodies directed at GPIb, IIb/IIIa, and von Willebrand factor (vWF). Blood can be collected in routine Vacutainer tubes and kept at room temperature up to 4 hours. The instrument can run two tests in sequence. A dysfunction of platelet activity caused by aspirin can be detected as a prolonged closure time with the collagen/epinephrine cartridge, while a normal closure time with the collagen ADP cartridge can be separately assessed. A constant vacuum of 30 mmHg/min is maintained in the system mimicking the pressure in a microcapillary in the human body.

Normal closure time is 100 seconds and the instrument can detect a closure time of up to 300 seconds. This is a limitation of this assay. Use of whole blood, simplicity, and automaticity are advantages of this test. The test usefulness in monitoring GPIIb/IIIa therapy requires further study.

In general, closure times are increased well beyond 300 seconds with GPIIb/IIIa antagonists.

CLINICAL STUDIES

The role of platelet function assay in determining optimal GPIIb/IIIa blockade has been studied in several clinical studies [6, 12–14].

The PARADISE study demonstrated significant variability between patients in the extent of platelet inhibition following a standard weight-adjusted abciximab dosing [13]. Nearly all patients achieved greater than 80% inhibition after bolus, but approximately 13% of the patients failed to maintain this level of inhibition during the infusion. The incidence of postprocedural adverse cardiac events was higher in patients in whom platelet inhibition was less than 80% 8 hours into infusion compared to patients with adequate platelet inhibition at 8 hours (46% vs. 7%).

In the GOLD study, the composite ischaemic endpoint occurred significantly higher in patients with less than 95% platelet inhibition (6.4% vs. 14.4%; $P = 0.006$) [6]. The extent of percent inhibition of platelet activation was found to be strongly correlated to ischaemic endpoint with an odds ratio of 0.44 for patients achieving greater than 95% platelet inhibition ($P = 0.019$).

In the Do Tirofiban And Reopro Give similar Efficacy outcome Trial (TARGET) a lower incidence of composite endpoint of death, myocardial infarction (MI), and urgent target vessel revascularisation (TVR) was seen in patients receiving abciximab compared to tirofiban [9]. This was likely due to lower incidence of maximal inhibition of platelet activation in the tirofiban-treated patients at 15–60 minutes into the treatment [15]. Flow cytometry and light transmission ergometry with EDP as the agonist were used to test the platelet function. Abciximab resulted in an average inhibition of 90–94% whereas tirofiban resulted in 61–66% inhibition ($P < 0.001$ at 15, 30, and 45 minutes) [15].

The PRIDE study, which used a double bolus of eptifibatide at a 180 μg/kg followed by 2 μg/kg/min infusion achieved a steady-state platelet inhibition of greater than 80% [16]. A double bolus regimen achieved an improved clinical outcome compared to the single bolus regimen [17].

In using GPIIb/IIIa agents in patients with thrombocytopaenia and those on oral anticoagulant (OA) therapy, a concern is excessive bleeding with standard dose of GPIIb/IIIa therapy. Utilising platelet inhibition monitoring with *Ultegra*-RPFA, reduced doses of GPIIb/IIIa agents have been used safely and effectively [18].

With increasing availability of data linking optimal inhibition of platelet activity to clinical outcome, it is likely that monitoring of antiplatelet therapy may help extend the use of GPIIb/IIIa therapy to more patients, without increasing adverse events.

In summary, antiplatelet therapy constitutes the standard of care for patients with ACS and those undergoing PCI. Many scenarios related to the patient, clinical situation, or other phenomena may require monitoring of the extent of platelet inhibition. Outcome data are becoming available which suggest a certain percent IPA may be optimal. With evolution of monitoring techniques the hope is that this class of drug can be extended to more patients without increasing bleeding risks. Among those currently receiving therapy, monitoring may improve efficacy and decrease bleeding rates.

Aspirin resistance

Aspirin resistance (as defined by the inability of aspirin to protect the patient from thrombotic complication, to cause prolongation of bleeding time, to reduce TXA2 production, or to produce an anticipated effect on one or more *in vitro* tests of platelet function) appears to be a true phenomenon despite the fact that no one drug is 100% effective. Variable platelet response has been described in patients with stroke, peripheral artery disease, and coronary artery disease (CAD). Proposed mechanisms for aspirin resistance have been transient expression of cyclooxygenase (COX)-2 in nascent platelets, extra-platelet source of TXA2 such as monocytes during ACS, and concomitant administration of non-steroidal anti-inflammatory drugs (NSAIDs), which may compete for the same binding sites as aspirin. Up to 5% of patients in a series of stable CAD patients were found to be aspirin resistant, and an additional 23% to be semi-responders based on the results of platelet aggregation induced by ADP and arachidonic acid [19]. The aspirin-resistant group had an increased incidence of death, MI, or cerebrovascular accidents during a two-year observation period [20]. In the future, platelet function tests may potentially be used to define aspirin responders.

Clopidogrel resistance

Similar to aspirin, considerable interindividual variability exists in patient response to clopidogrel using the ADP-induced platelet aggregation studies [21–23]. It has been suggested that concurrent administration of statins metabolised *via* CYP3A4 may interfere with the inhibitory effects of clopidogrel [21, 24, 25]. Many other drugs that are potentially metabolised *via* the CVY3A4 may also interfere with clopidogrel efficacy. Mukherjee *et al.* demonstrated no significant *in vivo* interaction between statin and clopidogrel [26]. The assessment of platelet inhibitory effect of clopidogrel can be made using flow cytometry [21, 27], light transmission aggregometry [22, 28], or the platelet works assay [24, 29], all of which use ADP for the assay. These studies illustrated the variable platelet inhibitory response to the standard administered dose of clopidogrel. These observations, irrespective of the methodology chosen to detect inhibition suggest that the response to clopidogrel therapy is heterogeneous with significant patient variability and resistance in some individuals [22].

MONITORING OF ANTITHROMBOTIC THERAPY

Anticoagulants are central in the management of both atherothrombotic and venous disorders. Unfractionated heparin (UFH) is the cornerstone therapy in such disorders, although its dominance is being challenged by more prevalent use of low molecular-weight heparins (LMWH) and direct thrombin inhibitors (DTI). UFH has a narrow therapeutic window, thus necessitating the monitoring of anticoagulant activity to optimise efficacy while maintaining safety. There may be less need for monitoring of anticoagulant activity of LMWH and DTI.

RATIONALE FOR ANTICOAGULANT MONITORING

Data from landmark trials of thrombolytics and anticoagulants in ACS patients have improved the understanding of the importance of achieving optimal anticoagulant levels. In the Global Utilisation of Streptokinase and Tissue Plasminogen Activator for Occluded Coronary Arteries I (GUSTO-1) trial, there was a linear relationship between activated partial thromboplastin time (aPTT) and the risk of haemorrhage when aPTT was more than 70 seconds. As shown in Figure 20.2, each 10-second increase in aPTT was associated with an approximate 1% absolute increase in moderate or severe haemorrhage, and a 0.07% increase in intracranial haemorrhage [30]. There was also an association with higher mortality when aPTT was less than 50 seconds or greater than 75 seconds. In the GUSTO-II trial, where a 20% increase in the dose of heparin resulted in a 5–10 second higher aPTT compared with GUSTO-I, the

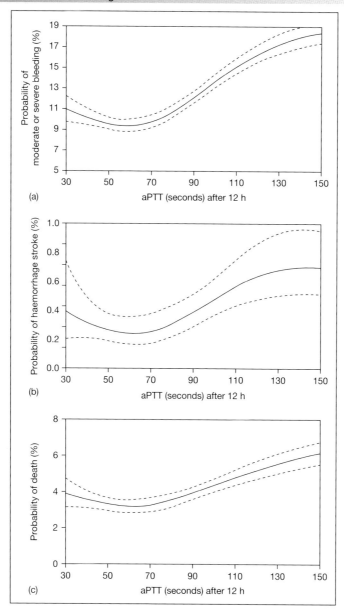

Figure 20.2 Activated partial thromboplastin times (aPTT) versus probability of (a) moderate or severe bleeding, (b) intracranial haemorrhage, and (c) 30-day mortality at 12 intravenous hours after enrolment among patients on heparin in the GUSTO-I trial. (Reproduced with permission from Granger *et al. Circulation* 1996; 93:870–878.)

risk of intracranial haemorrhage among patients treated with thrombolytics was doubled [31]. This incidence was reduced with the subsequent lowering of heparin dose in the GUSTO-IIb trial, whereby the aPTT at 12 hours was 65 seconds (compared with 85 seconds in GUSTO-IIa) among patients treated with thrombolytics [32]. The rate of intracranial haemorrhage was also reduced by one-half to 0.6%. Likewise, in the TIMI-9B trial, a reduction of intracranial haemorrhage risk was seen with reduction of anticoagulant doses [33]. Accordingly, the American

College of Cardiology/American Heart Association (ACC/AHA) altered the guidelines for management of acute MI in 1999 to lower UFH dosage to 60 U/kg bolus followed by 12 U/kg/hr infusion to target an aPTT of 50–70 seconds, in the setting of thrombolytic therapy [34].

In the setting of non-ST-elevation myocardial infarction (NSTEMI) ACS, a lower range of aPTT was also sufficient for optimal reduction of ischaemic events. In an analysis of the TIMI-3b study, aggressive anticoagulation with heparin to achieve aPTTs greater than 2.0 times control did not offer additional clinical benefit compared with lower aPTT levels (1.5 to 2.0 times control) among patients with NSTEMI ACS receiving intravenous heparin and oral aspirin. Thus, these data translate to an optimal standard aPTT range of approximately 50–70 seconds during management of patients with ACS. An even lower range may be acceptable when antithrombins are used in combination with potent antiplatelet therapies (though this has not been well characterised for medically treated patients).

Heparin

The standard method for monitoring heparin anticoagulation is the aPTT, a test that reflects the inhibitory effect of heparin on intrinsic coagulation pathway, thrombin, factor Xa, and factor IXa. APTT determination is usually made in the central laboratory using several commercially available instruments and one of many reagents, each with a different range of control values and a different aPTT–heparin level sensitivity relationship. It involves multiple steps, each of which can contribute to significant delays. This delay is typically about 2 hours. In a study from the University of Massachusetts, mean time of aPTT was 2 hrs and 6 min [35]. A survey of 79 hospitals participating in the GUSTO-I trial and data collected on 387 aPTTs showed the mean time from blood draw to availability of the result was 1 hr and 46 minutes [36]. Such delays can compromise care of patients who are at increased risk of life-threatening thrombosis and bleeding.

In addition to the delay, aPTTs obtained at central laboratories may also be subject to artefact related to the sampling technique and handling, as well as considerable variability between different reagents and laboratories. Sampling artefact may arise from poor venipuncture, insufficient blood collection, delay between sampling and measurement of results, and incomplete centrifugation [37, 38]. Moreover, there are substantial differences between reagent–instrument combinations [39], different reagents [40], and even among different batches of the same reagent [40]. There can be a substantial variability in heparin concentration in the serum for a given level of aPTT based on variability in the reagent used. In one study, where seven commercially available reagents were tested, the average amount of heparin required to double the baseline aPTT varied by two-fold [40]. The haematology and laboratory societies have not been able to develop a standard aPTT system analogous to the international normalised ratio for the prothrombin time (PT) [41]. In another study, using five different reagents, aPTT ratio corresponding to a heparin level of 0.2 U/ml by protamine titration varied from 1.8 to 4.2 [42]. Many hospitals have established a target aPTT range based on a target heparin level of 0.2–0.4 U/ml by protamine titration or 0.3–0.7 U/ml by anti-Xa activity.

Bedside 'point-of-care' testing

In general, bedside point-of-care (POC) testing has the advantages of being more convenient, giving rapid results, and requiring less nursing time in awaiting and retrieving results. It has the disadvantage of being less accurate, more expensive, difficult to control quality, more difficult to bill for, requiring more personnel training, and difficult to integrate into the hospital information system.

Numerous POC devices are currently available. Most of them measure multiple parameters as shown in Table 20.2. It is important to realise that different devices yield different values on the same blood sample [43]. Further, target activated clotting time (ACT) varies

Table 20.2 Point-of-care anticoagulant monitoring devices

Device	Main tests	Clot formation setting
Hemochron tube technology	ACT, PT, aPTT	Blood clots in a tube containing (ex. Response 401) magnet, and rotated in a magnetic field
Hemochron cuvette technology	ACT+, LR-ACT, PT, aPTT	Forced movement of unclotted (ex., junior II, signature, signature+) blood through a narrow channel
Hemotec ACT II, hepcon HMS	HR-ACT, LR-ACT, HMS, PT, aPTT	Mechanical plunger in and out of blood sample wells
i-STAT	ACT	Thrombin conversion sensed by a biosensor producing an electro-active compound
Rapid point coag	HMT, ENOX, ECT, PT, aPTT	Paramagnetic iron particles in oscillating magnetic field
Actalyke	ACT, MAX-ACT, PT, aPTT	Two-point electromagnetic detection of clot in a tube
CoaguChek	ACT, PT, aPTT	Capillary flow of unclotted blood

depending on the procedure. For example, CT surgery often requires target ACT of 400–600 seconds, whereas PCI requires ACT 250–350 seconds (depending on concomitant use of GPIIb/IIIa inhibitor). Dialysis and membrane oxygenators require target ACT of 180–200 seconds, and appropriate ACT level for removal of arterial sheaths is <175 seconds.

DEVICES FOR MONITORING UNFRACTIONATED HEPARIN

Hemochron whole blood coagulation systems (International Technidyne Corporation, USA)
Hemochron instruments can measure a variety of coagulant tests (see Table 20.2). They use either cuvette-based or tube-based platforms. The first type of machine uses three kinds of tubes that contain either celite, kaolin, or glass beads (e.g., hemochron response, Hemochron 401). The second type (cuvette-based) uses cartridges preloaded with silica, kaolin, and phospholipid (e.g., Hemochron Junior II, Hemchron Junior Signature, and Signature 1). Tube-based systems require about 2 ml of whole blood collected in glass tubes and manual shaking to mix the blood. The tube is then placed in a heating chamber at 37°C and rotated in a magnetic field. When blood clots it displaces a magnet in the tube, activating a switch. The time taken to displace the switch is the clotting time. The cuvette-based system utilizes a microcoagulation system that uses a disposable cuvette. A drop of fresh whole blood is placed on the cuvette, which then comes into contact with kaolin and the platelet factor substitute in the cartridge. The unclotted blood is mechanically moved back and forth in a capillary. The cessation of flow is detected by a change in light transmission. Different cartridges can be separately purchased to measure aPTT, ACT (ACT-LR or ACT 1), and PT.

Hemotec automated coagulation timer (ACT) II and Hepcon haemostasis management system (HMS) devices (Medtronic Hemotec Inc)
The Hepcon HMS is a microprocessor clot-timing instrument capable of measuring ACT, whole blood heparin concentration, and heparin dose–response. Different cartridges can be

used depending on the measurements desired (e.g., High-Range ACT, Heparin Assay, and Heparin Dose Response cartridges). Whole blood (about 400 μl) samples are placed in both wells of a cartridge containing kaolin as the activator. An automated plunger is then mechanically dipped in and out of the blood samples. As the sample clots, a fibrin web forms which impedes the descent rate of the plunger. This rate change is detected by optical photocells, and the clotting time is defined as the time to reach a pre-specified threshold of drop in plunger descent rate. The ACT II device uses the same principle, with the added advantage of being a portable POC system. Heparin concentrations measured by the Hepcon device correlated well with laboratory-measured plasma heparin levels, both before and during cardiopulmonary bypass ($r = 0.95$), unlike the weak correlation between ACT levels ($r = 0.35–0.59$) and plasma heparin levels during cardiopulmonary bypass [42].

Thrombolytic assessment system/Rapidpoint Coag (PharmaNetics Inc, Raleigh, NC)

The Rapidpoint Coag machine uses disposable test cards (e.g., heparin management test [HMT] card) containing small paramagnetic iron oxide particles (PIOP) in a flat capillary reaction chamber with reagents (e.g., celite). When one drop of whole blood (citrated or non-citrated) is added to the test card, the sample (~30 μl) is drawn into the reaction chamber dissolving the dry reagents. The PIOP begin to oscillate in a magnetic field, which slows down when blood clotting commences, and eventually stops moving when the clot entraps the particles. This movement is detected by an infrared photosensor which records the test completion time when the rate of PIOP movement drops. The HMT card can measure a broad range of heparin levels (1–10 U/ml). In fact, the HMT levels have been reported to have better correlation with heparin levels and anti-Xa levels compared with ACT levels [44, 45]. The effective range of HMT test is from 50–850 seconds (normal range is 89–169 seconds for citrated blood and 76–195 seconds for non-citrated blood) [46]. Similarly, PT and aPTT test cards can be used with a Rapidpoint Coag device to monitor PT and aPTT levels, respectively.

i-STAT Analyser (Abbot Laboratories, USA)

The bedside analyser uses disposable cartridges and is capable of measuring numerous laboratory tests, including electrolytes, creatinine, glucose, blood gases, and ACT levels. It uses celite pre-loaded cartridges to measure ACT of whole blood samples. The analyser uses an electromechanical microminiaturised sensor based on silicon chip semiconductor technology. The ACT cartridge contains preloaded celite, which activates the whole blood sample to convert to a thrombin substrate. The electromechanical biosensor detects this conversion, which produces an electroactive compound that is detected amperometrically. ACT values from the i-STAT device are relatively comparable to those obtained from the Hemachron 401 device [47]. However, the i-STAT ACT is not currently cleared for low ACT range applications.

CoaguChek System (Roche Diagnostics Corporation, Indianapolis, IN)

The CoaguChek is a portable hand-held instrument that can measure PT, aPTT, and ACT levels using disposable cartridges. A single drop of whole blood is placed onto the cartridge, which is preloaded with celite. Blood clotting time is determined by sensing the cessation of blood flow through a capillary channel *via* laser photometry. A laser beam through the blood sample is blocked when blood clots and this time is registered by the instrument. This system cannot measure ACT levels greater than 500 seconds, however, and thus is not as applicable during cardiovascular surgery [48]. The aPTT levels obtained with this device have conflicting correlation with central laboratory measured aPTT [49, 50]. This system may be more useful for at-home monitoring of PT in patients on long-term coumadin therapy [51].

Actalyke activated clotting time system (Helena Laboratories, Allen Park, MI)

Actalyke is a simple bedside heparin monitoring system that uses the whole-blood ACT method. It uses test tubes preloaded with reagents that are cross-compatible with the Hemochron System. Similar to the Hemochron system, it uses magnetic-displacement clot detection. However, it uses two-point clot detection, which enables detection of a clot at early fibrin formation, minimising testing error and non-heparin-related prolongation. In addition to the celite ACT test, this system also can perform the new MAX-ACT measurement, which utilises tubes that are preloaded with multiple activators (celite, kaolin, and glass beads). These particular tubes maximally convert all factor XII to XIIa for greatest heparin specificity, and may be less susceptible to changes associated with hypothermia and haemodilution as experienced with the traditional celite-ACT methods.

LOW-MOLECULAR-WEIGHT HEPARINS

Many clinical trials have shown equal or superior efficacy of LMWH over UFH in both arterial and venous thrombotic diseases. In particular, enoxaparin has consistently been proven safe and efficacious compared with UFH or placebo in medical therapy trials [52–56]. Unlike UFH, LMWH does not appreciably affect aPTT or ACT which are routinely used to monitor UFH therapy [57]. Central laboratory-run anti-Xa activity tests are available but have a long turnaround time which precludes their routine use during PCI or acute care settings. A POC test, Rapidpoint ENOX, recently became available to specifically evaluate clotting times in response to enoxaparin.

Rapidpoint ENOX test (PharmaNetics Inc, Morrisville, NC)

The Rapidpoint ENOX test is a 1-step assay, whereby all the components necessary to measure enoxaparin clotting time (aside from the patient's sample) are included in the test card's reaction chamber, to be used in conjunction with the Rapidpoint Coag analyser. A drop of the blood sample ($\sim$35 µl) is manually added to the appropriate well on the front of the test card. The test sample is then drawn into a reaction chamber *via* capillary action, rehydrating reagents and stimulating PIOP to move by an oscillating magnetic field in the test chamber. A specific factor Xa activator then rapidly activates factor X, which initiates the clotting process with formation fibrin strands that attach to and impede movement of iron particles. An infrared optical system monitors particle movement and indicates when a preset reduction in movement is achieved (corresponding to the test's endpoint which is reported in seconds). The ENOX test card is optimised for use with enoxaparin (clotting time range of 50–700 seconds) and should not be used to monitor UFH or other LMWH. Platelet inhibitors and thrombolytic agents do not affect the ENOX test, however, direct thrombin inhibitors have significant effects. ENOX times ranged from 106–160 seconds (mean $\pm$ 2SD) in 120 normal volunteers, and from 70–180 seconds (mean $\pm$ 2SD) among 166 unanticoagulated patients using citrated samples. Rapidpoint ENOX times correlated strongly to anti-Xa activities measured by the Stachrom Heparin Assays in both citrated and non-citrated whole blood samples [58].

The correlation of ENOX time to clinical outcome was evaluated in the ELECT study [59]. In this study, 445 patients received subcutaneous or intravenous enoxaparin during PCI and Rapidpoint ENOX time was correlated to clinical outcomes as shown in Figure 20.3. Mean procedural ENOX time was similar in patients with or without ischaemic events (461 vs. 425 seconds respectively). The nadir event rate was observed for ENOX times of 300–350 seconds. No significant association between ischaemic events and ENOX times were observed. Increased ENOX time during sheath removal were associated with increased bleeding risk. Based on this study and suggested anti-Xa activity of 0.8 to 1.8 IU/ml while using

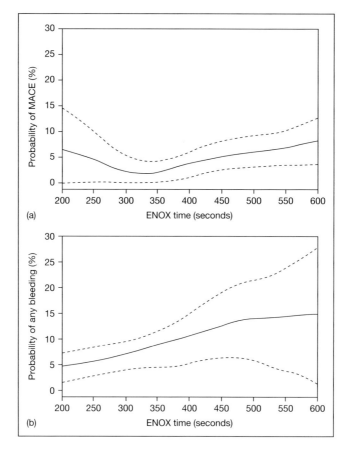

Figure 20.3 Results from the ELECT trial: (a) correlation of ENOX time to major adverse cardiac events (MACE), in-hospital death, myocardial infarction or urgent target revascularisation; (b) correlation of ENOX time to any bleeding events. (Reproduced with permission from Moliterno *et al. J Am Coll Cardiol* 2003; 42:1138.)

enoxaparin for PCI, Moliterno *et al.* recommended an ENOX time of 250–450 seconds for PCI and less than 200–250 seconds for arterial sheath removal.

DIRECT THROMBIN INHIBITORS

Direct thrombin inhibitors (DTIs) do not require a cofactor to antagonise thrombin activity; thus they directly inhibit thrombin activity on fibrinogen and also attenuate thrombin-induced platelet aggregation. Hirudin and its analogues (bivalirudin) have numerous other advantages over UFH and are increasingly being used for ACS and PCI, especially for patients with heparin-induced thrombocytopenia (HIT).

Anticoagulation levels with hirudin can be measured accurately with chromogenic-based substrate assays or ecarin clotting times (ECT). aPTT is inadequate for monitoring hirudin levels since the correlation is only linear for hirudin concentrations up to 1 mg/l (low normal therapeutic range) [60]. Furthermore, there is limited linear correlation between ACT and hirudin plasma levels, with high levels of hirudin concentrations (greater than 2 mg/l) associated with ACT levels beyond the detection limit [61]. Bivalirudin does appreciably affect aPTT, PT, and thrombin times in a dose-dependent manner, though over a limited range. However, the ECT provides a more accurate measurement of DTI activity than ACT.

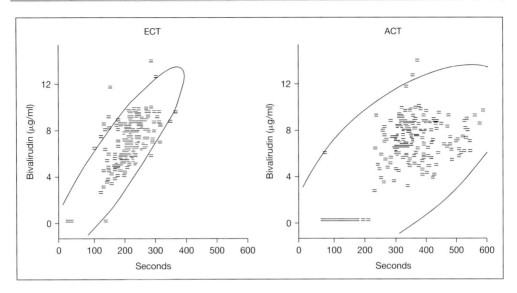

Figure 20.4 Considering samples from all time-points, the correlations between clotting time and bivalirudin concentration were $r = 0.90$ for ECT and $r = 0.71$ for Hemochron ACT. The ellipse shown on each graph represents the 90% density contour (confidence curve for the bivariate distribution). The ellipse becomes more circular in shape as the correlation decreases. (Reproduced with permission from Cho *et al. Am J Cardiol* 2003; 91:112.)

This test utilises ecarin (from the venom of *Echis carinatus*) to convert prothrombin to meizothrombin, which then catalyses the conversion of fibrinogen to fibrin (which is inhibited by DTI) [62].

Thrombolytic assessment system (TAS) ecarin clotting time (ECT) test cards (PharmaNetics Inc, Raleigh, NC)

The TAS ECT test card was recently authorised by the US for use in determining the anticoagulant effect of recombinant hirudin (r-hirudin) (Refludan) during cardiopulmonary bypass in patients who have HIT. This test card is a 2-step test that requires the patient's citrated whole blood sample to be first diluted with pooled normal human plasma. The diluted sample is then added to a pre-warmed ECT test card, which contains the dry ecarin (protein prothrombin activator from *E. carinatus* venom) reagent and PIOP. Ecarin catalyses the hydrolytic cleavage of the human prothrombin molecule, generating thrombin without the release of any zymogen fragment. Hirudin (and low-molecular-weight synthetic thrombin inhibitors) inhibits the formation of this type of thrombin (meizothrombin). The use of ecarin to activate prothrombin bypasses the coagulation cascade (activation of factors V–XII), and thus a deficiency in any of these factors will not be reflected in the results. ECT is measured in a similar fashion as the ENOX test cards deposited in the Rapidpoint Coag analyser, by assessing movement of the PIOP in an oscillating magnetic field. This instrument reports ECT in seconds and is sensitive to r-hirudin to 100 ng/ml. The normal range in 120 normal patients was between 41.6 and 55.3 seconds (mean + 2SD) [63]. This test card has also been reliably used in patients receiving bivalirudin. The TAS ECT correlated strongly with bivalirudin concentration (anti-IIa levels), whereas the Hemochron-measured ACT levels only moderately correlated with anti-IIa levels [62] as depicted in Figure 20.4. Evaluation of a larger number of PCI patients by the same group of investigators revealed that citrated ECT, non-citrated ECT, and ACT correlated well with bivalirudin concentration ($r = 0.96$, 0.93, and 0.90 respectively). Correlation with bivalirudin concentrations at therapeutic levels of bivalirudin was much lower. The correlation coefficient for ECT was 0.75 with citrated, and 0.59 with non-citrated sample, while it was 0.37 for ACT [64].

CLINICAL IMPLICATIONS

Rationale for monitoring heparin during PCI

Since the early days of PCI, large doses of heparin have been used to prevent thrombosis due to transient obstruction to coronary flow as well as endothelial disruption. Similar to coronary artery bypass graft surgery (CABG) the doses and levels of heparin used during PCI are above the level at which the heparin–aPTT response curve allows discrimination, and therefore ACT has become the standard monitoring test used at the point of care. Hemochron and HemoTec instruments are commonly used devices to measure ACT. Hemochron generally yields an ACT value that is 50 seconds longer than HemoTec derived value [65].

There are no randomised controlled trials comparing different doses of heparin during PCI. A number of observational studies prior to widespread use of GPIIb/IIIa inhibitor have shown that heparin effect as measured by ACT is associated with risk of thrombotic complications [66–69]. In one study, thrombotic complications of death and need for emergency CABG was associated with 60–80 second lower ACT values (measured using HemoTec device) compared to controls [67]. In another study, abrupt closure following percutaneous transluminial coronary angioplasty (PTCA) was associated with ACT values 30–40 second lower than control (measured by Hemochron device). Abrupt closure risk was twice the ACT value of 300 compared to 400 seconds [68]. These studies have led to the recommendation that heparin be titrated to an ACT value of at least 300 seconds with a HemoTec device and 350 seconds with a Hemochron device before angioplasty [70].

A lower ACT value of about 200 seconds achieved with a less aggressive heparin regimen of 70 U/kg or less in association with abciximab used in the Evaluation in PTCA to Improve Long-Term Outcome with Abciximab GPIIb/IIIa Blockade (EPILOG) [71] trial had fewer complications compared to the EPIC trial without any loss of efficacy [71]. Thus a lower dose of heparin is recommended when GPIIb/IIIa agents are co-administered [71, 72]. Further, abciximab alters the heparin level–ACT correlation such that ACT is prolonged by about 10% on average by concomitant abciximab administration [73]. In contrast, eptifibatide and tirofiban do not alter ACT level [74, 75].

Experience with bedside anticoagulant monitoring in clinical trials of PCI

Several trials evaluating multiple pharmacologic regimen during PCI have used POC ACT monitoring. This has made it possible to compare ACT levels and outcomes. In a pooled analysis correlating peak ACT to clinical outcomes from six large randomised PCI trials — Evaluation of Platelet Glycoprotein IIb/IIIa Inhibition for Prevention of Ischaemic Complications (EPIC) [7], Evaluation in PTCA to Improve Long-Term Outcome with Abciximab GP IIb/IIIa Blockade (EPILOG) [71], Evaluation of Platelet IIb/IIIa Blockade (EPISTENT) [2], Integrilin to Minimise Platelet Aggregation and Coronary Thrombosis-II (IMPACT-II) [76], Reopro in Acute Myocardial Infarction Primary PTCA Organisation and Randomised Trial (RAPPORT) [77], and Hirulog Angioplasty Study (HAS) [78]–ACT level at the time of device deployment was available for 5216 patients [79]. Peak ACTs were compared in 25-second intervals from 275–475 seconds. The majority of ACT was measured by Hemochron device (95%) and a small proportion by HemoTec device (5%). The seven-day incidence of death, MI, or any revascularisation and bleeding complications were calculated for each group and compared. When UFH was used alone, ischaemic complications were lower among patients with higher ACT values. The lowest events were observed for ACT values between 350–375 seconds, though more bleeding complications were noted. In patients receiving both abciximab and heparin no additional benefit was observed beyond ACT levels of 250 seconds.

Bedside aPTT monitoring in clinical trials of ACS

In the 41 000 patient GUSTO-1 trial, a prospective observational study was performed to evaluate patient outcomes according to the method of anticoagulant monitoring. Of the 28 172 patients that received intravenous heparin and had at least one aPTT measured, bedside aPTT measurement by a CoaguCheck Plus device was compared to aPTT measured by the central laboratory. aPTT was measured in 1713 patients by POC testing [80]. Patients who had bedside determination of aPTT were more likely to achieve target aPTT at 24 hrs (26% vs. 22%), had lower rates of bleeding, less drop from baseline to nadir haematocrit, less need for transfusion, a tendency towards slightly higher re-infarction rate, and a tendency toward a lower mortality. In the Platelet IIb/IIIa Antagonism for the Reduction of Acute Coronary syndrome Events in a Global Organisation Network (PARAGON) trial [81], aPTT was measured using a Hemochron Jr bedside device and heparin dose was adjusted to a target of 50–70 seconds. Median aPTT achieved was 62 seconds at 6 hrs and 50 seconds (25th to 75th percentile, 40–63 seconds) at 24 hrs [82], ranges that compared favourably with standard care approaches. Bleeding rates in the heparin control arm (5.5%) were likewise comparable to historical controls. The PARAGON experience shows that a bedside monitor used with an automated blinded system of heparin adjustment can achieve consistent therapeutic aPTT levels and low bleeding rates.

WARFARIN

Vitamin K antagonists have been the mainstay of oral anticoagulant therapy for >50 years for the prevention of venous thromboembolism, systemic embolism in patients with prosthetic heart valves or atrial fibrillation, acute MI in high-risk men, and stroke, recurrent infarction, or death in patients with acute MI. Their use is problematic because of a narrow therapeutic window, drug and diet interactions, variability in dose–response among individuals and difficult-to-standardise laboratory control.

Prothrombin time (PT) [83] is the most common test used to monitor warfarin therapy. PT responds to a reduction in three of the four vitamin K-dependent procoagulant clotting factors (i.e., II, VII and X) that are reduced by warfarin at a rate proportional to their half-lives. The PT assay is performed by adding calcium and thromboplastin to citrated plasma. Responsiveness of thromboplastin to reduction of vitamin K-dependent coagulation factors is measured by assessing its international sensitivity index (ISI).

PT monitoring of warfarin treatment is not standardised when expressed in seconds or as a simple ratio of patient's plasma value to that of a healthy control subject. International normalised ratio (INR), which accounts for the sensitivity of the given thromboplastin in relation to the WHO reference thromboplastin, is the correct way of expressing it [84–86]:

$$INR = (patient\ PT/mean\ normal\ PT)^{ISI}$$

There are problems with using this method which are summarised in Table 20.3.

INR is based on ISI values derived from the plasma of patients who had received stable anticoagulant doses for at least 6 weeks [87]. It is less reliable early in the course of warfarin therapy.

INR accuracy is also influenced by reagents of different sensitivities [88] as well as by the automated clot detectors now used in most laboratories [89–96]. The American College of Pathologists has recommended that laboratories should use thromboplastin reagents that are at least moderately sensitive (i.e., ISI <1.7) and reagent/instrument combinations for which the ISI has been established [95]. Concentration of citrate used to anticoagulate plasma affects INR [96, 97] such that higher citrate concentrations lead to higher INR values [96], and underfilling the blood collection tube spuriously prolongs the PT because of excess citrate.

Since warfarin therapy has a narrow therapeutic window several approaches have been developed to monitor warfarin therapy. These approaches include (a) anticoagulation

Table 20.3 Potential problems with and causes of erroneous INR

Problem	Description
1. Incorrect PT ratio from erroneous PT determination due to:	
a. Pre-test variables	Trisodium-citrate concentration, storage temperature and time, inadequate sample, variations in manual technique
b. Incorrect normal value	Non-use of MNPT, error in MNPT due to: (1) unrepresentative selection, (2) technical faults, (3) non-use of geometric mean
2. Incorrect ISI of local thromboplastin reagent from lack of reliability of ISI provided by manufacturer	Incorrect choice of IRP; poor distribution of coumarin test samples across treatment range, inadequate number of test samples in ISI calibration; incorrect transformation of PTR of test plasmas to INR
3. Drift of ISI since original calibration	
4. Instrument effects on INR at local site	
5. Lupus anticoagulant on some thromboplastin reagents	
6. Lack of reliability of INR system at initiation of warfarin therapy and in liver disease	
7. Relative lack of reliability of INR > 4.5	

management services, (b) POC PT testing that allows patient self-testing and self-management of dose adjustment, and (c) computer software programs to aid in dose adjustment. Tables 20.4 [98–101] and 20.5 [102–107] summarise the frequency of thrombosis and haemorrhage based on the mode of monitoring PT/INR.

Point-of-care INR testing

Point-of-care monitors measure a thromboplastin-mediated clotting time from a fingerstick sample of capillary whole blood or from unanticoagulated venous whole blood [108]. The result is then converted to a plasma PT equivalent by a microprocessor, and is expressed as a PT or INR. Each manufacturer typically establishes the conversion formula. Table 20.6 identifies monitors that are available. Numerous studies [109–118] have reported on the accuracy and precision of these instruments and on the patient's ability to obtain INR. POC instruments demonstrate greater differences compared to a standard plasma-based methodology when INRs increase above the therapeutic range [118, 119].

Although self-management by patients appears to be superior to usual care, it does not appear to be superior to AMS. In carefully selected and trained patients, home POC testing may be a suitable option.

One major reason for poor outcome in achieving target therapeutic range using usual care is poor dose management as currently practised [120, 121]. Use of computer programs to assist in dose management to achieve target therapeutic range has been tested in several studies [122, 123]. Computer programs typically calculate whether a dose adjustment is necessary from a user-defined table of trend rules for each therapeutic range. Contemporary computer programs perform as well as experienced medical staff of an AMS in achieving a target INR of 2.0–3.0, but they achieve significantly better control when more intensive therapy is required (i.e., INR of 3.0–4.5), and they achieve this result with fewer dose adjustments

Table 20.4 Frequency of major haemorrhage/thromboembolism in patients managed under a usual care model of management

Study/year	Patients (No.)	Patient years (No.)	Years of data collection	New or established patient	Indications	Haemorrhage† major	fatal‡	Recurrent TE	Definition of major bleed
Landefeld and Goldman [98] 1989	565	876	1977–1983	N	Ven & Art*	7.4	1.1	NA	Fatal or life-threatening potentially life-threatening (≥3-U bleed, hypotension, haematocrit ≤20)
Gitter et al. [99] 1995	261	221	1987–1989	E	Ven & Art	8.1	0.45	8.1	≥2-U bleed in ≤7 days; life-threatening bleed
Beyth et al. [100] 1998	264	440	1986–1993	N	Ven & Art	5.0	0.68	NA	Overt bleeding that led to loss of ≥2-U bleed in ≤7 days
Steffensen et al. [101] 1997	682	756	1992–1994	N	Ven & Art	6.0	0.9	NA	Fatal bleeding or requiring hospitalisation

* Ven & Art = mixed indications in the venous and arterial system; NA = not available; TE = thromboembolic event.
† Values given as percent per patient-year of therapy.
‡ Fatal haemorrhagic events also included with major haemorrhage.

Table 20.5 Frequency of major haemorrhage/thromboembolism in patients managed under an AMS

Study/year	Patients (No.)	Patient years (No.)	Years of data collection	New or established patient	Indica- tions	Target	Haemorrhage[†] major	fatal[‡]	Recurrent TE	Definition of major bleed
Forfar et al. [102] 1982	541	1362	1970–1978	N and E	Ven & Art	PTR 1.8–2.6	4.2	0.14	NA	Significant bleed requiring medical advice
Petty et al. [103] 1988	310	385	1977–1980	N and E	Ven & Art	NA	7.3	0.77	NA	Life-threatening bleed (GI, intracranial, sub-dural, or death); dis-continuing therapy
Fihn et al. [104] 1993	928	1950	NA	N	Ven & Art	PTR 1.3–1.5 1.5–1.8	1.7	0.2	7.5	Fatal/life-threatening bleed (CPR, surgery, angiography, irreversible damage, hypotension, HCT ≤20 ≥3 U of bleed
Van der Meer et al. [105] 1993	6814	6085	1988	N and E	Ven & Art	INR 2.4–5.3	3.3	0.64	NA	Fatal bleed: intra-cranial bleed, transfusion, surgery, all muscle and joint bleed
Cannegeiter et al. [106] 1995	1608	6475	1985–1987	N and E	Mech valves	INR 2.0–3.0	2.5	0.33	0.7	Fatal or bleed leading to hospitalisation
Palareti et al. [107] 1996	2745	2011	1993–1995	N	Ven & Art	INR 2.5–4.5	1.4	0.24	3.5	Fatal bleed; intra-cranial bleed, ocular bleed with blindness; joint, retroperitoneal bleed; surgery or angiography, ≥2 g bleed transfusion ≥2 U

PTR = prothrombin time ratio; INR = international normalised ratio; N = new; E = established; CPR = cardiopulmonary resuscitation; TE = thromboembolism; Ven = venous; Art = arterial.
[†] Values expressed as percent per patient-year of therapy.
[‡] Fatal haemorrhagic events also included with major haemorrhage.

Table 20.6 Capillary whole-blood (point-of-care) PT instruments

Instrument	Clot detection methodology	Type of sample	Home use approval
ProTIME monitor 1000 Coumatrak	Clot initiation: thromboplastin Clot detection: cessation of blood flow through capillary channel	Capillary WB Venous WB	No
Model 512 coagulation monitor CoaguChek plus CoaguChek pro CoaguChek pro/DM CoaguChek CoaguChek S	Clot initiation: thromboplastin Clot detection: cessation of movement of iron particles	Capillary WB Venous WB	Yes
Thrombolytic assessment system Rapidpoint coag		Plasma	
ProTIME monitor Hemochron JR	Clot initiation: thromboplastin Clot detection: cessation of blood flow through capillary channel	Capillary WB Venous WB	Yes
Avosure pro + Avosure pro	Clot initiation: thromboplastin Clot detection: thrombin generation detected by fluorescent thrombin probe	Capillary WB Venous WB	Yes
Avosure PT		Plasma	
Harmony	Clot initiation: thromboplastin	Capillary WB	Yes
INRatio	Clot initiation: thromboplastin Clot detection: change in electrical impedance as sample	Capillary WB Venous WB	Yes

[124–127]. A large study is currently in progress by the European Concerted Action on Anticoagulation randomising patients between a computer-controlled dosing arm and a manual arm using two software programs (DAWN AC, 4S Information Sys in Cumbria, UK, and PARMA, Instrumentation Laboratories in Milan, Italy).

NEWER ORAL ANTICOAGULANTS–XIMELAGATRAN

Ximelagatran is a prodrug of the active site-directed thrombin inhibitor, melagatran. It is absorbed in the intestines and biotransformed through two intermediates in the liver. It is an attractive option in many indications because of its predictable anticoagulant effect and hence lack of need for monitoring of therapy. In several trials it has been compared to low-molecular-weight heparin for prevention of postoperative venous thromboembolism with knee and hip surgery [128–131], with placebo for the treatment of venous thrombosis [132–134], with warfarin for long-term anticoagulation in non-valvular atrial fibrillation [135–137], and with placebo in long-term prevention of ischaemic events following ACS [138]. In all these trials it has proven to be either superior or not inferior to the corresponding control. The drawback is an elevation in liver enzymes seen in 4–10% of patients, typically occurring after 6 weeks to 4 months of treatment. At the present time this drug is not FDA-approved for clinical use.

FUTURE DIRECTIONS

Antiplatelet and antithrombotic agents have been separately shown to reduce the risk of adverse events during PCI and in medical management of patients. These therapies are now being used in combination in a significant proportion of patients. In attempts to improve efficacy and safety while broadening the population receiving these drugs, rapid point-of-care devices have been developed. Although no monitoring device has clearly been shown to improve clinical outcome, data are emerging that show the ability to correlate the extent of anticoagulation/antiplatelet effect with outcome. At the same time, evolution of device technology has improved such that correlation with central laboratory monitoring has a very high correlation coefficient. For the future, a therapeutic window will continue to be defined for each of these newer agents when used either as monotherapy or more likely as combination therapy.

REFERENCES

1. Boersma E et al. Platelet glycoprotein IIb/IIIa inhibitors in acute coronary syndromes. Lancet 2002; 360:342–343.
2. Randomised placebo-controlled and balloon-angioplasty-controlled trial to assess safety of coronary stenting with use of platelet glycoprotein-IIb/IIIa blockade. The EPISTENT Investigators. Evaluation of Platelet IIb/IIIa Inhibitor for Stenting. Lancet 1998; 352:87–92.
3. Topol EJ et al. Long-term protection from myocardial ischemic events in a randomized trial of brief integrin beta3 blockade with percutaneous coronary intervention. EPIC Investigator Group. Evaluation of Platelet IIb/IIIa Inhibition for Prevention of Ischemic Complication. JAMA 1997; 278:479–484.
4. A comparison of aspirin plus tirofiban with aspirin plus heparin for unstable angina. Platelet Receptor Inhibition in Ischemic Syndrome Management (PRISM) Study Investigators. N Engl J Med 1998; 338:1498–1505.
5. Inhibition of the platelet glycoprotein IIb/IIIa receptor with tirofiban in unstable angina and non-Q-wave myocardial infarction. Platelet Receptor Inhibition in Ischemic Syndrome Management in Patients Limited by Unstable Signs and Symptoms (PRISM-PLUS) Study Investigators. N Engl J Med 1998; 338:1488–1497.
6. Steinhubl SR et al. Point-of-care measured platelet inhibition correlates with a reduced risk of an adverse cardiac event after percutaneous coronary intervention: results of the GOLD (AU-Assessing Ultegra) multicenter study. Circulation 2001; 103:2572–2578.
7. Use of a monoclonal antibody directed against the platelet glycoprotein IIb/IIIa receptor in high-risk coronary angioplasty. The EPIC Investigation. N Engl J Med 1994; 330:956–961.
8. Umans VA, Kloeg PH, Bronzwaer J. The CAPTURE trial. Lancet 1997; 350:445.
9. Topol EJ et al. Comparison of two platelet glycoprotein IIb/IIIa inhibitors, tirofiban and abciximab, for the prevention of ischemic events with percutaneous coronary revascularization. N Engl J Med 2001; 344:1888–1894.
10. Chong PH. Glycoprotein IIb/IIIa receptor antagonists in the management of cardiovascular diseases. Am J Health Syst Pharm 1998; 55:2363–2386.
11. Mammen EF et al. PFA-100 system: a new method for assessment of platelet dysfunction. Semin Thromb Hemost 1998; 24:195–202.
12. Kereiakes DJ et al. Time course, magnitude, and consistency of platelet inhibition by abciximab, tirofiban, or eptifibatide in patients with unstable angina pectoris undergoing percutaneous coronary intervention. Am J Cardiol 1999; 84:391–395.
13. Steinhubl SR et al. Attainment and maintenance of platelet inhibition through standard dosing of abciximab in diabetic and nondiabetic patients undergoing percutaneous coronary intervention. Circulation 1999; 100:1977–1982.
14. Kereiakes DJ et al. Efficacy of abciximab induced platelet blockade using a rapid point of care assay. J Thromb Thrombolysis 1999; 7:265–276.
15. Kabbani SS et al. Suboptimal early inhibition of platelets by treatment with tirofiban and implications for coronary interventions. Am J Cardiol 2002; 89:647–650.
16. Tcheng JE et al. Clinical pharmacology of higher dose eptifibatide in percutaneous coronary intervention (the PRIDE study). Am J Cardiol 2001; 88:1097–1102.
17. O'Shea JC et al. Platelet glycoprotein IIb/IIIa integrin blockade with eptifibatide in coronary stent intervention: the ESPRIT trial: a randomized controlled trial. JAMA 2001; 285:2468–2473.

18. Mukherjee D *et al*. Clinical application of procedural platelet monitoring during percutaneous coronary intervention among patients at increased bleeding risk. *J Thromb Thrombolysis* 2001; 11:151–154.

19. Gum PA *et al*. Profile and prevalence of aspirin resistance in patients with cardiovascular disease. *Am J Cardiol* 2001; 88:230–235.

20. Grotemeyer KH, Scharafinski HW, Husstedt IW. Two-year follow-up of aspirin responder and aspirin non responder. A pilot-study including 180 post-stroke patients. *Thromb Res* 1993; 71:397–403.

21. Jaremo P *et al*. Individual variations of platelet inhibition after loading doses of clopidogrel. *J Intern Med* 2002; 252:233–238.

22. Gurbel PA *et al*. Clopidogrel for coronary stenting: response variability, drug resistance, and the effect of pretreatment platelet reactivity. *Circulation* 2003; 107:2908–2913.

23. Muller I *et al*. Prevalence of clopidogrel non-responders among patients with stable angina pectoris scheduled for elective coronary stent placement. *Thromb Haemost* 2003; 89:783–787.

24. Lau WC *et al*. Atorvastatin reduces the ability of clopidogrel to inhibit platelet aggregation: a new drug-drug interaction. *Circulation* 2003; 107:32–37.

25. Neubauer H *et al*. Lipophilic statins interfere with the inhibitory effects of clopidogrel on platelet function – a flow cytometry study. *Eur Heart J* 2003; 24:1744–1749.

26. Mukherjee D *et al*. Lack of clopidogrel-CYP3A4 statin interaction in patients with acute coronary syndrome. *Heart* 2005; 91:23–26.

27. Barragan P *et al*. Resistance to thienopyridines: clinical detection of coronary stent thrombosis by monitoring of vasodilator-stimulated phosphoprotein phosphorylation. *Catheter Cardiovasc Interv* 2003; 59:295–302.

28. Gurbel PA, Bliden KP. Durability of platelet inhibition by clopidogrel. *Am J Cardiol* 2003; 91:1123–1125.

29. Soffer D *et al*. Impact of angina class on inhibition of platelet aggregation following clopidogrel loading in patients undergoing coronary intervention: do we need more aggressive dosing regimens in unstable angina? *Catheter Cardiovasc Interv* 2003; 59:21–25.

30. Granger CB *et al*. Activated partial thromboplastin time and outcome after thrombolytic therapy for acute myocardial infarction: results from the GUSTO-I trial. *Circulation* 1996; 93:870–878.

31. Randomized trial of intravenous heparin versus recombinant hirudin for acute coronary syndromes. The Global Use of Strategies to Open Occluded Coronary Arteries (GUSTO) IIa Investigators. *Circulation* 1994; 90:1631–1637.

32. A clinical trial comparing primary coronary angioplasty with tissue plasminogen activator for acute myocardial infarction. The Global Use of Strategies to Open Occluded Coronary Arteries in Acute Coronary Syndromes (GUSTO IIb) Angioplasty Substudy Investigators. *N Engl J Med* 1997; 336:1621–1628.

33. Antman EM. Hirudin in acute myocardial infarction. Thrombolysis and Thrombin Inhibition in Myocardial Infarction (TIMI) 9B trial. *Circulation* 1996; 94:911–921.

34. Ryan TJ *et al*. 1999 update: ACC/AHA guidelines for the management of patients with acute myocardial infarction. A report of the American College of Cardiology/American Heart Association Task Force on Practice Guidelines (Committee on Management of Acute Myocardial Infarction). *J Am Coll Cardiol* 1999; 34:890–911.

35. Becker RC *et al*. Bedside coagulation monitoring in heparin-treated patients with active thromboembolic disease: a coronary care unit experience. *Am Heart J* 1994; 128:719–723.

36. GUSTO. *Gazette* 1992; 2.

37. Peterson P, Gottfried EL. The effects of inaccurate blood sample volume on prothrombin time (PT) and activated partial thromboplastin time (aPTT). *Thromb Haemost* 1982; 47:101–103.

38. Brandt JT, Triplett DA. Laboratory monitoring of heparin. Effect of reagents and instruments on the activated partial thromboplastin time. *Am J Clin Pathol* 1981; 76(suppl):530–537.

39. D'Angelo A *et al*. Effect of clot-detection methods and reagents on activated partial thromboplastin time (APTT). Implications in heparin monitoring by APTT. *Am J Clin Pathol* 1990; 94:297–306.

40. Bjornsson TD, Nash PV. Variability in heparin sensitivity of APTT reagents. *Am J Clin Pathol* 1986; 86:199–204.

41. Poller L, Thomson JM, Taberner DA. Use of the activated partial thromboplastin time for monitoring heparin therapy: problems and possible solutions. *Ric Clin Lab* 1989; 19:363–370.

42. Brill-Edwards P *et al*. Establishing a therapeutic range for heparin therapy. *Ann Intern Med* 1993; 119:104–109.

43. HUFFMAN, abstract presented at The American Society of Extra-Corporeal Technology (AmSECT) meeting.

44. Fitch JC et al. Heparin management test versus activated coagulation time during cardiovascular surgery: correlation with anti-Xa activity. *J Cardiothorac Vasc Anesth* 1999; 13:53–57.

45. Gibbs NM et al. Evaluation of the TAS coagulation analyzer for monitoring heparin effect in cardiac surgical patients. *J Cardiothorac Vasc Anesth* 1998; 12:536–541.

46. HMT Test Cards, package insert. Pharmanetics, Inc, East Walpole, MA, 2002.

47. Paniccia R et al. Evaluation of a new point-of-care celite-activated clotting time analyzer in different clinical settings. The i-STAT celite-activated clotting time test. *Anesthesiology* 2003; 99:54–59.

48. Giavarina D et al. Monitoring high-dose heparin levels by ACT and HMT during extracorporeal circulation: diagnostic accuracy of three compact monitors. *Perfusion* 2002; 17:23–26.

49. Ferring M et al. Point of care and central laboratory determinations of the aPTT are not interchangeable in surgical intensive care patients. *Can J Anaesth* 2001; 48:1155–1160.

50. Ansell J et al. Measurement of the activated partial thromboplastin time from a capillary (fingerstick) sample of whole blood. A new method for monitoring heparin therapy. *Am J Clin Pathol* 1991; 95:222–227.

51. Anderson DR, Harrison L, Hirsh J. Evaluation of a portable prothrombin time monitor for home use by patients who require long-term oral anticoagulant therapy. *Arch Intern Med* 1993; 153:1441–1447.

52. Cohen M et al. A comparison of low-molecular-weight heparin with unfractionated heparin for unstable coronary artery disease. Efficacy and Safety of Subcutaneous Enoxaparin in Non-Q-Wave Coronary Events Study Group. *N Engl J Med* 1997; 337:447–452.

53. Antman EM et al. Enoxaparin prevents death and cardiac ischemic events in unstable angina/non-Q-wave myocardial infarction. Results of the thrombolysis in myocardial infarction (TIMI) 11B trial. *Circulation* 1999; 100:1593–1601.

54. Efficacy and safety of tenecteplase in combination with enoxaparin, abciximab, or unfractionated heparin: the ASSENT-3 randomised trial in acute myocardial infarction. *Lancet* 2001; 358:605–613.

55. Levine M et al. A comparison of low-molecular-weight heparin administered primarily at home with unfractionated heparin administered in the hospital for proximal deep-vein thrombosis. *N Engl J Med* 1996; 334:677–681.

56. Samama MM et al. A comparison of enoxaparin with placebo for the prevention of venous thromboembolism in acutely ill medical patients. Prophylaxis in Medical Patients with Enoxaparin Study Group. *N Engl J Med* 1999; 341:793–800.

57. Linkins LA et al. In vitro comparison of the effect of heparin, enoxaparin and fondaparinux on tests of coagulation. *Thromb Res* 2002; 107:241–244.

58. Saw J et al. Evaluation of a novel point-of-care enoxaparin monitor with central laboratory anti-Xa levels. *Thromb Res* 2003; 112:301–306.

59. Moliterno DJ et al. A novel point-of-care enoxaparin monitor for use during percutaneous coronary intervention. Results of the Evaluating Enoxaparin Clotting Times (ELECT) Study. *J Am Coll Cardiol* 2003; 42:1132–1139.

60. Hafner G, Roser M, Nauck M. Methods for the monitoring of direct thrombin inhibitors. *Semin Thromb Hemost* 2002; 28:425–430.

61. Despotis GJ et al. The relationship between hirudin and activated clotting time: implications for patients with heparin-induced thrombocytopenia undergoing cardiac surgery. *Anesth Analg* 2001; 93:28–32.

62. Cho L et al. Correlation of point-of-care ecarin clotting time versus activated clotting time with bivalirudin concentrations. *Am J Cardiol* 2003; 91:1110–1113.

63. TAS ECT Test Cards, package insert. Pharmanetics, Inc, Morrisville, NC, 2002.

64. Casserly IP et al. Point-of-care ecarin clotting time versus activated clotting time in correlation with bivalirudin concentration. *Thromb Res* 2004; 113:115–121.

65. Avendano A, Ferguson JJ. Comparison of Hemochron and HemoTec activated coagulation time target values during percutaneous transluminal coronary angioplasty. *J Am Coll Cardiol* 1994; 23:907–910.

66. McGarry TF, Jr et al. The relationship of anticoagulation level and complications after successful percutaneous transluminal coronary angioplasty. *Am Heart J* 1992; 123:1445–1451.

67. Ferguson JJ et al. Relation between procedural activated coagulation time and outcome after percutaneous transluminal coronary angioplasty. *J Am Coll Cardiol* 1994; 23:1061–1065.

68. Narins CR et al. Relation between activated clotting time during angioplasty and abrupt closure. *Circulation* 1996; 93:667–671.

69. Bittl JA, Ahmed WH. Relation between abrupt vessel closure and the anticoagulant response to heparin or bivalirudin during coronary angioplasty. *Am J Cardiol* 1998; 82:50P–56P.

70. Popma JJ *et al*. Antithrombotic therapy in patients undergoing coronary angioplasty. *Chest* 1995; 108(suppl):486S–501S.

71. Platelet glycoprotein IIb/IIIa receptor blockade and low-dose heparin during percutaneous coronary revascularization. The EPILOG Investigators. *N Engl J Med* 1997; 336:1689–1696.

72. Lincoff AM *et al*. Standard versus low-dose weight-adjusted heparin in patients treated with the platelet glycoprotein IIb/IIIa receptor antibody fragment abciximab (c7E3 Fab) during percutaneous coronary revascularization. PROLOG Investigators. *Am J Cardiol* 1997; 79:286–291.

73. Moliterno DJ *et al*. Effect of platelet glycoprotein IIb/IIIa integrin blockade on activated clotting time during percutaneous transluminal coronary angioplasty or directional atherectomy (the EPIC trial). Evaluation of c7E3 Fab in the Prevention of Ischemic Complications trial. *Am J Cardiol* 1995; 75:559–562.

74. Dauerman HL *et al*. Activated clotting times in the setting of eptifibatide use during percutaneous coronary intervention. *J Thromb Thrombolysis* 2002; 13:127–132.

75. Casserly IP *et al*. Effect of abciximab versus tirofiban on activated clotting time during percutaneous intervention and its relation to clinical outcomes – observations from the TARGET trial. *Am J Cardiol* 2003; 92:125–129.

76. Randomised placebo-controlled trial of effect of eptifibatide on complications of percutaneous coronary intervention: IMPACT-II. Integrilin to Minimise Platelet Aggregation and Coronary Thrombosis-II. *Lancet* 1997; 349:1422–1428.

77. Brener SJ *et al*. Randomized, placebo-controlled trial of platelet glycoprotein IIb/IIIa blockade with primary angioplasty for acute myocardial infarction. ReoPro and Primary PTCA Organization and Randomized Trial (RAPPORT) Investigators. *Circulation* 1998; 98:734–741.

78. Bittl JA *et al*. Treatment with bivalirudin (Hirulog) as compared with heparin during coronary angioplasty for unstable or postinfarction angina. Hirulog Angioplasty Study Investigators. *N Engl J Med* 1995; 333:764–769.

79. Chew DP *et al*. Defining the optimal activated clotting time during percutaneous coronary intervention: aggregate results from 6 randomized, controlled trials. *Circulation* 2001; 103:961–966.

80. Zabel KM *et al*. Use of bedside activated partial thromboplastin time monitor to adjust heparin dosing after thrombolysis for acute myocardial infarction: results of GUSTO-I. Global Utilization of Streptokinase and TPA for Occluded Coronary Arteries. *Am Heart J* 1998; 136:868–876.

81. International, randomized, controlled trial of lamifiban (a platelet glycoprotein IIb/IIIa inhibitor), heparin, or both in unstable angina. The PARAGON Investigators. Platelet IIb/IIIa Antagonism for the Reduction of Acute coronary syndrome events in a Global Organization Network. *Circulation* 1998; 97:2386–2395.

82. Newby LK *et al*. An automated strategy for bedside aPTT determination and unfractionated heparin infusion adjustment in acute coronary syndromes: insights from PARAGON A. *J Thromb Thrombolysis* 2002; 14:33–42.

83. Ansell J *et al*. The pharmacology and management of the vitamin K antagonists: the Seventh ACCP Conference on Antithrombotic and Thrombolytic Therapy. *Chest* 2004; 126(suppl):204S–233S.

84. Poller L. Progress in standardization in anticoagulant control. *Hematol Rev* 1987; 225–241.

85. Ansell J *et al*. The prothrombin time in haemophilia and in obstructive jaundice. *J Biol Chem* 2004; 73–74.

86. Kirkwood TB. Calibration of reference thromboplastins and standardisation of the prothrombin time ratio. *Thromb Haemost* 1983; 49:238–244.

87. WHO, World Health Organization Expert Committee on Biological Standardization, in Technical Report Series No. 687. WHO, Geneva, 1983.

88. Lind SE *et al*. Clinically significant differences in the International Normalized Ratio measured with reagents of different sensitivities. SPAF Investigators. Stroke Prevention in Atrial Fibrillation. *Blood Coagul Fibrinolysis* 1999; 10:215–227.

89. Poggio M *et al*. The effect of some instruments for prothrombin time testing on the International Sensitivity Index (ISI) of two rabbit tissue thromboplastin reagents. *Thromb Haemost* 1989; 62:868–874.

90. D'Angelo A *et al*. Comparison of two automated coagulometers and the manual tilt-tube method for the determination of prothrombin time. *Am J Clin Pathol* 1989; 92:321–328.

91. Poller L, Thomson JM, Taberner DA. Effect of automation on prothrombin time test in NEQAS surveys. *J Clin Pathol* 1989; 42:97–100.

92. Ray MJ, Smith IR. The dependence of the International Sensitivity Index on the coagulometer used to perform the prothrombin time. *Thromb Haemost* 1990; 63:424–429.

93. van Rijn JL, Schmidt NA, Rutten WP. Correction of instrument- and reagent-based differences in determination of the International Normalized Ratio (INR) for monitoring anticoagulant therapy. *Clin Chem* 1989; 35:840–843.

94. Thomson JM, Taberner DA, Poller L. Automation and prothrombin time: a United Kingdom field study of two widely used coagulometers. *J Clin Pathol* 1990; 43:679–684.

95. Fairweather RB *et al.* College of American Pathologists Conference XXXI on laboratory monitoring of anticoagulant therapy: laboratory monitoring of oral anticoagulant therapy. *Arch Pathol Lab Med* 1998; 122:768–781.

96. Duncan EM *et al.* Effect of concentration of trisodium citrate anticoagulant on calculation of the International Normalised Ratio and the International Sensitivity Index of thromboplastin. *Thromb Haemost* 1994; 72:84–88.

97. Adcock DM, Kressin DC, Marlar RA. Effect of 3.2% vs 3.8% sodium citrate concentration on routine coagulation testing. *Am J Clin Pathol* 1997; 107:105–110.

98. Landefeld C, Goldman L. Major bleeding in outpatients treated with warfarin: incidence and prediction by factors known at the start of outpatient therapy. *Am J Med* 1989; 87:144–152.

99. Gitter M, Jaeger T, Petterson TA. Bleeding and thromboembolism during anticoagulant therapy: a population based study in Rochester, Minnesota. *Mayo Clin Proc* 1995; 70:725–733.

100. Beyth R, Quinn L, Landefeld S. Prospective evaluation of an index for predicting the risk of major bleeding in outpatients treated with warfarin. *Am J Med* 1998; 105:91–99.

101. Steffensen F *et al.* Major haemorrhagic complications during oral anticoagulant therapy in a Danish population-based cohort. *J Intern Med* 1997; 242:497–503.

102. Forfar J. Prediction of hemorrhage during long-term oral coumarin anticoagulation by excessive prothrombin ratio. *Am Heart J* 1982; 103:445–446.

103. Petty G *et al.* Complications of long-term anticoagulation. *Ann Neurol* 1988; 23:570–574.

104. Fihn S, McDonell M, Martin D. Risk factors for complications of chronic anticoagulation. A multi-center study; Warfarin Optimized Outpatient Follow-up Study Group. *Ann Intern Med* 1993; 118:511–520.

105. van der Meer F *et al.* Bleeding complications in oral anticoagulant therapy: an analysis of risk factors. *Arch Intern Med* 1993; 153:1557–1562.

106. Cannegieter S *et al.* Optimal oral anticoagulant therapy in patients with mechanical heart valves. *N Engl J Med* 1995; 333:11–17.

107. Palareti G *et al.* Bleeding complications of oral anticoagulant treatment: an inception-cohort, prospective collaborative study (ISOCOAT): Italian Study on Complications of Oral Anticoagulant Therapy. *Lancet* 1996; 348:423–428.

108. Muller E, Bergemann R. Economic analysis of bleeding and thromboembolic sequelae after heart valve replacement (GELIA 7): The Gelia study group. *Eur Heart J* 2001; (suppl):Q65–Q69.

109. Point-of-care prothrombin time measurement for professional and patient self-testing use. A multicenter clinical experience. Oral Anticoagulation Monitoring Study Group. *Am J Clin Pathol* 2001; 115:288–296.

110. Yano Y *et al.* Bedside monitoring of warfarin therapy by a whole blood capillary coagulation monitor. *Thromb Res* 1992; 66:583–590.

111. Weibert RT, Adler DS. Evaluation of a capillary whole-blood prothrombin time measurement system. *Clin Pharm* 1989; 8:864–867.

112. Gosselin R *et al.* A comparison of point-of-care instruments designed for monitoring oral anti-coagulation with standard laboratory methods. *Thromb Haemost* 2000; 83:698–703.

113. van den Besselar AM. A comparison of INRs determined with a whole blood prothrombin time device and two international reference preparations for thromboplastin. *Thromb Haemost* 2000; 84:410–412.

114. Kitchen S, Preston FE. Monitoring oral anticoagulant treatment with the TAS near-patient test system: comparison with conventional thromboplastins. *J Clin Pathol* 1997; 50:951–956.

115. Douketis JD *et al.* Accuracy of a portable International Normalization Ratio monitor in outpatients receiving long-term oral anticoagulant therapy: comparison with a laboratory reference standard using clinically relevant criteria for agreement. *Thromb Res* 1998; 92:11–17.

116. Cosmi B *et al.* Accuracy of a portable prothrombin time monitor (Coagucheck) in patients on chronic oral anticoagulant therapy: a prospective multicenter study. *Thromb Res* 2000; 100:279–286.

117. Prothrombin measurement using a patient self-testing system. Oral Anticoagulation Monitoring Study Group. *Am J Clin Pathol* 2001; 115:280–287.

118. Jennings I, Luddington RJ, Baglin T. Evaluation of the Ciba Corning Biotrack 512 coagulation monitor for the control of oral anticoagulation. *J Clin Pathol* 1991; 44:950–953.

119. McCurdy SA, White RH. Accuracy and precision of a portable anticoagulation monitor in a clinical setting. *Arch Intern Med* 1992; 152:589–592.

120. Samsa GP *et al.* Quality of anticoagulation management among patients with atrial fibrillation: results of a review of medical records from 2 communities. *Arch Intern Med* 2000; 160:967–973.

121. Ansell JE. Anticoagulation management as a risk factor for adverse events: grounds for improvement. *J Thromb Thrombolysis* 1998; 5(suppl 1):13–18.

122. Wilson R, James AH. Computer assisted management of warfarin treatment. *Br Med J (Clin Res Ed)* 1984; 289:422–424.

123. Ryan PJ, Gilbert M, Rose PE. Computer control of anticoagulant dose for therapeutic management. *Br Med J* 1989; 299:1207–1209.

124. Poller L, Wright D, Rowlands M. Prospective comparative study of computer programs used for management of warfarin. *J Clin Pathol* 1993; 46:299–303.

125. Ageno W, Turpie AG. A randomized comparison of a computer-based dosing program with a manual system to monitor oral anticoagulant therapy. *Thromb Res* 1998; 91:237–240.

126. Poller L *et al.* Multicentre randomised study of computerised anticoagulant dosage. European Concerted Action on Anticoagulation. *Lancet* 1998; 352:1505–1509.

127. Manotti C *et al.* Effect of computer-aided management on the quality of treatment in anticoagulated patients: a prospective, randomized, multicenter trial of APROAT (Automated PRogram for Oral Anticoagulant Treatment). *Haematologica* 2001; 86:1060–1070.

128. Eriksson BI *et al.* The direct thrombin inhibitor melagatran followed by oral ximelagatran compared with enoxaparin for the prevention of venous thromboembolism after total hip or knee replacement: the EXPRESS study. *J Thromb Haemost* 2003; 1:2490–2496.

129. Eriksson BI *et al.* Direct thrombin inhibitor melagatran followed by oral ximelagatran in comparison with enoxaparin for prevention of venous thromboembolism after total hip or knee replacement. *Thromb Haemost* 2003; 89:288–296.

130. Eriksson BI *et al.* Ximelagatran and melagatran compared with dalteparin for prevention of venous thromboembolism after total hip or knee replacement: the METHRO II randomised trial. *Lancet* 2002; 360:1441–1447.

131. Francis CW *et al.* Comparison of ximelagatran with warfarin for the prevention of venous thromboembolism after total knee replacement. *N Engl J Med* 2003; 349:1703–1712.

132. Eriksson H *et al.* A randomized, controlled, dose-guiding study of the oral direct thrombin inhibitor ximelagatran compared with standard therapy for the treatment of acute deep vein thrombosis: THRIVE I. *J Thromb Haemost* 2003; 1:41–47.

133. Fiessinger JN *et al.* Ximelagatran vs low-molecular-weight heparin and warfarin for the treatment of deep vein thrombosis: a randomized trial. *JAMA* 2005; 293:681–689.

134. Schulman S *et al.* Secondary prevention of venous thromboembolism with the oral direct thrombin inhibitor ximelagatran. *N Engl J Med* 2003; 349:1713–1721.

135. Petersen P, Grind M, Adler J. Ximelagatran versus warfarin for stroke prevention in patients with nonvalvular atrial fibrillation. SPORTIF II: a dose-guiding, tolerability, and safety study. *J Am Coll Cardiol* 2003; 41:1445–1451.

136. Halperin JL. Ximelagatran compared with warfarin for prevention of thromboembolism in patients with nonvalvular atrial fibrillation: Rationale, objectives, and design of a pair of clinical studies and baseline patient characteristics (SPORTIF III and V). *Am Heart J* 2003; 146:431–438.

137. Olsson SB. Stroke prevention with the oral direct thrombin inhibitor ximelagatran compared with warfarin in patients with non-valvular atrial fibrillation (SPORTIF III): randomised controlled trial. *Lancet* 2003; 362:1691–1698.

138. Wallentin L *et al.* Oral ximelagatran for secondary prophylaxis after myocardial infarction: the ESTEEM randomised controlled trial. *Lancet* 2003; 362:789–797.

Index